HEALTH

A Quality of Life

HEA

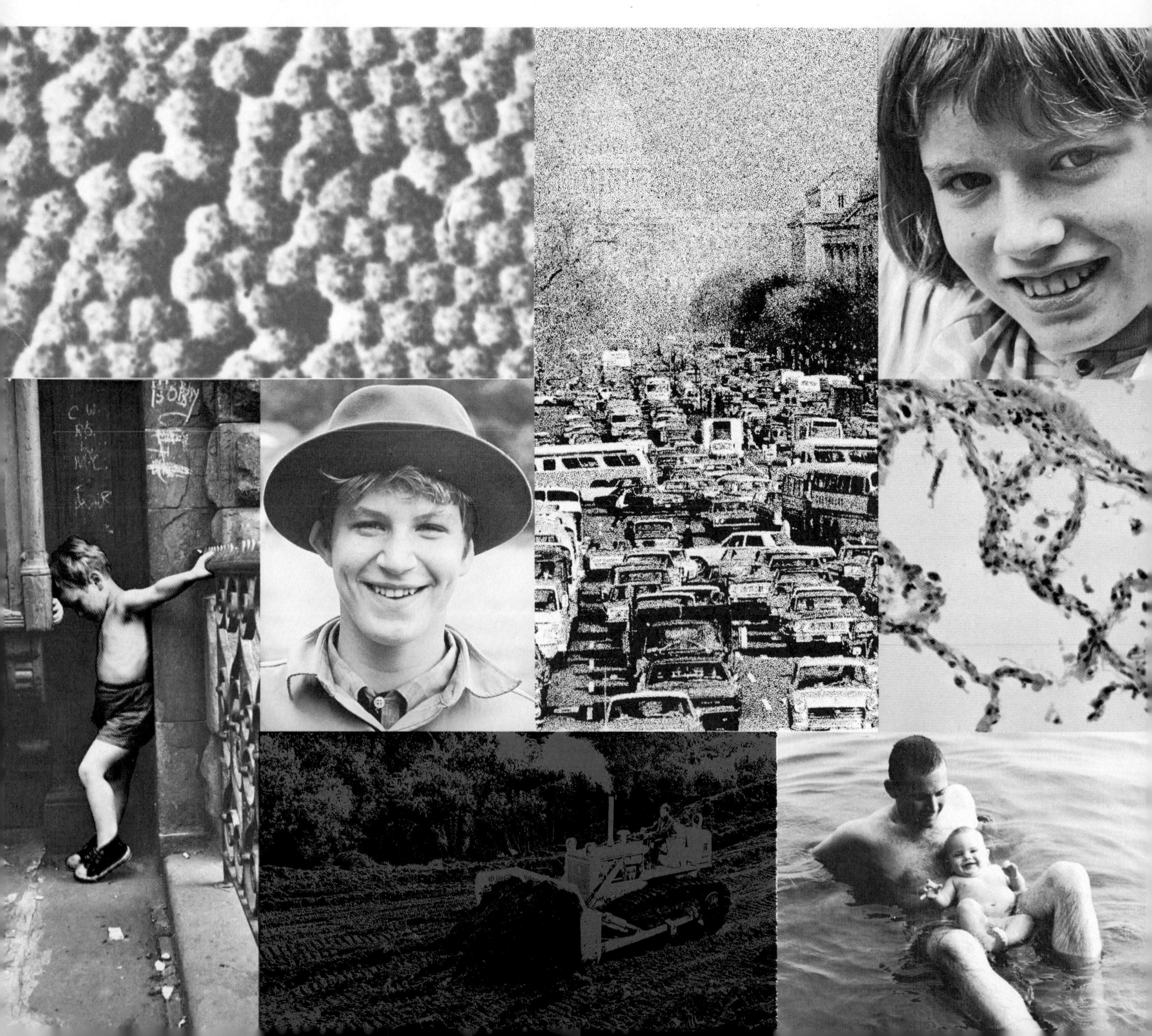

LTH

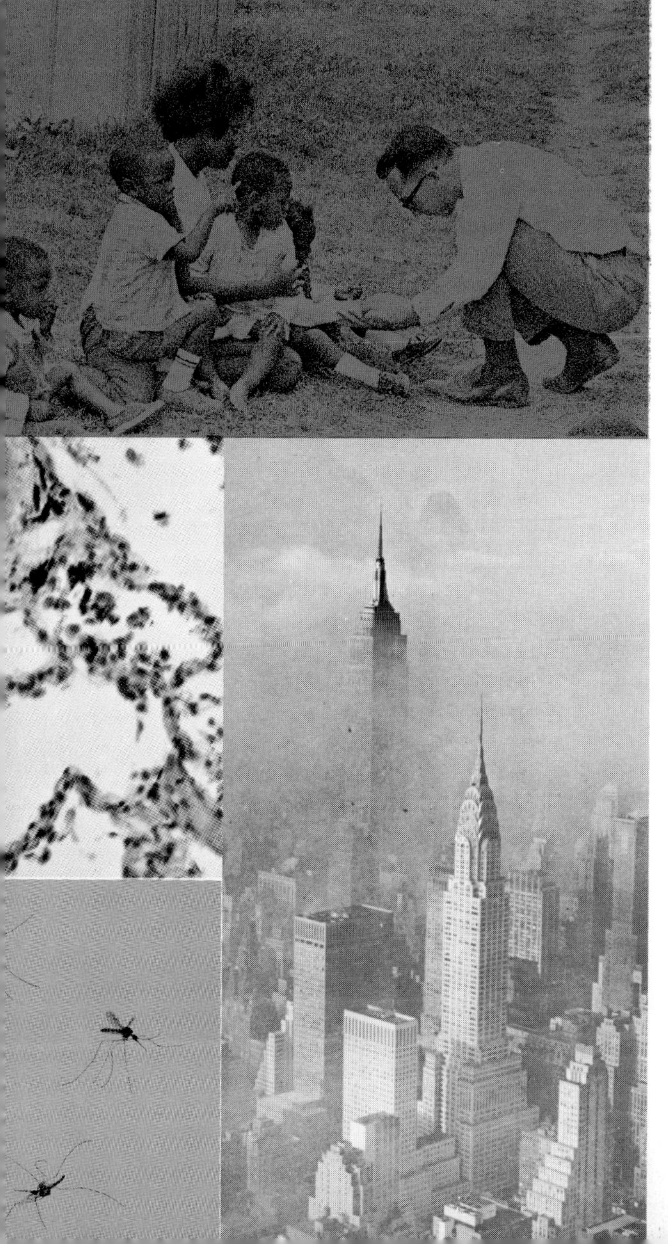

A Quality of Life

Second Edition

John S. Sinacore

Professor of Health Sciences
State University College
Brockport, New York

Macmillan Publishing Co., Inc.
New York
Collier Macmillan Publishers
London

Macmillan Publishing Co., Inc.
866 Third Avenue, New York, New York 10022
Collier-Macmillan Canada, Ltd., Toronto, Ontario

Library of Congress Cataloging in Publication Data

Sinacore, John S.
Health, a quality of life.

1. Hygiene, Public. 2. Hygiene. I. Title.
[DNLM: 1. Hygiene. 2. Public health. WA4
S615h 1974]
RA431.S5 1974 613 72-17962
ISBN 0-02-410700-X

Printing: 4 5 6 7 8 Year: 7 8 9 0

Preface

The purpose of this book goes beyond the reporting of comprehensive advances made in the health sciences. It gives candid discussion to some of the vital health issues of our times. Issues such as automobile safety, drug use and abuse, abortion, food faddism, sex values, and the nature of human sexuality are included. Honest, straightforward presentations of these often controversial topics are designed to assist the young adult in developing points of view in these important health areas. It is further hoped that this text will mark an end to those placid, innocuous writings that pretend these issues do not exist. The writing of this text is based on the premise that today's young adult does not gullibly accept an Alice-in-Wonderland approach to health studies, but would rather be prepared to confront the realities of life so that he may more appropriately deal with them. These realities include our society's unprecedented use of drugs for good and evil, the pollution problems reflective of our advanced technology, and societal neglect of these problems. They also include the revolutionary changes in the practice and delivery of medical care, along with other aspects of a rapidly changing environment. Like the animals who have preceded him, man's ability to adapt to his environment is vital to his survival. Through the text is found the theme that in an advanced society "the environment" is essentially man-made. Only the citizen well informed in the health sciences is appropriately prepared to make the individual, familial, and community decisions related to health affairs. He must also be aware of vested interests in our society whose primary concerns are not the public welfare. In these instances the individual may find that health protection must be sought through the actions of informed citizens and health-profession groups.

In addition to the updating of its contents this second edition has added discussions of new issues such as the feminist movement, the health-organic food movement, thanatology (the study of death), genetic diseases and genetic counseling, automobile recalls, nuclear power plants and their environmental implications, "Who are the drug abusers and why?," and the dramatic implications of recent research in the health and life sciences for man's future and well being.

The text is presented in seven parts. Part One consists of the introductory chapter, "On Health, Life, and Living." It seeks to define that quality called health and offers a philosophical statement on the relationship of health to life and living. It identifies personal, environmental, and hereditary factors inherent in the attainment and maintenance of qualities of health.

Part Two, "Mental Health," is concerned with the area of mental health, its nature, maintenance, its occasional breakdown, and rehabilitation. Included in this section are discussions of man's needed adaptations to civilization, research findings related to suicide, and our changing attitudes toward mental illness.

Part Three, "Gender and Family Living," is in many ways an extension and application of mental hygiene principles discussed in the previous section. Presented also is a chapter on human sexuality. It discusses concepts related to masculinity and femininity, sex values, the bases of sexual involvement together with other aspects of sexuality, and candid discussion of the feminist movement. Some of these concepts are further considered as part of a discussion on preparation for marriage. The physiology of reproduction, including prenatal development and care, is also presented. The issue of abortion laws and how they have been liberalized is discussed with the varying major arguments offered. The social, medical, and moral aspects of the complex abortion issue are also presented.

In Part Four, "Maintaining Health Status," the physical fitness needs of our society, their implications, and possible solutions are identified. In the broad areas of vision and hearing, the pros and cons of the use of contact lenses are presented as well as the nature and implications of hearing loss. Appropriate discussion of various aspects of dental and foot care is also included. In addition to basic nutrition and the values of a balanced diet, the changing nature of our nutritional problems is identified. Food faddism, the overuse of vitamins, the impact and contributions of food additives, the organic-food movement, and the complex problem of overweight are some of the topics included here.

In Part Five, "Disease Prevention and Control," some of the major communicable as well as constitutional and degenerative diseases are discussed. Emphasis is given to recent data and research findings related to conditions such as venereal disease, cardiovascular disorders, and cancer.

Part Six, "Health and Our Society," includes a discussion of the problem of health quackery. Means of evaluating health products and information are also offered. The rapid changes taking place in the financing and administration of medical care and their present and future implications are discussed.

The issue of drugs in this section does not focus solely on the addictive narcotic drugs, but prescription and nonprescription drugs as well. Included is a discussion of developing controversy related to drug advertisements. The psychedelic drugs, their use and misuse, are also presented. The writhings of the tobacco industry in the face of scientific evidence that condemns the cigarette as lethal are given due coverage. The use and abuse of alcohol and its inherent issues is also given appropriate attention.

Part Seven, "Community Health," is concerned with a description of public health organization in the United States. It also describes the nature of some of our global health problems and their significant implications for all people of the world.

This section is concluded with a discussion of recent research findings and their dramatic implications for man's near, if not immediate, future. It discusses the issues presented by the advances in genetic engineering, behavior control, and man's ever-increasing ability to replace worn-out parts of the body with organ transplants or artificial structures. Reflected, too, is the need for societal discussion for man's increasing ability to determine the nature, quality, and behavior of the human species.

J. S. S.

Table of Contents

Part One Introduction

Chapter 1 On Health, Life, and Living 3

The Attainment and Maintenance of Health / Environmental Factors / Personal Health Responsibilities / Health Status and One's Life Style / Heredity as a Health Factor

Review Questions 12

Part Two Mental Health

Chapter 2 The Bases of Mental Health 17

Man, Mental Health, and Civilization / Basic Needs / What, Then, Is Mental Health? / The Relationship of Body Systems to Mental Health / The Conscious and the Unconscious Mind / Psychological Stress / Anxiety as a Result of Stress / The Emotions / The Mental Mechanisms / Death—A Part of Every Life

Review Questions 35

Chapter 3 The Erosion of Mental Health 36

Psychosomatic Disorders / Neurotic Adjustments / Types of Neurotic Adjustments / The Psychoses / Suicide / Mental Health Specialists / Treating Mental and Emotional Problems / Mental Health Treatment Facilities / The Community Mental Health Center / Hospital Management of the Mentally Ill / Types of Admission / Our Changing Attitudes Toward Mental Illness

Review Questions 56

Part Three Gender and Family Living

Chapter 4 Human Sexuality 59

On Masculinity and Femininity / The Feminist Movement / Sex Values / Some Negative Bases of Sexual Involvement / On Sex and Love: A Positive Basis for Sexual Involvement / Sexual Outlets / Homosexuality / In Conclusion

Review Questions 73

Chapter 5 Preparation for Marriage 74

Motivations for Marriage / Love / Values / Personality Characteristics / Background / Economic Status / Sexual Considerations / Religious Matters / Role Expectations / The Engagement / The Premarital Physical Examination / On Having Children

Review Questions 87

Chapter 6 Human Reproduction 89

The Male Reproductive System / The Female Reproductive System / The Reproductive Process / Signs of Pregnancy / Prenatal Development / Prenatal Care / Breast Feeding / The Rh Factor / Childbirth / Multiple Births / The Premature Child / Abortion / The Legality of Abortion / The Morality of Abortion / Contraception and Family Planning / Some Aspects of Infertility / Genetic Counseling

Review Questions 118

Part Four Maintaining Health Status

Chapter 7 Personal Health 123

Physical Fitness / Physical Education Needs / Vision / Hearing / Dental and Oral Health / Problems of the Foot

Review Questions 151

Chapter 8 Our Shifting Nutritional Problems 152

Poverty, Hunger, and Malnutrition / Weight Control / Dieting / Quackery and Special Diets / Nutritional Misinformation / The Health Food–Organic Food Movement / Food Additives / Federal Legislation Relating to Food in the United States / Protecting the Public from the Faddist / The Need for Effective Nutrition Education / Problems Related to Food and Digestion / Basic Nutritional Needs

Review Questions 179

Part Five Disease Prevention and Control

Chapter 9 Man's Control of Communicable Diseases 183

Terminology of the Communicable Diseases / Disease-Producing or Pathogenic Organisms / Transmission of Infectious Organisms / Resistance and Immunity to Disease / Some Communicable Disease Problems / The Unfinished Task

Review Questions 209

Chapter 10 Constitutional and Degenerative Diseases 211

Cardiovascular Diseases / Stroke (Cerebrovascular Disease) / Hypertension (High Blood Pressure) / Rheumatic Fever and Rheumatic Heart Disease / Congenital Heart Defects / Varicose Veins / Cancer / Sites of Cancer / Treatment for Cancer / Cancer Research / The Outlook for Cancer / Neurological Disorders / Mental Retardation / Genetic Diseases / Other Constitutional Diseases

Review Questions 253

Part Six Health and Our Society

Chapter 11 Consumer—Beware! 257

Quackery: The Backwash of an Uninformed Public / Quackery's Areas of Gray / The Ethical (Prescription) Drug Industry / The High Price of Drugs on the Legal Market / Other Issues Concerning the Drug Industry / Protection of the Consumer / Evaluating Health Information / The Practitioners of Health Care / Nonmedical Specialists / Chiropractic / The Changing Nature of Health Care / Financing Cost of Health Care / Inequities in Health Care / A Look to the Future

Review Questions 297

Chapter 12 Drugs in Our Society 299

Modern Drugs and Their Contributions / Prescription Drugs / Nonprescription Drugs (or Proprietary Drugs) / Drug Abuse / Who Are the Drug Abusers and Why? / Stimulant Drugs / The Hallucinogenic Drugs / The Addicting Drugs / Drug Traffic / Various Approaches to the Problem / Alcohol. Who Drinks and Why? / Alcohol as a Drug / Alcoholic Beverages / The Effects of Alcohol on the Body / The Problem of Alcoholism / Treatment of the Alcoholic / A

Giant Step Forward / Man's Use of Tobacco / Why People Smoke / The Physiological Effects of Smoking / Cigarette Advertising / Attempts to Control Cigarette Advertising / The Decade Since the Surgeon General's Report / Prevention
Review Questions 345

Chapter 13 Man's Self-Created Environment 347

Air Pollution / The Pollutants / Air Pollution and the Weather / The Effects of Air Pollution / Industry and Air Pollution / Air Pollution Control / Water Pollution / Water Pollution Control / Federal Water Pollution Legislation / International Commissions / Research / Needed: Community Interest and Action / Land Pollution / Our Proliferate Pesticides / Pesticide Use and Exposure / Pesticide Effects on Wildlife / Toxicity of Some Pesticides / Pesticide Control / Research / Benefits of Pesticides / Proper Personal Use of Pesticides / Radiation / The Nature and Effects of Radiation / Sources of Man-Made Radiation
Review Questions 378

Chapter 14 Safety in Our Times 380

The Use of Epidemiology in Safety Research / Traffic Safety / The Automobile as an Accident Factor / The Life-Saving Interstate Highway System / The Driver / The Expanded Use of the Motorbike and Snowmobile / Home Safety / Types of Home Accidents for Various Age Groups / Industrial Safety
Review Questions 401

Part Seven Community Health

Chapter 15 Public Health Organization for Community Action 405

The Official Health Agency / Health Organization at the State Level / Health Organization at the Federal Level / The Voluntary Health Organization / The Hospital / The School / Nursing Homes / Humanizing Health Care / Health Careers and the Expanding Health Industry
Review Questions 420

Chapter 16 Global Health: Its Implications 421

Some World Health Problems / Diseases Found in Underdeveloped Countries / The World Health Organization / WHO Activities / UNICEF (The United Nations Children Fund) / Food and Agriculture Organization (FAO) / The Helping Hands / CARE / MEDICO / SS Hope
Review Questions 441

Chapter 17 Man's Moment of Decision 442

Genetic Cloning / Human Behavior Control / The Contributions of Space Medicine to Health / The Spare Parts Department / In Conclusion
Review Questions 453

Appendixes:

A Emergency First Aid 455

B Table: Nutritive Values of the Edible Part of Foods 485

Index 505

HEALTH

A Quality of Life

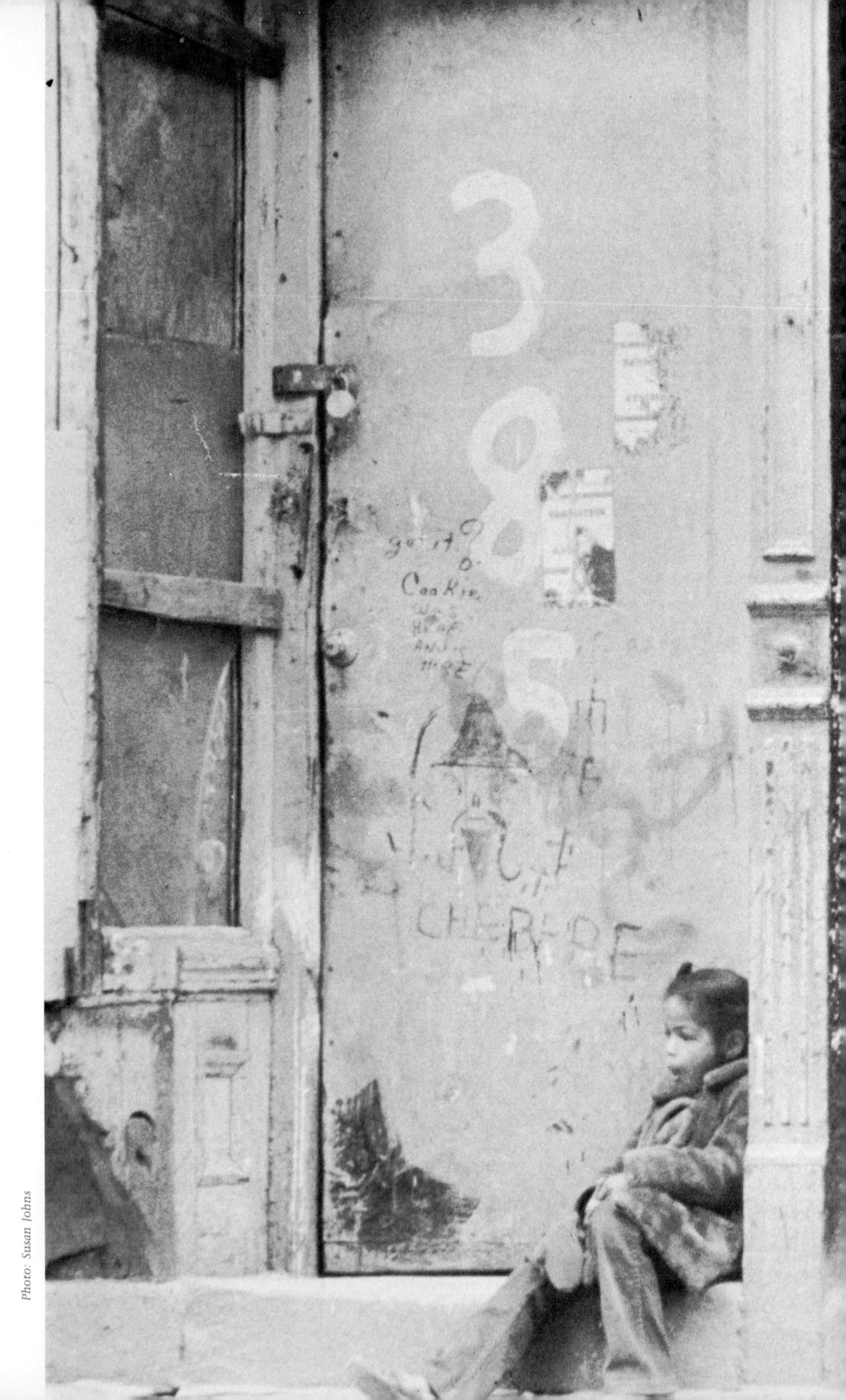

Photo: Susan Johns

Part One
Introduction

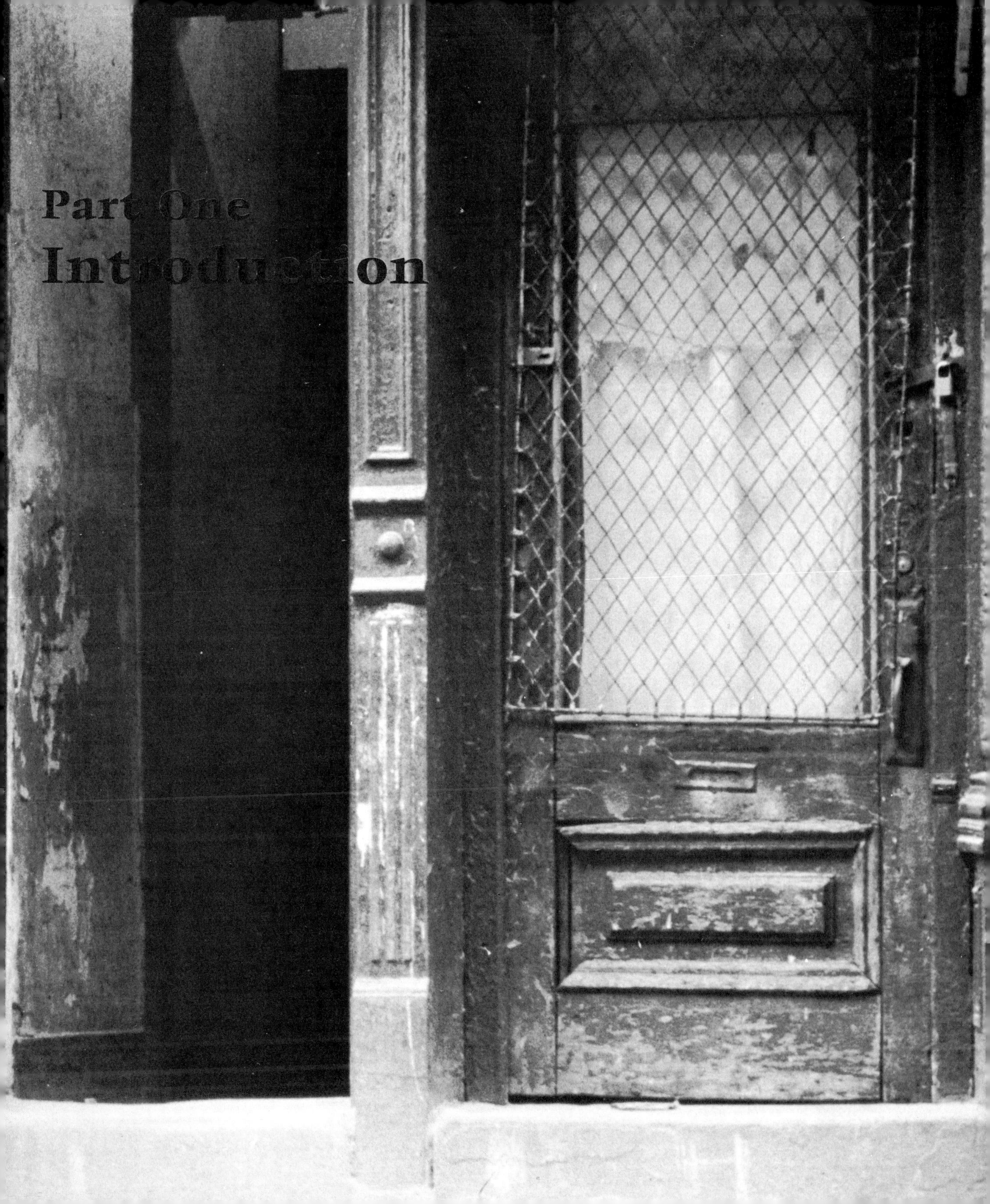

Chapter 1
On Health, Life, and Living

It seems only proper that it be stated at the beginning of this writing that man's strongest desires are not for health, but for life and living. He who would preoccupy himself with matters of health is at best a hypochondriac seeking to cloak himself from the rigors of living with a whimpering, self-inflicted incapacitation. Life, then, is best given to those willing to risk its living and possessing purposes that go beyond the self. The author Balzac on his deathbed pleaded with his physician to keep him alive for a few weeks so that he might finish his work. These would be weeks during which his body, ravaged with fever, would suffer excruciating torment. Yet at this moment he was reaching out for that fragment of health that would sustain him until his work was completed. Herein perhaps lies the crux of our story—health is not an end in itself, but a means of attaining life's purposes. So while we may conclude that health concerns do not deserve our *pre*-occupation, we do need to occupy ourselves with them to help assure the attainment of life's goals.

Traditionally, health has been viewed and measured in negative terms, namely the presence of disease, infirmity, or death. We have therefore in the past attempted to measure health by focusing on health failures. Dr. Forrest E. Linder, Director of the National Center for Health Statistics, a unit of the United States Public Health Service, recently reflected the limitations of this approach by stating:

> The health of a country's people has traditionally been measured by the rate at which they die: a decreasing death rate is taken as an indication of increasing health. In recent years, however, the concept of health has undergone significant changes. There is a new interest in the total quality of life rather than merely the length of life, in the positive elements of good health rather than merely the absence of disease and infirmity. As medical science advances, moreover, it becomes increasingly pertinent to know the extent and degree to which new knowledge and techniques are being applied throughout the population. The death rate, and indeed the entire battery of vital statistics that have long been collected by the states and the Federal Government, no longer yield enough information on which to base a sound national health policy.[1]

In view of man's advances in the health sciences, he can look forward to refining his definitions of health in positive terms. He will also be further developing means of attaining and maintaining levels of health qualitatively measured.

Already there are various means of measuring one's quality of health that do not fall into the all-or-none categories of life or death, disease or lack of disease. To cite several examples, a person's visual acuity could serve as such a measurement. Vision may vary considerably from person to person without illness being a part of the consideration. Nutritional status would also qualify as a standard which could include the iron level in the red blood cells. This could serve as an indication of the amount of iron taken in the diet and reflected in the person's ability to function. Other criteria could include one's physical fitness, levels of resistance to disease, fat levels in the blood, sensitivity to allergens, the

[1] Forrest E. Linder, "The Health of the American People," *Scientific American*, Vol. 214, No. 6 (June 1966).

degree of emotional stability, and body weight, among others.

There are a number of factors to assess people's levels of health and they will no doubt be increasing in number as medical knowledge expands and diagnostic techniques improve. Ideally, everyone in the population should undergo a periodic medical examination to determine his health status. The current shortage of physicians makes such a procedure impossible. There just are not enough physicians to perform such a broad-scale task. Some experimentation has been done in which the mechanics of the examination (vision testing, blood testing, blood pressure measurement, and many others) are performed by technicians or nurses with the test results then subject to review by the doctor. This procedure saves the physician time and permits him to review the test results of many more people.

A recent contribution along these lines has been made by Dr. Ernest L. Wynder. This physician was the first to produce evidence that cigarette smoking is a major cause of lung cancer, and now he is working on another first. Dr. Wynder has automated the medical examination at the Health Maintenance Center he directs. The person to be examined is initially asked to complete a 378-item questionnaire on his own and his family's medical history. With the aid of technicians, the person goes through a medical assembly line with blood and urine samples tested, and with electrocardiograms taken. The results are checked through a computer with any suspected abnormalities double checked. The entire procedure is completed in one hour. The physician reviews the report of the examination and makes any necessary recommendations. If the examinee has a smoking, an overweight, or a physical fitness problem, he may be assigned to one or more of the center's intervention clinics. Here he may be placed on a diet or on an exercise regimen, or asked to attend a smoking withdrawal clinic. The objective is to correct any patterns of living that will ultimately prove destructive to the individual. The question raised is that it may be necessary to reexamine medical care procedures and their organization if the mere measurement of personal health is to become a reality.

The Attainment and Maintenance of Health

As the information, technique, and technology of the health sciences, including the medical sciences, become more sophisticated, the means of attaining and maintaining desirable levels of health will become more complex—as well as more effective. Generally, in the past, the level of health a person achieved was considered to be pretty much a personal matter. The attitude implied that it was the prerogative of the individual to decide how healthy he wanted to be. While this was never completely true in the past, it is even less so now. Increasingly a person's level of health is becoming more dependent on other facilities, conditions, and people. The individual is less a master of his fate than he ever was, and the trend can be expected to continue.

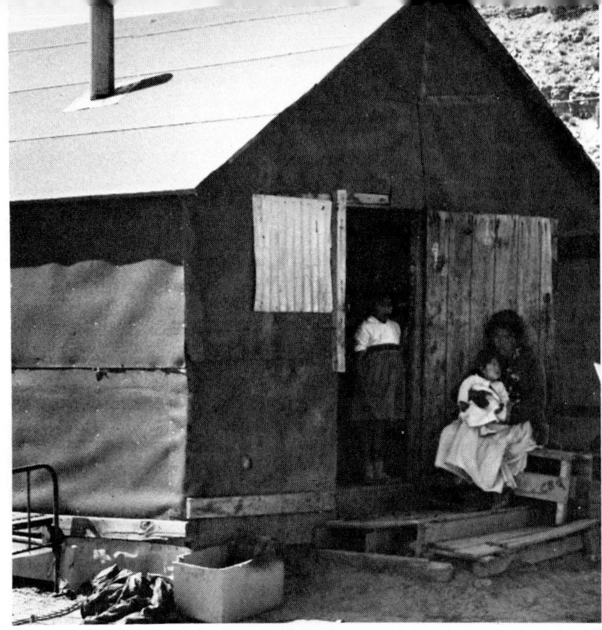

Fig. 1-1. The availability of health services is as important as other environmental factors in the maintenance of health. (Gerry Souter/ VAN CLEVE)

Environmental Factors

We, as professionals in the field of public health, can lay out a wide range of concerns that involve those yet unborn, as well as those who drive, eat, fly, drink, and work, and even those who are lingering in the very shadows of life, soon to disappear. "Consumer protection" is the phrase we have been using for many years. But who "consumes" a drug before birth, who can be said to "consume" urban noise, who "consumes" the errors in laboratory analysis, who is a "consumer" in a substandard nursing home, or who is *not* a "consumer" of polluted air and water? We might conclude from this that it is not a "consumer" who has captured our attention, but the quality and integrity of life itself.[2]

While man is still privileged to bring on his own lung cancer through cigarette smoking, he has little control over the pollutants in the air he breathes if he lives in an urban area. He relies on the health department to safeguard the water he drinks and the food he eats. He must to some extent rely on the "other driver" for his safety while on the highway. How well-made and therefore how safe are his car and tires may determine his life expectancy. Yet, how much control can he exert over private industry to guarantee his safety? Man therefore can no longer go it alone, so far as his health is concerned. Where broadly based environmental factors or problems arise, man's only control of them can be through interested, well-informed citizen groups and those organizations in the community that have health responsibilities. In the absence of these alternatives, he must eat the food, drink the water, breathe the air, and drive the cars provided him.

The National Health Survey (a continuous study conducted by the United States Public Health Service to determine the health status of the nation) has shown that there is a "positive" relationship between poor health and low income. It has also indicated that the low-income groups receive less medical care in spite of greater need. It is, of course, not always possible to ascertain if the low income caused the poor health or vice versa. It can, however, be concluded that the ability to secure medical care is related to the person's earning power and therefore the ability to maintain health. The availability of health services is rarely viewed as an environmental factor. Yet it is an essential element for the maintenance of health and a segment of man's surroundings that must be considered important. The dental health of a community without a dentist cannot be expected to compare with that of one well supplied with dental services. Likewise, the community without medical services would find its health status considerably lowered. Its people would lack the protection of vaccines for smallpox, polio, diphtheria, and whooping cough, to mention a few. Routine cases of appendicitis could mean death. We could easily regress to the level of primitive societies where life is a struggle for existence. In a more sophisticated society such as our own, the question is not one of having or not having dental and medical services. Rather it is a question of their extensiveness, their quality, and their accessibility to all in

[2]Dr. James Goddard, "Public Health and the Consumer." Delivered at the 63rd Annual Health Conference, May 24, 1967.

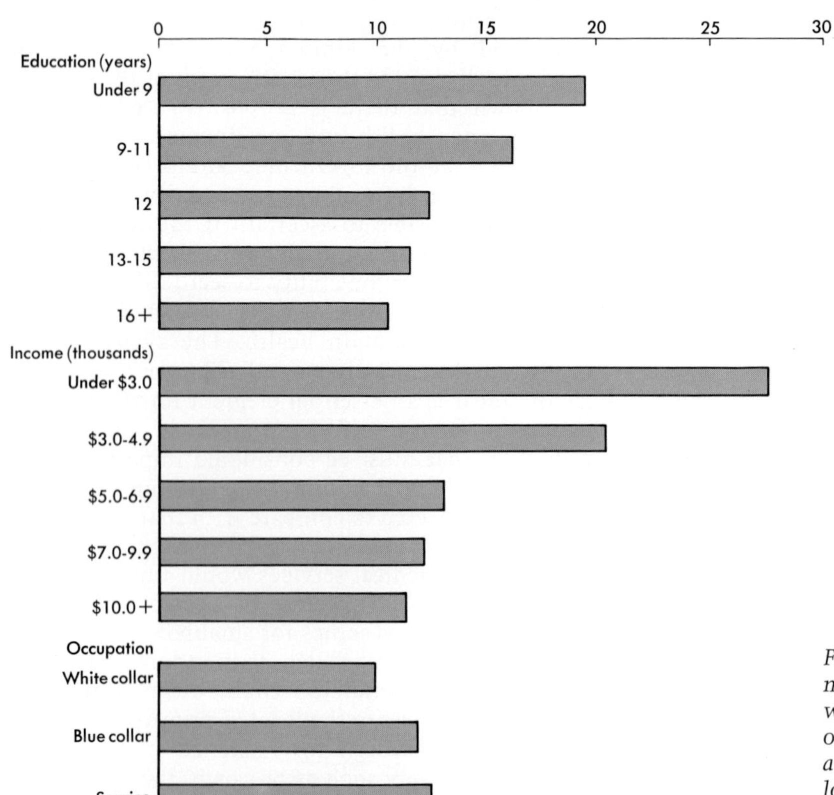

Fig. 1-2. Total impact of illness is measured by the number of days on which people missed work or school or otherwise had to reduce their usual activities. The graph shows that lower-income people have more "restricted-activity days." (Adapted from unpublished data from the National Center for Health Statistics.)

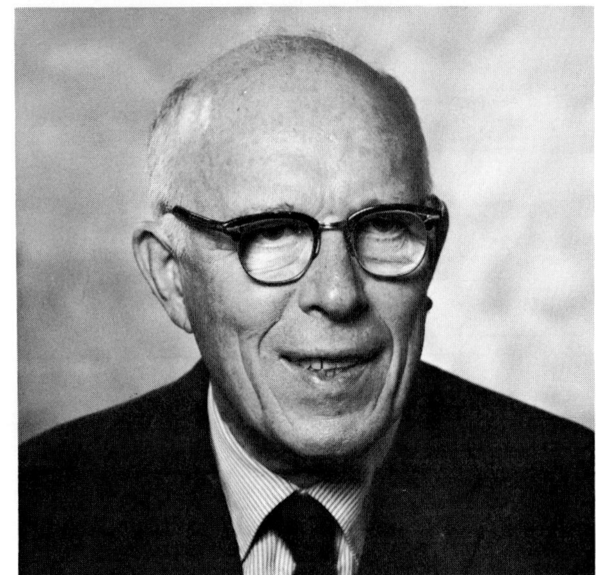

Fig. 1-3. René Dubos, Ph.D., Professor Emeritus, The Rockefeller University, is a renowned researcher and spokesman for the health sciences.

the community. A person who suffers a heart attack has a better chance of survival if it occurs in a community that has prompt, well-equipped ambulance service and whose hospitals are well prepared to deal with these emergencies. As important, though less dramatic, is the community's preparedness to function in the area of medical rehabilitation. Having the personnel and facilities to return a person suffering an infirmity to useful living could prove as important as saving his life.

Personal Health Responsibilities

The modern American . . . claims the highest standard of living in the world, but 10 per cent of his income must go for medical care and he cannot build hospitals fast enough to accommodate the sick. He is encouraged to believe that money will create drugs for the cure of heart disease, cancer, and mental disease, but he makes no worthwhile effort to recognize, let alone correct, the mismanagements of his everyday life that contribute to the high incidence of these conditions. One may wonder indeed whether the pretense of superior health is not itself rapidly becoming a mental aberration.[3]

While we are to a greater extent looking outward to the community for means of attaining and maintaining health status, we have by no means outgrown our need for personal health responsibilities. Advances in the health sciences make it important for the individual to keep informed of these developments so that he may modify his behavior in accordance with their findings. As a nation we have always enthusiastically supported research. The results of research have been met with equal enthusiasm if they take the form of a vaccine that will prevent disease or a drug that will cure it. If research results indicate that cancer can be prevented by not smoking or some accidents by not speeding, the enthusiasm somehow wanes. Part of the explanation of this is our built-in resistance to change. An additional factor involved is that when we are asked to give up something we enjoy doing, we then have to make a value judgment as to whether the possible results justify the change. Certainly, in some instances we will continue a pattern of behavior even though it contradicts what is considered the healthy thing to do. A fireman who charges into a flaming house to save the life of another is not doing the healthy thing—he has other motivations.

Research results that produce health information are also ignored because people view "the magic pill" or the "miracle drugs" as the only kind of contribution to be made by health research. This attitude probably prevails because concerted efforts have not been made to inform the populace of health research informational findings and of their significance to the individual. The attitude has also persisted that new health information is for the physician or other health professionals but not for the lay public. The result has been that the American public does not enjoy a high level of health information. This conclusion was borne out by the National Health Test conducted by CBS.

[3]René Dubos, *Mirage of Health* (New York: Doubleday, 1961), p. 31.

It is somewhat ironic to note that the broadcasting system whose fine efforts went into the development and administration of this examination is also part of a pattern of mass media that have contributed to the low scores registered on this health test. The mass media in the United States have long been known as sources of misleading or outright false information in the health area. This was substantiated by a study conducted by medical students at Wayne State University School of Medicine who

> found that during a typical 130-hour week on one commercial television channel health-related content was used 7.2 per cent of the time, including both actual programs and commercials, and that only 30 per cent of the information was "useful." The study cited as examples of misleading health information in commercials the claim that a cough medicine was as strong as codeine, and a commercial implying that a medicated foam might cure psoriasis, which has no cure.[4]

(This matter is further discussed in the chapter on consumer health education entitled, "Consumer—Beware!")

In Europe, if a health measure is to be put into effect, health officials make an announcement of it and proceed to implement the program. In the United States, before action can be taken on a recommended health measure it must in one form or another have the approval of the people. Vital public health decisions are thus being asked of a public that is not nearly as informed as it should be for this responsibility. One need only view a public forum on the fluoridation of drinking water to see an unfortunate result of these circumstances. The meeting often becomes mired in distortions, untruths, and inappropriate flag-waving reflecting a resounding lack of good old American know-how.

In addition, the individual is called upon daily to make a number of personal health decisions that will affect his well-being. He must decide if and when to seek medical help, whether or not to use self-prescribed drugs, and the nature of his diet, to mention just a few. It has, for instance, been estimated that half of all blindness and a great deal of impaired vision are due to the failure of people to perform some comparatively simple functions. Glaucoma, a leading cause of blindness in this country, can be controlled in most cases by early detection and treatment. Strabismus (cross-eyed condition), a cause of one-eyed blindness, is usually permitted to advance to have its deleterious effects on children because parents waited for them to "outgrow" the condition. Similarly, a great deal of hearing loss that now occurs is either preventable or results from improper treatment. The lack of sophistication with regard to the basic care and preservation of vital senses seems to be a rather extraordinary complacency of our society.

Fraudulent consumer health practices are also as prevalent today as they ever have been. The sale of cancer and arthritis cures, the half a billion dollar business of food faddists and weight-reducing quackery are but a few examples of practices that are monetarily wasteful and many times dangerous to

[4] "Bad Health Information on TV," *Today's Health* (June 1972), p. 7.

health. In addition, a real lack of sophistication exists with regard to the utilization of medical care services and facilities. The distinction between medical, paramedical, and sectarian practitioners is not clear to many people.

Statements by various health authorities indicate health knowledge deficiencies related to a number of health problems. Dr. Leona Baumgartner, former Health Commissioner of New York City, stated at a three day conference sponsored by the National Health Council:

> There is widespread evidence that the health professions are not communicating what they know about control and prevention of certain diseases to the public. We can cure an estimated one-half of all cases of cancer today by finding them soon enough, and doing for them what we already know how to do.[5]

An estimated 1500 children under the age of fourteen die each year from accidental poisoning. American health authorities estimate that 95 per cent of all childhood poisonings can be prevented. Dr. Howard M. Cann stated:

> Poison control centers need to place more emphasis on the prevention of accidental poisoning. The lag in promoting preventive activities may be explained by the lack of effective techniques and materials. A vigorous community education program, as a cooperative poison control center and local health department venture, has not been fully exploited. . . . Local, state and national groups must cooperate in coordinated and concentrated preventive activities.[6]

The American Diabetes Association reports that there are two million undetected cases of diabetes in the United States. These are people who have the disease but do not know it, either because they show no obvious symptoms or do not know what the symptoms are and consequently ignore them.

A conclusion reached as a result of a Harris poll conducted for the Blue Cross Organization is that,

> Most people apparently know considerably less about their own health and the nature of disease than they think they do. The Harris Organization interviewed 1,609 adults around the nation, asking them first how well-informed they thought they were, and then asking specific questions about health matters. Sixty six percent of those surveyed said they were well informed, and only 28 percent felt they didn't get enough information about health. Sixty-five percent said they could recognize the symptoms of the most important illnesses. But when the survey got down to asking specific questions, the results were quite different. Thirty percent could not name even one of the seven danger signals of cancer; 17 percent could name only one; and only 13 percent could come up with four or more. Similarly, only half the total could volunteer more than one symptom of a heart attack or other heart condition and 27 percent were unable to think of any at all.[7]

[5]Leona Baumgartner, M.D., former Health Commissioner of New York City, in a speech to the National Health Forum as quoted by *The New York Times*.

[6]Howard M. Cann, "Poison Control and Prevention," *Currents in Public Health*, Vol. 1, No. 2 (May 1961), Ross Laboratories, p. 3.

[7]"Serious Gaps in Health Knowledge," *Today's Health* (April 1972), p. 7.

PEANUTS
Tm. Reg. U.S. Pat. Off.—All rights reserved
© 1972 by United Feature Syndicate, Inc.
YES, MA'AM, I'D LIKE TO TALK TO THE DOCTOR...
11-3

NO, I FEEL FINE... I'D JUST LIKE TO TALK TO HIM FOR A MINUTE...

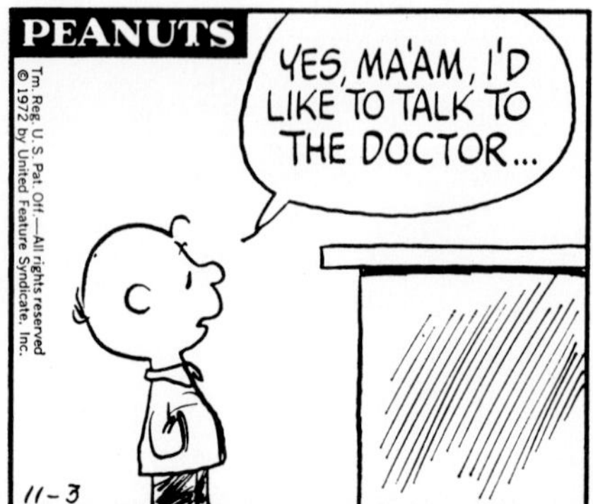

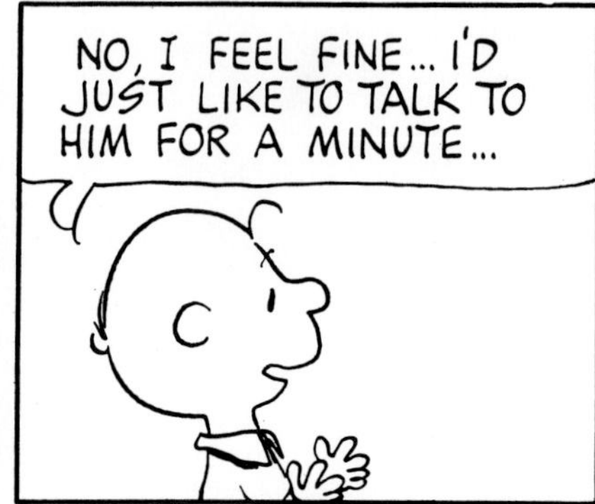

These are but a few examples of the innumerable statements made by health authorities citing a lack of health knowledge as a strong contributory factor to our health problems.

Health Status and One's Life Style

It is becoming increasingly evident that how one lives will strongly effect one's quality of health and life expectancy. For example, at the present time the leading cause of death and disability in the United States is heart disease—a disease of "civilization." What are the major risk factors associated with the condition? Cigarette smoking, lack of exercise and overweight, or other factors related to poor nutrition. In essence a great deal of heart disease could be prevented if people were to change their life-styles and eat properly, exercise adequately, and avoid cigarette smoking. The usual pattern is to respond to heart disease with surprise and dismay, when in fact it had been made practically inevitable by the manner in which the person lived. If the person survives his first heart attack, then he begins hopefully to reorder his way of living—literally under the threat of death.

In the epidemic incidence of alcoholism, drug addiction, emphysema, and lung cancer, we find other examples of how the manner in which one lives affects his health status. The overuse or inappropriate use of alcohol, drugs, and cigarettes serve as the vehicle for serious societal health problems. When the individual lives in an environment that encourages the misuse of these substances, it becomes clear that his decisions on these matters are not made in a vacuum.

A factor further complicating these problems is that our medical care system is therapeutically and disease-oriented. It sits back waiting for people to become ill, then goes into action attempting to correct the problem. The difficulty is that with many modern-day health problems (i.e., heart disease, alcoholism, drug abuse, emphysema, or lung cancer) the person is either already seriously damaged by the time he is seen by the physician or the physician has no effective "cure" for the problem. We have in essence painted ourselves into a corner developing life-styles that often include substance use and other factors that predispose us to serious health problems that our medical care system cannot effectively handle.

> For our cigarette users we build heart, cancer and respiratory disease institutes. For our alcoholics, addicts and venereal disease sufferers, we build diagnostic and rehabilitation centers, with mental hospitals and correctional institutes held in reserve. All of these with so little thought or research given to support the thesis that if our youth were given relevant information systematically and professionally, at a time in their lives when it could be of some value, they might very well solve the majority of these problems themselves with that selfsame common sense that we do not give them credit for having. I propose to you, that if a solution to these medical problems does not come by the positive decisions of an enlightened youth, the solution is not likely to come at all.[8]

[8]Ronald G. Vincent, M.D., "The Physician's Role in the Health Program," *New York State Journal of Health, Physical Education and Recreation*, Vol. 22, No. 3, p. 28.

I SEE...

IF I GO BACK OUTSIDE, AND CATCH A COLD, THEN MAY I TALK TO HIM?
SCHULZ

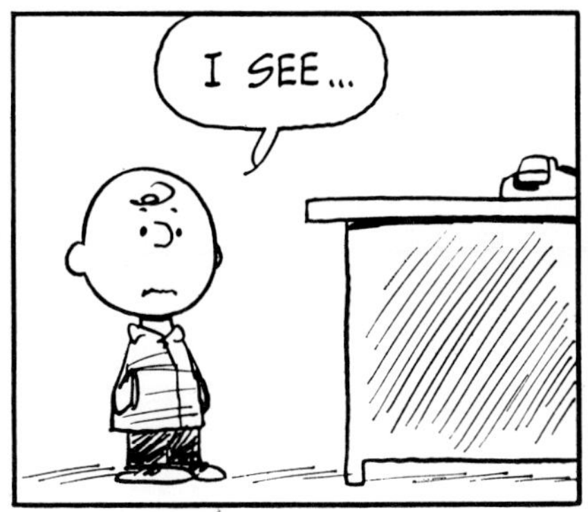

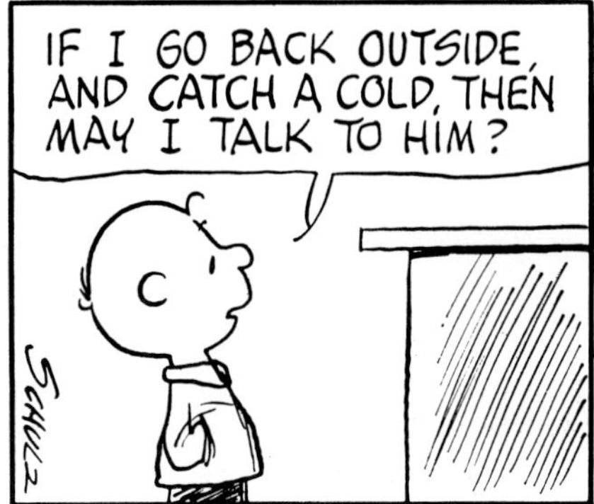

Fig. 1-4. "I'd Like to Talk to the Doctor." Peanuts cartoon by Charles M. Schulz. (© 1972 by United Feature Syndicate, Inc.)

It would seem that no health problem is under control until it can be prevented. This principle even applies to the problem of venereal diseases where effective treatment is available, but where the epidemic of VD still rages out of control. Since life-styles are learned—not born—it becomes necessary to inform people at early ages of the advantages and consequences of various life-styles. Obviously this kind of education should not belatedly occur in the intensive care unit of a hospital.

It may be that the health professions of the future will be oriented more toward developmental processes than diseases. Indeed, this is already taking place as the new knowledge of genetics, biochemistry, immunology, and microbiology provides more techniques by which we can understand each human being more fully, anticipate the developmental hazards to which he may be predisposed, and hopefully intercept these hazards. In the process, medicine will need to shift some of its institutional base from the hospital to the community in order to observe people who are considered healthy. And in the process, the health professions will come to scrutinize more carefully whether we are applying the knowledge we already have.[9]

While the health professions are reorienting themselves from a disease and therapeutic orientation to one embracing the concepts of health and prevention, each individual needs to assess his own health values. He must do this, recognizing that if he makes mistakes there may be no one available who is capable of correcting them.

[9]Julius B. Richmond, M.D., "Human Development," *The Health of Americans,* ed. Boisfeuillet Jones (Englewood Cliffs, N.J.: Prentice-Hall, 1970), p. 7.

Heredity as a Health Factor

One cannot overlook the hereditary factor in any discussion of health. As every physician knows, a family history is as important as the individual's medical history. We are, after all, the products of our parents and to some extent our grandparents and great-grandparents. Their genes in varying combinations become our genes—both the desirable ones and the undesirable ones. Physicians are often on the alert for the appearance of disorders in an individual simply because the disorder appeared with such frequency in the family. We know for instance that there is a genetic factor associated with diabetes. If this disorder has been present in the family (particularly on both sides of the family), the physician knows that there is a greater possibility for this disease to appear in this patient. Because the tendency for diabetes is passed on by a recessive gene, a minority in the family will be thus affected. It will be in this case a larger minority than normally found in a family group.

The advances made in the medical sciences has increased the survival rate as well as the degree of comfort of those who have disorders that are genetically influenced. The life expectancy of the diabetic has been extended. Epilepsy is largely controlled now by drug therapy, and so it goes for a number of other such disorders. The once hopeless reaction to genetic-borne diseases has changed rather radically. There are some, however, who have viewed this progress with jaundiced eye. They point out that the increased survival rate of people with these disorders results in their reproducing increased numbers of individuals to whom these deficiencies would be transmitted. The claim is made that advances in the medical sciences will effect some short-term gains in dealing with these genetic conditions, but in the long run will result in disadvantages to man. Others feel that the continued advances in medical science will result in man's complete control of these deficiencies and render them inconsequential factors.

Man's genetic endowment does not stand alone. Its interaction with his environment will determine his development.

> Modern man is now busily at work altering his environment, and he is doing this at what appears to be an ever-increasing rate. He is synthesizing new chemical compounds with which life has never before been confronted, using some as drugs, putting others into atmosphere as wastes, and spreading still others on crops as insecticides. As a result of modern medical and public health practice, vast numbers of people are being injected with new chemical and biological preparations. Some of these alterations of the genetic endowment may, under certain conditions prove to be undesirable or harmful. It is one of the basic tasks of human geneticists to discover what these alterations are likely to be, and how the unwanted ones could be avoided.[10]

Health used to be regarded as a gift from the gods. It is still an entity that is not well understood, one that people alternately drink to, pray for, take for granted, abuse, or become hypochondriacs about. It is time for some objectivity. Under the focus of the health sciences it has now been assessed that health is measurable, qualitatively and quantitatively. The varied hereditary and environmental health factors singly, in combinations, or in interaction with each other are being studied with regard to their positive and negative health contributions. Maintaining and raising levels of man's health can now be planned and educated for and the results measured and evaluated. This is not to imply that the sciences concerned with the study of health have attained an ultimate in their field. But they have begun.

[10] "Inside The Factory That Moulds Man," *World Health* (August–September 1966), p. 9.

Review Questions

1. What are the bases of your concern for your health?
2. How have the advances in the health sciences changed the traditional criteria for measuring the quality of health?
3. How have some environmental factors complicated man's quest for a long and healthful life?
4. Discuss those elements of man's environment that contribute to his health status.
5. Research that produces new health information is often not applied as enthusiastically as a new drug or vaccine. Explain.
6. The level of health knowledge of the American public leaves much to be desired. Cite evidence to support this statement.
7. "Man's genetic endowment does not stand alone. Its interaction with his environment will determine his development." Explain.

8. Having effective treatment for a disease condition does not guarantee control of it. Explain.
9. Explain why the health professions need to reorient themselves from a posture of offering treatment after the fact to one of promoting health and preventing health problems.
10. How can altering one's life-style affect one's health status?

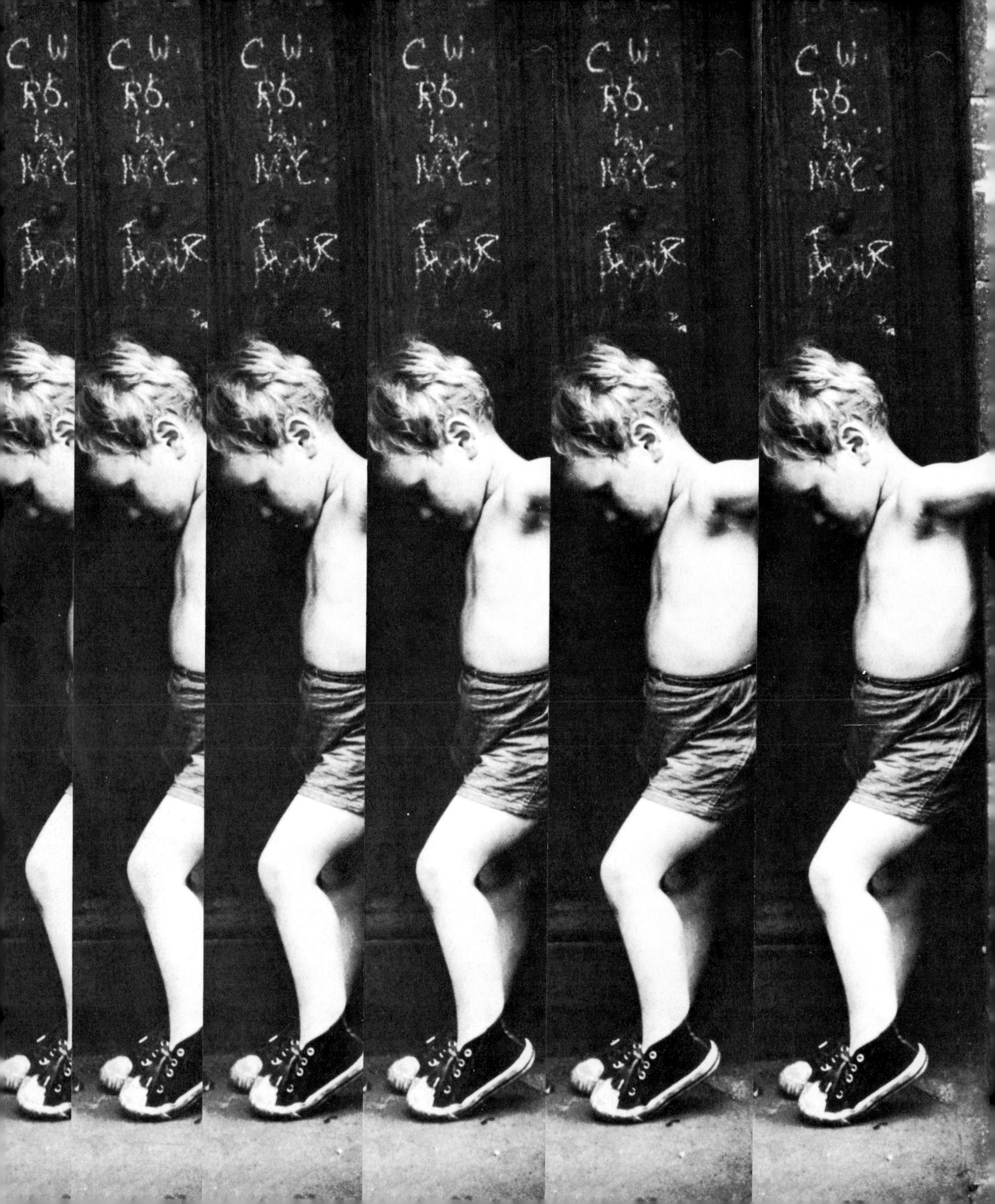

Part Two
Mental Health

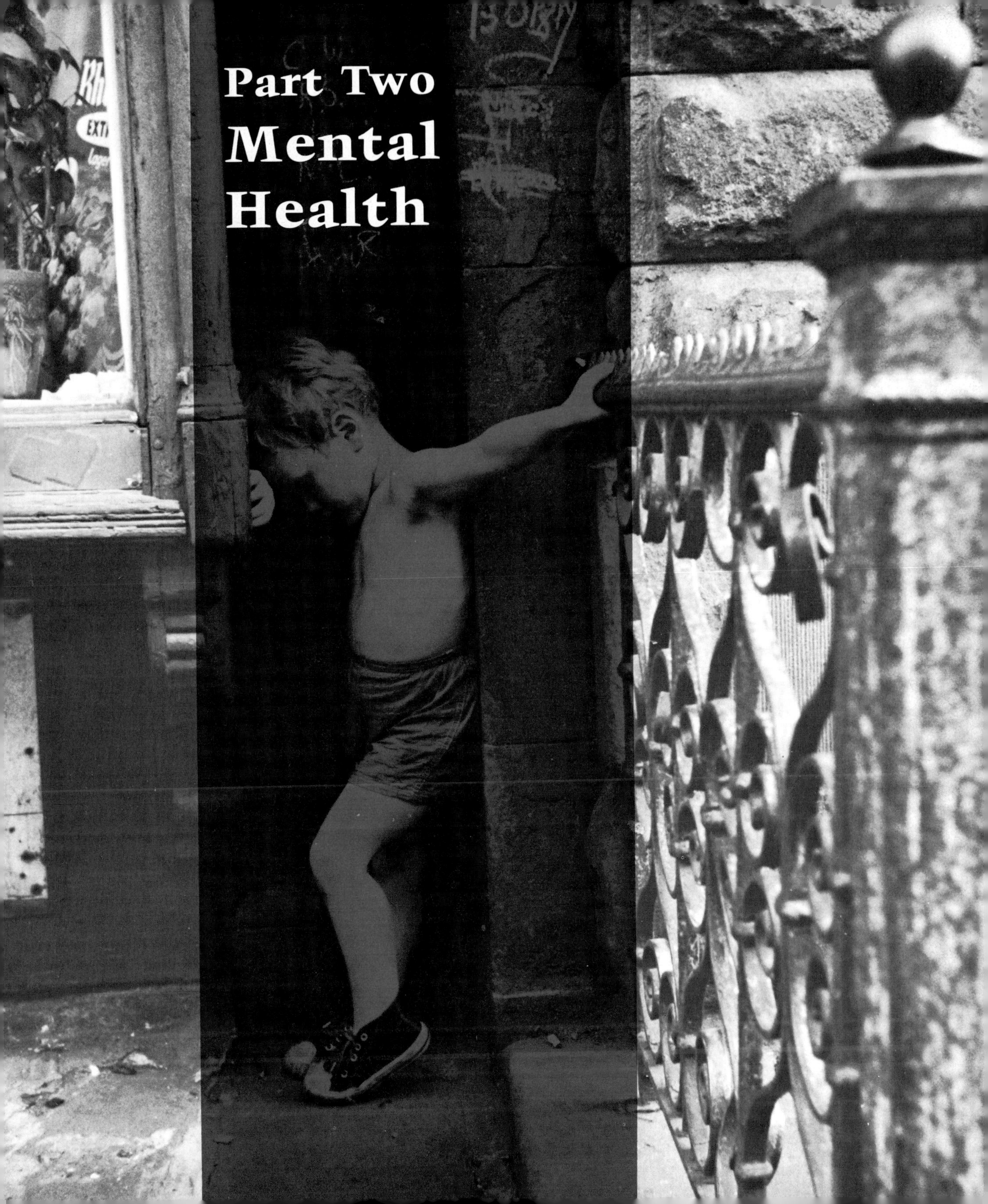

Chapter 2
The Bases of Mental Health

All our lives long, every day and every hour, we are engaged in the process of accommodating our changed and unchanged selves to changed and unchanged surroundings; living, in fact, is nothing else than this process of accommodation; when we fail in it a little we are stupid, when we fail flagrantly we are mad, when we suspend it temporarily we sleep, when we give up the attempt altogether we die. In quiet, uneventful lives the changes internal and external are so small that there is little or no strain in the process of fusion and accommodation; in other lives there is great strain, but there is also great fusing and accommodating power; in others great strain with little accommodating power. A life will be successful or not, according as the power of accommodation is equal to or unequal to the strain of fusing and adjusting internal and external changes.[1]

Man, Mental Health, and Civilization

Consider the simplicity of life for primitive man. He preoccupied himself with such basic matters as hunting, fighting, sleeping, and reproducing. It was an uncomplicated existence with a low incidence of "nervous breakdown." Civilization has made things much more complex and the satisfaction of needs more indirect. In order to obtain food, man does not hunt, but must train himself to acquire marketable skills that will earn the money to buy food. Man's instincts to fight have also been modified. Provocation does not now call for a direct punch, but for due process of law, a carefully worded verbal retort (lest we be sued for libel), or a nasty letter to the editor. The man who resorts to fisticuffs is behaving like the animal he *was* rather than the human being he is supposed to be.

Man's evolution is based on the fact that he has lost his original home, nature—and that he can never return to it, can never become an animal again. There is only one way he can take: to emerge fully from his natural home, to find a new home—one which he creates by making the world a human one and by becoming truly human himself.[2]

The reproductive function has probably become the most complicated of all. This now requires marriage and the setting up of a home, which immediately embroils the individual in the most complex of legal and economic systems. Religious factors of even finite proportions related to the marriage become major considerations. Social customs surrounding the wedding further enmesh the original intent.

Sleep, which was once a simple reaction to fatigue to the active precivilized man, is now often thwarted by tension and too often pill-induced.

While all this may have some negative undertones, there is a positive side. As stated by Dr. Karl Menninger, an eminent psychiatrist:

It is only when resistance is placed in the course of an electric current that heat and light are developed. And it was only by the imposition of certain repressions that

[1] Samuel Butler, *The Way of All Flesh* (New York: New American Library, 1960), p. 280.

[2] Eric Fromm, *The Sane Society* (New York: Rinehart, 1955), p. 25.

the interests of mankind became extended to their present and ever-increasing range.[3]

The maze that is civilization, then, requires a modification of man's aggressive instincts and behaviors if chronic frustration and unhappiness are to be avoided. Like the mouse in the maze, overly direct actions merely result in hitting one's head against a solid wall. The more indirect routes dictated by civilization can result in a life with greater meaning and abundance. The adaptive changes required in a technological society are factors that man is challenged to meet in order to continue his progress.

Civilized man is in a great period of transition. He is in the process of adapting to a new self-created environment, an environment that has new elements related to both his physical and psychological self. That this adjustment should create some visible stresses and strains is to be expected. We are living in an era of such fundamental change that man's very soul seems to be the object of public discussion, if not criticism. Nothing is sacred. The very pillars of societal or individual strength appear to be crumbling.

> Faith has been replaced by a shallow rationalism, spiritual values by utilitarian ones, pride in one's work by interest in the profit it brings, tradition has been divested of its glory by historical criticism, and social conventions are for many no more than an object of ridicule.[4]

[3]Karl A. Menninger, *The Human Mind* (New York: Knopf, 1937), p. 130.

[4]Oswald Schwarz, *The Psychology of Sex* (Pelican Books, 1962), p. 242.

How does one play a game without rules? There will be those who will be intimidated by this lack of structure and be tempted to blame the previous generation for a chaotic state of affairs, as if a single generation could be responsible for man's current state—a development that has taken thousands of years.

Others will try to escape from it through the world provided by drugs. Some will try to return to the land, to live as their ancestors did, attempting to forget civilization and the technology it has wrought with its destruction of past values and social structures. It may be a futile attempt to escape the reality of things or merely a respite while one conducts an inner search for one's fundamental values. Basic in all this is that element of hope that marks the difference between animal and man. Life and living *happen* to an animal. He eats when he is hungry, he sleeps when he is tired, and mates during nature's predetermined time of year. With man, life is not so much a happening as it is something that he makes happen. *Man is the maker of his own destiny.* Those who are not faint of heart will come forward and build the new social structure based on greater human understanding.

Basic Needs

Each human being has fundamental physical and psychological needs. These are fundamental to the survival and development of the individual as an organism and a personality. The child that does not receive love from its mother may become as emo-

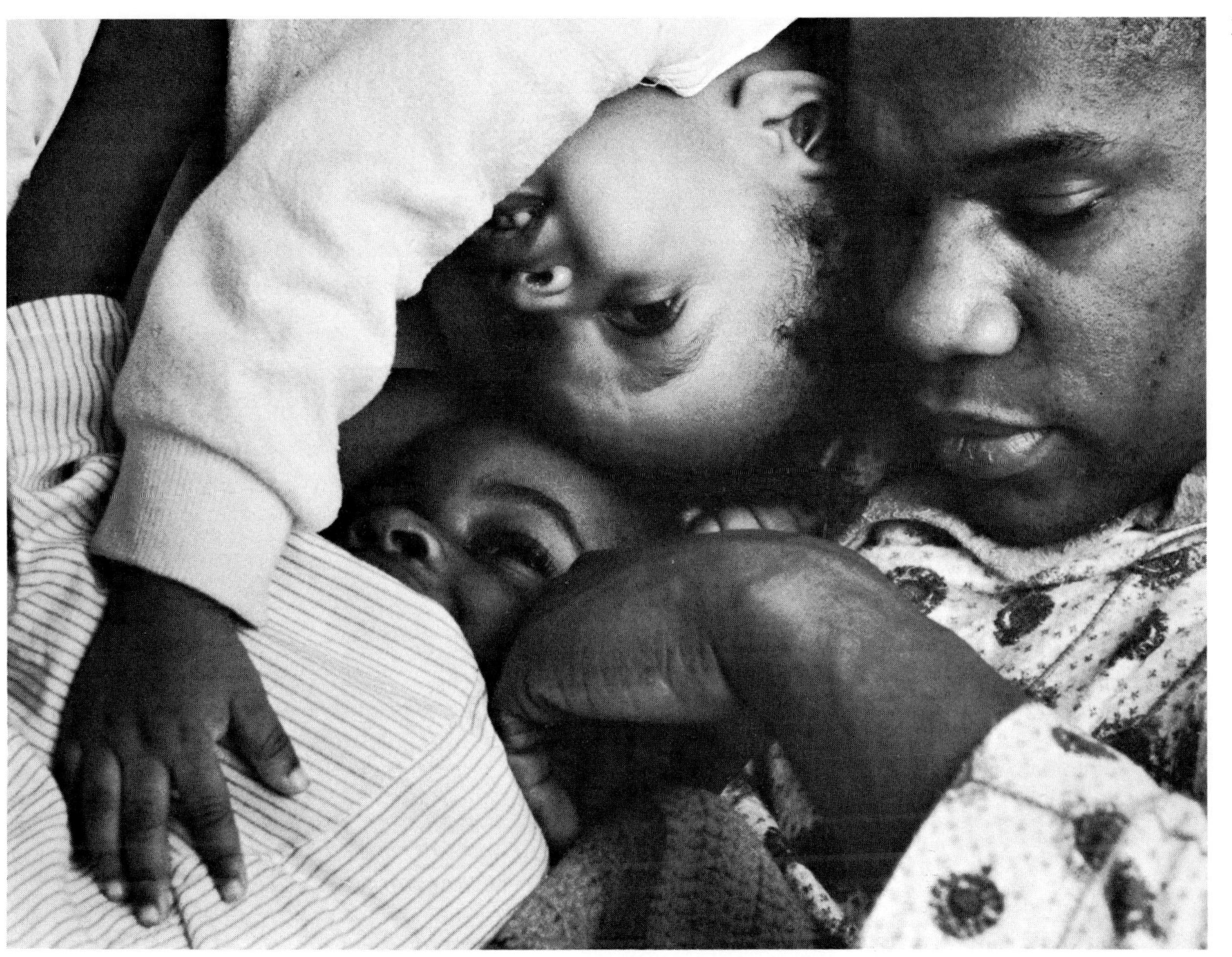

Fig. 2-1. Emotional needs are based initially on receiving love, affection, and acceptance from parents in the early years of life. (Ken Heyman)

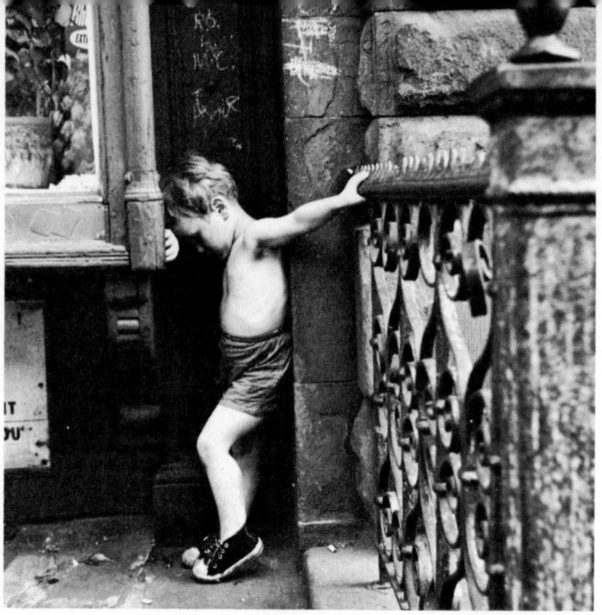

Fig. 2-2. *Some people are so convinced of their inability to perform certain tasks that they inevitably fail.* (*Ken Heyman*)

tionally deprived as one not receiving enough food is physically deprived.

Basic needs of a physical nature revolve around needs for air, sleep, food, and sex. We would not survive in an environment that lacked air for more than a few minutes. We spend approximately a third of our lives satisfying our need for sleep. The need for food serves as a prime motivator for a person developing marketable skills so that he can purchase this commodity. Sex needs are the ones most likely to be frustrated or sublimated because our culture has certain taboos with regard to sexual activity and because personal values of some people lead them to sublimate this drive until marriage.

Physiologists feel that the disruption of the functioning of any system of the body creates a basic physical need because the life of the organism can be endangered. A lack of oxygen or the inability of blood to clot could serve as two of many possible examples.

Emotional needs are based initially on receiving love, affection, and acceptance from parents in the early years of life. It has been dramatically demonstrated that infants who are separated from their mothers or a mother substitute for extended periods of time become extremely dispirited. They not only exhibit obviously poor mental health but can also become physically ill by this deprivation. Delinquency and varied emotional problems are related to the failure to receive normal love and affection at an early age. This emotional barrenness may cause the individual to grow up with a distrust for other people and the inability to give or receive love.

As the child grows older, added to the needs of love, affection, and acceptance by parents, are needs for achievement and the development of status. The need to achieve is basic to our ego development. The means of satisfying these needs are of course many and varied. Some individuals have talent academically, others develop creative skills with paints, music, or dance, and some demonstrate multiple talents. Actually, the important thing is not so much the profoundness of the achievement as it is the satisfaction one derives from the experience. For instance, who is to say that the solving of a complex mathematical problem is a greater accomplishment than the successful growing of a beautiful rose?

Need for status is related to, and sometimes grows out of, the fulfillment of the psychological needs, namely love, affection, acceptance, and achievement. The person needs initially to have status in his family group; later in his development this need is extended to his peer group. As an adult, the person seeks added status in his or her field of endeavor. When a person's status is threatened, the assertive question, "Just whom do you think you are talking to?" may be heard or actions reflecting the question may be seen. This kind of response and its frequency reflect how important status needs are to the individual. Very often the desire for status will lead to the acquisition of material possessions that are not really needed but become psychological trophies for the individual (the expensive car, the mink coat, the bizarre wardrobe). Some relegate themselves to the level of pseudosophisticates in attempts to reflect cultural qualities they do not possess.

Maslow,[5] in his theory of hierarchy of human needs, states that people have physical needs that lead to personality growth and toward self-actualization. Maslow states that these needs must be successively satisfied. The organism seeks to satisfy the lower-level needs such as hunger before it becomes concerned with higher-level love needs. The epitome of personality development, according to Maslow, is the self-actualizing person. This person is dedicated to a profession, cause, or science. The self-actualizing person is dedicated not for the recognition or other rewards his work may bring him. He follows his dedication to wherever it may lead him, even though it may result in disapproval from others, or even persecution. Darwin, with his theory of evolution, and Pasteur, with his germ theory of disease, stirred up a great deal of controversy. These men did not, however, waver in their dedication and their work. This Maslow regards as self-actualization.

Maslow also states that the person whose basic needs have been met early in life develops a strong personality structure. He is then capable to a much greater extent to weather opposition, rejection, and other negative conditions later in life. In planting a small tree one takes every precaution to protect it from the elements so that it will develop strong roots and have a good start in life. The transfer of this principle from trees to man on occasion falls short. This is exemplified by the father who feels he must subject his son to "rough" treatment in order for the boy to grow up to "be a man." The physical and emotional violence directed toward the youngster is comparable to stomping on the young tree and shaking it from its roots. Growth is not a response to overzealous, misconceived actions, but a reaction to nature's slow, positive, and constructive elements.

The ability to satisfy our psychological needs is reflected in our self-concept. How a person views himself is quite crucial to his mental health and to his effectiveness. Some people are so convinced of their inability to perform certain tasks that they inevitably fail. The coach's locker-room pep talk is often aimed at improving the self-concept of his team. As we know, this can at times prove an effective antidote to an uninspired group. However, we must also be realistic enough to realize that all cannot be accomplished by merely the will to do. A certain amount of talent is also necessary. A person whose self-concept is on a healthy level is one who is confident of his decisions, has set fairly specific goals, understands his values and ideals, and is comfortable with regard to opinions of others about him.

It is important to know that self-concept is learned. One's concept of self is strongly influenced by his childhood interrelationships with parents and siblings. The child becomes more and more aware of how he is being appraised by others. If these appraisals are positive, feelings of worth then develop. If the appraisals are derogatory, then the person is made to feel undesirable, worthless, and inferior. One's self-concept is always subject to change throughout life. Greater changes usually occur during childhood

[5] Abraham H. Maslow, *Toward a Psychology of Being* (Princeton, N.J.: Van Nostrand, 1962).

as compared with the adult years. One of the important responsibilities of parenthood is to help children to grow up feeling accepted in an environment reflecting warmth and affection. In addition, each of us has the opportunity to make a contribution in dignifying every human life we come in contact with. Self-concepts are made, not born.

What, Then, Is Mental Health?

Mental health is sometimes mistakenly viewed as an absolute, something that a person either has or does not have. Actually it is more of an ideal that people strive for with varying degrees of success. It is reflected in our abilities to assume responsibility, to solve problems, to make decisions, to find satisfactions and happiness, and to live effectively with other people. To be sure, all people enjoy successes and experience failures in attempts to accomplish the difficult and to resolve conflicting drives and goals. Our level of mental health can be measured by our ability to take advantage of the buoyancy provided by success and to survive the depression of failure.

Many view the "well-adjusted" person as being mentally healthy. This is a person who has struck a suitable balance between himself, his needs, and his environment. Because there is a constant change taking place in our internal as well as external environment, adjustment is not a static condition but one that is in a constant state of flux. The only people who are permanently adjusted are those in cemeteries; the rest of us have to work at it constantly.

Leading psychologists and psychoanalysts have varying concepts with regard to what constitutes a well-adjusted or mentally healthy person. William Blatz, a well-known child psychologist from Canada views self-reliance as the most important characteristic of the healthy personality. This means the ability to accept the consequences of one's decisions and actions. Alfred Adler, a psychologist who once worked with Freud, regarded social feeling or the ability to identify with mankind as a barometer of mental health. Otto Rank, an early psychoanalyst, viewed creativity as the important criterion in evaluating healthy mindedness. He felt the person who was not afraid to be different and to assert his indivuality was self-assured. Sidney Jourard, psychologist, views a healthy personality as one that is "able to gratify his needs through behavior that conforms with both the norms of his society and the requirements of his conscience."[6] Herbert Carroll feels that mental health depends upon the development of a mental hygiene point of view that would include:

1. Respect for one's own personality and for the personalities of others.
2. Recognition of limitations in the self and in others.
3. An appreciation of the importance of the causal sequence in behavior. (All behavior is caused; it does not just happen.)
4. A realization that behavior is a function of the whole individual.

[6]Sidney M. Jourard, *Personal Adjustment* (New York: Macmillan, 1961), p. 17.

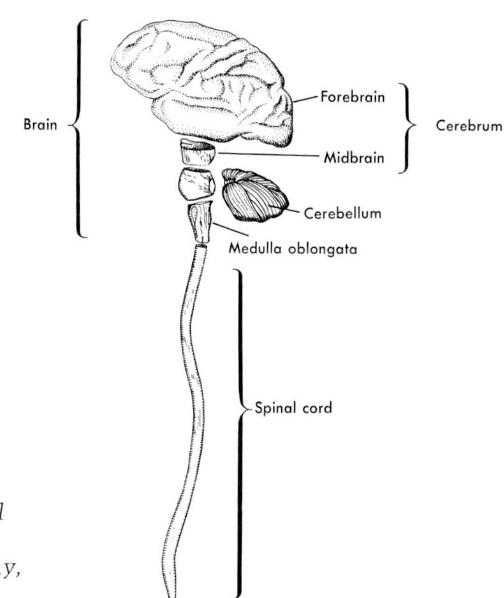

Fig. 2-3. The major sections of the central nervous system. (Adapted from Morris, Human Anatomy, *The Blakiston Company, N.Y.)*

5. An understanding of the basic needs that motivate behavior.[7]

Though there is not a universally accepted definition of what is mental health or a healthy personality, the foregoing provide us with some guidelines.

The Relationship of Body Systems to Mental Health

THE NERVOUS SYSTEM

The nervous system acts as the controlling and communications center of the body. It is responsible for conscious and unconscious thoughts and all of the voluntary and involuntary muscular movements of the body. It regulates such vital processes as circulation, respiration, and digestion.

The nervous system is divided into two main divisions, namely, the central nervous system, made up of the brain and spinal cord, and the peripheral nervous system. The latter is composed of 12 pairs of nerves (cranial) arising from the brain, 31 pairs of nerves arising from the spinal cord, and the nerves of the autonomic nervous system.

The brain, in acting as the control center, responds to the many and varied impulses that reach it. It can respond to various sensory impulses (sight, touch, sound, smell, and taste) all at the same time. Consider the varied impulses being received by the brain when one sits down to dinner with friends. Distinguishing between the brain or brain function and the mind is a fascinating topic that this text will leave for further student conjecture and investigation.

The largest part of the brain is the cerebrum. This is the area where experiences are stored (memory) and where they are associated with one another. Reason, judgment, and emotions emanate from this area. Our speech center as well as centers for hearing, smell, balance, and vision are located here.

The cerebellum is the second largest portion of the brain. Its functions relate to effecting muscular coordination. What appears to be a simple act, like that of picking up a pencil, requires the coordination of a large number of muscles and the relating of distance to rate of movement. Disorders that affect the cerebellum will not cause paralysis but will result in tremors, a staggering gait, and other evidence of poor muscular coordination.

A third part of the brain is the brain stem, made up of the midbrain and the medulla. The medulla controls such functions as breathing and heartbeat, as well as affecting digestion and body metabolism. The midbrain acts as a relay station for impulses traveling to the cerebrum. It also serves as the place from which several cranial nerves emanate.

The spinal cord, the other portion of the central nervous system, serves as the trunk line to the brain.

The 12 pairs of cranial nerves and 31 pairs of spinal nerves of the peripheral nervous system have the basic function of feeding impulses to the central nervous system. The second cranial nerve, for instance, originates in the retina of the eye and termi-

[7]Herbert A. Carroll, *Mental Hygiene* (Englewood Cliffs, N.J.: Prentice-Hall, 1956), p. 13.

nates in the optic lobe of the brain. The 31 pairs of nerves that emanate from the spinal cord keep the brain in touch with the various other parts of the body.

The Endocrine System

The endocrine glands are ductless glands that secrete chemical substances called hormones. These substances are secreted directly into the bloodstream where they are carried to all parts of the body. The hormones of the endocrine glands can have profound effects on certain tissues. The tissue upon which a specific hormone acts is called a target tissue. Hormones also have an effect on other endocrine glands and can either stimulate or inhibit their actions. The hormones of the endocrine system have a strong influence upon both the physical and personality development of the individual, affecting growth, behavior, and varied body processes.

Pituitary. The pituitary gland, located in the brain, is sometimes referred to as the master gland because of its influence on other endocrine glands. The pituitary secretes a number of hormones among which is one affecting growth. If there is an excessive secretion of this hormone during childhood, giantism results. Should the excesive secretion occur during the adult years, a disorder known as acromegaly develops. Although the person does not grow taller, he develops abnormally large hands and feet with a characteristic change in facial features. Should there be a deficiency of growth hormone of the pituitary in childhood, then the opposite condition, dwarfism, occurs. The mental ability of these persons will not be affected but will remain normal.

The pituitary gland also secretes a hormone that has an influence on the gonads. The amount of this hormone produced can cause either early or late puberty. The pituitary also has an effect on the rate of metabolism in the body and together with the hormone thyroxin can affect the accumulation of fat. In animal experiments, the removal of the pituitary causes an aggressive animal to become a very docile one. Animals deprived of their pituitary glands are also unable to produce sperm or egg cells.

Thyroid. The thyroid gland, located at the base of the neck, secretes the hormone thyroxin. The basic function of this hormone is to control the rate of metabolism in the body. The thyroid gland that is secreting an insufficient amount of the hormone tends to make the person sluggish, apathetic, and possibly emotionally depressed. Serious thyroid deficiencies in childhood result in a disorder known as cretinism. Retarded mental development and stunted growth are typical. When the thyroid deficiency occurs in the adult years, it causes a condition known as myxedema, which results from the atrophy of the thyroid gland. This disorder is characterized by a slowing down of both the mental and physical processes; the skin becomes dry and there is an accompanying loss of hair and teeth. Obesity is a common complication of myxedema, which can be corrected by the administration of thyroxin. The overactive thyroid gland secreting an excessive amount of the hormone thyroxin tends to have an accelerating affect on the person. Nervousness, excitability, and anxiousness are typical. Loss of weight, increased body temperature, and emotional instability may also occur. The condition is sometimes treated by the use of antithyroid drugs or by the surgical removal of part of the thyroid gland. Simple goiter is also a complication of the thyroid when there is a deficiency of iodine in the diet. This results in an enlargement of the gland in the neck. The prevention of the condition is through the administration of iodized salt.

Parathyroid. The parathyroid glands are usually four in number and are embedded in the thyroid tissue. Their primary function appears to be that of maintaining the proper calcium and phosphorous ratio in the blood and tissues of the body. A decrease in the parathyroid hormone is most commonly caused by accidental removal or injury of the glands in an operation on the thyroid, causing irritability, muscle weakness, and spasms. Excessive secretion of the parathyroid results in the formation of kidney stones and the decalcification of bone.

Adrenal. The adrenals are found on either side of the body above the kidneys. The inner portions of the adrenal glands secrete the hormone adrenalin that prepares the body for emergency action. The functions of the adrenal cortex are not well understood. Its absence is known to cause death; an oversecretion of its hormone causes a precocious sexual development in the boy prior to puberty and has a masculinizing affect on the female.

Gonads. The gonads' major function is the reproduction of sex cells. The testes produce sperm cells while the ovaries produce the egg cells. The gonads also secrete hormones that promote the development of secondary sexual characteristics such as the deeper voice and the beard. In the female the sex hormones result in the development of mammary glands and the feminine characteristics of the female body. They also serve to control menstruation, pregnancy, and lactation. The proper functioning of these glands has rather obvious implications for personality development. The person who feels inadequate sexually and unable to fulfill the role of "male" or "female" will no doubt face a number of emotional problems.

The Conscious and the Unconscious Mind

The psychological workings of the conscious and unconscious minds may be compared with the physiological functioning of voluntary and involuntary muscles. The actions of voluntary muscle tissue and the conscious mind are quite obvious and aboveboard. The involuntary muscles of the digestive tract and circulatory system, like the unconscious mind, are much more subtle in their functioning. We are unaware of their actions until something calls our attention to them—often as a result of a malfunction.

The unconscious serves to store the memory of past experiences. Recently experimentation has demonstrated that this function, previously regarded as just psychoanalytic theory, is true. Electrically stimulating various portions of the temporal complex with electrodes resulted in a conscious person's recalling periods of past experience. He relived the experience by hearing and seeing it with all the emotions initially related to it. The experience could be made to reappear with the reapplication of the electrodes.

There is evidence that unconscious thoughts influence our behavior, feelings, and decisions. These thoughts are sometimes "seen" in dreams or in purposeful forgetting. However, like the iceberg, most of it lies submerged and its great influence on us remains unrecognized.

A nine-year-old was judged by all who knew him to be very "good." He was extremely obedient to his parents and affirmed his love for his father in almost every conversation with anybody. He related this dream to the author:

"I dreamed that I was a soldier, and we had a very mean and cruel officer. One day, when nobody was around, he was beating up a very nice lady. I took my machine gun and shot him a million times. He fell into a lot of little pieces when I was finished."

One does not have to be a professional interpreter of dreams to suspect that the officer was a symbolic version of his father, toward whom the boy had strong but repressed hostility, while the "nice lady" was his mother, to whom he was very attached.[8]

The unconscious is often viewed in negative terms functioning to repress needs that the individual is afraid or ashamed of. In healthier personalities it can serve as a positive, creative source. When the unconscious is not preoccupied with the business of repression and inhibition, it is free to permit the surfacing into the conscious mind innovative ideas, solutions to problems, insights into oneself and others, and an otherwise surging forth of one's positive potentials.

Freud, basically responsible for the psychoanalytic theory with regard to the unconscious mind, felt that people tend to react in two ways, namely in relation to their environment and in relation to themselves. He therefore tended to categorize people's thinking into three component parts, which he called the id, superego, and ego. The "id" he described as that force of basic, primitive, uncivilized, and uninhibited drives related to man's nature, such as sex drives, infantile needs, and basic wants. As parts of the id these demand gratification without concern for the welfare of the individual or others.

Freud[9] regarded the superego as the conscience of the individual, acting to distinguish right from wrong. The superego has the function of impelling the individual to conform with or uphold those values that he learned early in life from parents and other authoritative figures. The superego tends to make the individual conform to the cultural pattern of which he is a part.

The ego was conceived by Freud as being a mechanism that merges the id and the superego. It accepts the basic drives and instincts of the id and on the other hand accepts the regulations of the culture that

[8]Sidney M. Jourard, *Personal Adjustment* (New York: Macmillan, 1967), p. 51.

[9]Sigmund Freud, *The Basic Writings of Sigmund Freud*, translated by A. A. Brill (New York: Modern Library, 1938).

Fig. 2-4. Emotional first aid. (James Foote)

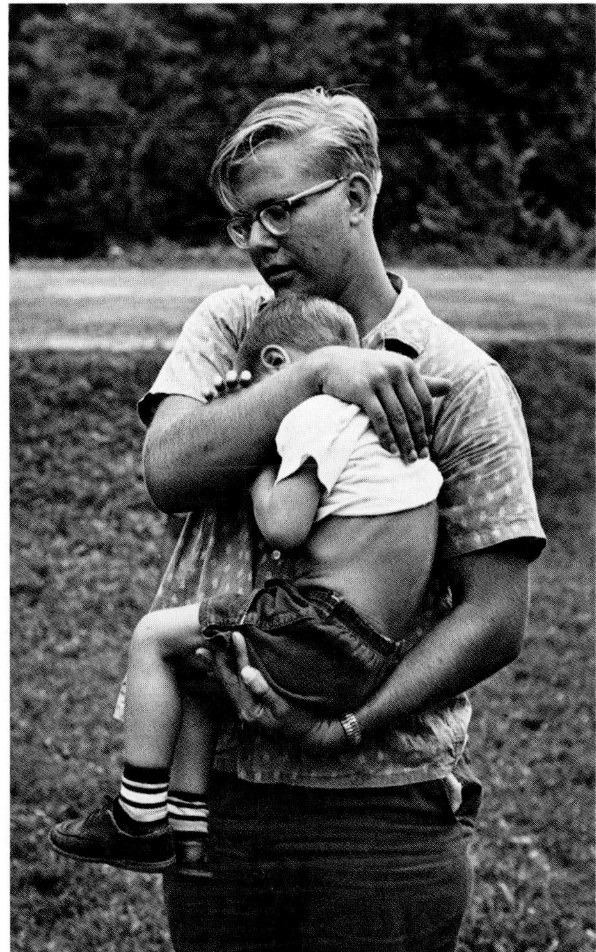

the superego imposes. It functions as an intermediary, regulating the forces between the id and superego, particularly in reaction to the environment and reality.

Psychological Stress

A person's ability to function can be inhibited by physical stresses such as undue fatigue, nutritional deficiencies, illness, and injury. A person can be debilitated to a similar, if not a greater, extent by psychological stress. The origins of psychological stress are often not clear to the individual, and as a result it is difficult for him to take actions of a preventive or corrective nature. The sources of psychological stress are often quite varied and can arise from any part of the environment. There can be social or cultural stress as related to poverty or social status. There are many stresses that can be developed right in the home as a result of interactions between parents and children. Disciplinary actions reflecting disapproval or rejection can many times develop stressful situations. A source of stress may be the individual himself, who finds it difficult to make decisions and who does not adapt easily to change. Because stress tends to have a wearing effect on the personality, it becomes important that stressful situations be resolved within relatively short periods of time. While stress of a mild nature can act as a stimulant to help the person become more productive, in greater amounts it may cause a person to direct his attentions toward relieving the discomfort involved rather than solving the problems that are causing the stress in the first place. The person who has a "safety valve" for the accumulated tensions developed by psychological stress has a much better chance of surviving these kinds of conditions. The person with a recreational outlet or hobby has found a means of diverting the excess energies thus developed. Where these diversions do not exist, the "safety valve" then may consist of the improper use of alcohol, drugs, or other damaging substances.

It is difficult if not impossible to separate the physical from the psychological. What affects one invariably affects the other. When a child scrapes a knee, "treating" the child's emotional reaction to the injury may be as important as the care of the injury itself. This is not to imply that the child should be coddled. In fact, just the opposite type of reaction may be appropriate in some cases. It does mean that emotional feelings should be considered along with the physical.

It should also be recognized that real physical disorders and pain can be produced by psychological stress. Any person under tension is reacting not only mentally, but physically as well. In response to these situations there are secretions from the adrenal glands, the pituitary gland, and increased thyroid activity. There is oftentime involvement of the gastrointestinal tract, as indicated by the relationship of ulcers to long term tensions. The acid production of the stomach is significantly increased during such periods of stress with resultant erosion of its lining. The physical reactions to stress are many and varied and could involve the cardiovascular system, with resultant cardiovascular disease, as well as the respiratory tract, with allergies and asthma being common reactions.

Anxiety as a Result of Stress

Kaplan describes anxiety as a "state of dread or apprehension characterized by an uncomfortable, vague, diffuse feeling of uneasiness.[10] All people have experienced anxieties of varying intensities at one time or another. Anxiety can have a wide range from the comparatively mild feelings experienced by the athlete before an athletic contest to the other extreme of real terror. Most kinds of anxiety prove to be helpful. The anxiety experienced by the runner before the race actually helps him to perform better. Controlled levels of anxiety tend to serve as stimulants to better performance. However, as with fear, if anxiety reaches a point where it becomes so distressing that the individual then becomes preoccupied with relieving it, he cannot attend to the other tasks about him. The biggest difficulty with anxiety arises when the person cannot identify its source. The person has anxious feelings and does not know why. These feelings are at times related to the workings of the superego serving as the conscience and emanating from the subconscious. This state of mind if continued over a long period of time can tend to be quite handicapping and may result in a number of neurotic reactions. We will have more to say about this later.

[10] Louis Kaplan, *Foundations of Human Behavior* (New York: Harper & Row, 1965), p. 212.

The Emotions

The three basic emotions have been identified as anger, love, and fear. Our ability to control emotions has a great deal of bearing on how well we will be able to function. It has been found that moderate levels of emotion stimulate us to think more clearly, react faster, and achieve higher levels of accomplishment. Emotions also enrich our lives when we experience the warmth of love and affection which gives a crescendo to living that would not otherwise be there. Emotions also serve to unite people even when they are experiencing an emotion like fear. A group of people trapped in an elevator develop a feeling of comradeship as a result of experiencing fear together. Each section of the country has its small commercial airline with borderline efficacy that seems to inspire in their passengers a camraderie not found in airlines with more sophisticated operations.

Intense emotion can have the effect of interfering with mental activity and break down our efficiency in various endeavors. For example, the lawyer who loses his temper in the courtroom is no longer capable of properly conducting his case. The adept fencer similarly swings wildly and ineffectively. Our ability to harness our emotions, therefore, is important to our effective functioning.

Emotions will often involve a number of physiological as well as psychological changes in the individual. The autonomic nervous system, for example, is concerned with the control of the parts of the body that function involuntarily. These include blood vessels, the heart, glands, and involuntary muscles. This system is made up of a series of nerve cell collections or ganglia. These ganglia lie along either side of the spinal cord and are connected to it by means of fibers. Some ganglia are located in the brain and control the tear glands and pupils of the eye. In an emotional state the autonomic nervous system prepares the body for a "fight" or "flight" reaction. It does this by diverting circulating blood to heart and skeletal muscles. Lung function is increased, the pupils of the eyes become dilated, and the skin becomes moistened with perspiration. The adrenal glands secrete adrenalin, which serves as a general body stimulant, and the liver releases sugar to serve as a source of additional energy. All systems are go!

A difficulty that can arise is that the emotional reaction may have been stimulated by a situation where a violent reaction is not appropriate. Many a person who is about to speak to a large group has experienced the increase in heartbeat and respiration as well as the clammy perspiration of nervousness. While the individual is geared for action, the situation calls for polite discussion. The emotional response then improperly prepares the person for the "emergency" situation. Some people have questioned whether fear and anger are emotions that serve an advantage or disadvantage to a person living in a highly technical society. The suppression of our emotions of fear and anger are in many respects related to headaches, backaches, tics of various types, and high levels of anxiety.

We also live in a competitive society where the fear of failure runs high. It is imperative that the

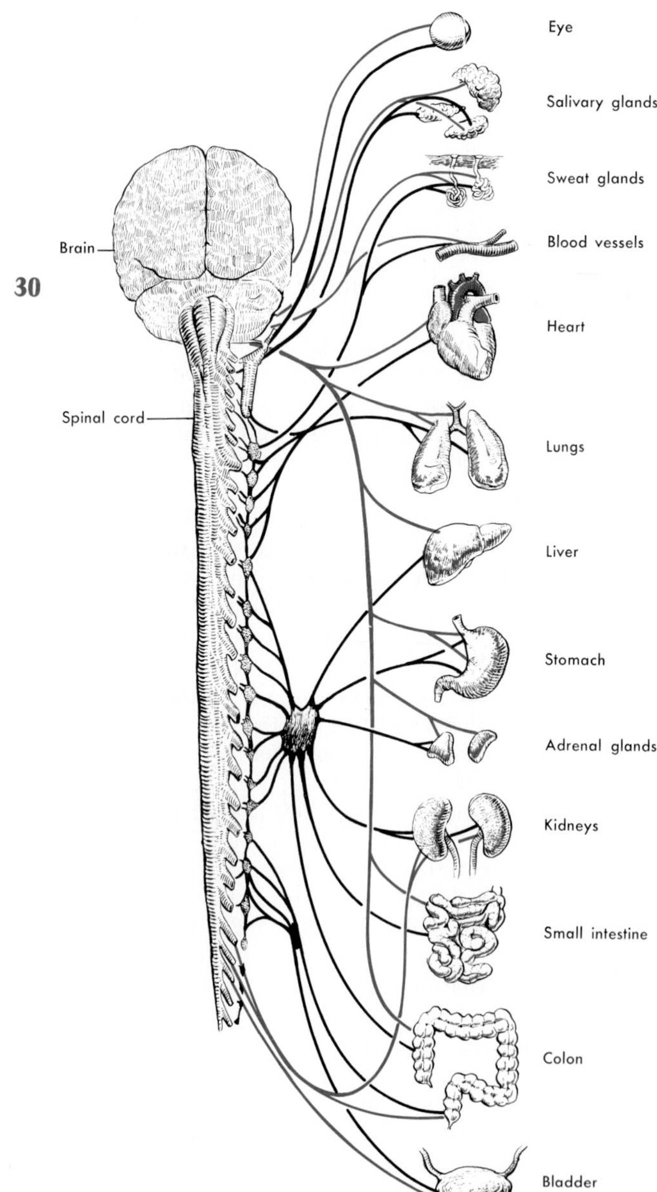

Fig. 2-5. The autonomic nervous system is made up of neurons that carry impulses to and from the organs, glands, and blood vessels of the body. The impulses operate automatically, causing bodily reactions that are not under the direct control of the individual. (Adapted from Clifford T. Morgan, Introduction to Psychology, *McGraw-Hill, N.Y.)*

individual become somewhat insulated against failure because he will experience a measure of this in the many highly competitive situations in which he will find himself. The real test of personality may not necessarily be measured in terms of degrees of success so much as it might be determined by the ability to deal realistically with failure. This ability might prove to be the ultimate success.

In a recent pole-vaulting event all contestants were eliminated save two. One of the men attempted to clear the new height the bar had been raised to and missed. His competitor noticed a flaw in his form that led to his missing his vault and informed him so. On the succeeding try he cleared the bar and won the event. By all standards in our competitive world the man who had placed second had failed. What would seem to be the greatest irony to many is that he contributed to his own "failure." "What is a man profited, if he shall gain the whole world, and lose his own soul?" Stated positively—if a man loses the world but gains his soul, has he really failed or has he in fact succeeded? It represents at the very least a selfless rather than a selfish act. It is also a religious concept too often forgotten in an egocentric, materialistic society.

The Mental Mechanisms

Mental mechanisms are means that we utilize to cope with anxiety. These mechanisms can be classified in three groups reflecting the kinds of actions that are taken in each, namely attack, flight, and compromise. The person in attack exhibits aggressive behavior that may be either physical or verbal in nature, directed at the source of frustration or a substitute for it. In flight, the person seeks to escape the situation or attempts to ignore it. In compromise, he decides to look at the problem once more and to live with it. These mechanisms tend to be generally used by people as a way of making life more comfortable by relieving anxiety. They can, of course, be symptomatic of personality difficulty when they are extensively used or when they are used rather rigidly and in fixed patterns. Usually mental mechanisms are unconscious in nature so that the person may be unaware he is employing them.

Daydreaming is a rather universal mechanism that is used by just about everyone from childhood on. It serves as a simple escape from situations that are unpleasant, boring, and perhaps even frustrating. It tends also to act as a bit of emotional relaxation. The "conquering hero" type of daydreaming is one in which the individual achieves the epitome of success. The boy pictures himself as the outstanding athlete or actor or whatever his unresolved dream might be. The girl might see herself in possession of great beauty, money, or fame. The "suffering hero" type of daydream is one that is of the opposite variety. In this the dreamer sees himself as the victim of neglect, abuse, and mistreatment. This type of daydream might follow punishment that the individual feels is unjust. Daydreams that focus on success can many times have positive results. When they are not too unrealistic, they can often serve as goals and encourage constructive planning. The mechanism can serve useful purposes as long as it is not used to excess.

Regression is the return of the individual to a more infantile manner of behavior. The person who resorts to childish acts when he does not get his way or cannot face problems on the adult level is regressing. A temper tantrum is a common type of regressive action. Those people who find it difficult to assume the responsibility and the tasks of their age group will many times revert to the dependency level and irresponsibility of younger years. If overused, regression may serve to make the person more dependent, indecisive, and overly cautious with regard to change.

Compensation is the mechanism whereby someone may offset his ability and success in one area against his failings in another. A person who feels he lacks status may seek to gain recognition through the purchase of an expensive item such as a car, suit, or dress as a means of compensating for his feelings of inadequacy. The person who tends to overcompensate for his feelings of inadequacy may become overly aggressive and domineering, and develop a fanatical need for power. On the other hand, compensation has its positive aspects as well. Some people who engage in community projects of various types are many times making a fine contribution, but are also compensating for unhappiness or boredom at work or at home. This kind of compensation might have a wholesome influence not only on the individual but on the community as well.

Substitution is a mechanism by which we tend to substitute one goal for another. A person may desire to own a very expensive car, but the reality of his bank balance motivates him to substitute the buying of a less expensive one. Where the person finds that he does not have the capability to perform well in a given activity or profession, he may decide to shift to one in which he can do better. This is a kind of substitute compensation. Substitution as a mechanism works out well only when the substitute goal is closely enough related to the desired one. Otherwise it is not really acceptable to the person. An inadequate substitution gives relief that is only temporary in nature, and the anxiety that stimulated the mechanism in the first place will recur.

Suppression is the process of consciously hiding thoughts and feelings. Unexpressed fear, hostility, or even laughter, may interfere with the ability of the person to do routine things such as to read with comprehension, play the piano, repair machinery, and so forth. The ability to suppress thoughts and feelings and thereby to delay their expression can be a desirable thing. It may be inappropriate to laugh or express fear at a given moment. Delaying their expression could spare the feelings of others who might feel they were being laughed at, or whose levels of fear were already reaching, for them, unmanageable proportions.

Repression is similar to suppression except that it is unconscious in nature and the person does not have conscious control over this mechanism. It serves to push into the unconscious shameful or guilt-ridden thoughts, memories, or painful and distasteful experiences. A person who has witnessed a serious automobile accident or a soldier who has seen death will many times repress these painful, unpleasant thoughts. Repressed thoughts are often the bases of anxiety that we do not understand. A person may see an object or be in a situation that reminds him of an incident that has been repressed. This may cause a degree of anxiety that the person has difficulty understanding. The unconscious thought would have to be uncovered in order for the person to become consciously aware of the relationship.

Repression is generally regarded as an unhealthy mechanism because unconscious motives are sometimes unhealthy ones. When one permits himself to identify his needs accurately, then he can set about to deal with them. When for one reason or another a person is afraid, ashamed, or in conflict with regard to a basic need, he represses it. The need or what to do about it then remains chronically unfulfilled. Conscious reminders of the need develop in turn feelings of anxiety, fear, or guilt. Repression, then, is an attempt to hide a problem and therefore an unsuitable means of solving it. One's biological sex drive and what is socially and morally acceptable present such a conflict.

Sublimation is the means by which instinctive and unacceptable impulses are transformed into socially useful goals. Primitive or aggressive impulses can be channeled into activities such as sports, art, literature, or religion. The mechanism of sublimation can serve an important function in the development of sound character and personality. Where sublimation is not possible, the personality finds itself in constant conflict.

Reaction-formation is exemplified by the submissive person who is actually covering up aggressive tendencies. Excessive amiability may be a facade for hostility. Reaction-formation, then, is a defense against the anxiety developed by disturbing and socially unacceptable feelings or impulses. The overly aggressive person may be covering up real feelings of insecurity. The overprotective mother who is obsessed with concern for her child's health and safety may actually be repressing hostility toward the child. This kind of false behavior usually becomes rather obvious. The mechanism does not reduce the tension caused by the conflict and somehow the underlying feelings seem to permeate the personality.

Fixation is the cessation of the development of the personality or a facet of it at an incomplete stage. There is normally a progressive development of the personality, not only in the psychosexual aspects, but in the ability to control emotion, to deal with frustration, and to assume responsibility. Why this process is arrested is not always understood. An example of this may be seen where child-parent ties persist for too long and the mother makes a son overly dependent upon her. His relationship to her remains childlike and he never reaches true adulthood.

Identification is a mechanism whereby the individual identifies with another. The girl may identify with a favorite actress, the small boy with a baseball player. The overevaluation of the abilities and attributes of these idealized figures usually occurs. The use of celebrities for commercials is based on their being viewed by many as being all-wise and near perfect. A second variety of this mechanism is in the association of one individual with another. On meeting a person, we may find we have a distinct impression of what the person is like and react accordingly. Because there has been no time to get to know the personality, we have actually identified him with someone we knew previously and attributed to him the characteristics of the other personality for better or for worse.

Rationalization is one of the most commonly used mechanisms. This is a means whereby a person gives a plausible reason for his behavior rather than the actual reason. The person who rationalizes is unconscious of his motives, and is not making a deliberate attempt to distort the truth. Rationalization makes the person feel better about playing golf instead of mowing the lawn, or helps the person feel guiltless about going to a dance instead of studying. He might rationalize these situations by indicating that he has been working too hard and is in need of a recreational outlet. If rationalization is used beyond the degree of moderation, the individual may rationalize his way out of many of his basic responsibilities.

Projection is a means of shifting blame and responsibility for an act or a thought to someone else. The person who fails the course blames the instructor, or the salesman having difficulty selling blames the product. Another form of projection is scapegoating, whereby the blame for situations may be focused or projected on to other groups in the community. A weak minority tends to serve this negative purpose well. Even though projection may many times relieve anxiety, it often carries with it a sense of guilt that can lead to a need for self-punishment.

These internal mechanisms which are used universally are generally unconsciously selected and used automatically by the personality. Because they help to manage anxiety, aggressive impulses, and frustration, they make life a good deal more bearable during difficult times. The manner and extent to which they are used can serve as barometers of a healthy personality.

Death—A Part of Every Life

Death is an inevitable part of every life. It is a normality of life, just as every sunset must follow a sunrise. It has often been stated that "nothing is more certain than death and taxes," yet there are in our society many inappropriate responses to death. Death is often denied or repressed and the thought of it, resulting in an inability to cope with it when it occurs. The hysterical reactions of friends and relatives as well as the frantic, fruitless efforts of health professionals do not enrich one's last moments. When the death of an individual is expected *and* inevitable, it is time for solace and compassion.

In years gone by, the family would be called together when "grandfather" lay on his deathbed. It was a time to tidy up one's affairs, a time for sorrow and final goodbyes. When the man died it was in the company and comfort of family and friends. With the advent of "civilization," grandfather dies in the sterile environment of the hospital under the glaring lights of the intensive care unit surrounded, punctured, and manipulated by gadgetry designed to save life rather than to delay death long after the individual is prepared to accept it. The family is herded oftentimes in a waiting place down the hall so that they may not interfere with hospital procedure. Dying with dignity should be the last humane act permitted and should not be lost to the superfluous efforts of technology.

As stated by Reverend Carl Nighswonger, "In 12 years of hospital chaplaincy, I have yet to find a family that could cycle their grief according to the hospital schedule. . . . How much better it would be when the doctors give up, if the patient could be moved to a dimly lit, quiet room where the family could sit at his bedside and hold his hand."[11]

The physician and health professionals are trained to sustain life. It is understandable that to them death is viewed as being synonomous with failure. The technology now available to the physician is no doubt in many instances life saving. The decisions become more difficult when it becomes questionable whether "the machinery" is sustaining life or delaying death. To sustain a vestigial fragment of life obviously misses the point.

In an effort to remove the dying process from its depersonalizing, technological context and to give it back to humanity, a new medical subspecialty has evolved called thanatology (The Study of Death). At the Billings Memorial Hospital in Chicago, health professionals are offered a course on The Dynamics of Death and Dying. The objectives of the course

[11] "Death: Making It Easier for Patient and Family," *New York Times*, May 9, 1971.

are to make the health professional more aware of the psychological adjustments a person makes to his impending death. The health professional is thus trained to help the patient during this difficult period. Physicians who undergo this training seem more capable of handling their own emotional reactions to their patients with regard to their life expectancy and to help prepare them psychologically for life's final act.

Review Questions

1. Describe what you would consider to be the "well-adjusted person."
2. What are man's basic physical and emotional needs? How are these best fulfilled?
3. What does Maslow regard as self-actualization?
4. "Self-concept is learned." Describe those influences that contribute to the development of one's self-concept.
5. Distinguish between the conscious and the unconscious mind. How does Freud describe the unconscious mind?
6. What are the relationships of the autonomic nervous system and bodily responses to emotion?
7. Why are man's emotional responses sometimes inappropriate in our current level of civilization?
8. The test of personality is often measured by its ability to deal with failure. Explain.
9. Describe how anxiety can be helpful to the individual.
10. Describe the nature of the mental mechanisms and the purposes they serve.
11. Give examples of mental mechanisms that you have observed others using.
12. What are some of the relationships between the proper functioning of the endocrine system and mental health?
13. How has civilization affected man's behavior? What kinds of adaptation does it demand of him?
14. What are the objectives of the new medical subspecialty called thanatology?

Chapter 3
The Erosion of Mental Health

In the preface of his book *The Human Mind,* Dr. Karl Menninger wrote, "Many readers have said to me: 'I almost imagined I had some of those abnormal conditions myself.' To such persons I usually reply quite gravely: 'I hope so.' For if one has a mind at all, his mental processes are subject to some of the faults and failings that characterize the human mind. If someone does not find himself at all in this book, it is either that he is not human or that some pages have been left out (or torn out). That curious emotional defense which impels some people to believe themselves exempt from all failure, from all weakness, from the taboo of 'abnormality' is perhaps the greatest enemy of healthy mindedness."[1]

Psychosomatic Disorders

The notion that the physical and the mental are two separate entities that have nothing to do with each other is poorly based. One need only watch a person cry. The tears are an obvious physical reaction to an emotion. There is not a gland or system of the body that cannot be influenced by emotion. This entity of mind and body is a human reality—we are made that way. It serves us well since it gives us a wholeness we would not otherwise enjoy. Because of this interrelationship, we are at times bothered by psychosomatic disorders; that is, physical disorders that are psychologically induced.

[1]Karl A. Menninger, *The Human Mind* (New York: Knopf, 1937), p. viii.

In reaction to anger, the body responds with the constriction of blood vessels, thus diverting blood to the skeletal muscles in preparation of the "fight" reaction and thereby raising the blood pressure. Where we have people who repress this emotion of anger, we find that the blood vessels remain constricted instead of returning to normal, resulting in chronic high blood pressure. Many people of this type give a rather calm outward appearance and are often referred to as "inside burners." There is evidence to indicate that when a person suffering from this condition is placed in a different psychological situation the condition is relieved. The modification of a chronic source of irritation and tension such as an unsuitable job or an incompatible marriage has a corrective reaction.

It is commonly thought that ulcers occur only in those personalities that are hard-driving go-getters. The easy-going and passive person, however, is also vulnerable to this disorder. In cases where an individual is overly dependent on another (such as a parent or spouse), if this relationship is threatened, enough anxiety is produced to cause physiological changes to take place in the digestive tract. Personality type is not so much a factor in ulcer development as is the excessive amount of anxiety that the person experiences.

Colitis is another malfunction of the digestive system sometimes related to emotional causes. The condition interferes with the digestion of food and disturbs the functioning of the bowels. Case histories of patients with colitis sometimes show that in childhood there was a mother whose domineering, antagonistic attitudes set up conflicts in the individual. The person therefore tended to grow up with a sensitivity to rejection or humiliation. Even minor failures resulted in emotional reactions that were out of proportion to the cause. The result is a sick colon.

It is thought that some cases of asthma are likewise psychologically induced. Attacks of asthma seem to be related to a child's fear of loss of mother love or psychological rejection. It is noted that many children and adults who suffer from asthma are overanxious and emotionally insecure. It must also be recognized, however, that some cases of asthma appear to be basically physical in cause.

Neurotic Adjustments

Neuroses are undesirable means whereby the individual deals with anxiety that has been produced by frustrations and conflicts. There are a number of basic differences between a neurotic adjustment and a psychotic one. Neurotic adjustments are not only less serious than psychotic ones but are always functional (psychological) in nature, whereas psychotic reactions may sometimes be organically caused. In a number of psychotic reactions there is actual physical damage to the brain that precipitates the reaction. In the neurotic there also does not occur the kind of personality disorganization that takes place in the psychotic. While the neurotic may misinterpret reality, he does not replace it as the psychotic does. The neurotic person has an awareness that something is wrong, whereas the psychotic individual has replaced reality with fantasy. Freud described neurosis as a situation in which we are dealing with scars, whereas the psychosis is one where we are dealing with bleeding wounds. One description distinguishing between the two is illustrated by the statement that the psychotic believes two plus two equals five, whereas the neurotic knows that two plus two equals four, but it bothers him.

Many psychologists feel that the bases for neurotic reactions are developed in childhood and that they are particularly related to parent-child relationships. As stated by Kaplan:

> The typical family patterns encountered are those in which protective anxious parents prevent the child from growing up. Perfectionistic parents make the child feel that he can do nothing right. Overly strict parents make him feel mistrusted or ashamed of his natural impulses, and rejecting parents make the child feel worthless and unloved.[2]

Because neurotic reactions are motivated by unconscious thoughts, the individual is perplexed by them and will many times take inappropriate actions in dealing with them. The person who goes from one doctor to another hoping to find a cure for his physical ailments (that are psychologically caused) usually will not cooperate with the doctor because the physical symptoms he is exhibiting hide his real emotional problem. Because he is not conscious of all the factors involved in his condition, the neurotic is in a sense on a merry-go-round. He consciously

[2]Louis Kaplan, *Foundations of Human Behavior* (New York: Harper & Row, 1965), p. 270.

 seeks to relieve the symptoms of his neurosis while unconsciously he wants those symptoms to persist because they hide the real problem that he feels incapable of facing.

Types of Neurotic Adjustments

Anxiety Reaction. Anxiety is a feeling of apprehension or dread that something unpleasant is going to happen. Under normal circumstances, the person realizes why he is experiencing the feeling of anxiety. A person may have anxious moments about losing his job if he hears that his company has to cut back on employees. A mother may become concerned about her child who she knows has been exposed to a serious disease. Anxiety, however, is neurotic when there is no apparent cause for its occurrence or where a very slight cause results in a highly exaggerated response. The latter is exemplified by a person who has a pain in his chest and imagines that he is having a heart attack, or the person with a slight cold who is sure that it is pneumonia. When the reason for anxiety is not apparent, it is usually because it is due to a repressed and usually unacceptable emotion. The closer the repressed emotion comes to making its way into the consciousness the greater is the anxiety developed. Anxiety can cause a number of physical symptoms and reactions such as headaches, indigestion, chronic fatigue, dizziness, constipation, and loss of appetite. The anxious person usually has difficulty sleeping and when he does get to sleep he is many times bothered by fearful dreams. This person usually seeks a physical explanation for his distressing mental state. The person generally reflects feelings of apprehension and helplessness and is quite indecisive. He also lacks confidence, feels chronically fatigued, and will often complain about the inability to concentrate.

Dissociative Reaction. In this reaction the person disassociates or separates himself from his personality. One of the most common of these reactions is amnesia. When a person faces a problem that overwhelms him, forgetting his identity and therefore his problem becomes one means of escape. How well amnesia serves the person is indicated by how unperturbed the individual is in regard to his loss of memory. In this condition, the person will forget who he is or even assume a different identity and will not recall people or factual events related to his past. It must be remembered that amnesia is not purposeful forgetting. The reaction is quite unconscious and beyond the conscious control of the individual. While most dissociative amnesias last a relatively short time, some can blot out a person's entire previous life. The fictional story of *Dr. Jekyl and Mr. Hyde* exemplifies this mental condition. Another example is *The Three Faces of Eve,* which is an actual case of multiple personality where three quite different personalities occupy the same body and predominate it at different times. Most cases of amnesia, however, are not as dramatic as *Dr. Jekyl and Mr. Hyde* nor as involved as *The Three Faces of Eve.* Quiet, neurotic forgetfulness better describes most cases of this type.

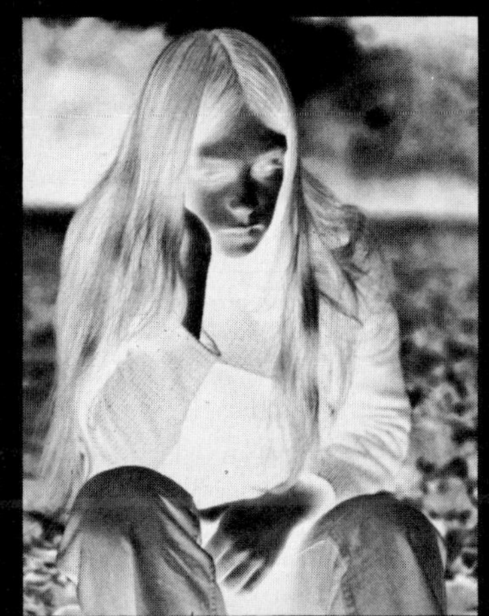

Conversion Reactions. A conversion reaction or conversion hysteria, as it is sometimes referred to, can oftentimes be quite dramatic. A sudden loss of vision or hearing, paralysis of an arm or leg, or the loss of sensation in the skin can be typical types of reactions. After a thorough physical examination, it is found that the person has nothing organically (physically) wrong with him. The basic difference between this type of disorder (psychogenic) and a psychosomatic one is that in the latter the psychological stress results in the development of a physical disorder. The symptoms that develop in a conversion reaction provide to some extent the solution to a problem facing the person. The soldier who in the army is trained to kill may find himself unable to pull the trigger as a result of a paralysis of his arm. This occurs because of the conflict created with his early upbringing that indicated "Thou Shalt Not Kill." The girl who is about to marry someone that she does not really love may suddenly find her legs paralyzed and unable to walk down the church aisle. People who tend to be most prone to the development of these neurotic reactions are persons who are generally immature, self-indulgent, and self-centered. Lesser kinds of conversion reaction involve twitches and spasms of the muscles of both the face and limbs. It can also include the experience of imaginary symptoms of illness to the point where the person actually feels pain. The solution to these problems of course does not lie with aspirin or other such medication but with psychotherapy and with the person's understanding of his problems. It also illustrates how fallacious self-diagnosis and self-treatment can be where these kinds of conditions are involved. Where unconscious motivation is a factor, the person cannot be in a position to diagnose the nature of his difficulty objectively.

Obsessive Compulsive Reaction. If a person has a repressed thought or emotion, he may occupy himself with an obsessive thought or a compulsive act which takes the form of a ritual. When the mind occupies itself with these obsessive or compulsive functions, it does not have the opportunity then to think of the distasteful thought that it is trying to keep repressed. Obsessive compulsive acts have a wide range in terms of activity, thoughts, and significance. Just about all people have found themselves experiencing the compulsion to double-check the front door that they know is locked and the alarm clock that has obviously been set. Likewise, we have all experienced obsessive thoughts like the inability to get a certain jingle or tune out of our minds. While these obsessive thoughts or compulsive acts have, at worst, nuisance value, more intense forms of these behaviors can prove to be real handicaps. In some instances, people develop rather elaborate rituals or ceremonies. There is a case of one woman who when retiring to bed would fold her clothes very meticulously and in a complicated manner. Her preparations to retire usually took two hours. There have been instances where people have spent their time traveling on a train counting telephone poles from one major city to another hundreds of miles apart. Some people find themselves arranging furniture and the accessories of a room in a very fixed pattern and in minute detail. The slightest change in position of any object in the room causes intense feelings of anxiety and even panic in the person. People most prone to the development of these types of reactions are those who would be described as hair splitting and stubborn, submissive and yet in need of asserting their importance. They are usually overconscientious in tasks that they perform and are intolerant and highly critical of others. Kleptomania, the compulsive urge to steal, pyromania, the compulsion to set fires, are more serious forms of obsessive compulsive reactions.

Phobic Reaction. A phobia is an intense fear of a specific thing or situation that is of no real danger to the individual. A person with claustrophobia, who is afraid to enter the confined space of a crowded elevator exemplifies this. Should he enter that elevator, he would probably panic and even faint. While all people have fears, generally these fears are based on a real threat or at least a potential threat. Phobic fear is based on a fear reaction when no real cause for it is observable. The principal causes of phobias are traumatic experiences that a person may have had and forgotten. Anything that reminds the individual unconsciously of that experience would stimulate a phobic reaction. A person may also be conditioned as a child to fear certain situations or things. The mother, for instance, who has a phobic fear of mice could very well condition her daughter to react likewise. In many instances, the real cause of a phobia is repressed so that it is unknown to the sufferer. The precipitations of phobic reactions may be unconscious forbidden tendencies or impulses that the individual is trying to repress. Anything, then, that is symbolic of any such tendency or impulse will stimulate a phobic reaction which serves to punish the individual for the forbidden thought. Phobias are many in number and examples of a few follow:

Acrophobia, fear of high places.
Agoraphobia, fear of open places.
Algophobia, fear of pain.
Hematophobia, fear of the sight of blood.
Hydrophobia, fear of water.
Mysophobia, fear of contamination.
Nyctophobia, fear of darkness.
Photophobia, fear of strong light.
Toxophobia, fear of being poisoned.
Zoophobia, fear of animals.

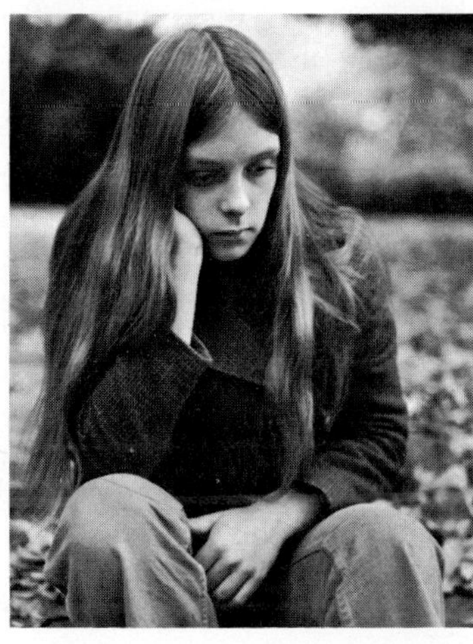

Fig. 3-1. Depression is a very common reaction to life's disappointments. It becomes a chronic disability when it fulfills neurotic needs. (Susan Johns)

Phobias are of varying intensities and quite common. When they begin to interfere with one's work and activities, then it is time to seek professional help to correct them. Because phobic reactions are often unconsciously stimulated, individuals should not attempt to correct them themselves. One college student suffering from claustrophobia asked his classmates to put him in a dumbwaiter, lock the door, and not open it regardless of his reactions. This was his erroneously conceived approach to solving the problem by fighting it directly. Upon placement in the dumbwaiter, he panicked and fortunately his screams did induce his colleagues to open the door, although by the time they did he had already fainted. The experience did nothing more than aggravate the condition for the individual. The treatment of a phobia lies within the realm of the professional and not the amateur. People who like to play pranks with the phobic fears of others are in essence playing with fire. The hysteria that may be triggered by aggravating a phobic reaction can lead to even more intense psychological problems.

Depressive Reactions. Neurotic depression lies somewhere between normal discouragement or grief and the intense psychotic depression that is accompanied by suicidal desires. We are all familiar with the reactions that take place when the individual experiences a deep personal loss. However, after a period of time the depression following this kind of event is lessened as the individual gets back to the routine of living. In neurotic depression, the feelings that develop occur without any apparent cause. In other instances, a minor disappointment triggers a reaction that is completely out of proportion to the event. In neurotic depression, the person has the feeling of being unloved and a failure. The depression will usually be of long duration basically because it is fulfilling a neurotic need. The depression in this instance is a symptom and is in essence an indirect expression of a repressed feeling of guilt or hostility. Depression is considered a most common mental disorder.

The Psychoses

The psychoses refer to a broad range of mental illnesses that have wide variations in terms of their severity, duration, and nature. As mentioned earlier, they are basically characterized by personality disintegration and loss of contact with reality.

The following discussion of mental disorders we hope will lend some understanding of the breadth and nature of mental illness. The broadly based classifications of mental illness referred to are intended to serve as a guideline to understanding. They are not intended for the overzealous, amateur diagnostician who is invariably found in every group and who enthusiastically categorizes friend and foe alike as having one type of mental illness or another . . . like a hypochondriac turned outward.

Schizophrenia is the most common of the mental illnesses. It is sometimes erroneously referred to as split personality, when it really is a disintegrated personality. Although schizophrenia is referred to as a single disorder, psychiatrists feel that it is actually a grouping of disorders. Most cases of schizophrenia have their onset during the adolescent or early adult years. A rather small percentage occur between the thirties and middle age. The early signs of schizophrenia are evident many years before the person undergoes the actual breakdown and often these signs go unnoticed. In these people there develops a general tendency toward greater withdrawal, feelings of unworthiness, and increased sensitivity to being rejected and unloved. There is a continual development toward a lack of response to people and activities about them. There appears to be a kind of drifting into an unresponsive state. Oftentimes there is a great and abnormal preoccupation with such abstract things as life, good, evil, and God. In some cases, the schizophrenic loses his identity, sometimes thinking that his body no longer belongs to him and that he is literally beside himself. The reactions that are stimulated by the hallucinogenic drugs are considered to be very much like those experienced by the schizophrenic. Recent experimentation has shown that a substance very similar to mescaline, a hallucinogenic drug, was isolated from the urine of most schizophrenics. This has led to the conjecture that possibly schizophrenics form hallucinogens because of defective body chemistry and are in effect on a permanent hallucinogenic kick. Statistics show that the incidence of schizophrenia is 1 per cent (1 in 100) in our population. However, where there has been some schizophrenia in the immediate family, the incidence is 14 per cent (1 in 7). This does not mean that the condition is inherited; it does imply that the person may inherit a weakness which if abused could result in the greater tendency to develop the illness. It has also been noted that in the use of LSD, those individuals who experienced permanent mental illness were usually those who had genetic inclinations along these lines. Individuals with such a genetic weakness can with the use of a hallucinogenic drug create enough stress to "tear the fabric" and cause permanent mental illness.

For the purposes of diagnosis, greater understanding, and treatment, schizophrenic reactions have been subdivided into four major groups:

Simple Type. Simple schizophrenia is characterized by indifference and apathy. The person develops the attitude that it is much more comfortable *not* to try and lives essentially through his daydreaming. Vagrancy, prostitution, and delinquency are frequently "occupations" of the simple schizophrenic.

Hebephrenic Type. Hebephrenic schizophrenia is probably most closely related to the layman's conception of insanity. The behavior is characterized by inappropriate laughter, smiling, and smatterings of hallucinations and delusions. The person's speech is quite incoherent and illogical. The person's personal habits with regard to cleanliness and sanitation tend to deteriorate. The auditory hallucinations of hebephrenics are often related to God and religion. When the patient hears the voice of God, psychiatrists feel that this is in essence the voice of conscience reflecting feelings of guilt. In many instances, the patient will regress to an infantile level which he creates and in which he seeks protection.

Catatonic Type. The behavior of the catatonic schizophrenic varies from one extreme to the other. In some instances, the patient may remain in a fixed position without movement for days and even weeks on end. During these periods of catatonic stupor, the patient is conscious and though he shows no reaction to activities around him, he is aware of their presence. The waxy and statuelike positions assumed by these patients is typical of the catatonic condition. On the other hand, the catatonic also experiences periods of wild excitement. He becomes very aggressive, hostile, and destructive. He may attack people, smash objects, and tear clothing. Speech during these wild periods of time is meaningless. The catatonic reflects a negativism and an antagonism that result in his not eating or sleeping, to the point of physical exhaustion. Developing catatonia is sometimes seen in introvertive individuals who will sit quietly, sullenly, and motionless in a room for long periods of time. These persons usually show unstable temperaments and a characteristic exhibition of fits of anger.

Paranoid Type. The paranoic schizophrenic is characterized by delusions of persecution and grandeur. It seems that the disorder develops slowly and appears somewhat later in life than other schizophrenic reactions. The paranoid appears frustrated with regard to his abnormal need for achievement or status. He concludes that others have schemed and are scheming to keep him from success. He will trust no one, particularly those he is most closely associated with, such as members of his family. In some cases, he develops the feeling that people want to destroy him and he may in "self-defense" kill them first. Not all paranoic patients, however, are dangerous. The feelings of inferiority that these people experience are usually compensated for by the psychotic belief that they are God, Napoleon, or some other omnipotent figure.

Schizophrenia has the highest frequency rate accounting for approximately one-fifth of all admissions to mental hospitals in the United States. Because it is a chronic kind of mental illness that psychiatrists have had the most difficulty in treating, approximately one-half of all patients in mental hospitals today suffer from this ailment. Research that will identify more specifically the nature of the illness is needed before we can significantly reduce its incidence and duration.

Manic Depressive Psychosis. It is quite normal for people to experience changes in mood. We tend to be in a pleasant mood when things are going well and become rather unhappy when we fail in one task or another. Changes in a person's mood tend to be fairly predictable in terms of their variance and what causes them. However, when a person's moods are extreme, ranging from very high elation and hyperactivity to severe depression, particularly without apparent cause, then something is wrong. Manic depressive reactions do not have the effect of causing personality deterioration or disintegration, as occurs in schizophrenia. Rather they seem to be an exaggeration of normal behavior. In the manic stage of this condition, the person becomes quite elated and talks very rapidly, sometimes so rapidly that he becomes incoherent. The person in this stage has all kinds of energy and everything seems completely simple. He feels he can speak almost any language, solve any of the great world problems, and may sign checks for fantastically large sums. He feels he has little time for sleep, and in spite of great activity shows little sign of fatigue. He resembles a car that has been thrown out of gear with the motor racing. While it is making a lot of noise, it is not really going anywhere. The manic who begins to express his antagonism for others may lose what little control he has over himself and do others bodily harm.

In the depressive stage of the condition, the depression may range from a mild state to a very severe one. Rather intense feelings of guilt are usually present during the depressed state, along with feelings of hopelessness, confusion, and dejection. In the depressive stage, people sometimes express feelings of being in need of punishment and think about, or even attempt, suicide. In manic depression, the patient may alternate between manic and depressive phases. In other instances, the person may experience just the manic or just the depressive phase. The incidence of recovery from this condition is quite high. It does not appear to be as serious an illness as schizophrenia. In schizophrenia, the patient gradually withdraws from reality, whereas in manic depression there seems to be an accumulation of frustration which suddenly bursts forth and may prove to have catharsis value. It is felt that manic depression generally results from too much stress for too long a period of time. Some authorities feel that gifted people with a certain amount of mania have an increased drive that makes it essential that they work long hours and therefore accomplish many and great things during their lifetime. The difference, then, between a great contribution and mental illness could at times be a small area of gray. It is perhaps analogous to the race driver who makes a turn at a maximum safe speed and therefore wins the race, as compared to the one who goes just a little too fast and crashes. Other authorities feel that there may be a genetic factor associated with manic depression. In his study of identical twins, Dr. Franz Kallman of Columbia University found that if one twin suffered the disorder, the chances were 85 to 90 per cent that the other twin also suffered from manic depression. Dr. Kallman concluded that at least one type of manic-depressive psychosis has all the markings of a hereditary disease. Scientists are now attempting to find biochemical causes of the illness and ultimately its correction.

Organic Psychosis. Mental illness can be caused by a number of physical factors. The most common is probably that caused by cerebral arteriosclerosis. The narrowing down of the arteries by deposits that accumulate along their walls reduces the amount of blood carrying food and oxygen to brain tissues. The result is that many older people suffering from this condition show signs of confusion, incoherency, forgetfulness, and bewilderment. There are fairly large numbers of older people in mental hospitals because of cerebral arteriosclerosis. Paresis is another example of organically caused mental illness. The spirochete that causes syphilis attacks nerve tissue and ultimately migrates to the brain. In spite of an increased incidence of syphilis, fewer new cases of paresis (brain damage due to syphilis) now occur, because of effective treatment with penicillin.

Large amounts of bromides act as toxins in the body and can cause psychotic conditions. People who douse themselves with some of the patent medicines containing bromides can run this risk. Discontinuance of intake of the substance will return the person to normality.

Alcohol intake by the chronic alcoholic will cause Korsakoff's Psychosis, which is a reaction to a toxic level of alcohol in the body over a prolonged period of time.

Suicide

The destruction of human life, whether it is due to the mass homicide of war, disease, accidents or suicide, represents an unacceptable circumstance. Suicide represents the most unacceptable for it generates guilt, despair, and bewilderment mixed with a sense of failure and helplessness. It stands in stark contradiction to a basic democratic ethic, namely the value of human life. Historically some societies responded to suicide with crude vengefulness. The bodies of suicides were dragged through the streets or impaled on stakes for public view. His property was confiscated and burial denied in church and city cemeteries. In the last century or so the suicide was viewed not as a criminal but a lunatic, which represented but a slight improvement, in view of the maniacal attitudes toward the mentally ill. In recent years these attitudes are changing in more positive directions with the suicide being recognized as a person in difficulty and if the person were helped the suicide would be prevented.

Emil Durkheim, a French sociologist and suicidologist, has asserted that suicide is the result of society's strength or weakness of control over the individual. Durkheim describes three basic types of suicide, each being the result of man's relationship to his society. "Altruistic" suicide is the first type he describes where there are social pressures to commit suicide under certain circumstances. The Japanese who committed hara-kiri serve as examples of altruistic suicide. Hindu women were expected to cremate themselves on the funeral pyres of their husbands. The death of a Gallic chief required that his slaves, servants, and followers join him in death. In the above circumstances the person killed himself because *it was his duty* to do so and he was dishonored and punished if he did not.

"Anomic" suicides are described by Durkheim as those occurring when the relationship between an individual and his society is suddenly destroyed. The shocking and unexpected loss of a close friend, or fortune, or position might precipitate suicidal actions. Surprisingly, sudden wealth can also cause the suicide of some people. Serious social readjustment either in the form of sudden growth or unexpected catastrophe can apparently set off self-destructive inclinations in some people.

"Egoistic" suicide, a third kind described by Durkheim, is the form most commonly seen in the United States. The individual in egoistic suicide has few ties with his community and tends to have no strong attachments to church, home, or the political life in society. In essence he is uninvolved.

Approximately 25,000 suicides occur in the country each year. An additional 175,000 to 200,000 make unsuccessful attempts to kill themselves. About 2 million people in the country have made at least one attempt at suicide. These statistics with regard to suicide attempts and incidence are probably conservative estimates. Suicides are often disguised and certified as accidents because of the stigma associated with it or because insurance policies do not cover suicide. The circumstances of death are many times unclear so as to make it difficult to determine if death was caused by an accident or suicide. It is estimated that the underreporting of suicide may be as high as 200 per cent.

Youthful suicide is causing increasing concern in the United States. It has risen in prominence as a cause of youthful death in recent years. Research at the University of Southern California School of Medicine[3] reveals the profile of the suicidal adolescent often involves problems relating to family. A large percentage of these adolescents had one or both parents missing from the home because of death, divorce, or separation. Many had parents who were married more than once. Those with stepparents were not adjusting well to the newcomer. Many had both parents working or in one-parent families, the one parent worked. A large percentage lived with persons other than their parents. Poverty also seemed to be a factor with regard to suicide. A young person who is suicide-prone is attempting to cope with the stresses and strains of growing up without the support of important family relationships.

As a society we have attempted to sweep suicide under the rug and pretend that it does not exist—then alternately express surprise and shock when it does occur. The lack of discussion of this topic has made it possible for a number of misconceptions about suicide to establish themselves in the public thinking. Some of the more common ones follow:

1. *People who talk about suicide won't commit suicide.* It is estimated that up to 80 per cent of people who commit suicide have communicated their intention to do so. Persons who hint or threaten suicide should be taken seriously and help sought for them.
2. *Suicide happens without warning.* In addition to verbal warnings persons may communicate suicidal intent by writing a will, leaving a note, or giving expensive gifts without apparent reason. It must also be added that most suicides are not impulsive acts but premeditated.
3. *Suicide and attempted suicide are the same class of behavior.* While 5 to 10 per cent of those who attempt suicide unsuccessfully will later succeed, most people attempting really want to live. They use this desperate means of drawing attention to themselves and their problems, hoping someone will come forth to prevent the suicide and help them to correct their problems.

[3]Joseph D. Teicher, M.D., "Children and Adolescents Who Attempt Suicide," *Pediatric Clinics of North America,* Vol 17, No. 3 (August 1970).

4. *Suicide involves only a specific class of people.* Suicide is neither "the curse of the poor" nor "the disease of the rich." All levels of society are rather equally represented in its statistics.
5. *All suicidal individuals are mentally ill, with suicide always the act of the psychotic person.* Studies of suicide notes indicate that many are logical and rational and not psychotic. So, while some suicides may be psychotic, others are just extremely unhappy people.
6. *Suicide is inherited.* In studies reported on twins there is not a single case where both twins committed suicide, although there are a number where one twin has committed suicide and the other has not. There is no evidence that suicidal behavior is inherited as the color of one's hair or eyes.
7. *Once a person is suicidal he is suicidal forever.* A person's desire to kill himself may last for only a short period of time or until he is helped to face and overcome his problems.
8. *Improvement in a suicidal patient means the danger is over.* It has been noted that with depressed patients the greatest risk of suicide is during the period of improvement. The patient may regain sufficient drive and energy to take his life at this time.
9. *Only a psychiatrist or mental hospital can prevent suicide.* While psychiatrists and mental hospitals can be most helpful, there are a variety of religious, lay, and community groups making up the developing suicide-prevention movement.

Is it possible to identify the potential suicide? Almost everyone seriously considering suicide gives indications of his interest. Some indications are rather obvious; in other instances they may be subtle. The suicide decision is usually not an impulsive one, but a premeditated one. The person is disturbed and very often depressed. He (she) feels hopeless about the direction his life is taking and feels helpless to do anything about it. This pessimism in combination with depression can serve as initiators of the act.

There are often verbal threats and cries for help such as "You won't have to put up with me much longer." "They'll miss me when I'm gone." "This is the last straw—I wish I were dead." "I'm good for nothing." "I'll show them!"

Other common signs include withdrawal, loss of initiative and motivation, loneliness, disturbed sleep, loss of appetite, inactivity, a drop in academic performance. More subtle signs might include boredom, antisocial behavior, restlessness, defiance.

Obviously any *one* of the above signs by itself is not an indication of suicidal intent. A changed pattern of behavior including a number of the above *is* cause for concern.

An increasing number of suicide prevention centers are being established in communities and college campuses across the country. They are manned by mental health professionals as well as carefully selected lay personnel. Such centers are usually available for services twenty-four hours a day. Such a center in the city of Los Angeles averages 500 persons contacting it each month. Their help is as close as the nearest telephone, since they have "hot lines" manned 24 hours a day by lay personnel who can be of immediate help to a person calling for help.

No one knows what it is like to be dead. At best, one can only imagine what it would be like if one were alive to watch—an invisible personality—at one's own funeral. Often such an attractive fantasy intoxicates the suicidal mind, and tips the scale to death. But until the very moment that the bullet or barbiturate finally snuffs out life's last breath—while the ground is rushing up—the suicidal person terribly wants to live. No doubt, he also wants to die. But it is an ambivalent wish—to die and to live. Until he dies, a suicide is begging to be saved. Before his death, the suicidal person leaves a trail of subtle and obvious hints of his intentions. *Every suicide* attempt is a serious cry for help. This cry can be heard, and suicide can be prevented.[4]

Mental Health Specialists

The Psychiatrist is a medical doctor who specializes in the treatment of mental and emotional disorders. In addition to the M.D. degree, three additional years as a resident physician in an institution where mental illness is being treated is required. After two additional years of experience in the area of specialization, the physician must pass an examination by the Board of Psychiatry and Neurology of the American Medical Association, The American Psychiatric Association, and the American Neurological Association.

[4]Edwin S. Shneidman and Philip Mandelkorn, *How to Prevent Suicide*, Public Affairs Pamphlet #406, p. 6.

The Psychologist is an individual without a medical background who concerns himself with applying scientific methods to the study of human behavior. If he is a *clinical psychologist,* he has earned a Ph.D. and has completed a supervised internship at a psychiatric clinic. If the clinical psychologist meets the standards set by the American Psychological Association, he is then qualified to diagnose and treat behavior disorders, usually through testing and other psychological diagnostic devices.

The Psychoanalyst can be either a psychiatrist or a psychologist who devotes his time primarily to psychoanalysis, which is a method of studying the emotional problems of a patient with the purpose of alleviating them.

The Psychiatric Social Worker usually has a master's degree in social work and then concentrates on psychiatric case work. Field work in a mental hospital, clinic, or family service agency is part of the training of the psychiatric social worker. After graduation, this professional will work in one of those three settings. The National Association of Social Workers sets accreditation standards for its members.

The Psychiatric Nurse is a graduate nurse with additional training in the care of the mentally ill.

Treating Mental and Emotional Problems

Psychotherapy is the treatment of mental and emotional problems by psychological means. The

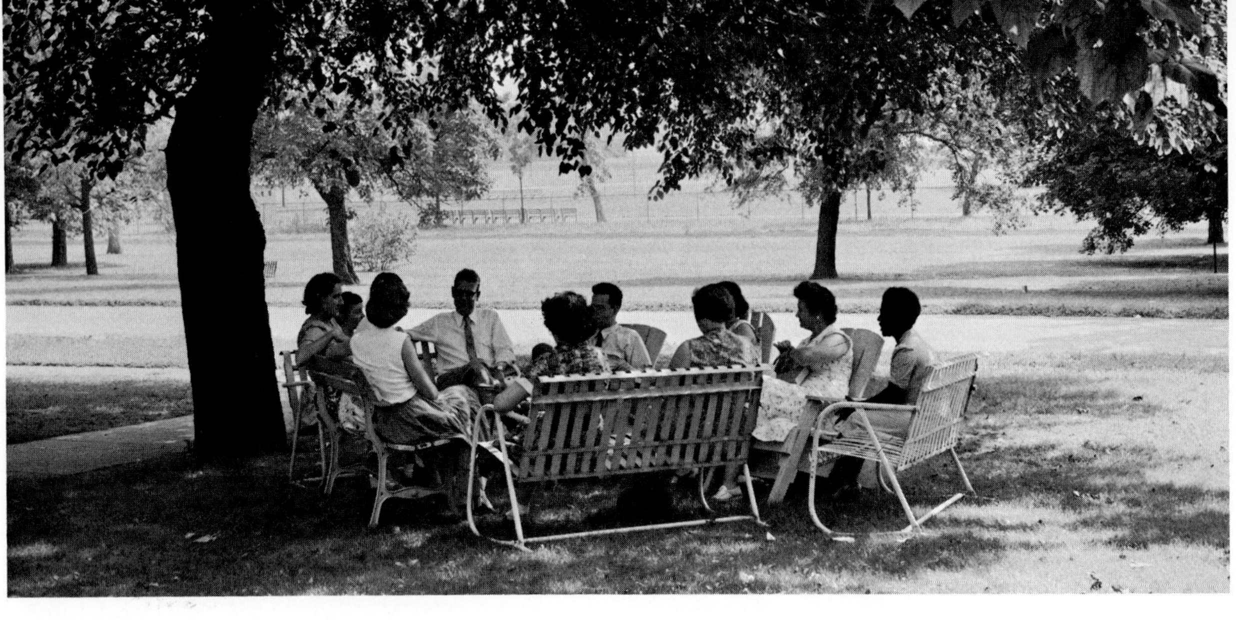

 therapist meets with the patient and through verbal exchange determines the nature, cause, and possible solution of the patient's problem. Psychotherapy is often of a supportive variety, where the patient is given reassurance and emotional support in facing his problems.

When the therapist deduces that repressed thoughts and emotions are underlying factors in the person's problems, he attempts to bring these factors to the surface or to the conscious level. He may do this through dream analysis and free association. In free association the person responds to a stimulus, such as a word or picture, with the first thing that comes to his mind. These responses give clues as to the nature of the repressed thoughts. Dreams often reflect unconscious thoughts and their analyses sometimes prove helpful in the better understanding of the patient. Hypnosis may also be used as a means of overcoming patient inhibitions and amnesia with regard to his past. Under hypnosis, the patient is very suggestible and responds more easily to the questions and suggestions of the therapist. It helps the therapist to discover the causes of the person's difficulty and to give guidance for the reeducation of the personality. Often, the closer the therapist gets to uncovering the repressed thoughts or feelings, the more uncomfortable the patient becomes. As in the case of the dentist, the closer he gets to finishing the drilling on a cavity, the more painful it is. As some people proceed through the therapy, they may decide to stop seeing the therapist because they are being "upset." This is often an indication that the therapy is proving successful and moving toward the root of the problem. Psychotherapy is in many ways a learning process. The person is learning about himself and how to react more appropriately to life situations.

Group Therapy. The therapist will often bring a number of people together for group therapy. Here patients have an opportunity to react to each other as well as to the therapist. The situation itself is helpful to the patient as well as the therapist, for it gives the therapist the opportunity of seeing the patient in a different setting which invariably reveals other facets of the personality he is dealing with.

Sensitivity Training. There is a wide range of activity that may be classified as "sensitivity training." Encounter groups represents one of these. These are often candid confrontations with the person made to acknowledge his rationalizations. Drug and alcoholic patients are often involved in such encounter groups to assist them in acknowledging the real reasons they use drugs. Various forms of nonverbal communication may also be used as part of this approach. Care needs to be taken in the use of this approach lest the abrasive confrontation prove to be psychologically destructive rather than constructive. It is a technique best left to the highly qualified and experienced rather than to amateur psychiatry.

T-Groups represent another form of sensitivity training. It tends to focus on how people feel rather than on how they think. It encourages people to be open and candid about how they feel about others. The theory is that criticism will develop honesty, self-understanding, and trust in others. Because it can also result in conflict, expert leadership is neces-

Fig. 3-2. *Group therapy in a relaxed setting. Here a person has the opportunity to interact with others and gain insight into his own behavior. (N.Y.S. Mental Hygiene; Photo by Julian A. Belin)*

sary for such groups. A person lacking ego-strength could find such a group session to be threatening and emotionally destructive. Widespread use of these techniques has caused some concern where groups are led by people not prepared to cope with the emotional responses they may turn loose in the group.

Psychodrama or Role Playing is a technique whereby patients act out their problems. As a result they often gain some insights with regard to their solution. Closed circuit television is sometimes used to play back the psychodrama to the persons involved. A person watching himself on television often "sees" himself for the first time. It has often resulted in the development of a more positive self-concept.

Play Therapy is another form of psychotherapy, one that is used with children. How a child feels about various members of its family, for example, may be revealed by its play reactions to dolls that represent mother, father, brother, or sister. Repressed thoughts are often communicated via this approach.

Drug Therapy. The two basic types of drugs used in drug therapy are tranquilizers and psychic energizers (stimulants). Tranquilizers such as chlorpromazine and reserpine (there are many brand names for them) are used mostly for psychotic patients with schizophrenia and manic-depression as well as for acute alcoholics. These drugs have a quieting effect, blunting the exaggerated threats commonly experienced with psychotic patients. The stimulants or antidepressants are used for depressed patients and alchoholics with success in counteracting these depressed conditions. Drug therapy is used in conjunction with psychotherapy, and in many instances, even when drugs are used alone, they prove helpful to the patient and his management.

Shock Therapy was much more widely used before the introduction of drugs. In one form of this therapy, insulin is administered to reduce the blood level of sugar and cause the patient to go into a coma. In another form of this therapy, a small electrical current is passed through the patient's brain for several seconds causing a convulsive reaction. The use of shock therapy has declined since the 1950's when antidepressant drugs such as thorazine and marplan came into expanded use. Shock therapy to treat depression gets faster results than psychiatric counseling and drug therapy. When carefully administered, it is reported to be effective in a vast majority of the depression cases within days and surely within a month. Shock therapy is very often used in conjunction with psychotherapy and/or drug therapy.

Mental Health Treatment Facilities

Until the early nineteen fifties, the only places of treatment available for people with serious mental illness were the state mental hospitals, Veterans Administration hospitals, and small private hospitals for those who could afford them. In recent years, general hospitals have increasingly developed psychiatric wards. The development of drug therapy for the mentally ill person has helped to make this possible because it affords greater control of the patient. Patients who stay at general hospitals are usually those requiring short-term care.

On being admitted to a state mental hospital, the patient is generally given a course of intensive treatment which could include drug therapy, psychotherapy, and possible shock therapy. How long this intensive care lasts depends on how well staffed the hospital is. Because of the shortage of personnel in this area, some mental hospitals will have a doctor-patient ratio of 1 to 100 or worse. This ratio needs to be reduced if intensive care is to be given over longer periods of time to ensure a greater percentage of successful therapy. Many state mental hospitals that are properly staffed can discharge up to 75 per cent of their patients within three months after admission and 85 per cent within a year. Some of these patients will not require any further treatment. Others will need to follow a prescription of psychiatric drugs for several months or several years. In other instances, psychiatric clinics in the community will provide follow-up services to support the patient through further rehabilitation.

The community psychiatric clinic is staffed by a team consisting of a psychiatrist, a clinical psychologist, and a psychiatric social worker. In addition to follow-up treatment given to a patient from a hospital, many of these clinics will provide treatment for individuals not requiring hospitalization. These clinics often serve a preventive function by giving early assistance to those with emotional problems. Where emotional problems are not permitted to fester, they do not develop to the point where hospitalization becomes necessary. Persons may be referred to an out-patient clinic of this type by a physician or another community agency such as the school. In other instances, a person may initiate treatment by merely walking in and asking for it. The treatment cost for the patient at most of these clinics is usually nominal, with payments scaled according to the patient's ability to pay. In a number of states the community psychiatric clinic is liberally subsidized by the state government.

Veterans Administration hospitals treat veterans with service-connected mental disorders. Where a veteran is mentally ill with a disorder that is not service-connected, he can be admitted to these hospitals if he is indigent. There are approximately sixty Veterans Administration hospitals in the United States. These hospitals are usually more completely staffed and better equipped than state mental hospitals and as a result can often provide more thorough treatment.

The Community Mental Health Center

In 1963 the Community Mental Health Centers Act was passed. This legislation was introduced at the request of the late President John F. Kennedy. The legislation authorized federal funds to states for the construction of community mental health centers. These centers are designed to provide a wide range of services for the mentally ill and to keep them in the communities where they live. Too often sending a person to a mental hospital a distance away from home cuts him adrift from family, friends, and job, thus superimposing an additional problem on the one the patient already has. President Kennedy believed that community mental health centers would help reduce the number of mental patients by at least half by providing services that would focus on diagnosis, care, rehabilitation, and emergency service that would be available both day and night. It is felt that the cost of per patient care would also be reduced by such a center. At the present time the cost of patient care per day in a psychiatric ward would be six times that in a public mental hospital. Psychiatric care at a local general hospital averages a period of two or four weeks, whereas in a public mental hospital the stay averages six months. The nature of a community mental health center will vary from community to community. The functions of the center would include prevention as well as treatment. Basically all such centers will offer the following services:

Inpatient Services. This unit would offer treatment for a limited time to patients needing 24-hour care, including provision of 24-hour emergency service, after which other arrangements would be made, such as day hospital, outpatient clinic, or if indicated transfer to a state hospital which, it is hoped, would offer specialized care.

Outpatient Services. Various kinds of individual and group treatment programs, including 24-hour emergency services, would be provided for adults, children, and families when needed, without a waiting period.

Partial Hospitalization. Space and activities would provide day care and treatment for patients able to return to homes and families evenings and weekends. Night care and treatment would be provided patients able to work or attend school, but in need of further care or without suitable home arrangements.

Community Services. Members of the center staff would provide consultation to professional personnel in the community, such as nonpsychiatrist physicians and clergymen and to community agencies, such as schools, public health departments, courts, police and welfare departments, and voluntary health, welfare, and recreation agencies concerning emotional problems of individuals with whom they deal.

Diagnostic Services. These would provide extensive examination of emotionally disturbed and mentally ill persons and screening of patients prior to admitting them to the appropriate service within the center.

Rehabilitative Services. Vocational, educational, and social programs would aid those who need such care, including former hospital patients.

Precare and Aftercare Services. These would place patients needing such care in foster homes or halfway houses, and would include home visiting.

Training. The center would provide training for all types of mental health personnel.

Research and Evaluation. The center would carry out research into mental illness, or cooperate with other agencies in research.[5]

It is hoped that with the more effective use of what we already know about the care of the mentally ill, treatment time may be significantly reduced, along with hospital and medical costs. The develop-

[5]The Comprehensive Community Mental Health Center, U.S. Dept of Health, Education and Welfare, PHS publication No. 1137 (April 1964), p. 11.

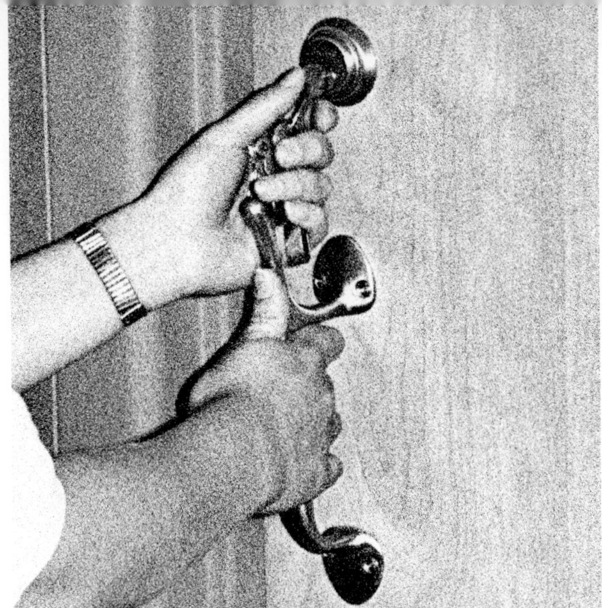

Fig. 3-3. The indignity of locking in mental patients is fast disappearing. (Clarence Bassett)

ment of health insurance that would include mental health care could then become a feasible reality.

Hospital Management of the Mentally Ill

In the past, mental "hospitals" were such in name only. They were essentially institutions where the mentally ill were locked up and detained. Within recent years, mental hospitals have been developing a more liberal policy with regard to patients, and more and more of these institutions have been adopting an open-door policy. At the present time, at least two-thirds of the mental hospital population enjoys the freedom, as well as the dignity, of the open ward. The time that was spent by nurses locking and unlocking doors is now directed toward more positive measures. Hospitals have recorded rather dramatic changes in the attitudes of their patients when the bars came off the windows and the doors were unlocked. This approach in itself has created a better therapeutic atmosphere. It is recognized, of course, that patients in some of the acute phases of illness need to be secluded for their protection as well as that of others. This open-door policy has also made it more possible for patients to leave the hospital and continue treatment in outpatient clinics. The patients have also been encouraged to go home for visits during week ends to help maintain family ties and relationships. It is felt that this greater flexibility in hospital management has helped to decrease the average length of hospitalization of the mental patient.

Types of Admission

There are four basic ways in which a patient may be admitted to a mental hospital. The first is the *informal admission:* the patient merely enters the hospital and indicates that he feels he needs help. Under this type of admission, the patient is free to leave at will. At the present time, there are comparatively few states that permit this type of admission. In *voluntary admission,* the patient again approaches the hospital, indicating that he is in need of help, signing a paper asking for treatment as well as hospitalization. He can leave the hospital whenever he chooses, provided he gives the hospital notice of intent to leave several days before. An increasing number of states have developed a voluntary admissions policy. Many, however, still do not have such a policy and require commitment of the patient. *Commitment by medical certification* occurs, in the usual case, when a relative approaches a doctor, indicating that he believes a member of the family to be mentally ill and in need of treatment. After examination of the patient, if the physican feels that the person should be hospitalized he will sign a certificate to that effect. In some cases the medical certificate for admittance can be given by the admitting physician at a mental hospital. In *legal commitment,* the patient is brought before a judge for a sanity hearing. The judge will often ask a medical doctor to act as his adviser, to hear testimony, and to help him come to a decision with regard to hospital treatment. The physician, unfortunately, is not always a psychiatrist; in fact, in most cases he is *not.*

Our Changing Attitudes Toward Mental Illness

There was a time when the mentally ill person was locked in a cell and was the recipient of much physical abuse. He was the object of ridicule and was regarded as something to be ashamed of. That this kind of care came from so called "sane" people represents a colossus of contradiction. Ignorance invariably stimulates fear of the unknown. Clifford Beers' manuscript, *A Mind That Found Itself,*[6] described his own experiences as a mental patient and drew early attention to the need for the better understanding of mental illness and the mentally ill person. His writing set off the Mental Hygiene Movement, which stressed prevention of mental illness as its goal. It also sought to correct the distorted idea that it was a disgrace to be or to have been mentally ill. In his writings, Beers indicated that mad men were too often man-made. He felt that mental "hospitals" that deprived the person of his dignity and rights were just as disturbing to the mentally ill person as they would be to a well person. Although many of our mental institutions may now be called hospitals, there are a number, even today, that are in need of great improvement.

Present-day attitudes toward the person with an emotional problem are improved, but by no means perfect. There persist fallacious ideas with regard to mental illness that distort reactions to it. Many unfortunately still believe that a mentally ill person is usually a wild, dangerous lunatic. It is undoubtedly safer to be on the ward in a mental hospital than in a room where two "normal" people have lost their tempers. Mental illness is still not a completely socially acceptable disease, although giant strides have been taken in this direction through public education. A reason for the inability to accept the mentally ill person as sick is that he does not behave the way "sick" people do. The sick person usually expresses some feelings of helplessness, and in response is helped and cared for. The mentally ill person often does not realize that he is ill and therefore does not ask for help and does not expect any. If help is forced on him, he begins to feel abused, which is a reaction that any one of us would have.

A further complicating factor in dealing with the mentally ill is that families cling to the irrationality that mental illness constitutes a shameful disease. This attitude not only inhibits the seeking out of treatment but blunts its effectiveness as well. The patient, after receiving treatment, returns to family, friends, and job, and acceptance of the former mental patient by those closest to him becomes important if he is to be helped to continue his recovery and make a good readjustment to normality. In response to negative attitudes toward mental illness, Dr. Karl Menninger once stated that many patients recovered from their mental illness, but not from their diagnosis.

Mental illness has become a highly treatable disorder. When mental hospitals are fairly well staffed, 75 per cent of the patients admitted are discharged

[6]Clifford Beers, *A Mind That Found Itself* (New York: Doubleday, 1948).

within a three-month period. While we certainly do not know all the answers as far as mental illness is concerned, current treatment can prove to be quite helpful. The difficulty at the present time is that there is a lack of mental health facilities as well as personnel. The shortage of psychiatrists and other mental health professionals is critical. As a society we are just beginning to come to grips with one of our major health problems—mental illness. We need to develop more realistic, less prejudicial attitudes toward these disorders. We must be willing (we are certainly able) to invest in the facilities and in the training of the professional personnel so urgently needed. Research in this area also needs to be significantly increased if newer and more effective preventive and treatment procedures are to be developed.

Review Questions

1. How do psychosomatic disorders exemplify the unity of the physical and the mental? Give some examples.
2. What are the reasons for neurotic adjustments? How can unconscious thought complicate the understanding of neurotic reactions?
3. Distinguish between a psychosomatic disorder and a conversion reaction.
4. What is a phobia? Describe the dangers inherent in playing pranks with the phobic fears of others. Why do phobic reactions often require professional help to overcome?
5. Though schizophrenia and manic-depression are both psychotic conditions, there are marked differences between them with regard to their nature, prognosis, and possibly their causes. Explain.
6. Distinguish between the functional and organic psychoses. Give some examples of the latter.
7. Suicides are not as spontaneous and as singularly caused as they are often considered to be. How would you support the aforementioned thesis?
8. Define: (1) psychiatrist, (2) psychologist, (3) psychoanalyst, (4) psychiatric social worker, (5) psychiatric nurse.
9. Describe the types of therapy currently used with the mentally ill.
10. Mental illness is a highly treatable disorder. Explain.
11. The mentally ill are people! How does the open-door mental hospital contribute to the dignity as well as the recovery of the person with a mental disorder?
12. Describe the various types of admission to a mental hospital: (1) informal, (2) voluntary, (3) commitment by medical certificate, (4) legal commitment.
13. Describe the changes in attitude taking place in our society toward the person with an emotional problem.
14. What are three basic types of suicide and their sociological rationale?
15. Why are there so many misconceptions about suicide even as late as the twentieth century?

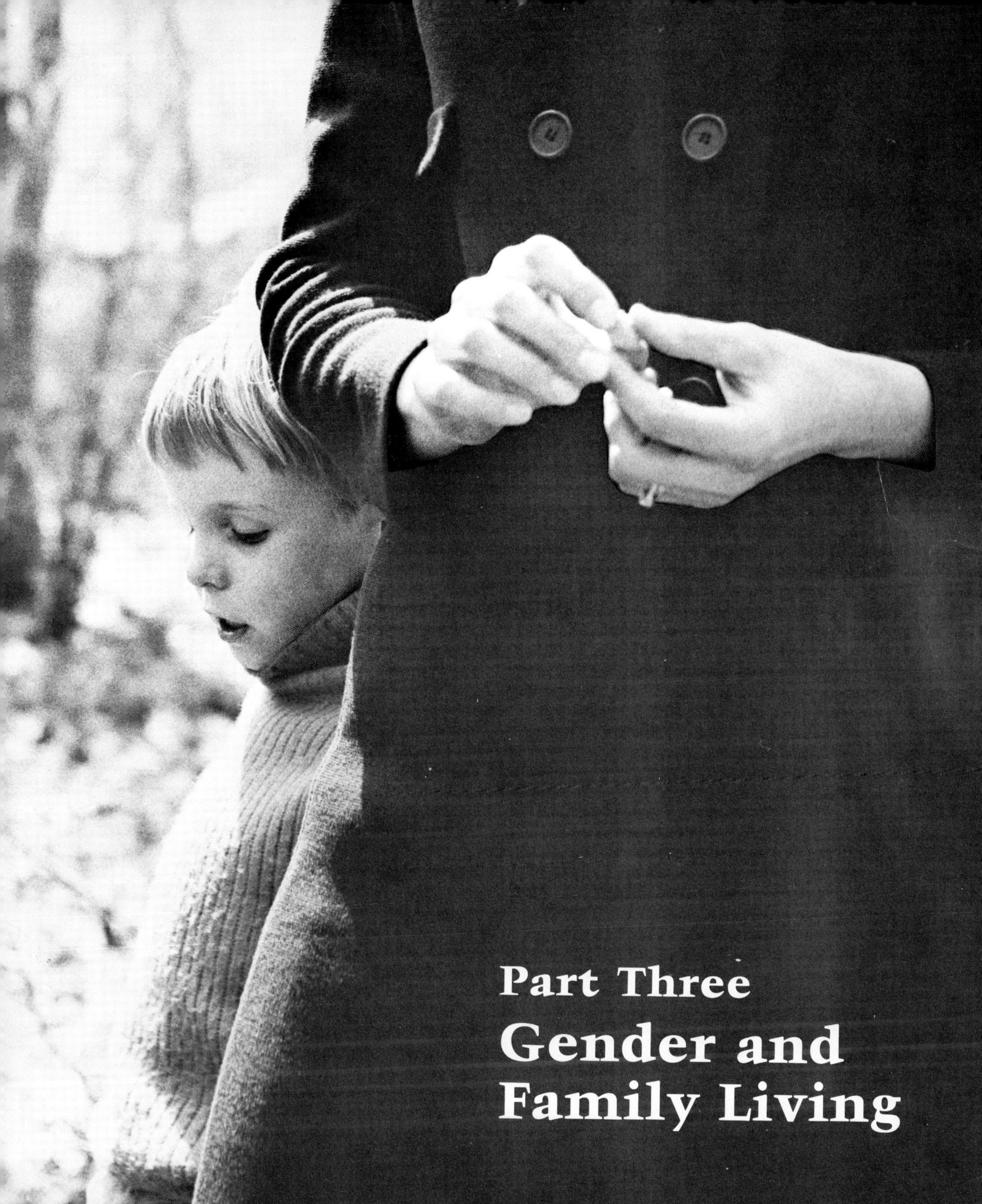

Part Three
Gender and Family Living

Chapter 4
Human Sexuality

"Sex is not something we do but something that we are."[1] Our first identification when we enter this world is invariably in terms of "It's a girl!" or "It's a boy!" Unmistakably it is an identification of *being*.

In the past and even the present, sexuality is often viewed as being solely related to the sex act. The notion persists that in the absence of sexual intercourse sexuality does not exist. It does, for we cannot divorce ourselves from the hormones that run through our blood vessels. Sexuality is, in fact, one of the fundamental aspects of our personality. It defies categorization as something apart. To view sex as purely a physical phenomenon is to lose sight of its broader, more significant meanings. As stated by John L. Thomas:

> Past and present experience suggests that a major source of difficulty in dealing with sex—and all known societies have had their difficulties—is the tendency to take a partial or topical view of it, to see it in terms of only one of its dimensions, and to value only one of its many aspects.[2]

Viewed within its broader concepts, sexuality is, then, one of the most important and fundamental aspects of life. It gives us our initial identification and is reflected in our thinking and behavior. It further colors our choice of occupation, social activities, mode of dress, in fact, our entire view of life and life's activities. Our ability to accept our sexuality and to deal with it properly is basic to our happiness and mental health.

On Masculinity and Femininity

Interpretations of what is masculine or feminine vary. A woman with a husky voice may be categorized by some as having a masculine-sounding voice. Others would consider her to have a seductive quality—and quite feminine! Determining what represents maleness and femaleness by biological standards is quite simple, because these characteristics are genetically rooted and physical in orientation. Femininity and masculinity, on the other hand, are learned and psychological in context. Cultural influences play significant roles in the determination of standards here. In our society, emotional and intuitive qualities and sensitivity for the arts would be classified as feminine in nature. There are societies, however, where these would be masculine qualities, where unemotional, calculating, reasoned reactions would be considered feminine qualities. Cultural standards in this area can exhibit wide differences substantiating the thesis that behavior here is learned.

Though the foregoing may sound confusing, it is not particularly disturbing to the individual who never or rarely leaves his environs. He or she can reject the standards of another society as being wrong, undesirable, or placed in the "that's interesting, but . . ." category. When the individual is in a

[1] Mary S. Calderone, "Sex and Social Responsibility," *Journal of Home Economics*, Vol. 57, No. 7 (September 1965).

[2] Father John L. Thomas, "Sexuality and the Total Personality," *SIECUS* (*Sex Information and Education Council of the United States*) *Newsletter*, Vol. 1, No. 3 (Fall 1965).

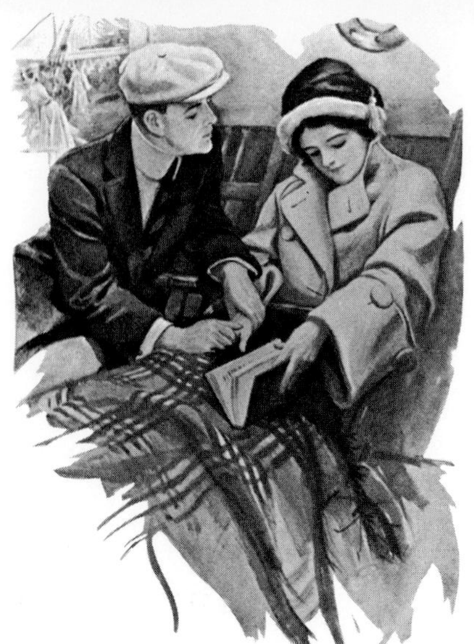

Fig. 4-1a. "The Proposal."

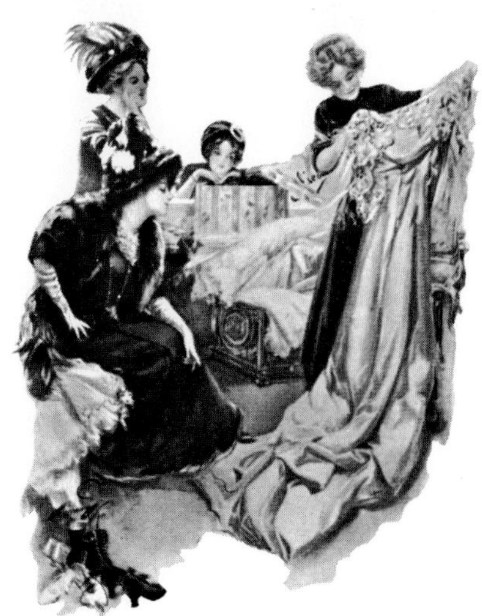

Fig. 4-1b. "The Trousseau."

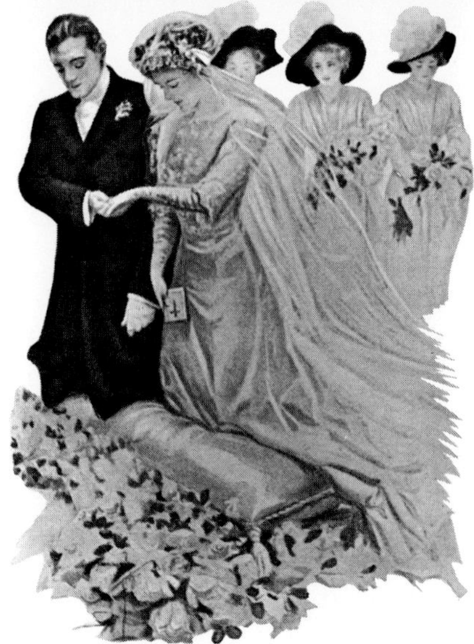

Fig. 4-1c. "The Wedding."

society such as our own, where the standards for feminity and masculinity are undergoing change, the bases for some adjustments present themselves.

In the past in our society, the epitome of femininity was exemplified by the woman who was coy and demure and cultivated ineffectualness and inferiority to man. A woman who dared challenge a man intellectually or professionally during that era was at the very least "no lady!" These concepts of femininity have been rapidly undergoing change. Now over 50 per cent of the women who are college graduates are working professionally and quite successfully. Women are also seeking equality in their interactions with the opposite sex, professionally, socially, and in marriage. They would rather leave the "dumb Dora" role to those who enjoy the pretense or to those who genetically were not given a choice.

The concept of "virginity" is also being questioned. Traditionally, it has been thought that the presence of the hymen (a thin fold of perforated, elastic, mucus membrane) covering the opening to the vagina represented "virginity." It is now known that the hymen may be present in the nonvirgin and absent in the virgin. It might be appropriate to ask at this point, just what is "virginity"?

Early Christian teaching epitomized virginity as a state preferable to marriage, with sex even in marriage being related closely to sin. Today, in some primitive societies, the unmarried girl walks carefully and gingerly lest she destroy her hymen and thereby her eligibility for marriage. The "modern" girl on being asked to prove her "virginity" with physical evidence, would justifiably react with outraged indignation. Because there is no equivalent state for the male, it represents the employment of a double standard. If virginity cannot be defined in physical terms, what, then, does it represent? For those *pre*occupied with the thought, it could be symbolic of a perfectionism that no woman is capable of. In more positive terms, some might define it as a state of mind, a faith in or loyalty to a marriage or lover. Suffice it to say that those who demand "evidence" of such faith have themselves lost it.

Developing outcomes of the reevaluation of our standards of femininity appear to be greater companionship in marriage and greater socialization of the sexes. The woman sees in the newer developing concepts of femininity greater intellectual and social freedom and the opportunity of being, to a much greater extent, herself.

Definitions for masculinity are also undergoing change in our culture. Historically, masculinity referred to muscular strength and the ability to protect. The "Prince Valiant" swinging his singing sword could serve as the model of manhood defending spouse and country. Wars are no longer fought with swords, and rifles are already obsolete. The scientist, the engineer, and the technician prepared to push "the button" are the present day Prince Valiants. They do not swagger, and they may have trouble picking up, much less swinging, a heavy sword. Although muscular strength and skills are still admirable qualities, their identification with masculinity is waning.

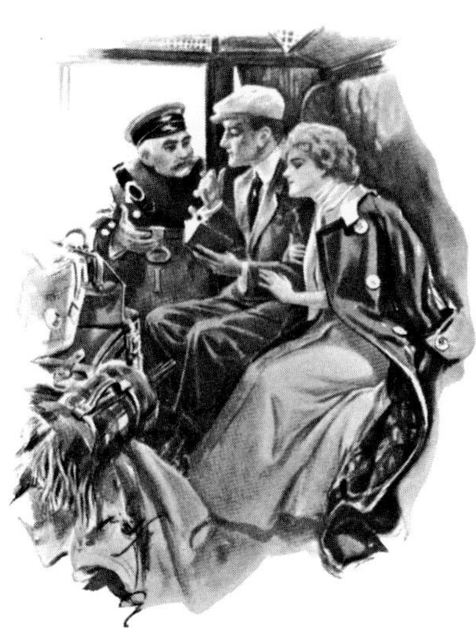
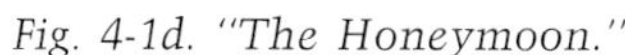

Fig. 4-1d. "The Honeymoon."

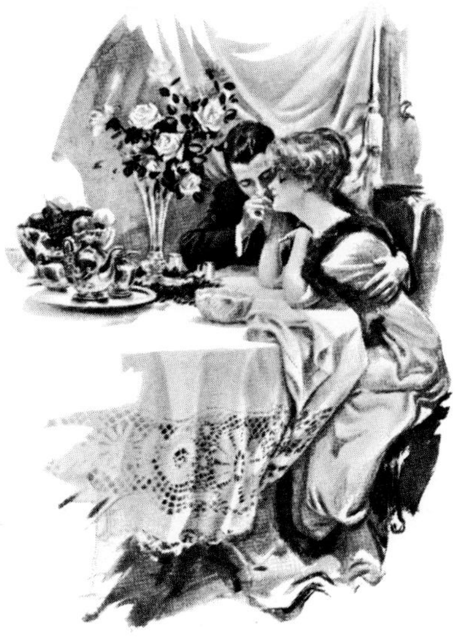

Fig. 4-1e. "The First Evening in Their Own Home."

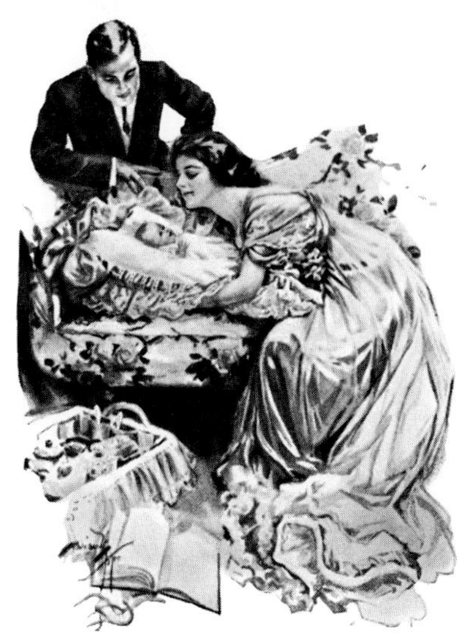

Fig. 4-1f. "Their New Love."

Fig. 4-1. "The Greatest Moments in a Girl's Life.": Those who can identify with the values expressed in these pictures will find it interesting to discuss the matter with those who cannot. (Reinthal & Newman, Pubs., New York)

The male clinging to the more traditional concepts of masculinity and femininity may feel threatened by the changes taking place. The more aggressive female who does not recognize his concepts of masculinity can emasculate him. He can retreat to the coy, demure, "old fashioned" girl, or to the solace of equally bewildered, sympathetic males.

The male who will not have difficulty in this era of change is he who can develop his masculinity around other kinds of strengths. These are inner strengths that give him the courage to admit his mistakes and not be shattered by them; that render him unafraid to make himself be heard; that make him dedicated to his work and help him influence the course of events around him. This self-actualizing male is one who is not a "yes man" at work or a nonentity at home, but one whose moral strengths and values make him a masculine model for a son to identify with and for a woman to love.

The Feminist Movement

"We hold these truths to be self-evident; that all men *and women* are created equal."[3]

"Women are helpless . . . because men control the basic mechanisms of society."[4]

"The average man, including the average student male radical wants a passive sex object cum domestic, cum baby nurse, to clean up after him while he does all the fun things and bosses her around—while he plays either big-shot executive or Che Guevara and he is my oppressor and my enemy."[5]

"There is no way out of such a dilemma but to rebel and be broken, stigmatized and cured. Until the radical spirit revives to free us, we remain imprisoned in the vast gray stockades of sexual reaction."[6]

"Heaven has no rage like love to hatred turned,
Nor hell a fury like a woman scorned."[7]

The message coming through is quite clear: women do not want to be regarded as second-class citizens. At the present time women make up about 9 per cent of all professional groups. Women constitute 7 per cent of the doctors, 3 per cent of the lawyers, and 1 per cent of the engineers. Starting salaries for women in these fields are lower than for the men. The average full-time salary of a woman is about half of that of a man. Financial independence is thus a primary goal of the women's liberation movement and lack of it a primary gripe.

The fury that has been generated around the issue goes beyond pure economics. A great deal of resent-

[3]The Declaration of Sentiments—The first Women's Rights Convention held in 1848 at Seneca Falls, New York. Leaders were Lucretia Mott and Elizabeth Cady Stanton.

[4]*Time Magazine,* August 31, 1970, p. 14.

[5]Ibid., p. 14.

[6]Kate Millett, *Sexual Politics* (Garden City, N.Y.: Doubleday, 1970), p. 233.

[7]William Congreve, *The Way of the World,* Act III, Scene 8.

ment revolves around the woman being regarded as a thing, a sex object, a housekeeper, an intellectual inferior, and generally a subsidiary to that of the man. The current drive for women's rights received great impetus in 1963. At that time Betty Friedan published a book entitled *The Feminine Mystique,* which exposed the vacuumlike existence of the suburban housewife. However, lest one be misled into thinking independent women are a new breed in our society, historically even in the ancient Hebrew civilization where women were expected to fulfill their roles only by caring for the house and bearing and rearing children the influence of such women as Sarah, Rebekah, and Jezebel had to be reckoned with. Mary Astell, during the seventeenth century in England, was one of the first women to publicly denounce the unfair treatment and low status of her sex and Mary Wollstonecraft's *Vindication of the Rights of Women*[8] attempted to put an end to the theory of female inferiority by arguing for education of women in all matters. More recently, Kate Millett expressed in her book *Sexual Politics* a rage some suspect was based strongly on her own family experience which was then translated into societal concern. Kate Millett and others who have taken up the cry for women's rights have hit responsive chords in many. The term "male chauvinist" became not only a common expression, but a battlecry for women and a thrust at any male who exhibited any signs or symptoms of male supremacy.

[8] *Vindication of the Rights of Women* (Philadelphia: Mathew Carey, 1794).

There have been comparisons made between the women's liberation movement and the struggles of the black population for equal opportunity. A basic difference, however, is that while blacks represent about 10 per cent of the population, women constitute 51 per cent and therefore a majority. There has been a reluctance on the part of black women to join the women's liberation movement. In some instances black men are just beginning to emerge as provider and champions of their families. The black woman also recognizes that building up a man's ego is an inherent part of overcoming the racial oppression and emasculation he has suffered for centuries. This they regard as a more important issue than women's liberation. Many black communities have been matriarchal ones with the woman assuming, virtually alone, the role of breadwinner, housekeeper, and mother. She is seeking help and greater companionship from the male and is not anxious to discourage that at a time when it is developing.

Practically all women liberationists are agreed on such issues as equal pay for equal work, an opportunity to fill jobs traditionally reserved for men only, abortion reform, child-care centers to free mothers for work, more equitable income tax laws, and male respect. The more radical feminist groups see their mission as one of destroying the patriarchal system—to be replaced presumably by the only other alternative an equally unequal matriarchal system. This represents not so much a change in the system, but rather *who* is in charge of it. A basic difference one sees therefore in the feminist movement is that while most are calling for equality, some are seeking power to shift their current inequities onto others. The latter is hardly a quality found in just some women; some men have also sought power for the same discriminatory purposes. Suffice it to say that the acquisition and the abuse of power is unfortunately at times a human quality—but not a humane one.

Should the women's liberation movement succeed, the following would be some of the outcomes. The woman would assume many more positions in the ranks of the professions, in administration, and in the political arena. She will therefore become more independent financially, have a greater range of choices as to what she may choose to do with her life and have greater impact on influencing the course of events around her. She may choose not to marry, preferring a career. Fear of being called an "old maid" will become an anomaly of the past. She may choose to be a wife, mother, or professional or she may choose a combination of all three.

The man on the other hand may also benefit from the change. He may not have the pressures of being the sole or even the major source of income for the family. He may therefore have greater choice in the kind of work he selects, which may pay less, but is more satisfying to him. He may be free to spend more time with his children and thereby truly share the responsibility of raising them as is done in Sweden. Gloria Steinem, editor of the feminist magazine entitled *Ms,* is credited with saying that ideally men and women should not reverse roles, but they should be free to choose their roles according to their individual talents and preferences. It is felt that role reforms will change the sexual hypocrisy we have now.

> No more sex arranged on the barter system, with women pretending interest, and men never sure whether they are loved for themselves or for the security few women can get any other way. . . . No more men who are encouraged to spend a lifetime living with inferiors; with housekeepers, or dependent creatures who are still children. No more domineering wives [and] emasculating women . . . all of whom are simply human beings with all their normal ambition and drive confined to the home. No more unequal partnerships that eventually doom love and sex.[9]

Women will also have an impact on the current order of things in religion. In the past, organized religion cast women in very secondary roles. Male clergy have viewed women as unworthy, temptresses, and at best those who would perform the more menial tasks of the organization. It is not unreasonable to assume that the not too far distant future would produce women serving as priests and rabbis. Some are already serving as Protestant ministers. As the black man strove for greater equality he challenged that perhaps God was black. Who is to say that God is not female!

Studies have shown that societies that were most peaceful were those where sex roles were not polarized—a society where men were not expected to be the aggressive warriors and women the subservient peons. Rather, differences in dress and occupation were minimal, with men and women as true partners. The feminist movement, which started out

[9] *Time Magazine,* August 31, 1970, p.22.

with a warlike attitude, may have as its outcome a more peaceful society, where men and women will have freedom of choice as the kind of life they see for themselves.

Sex Values

We live in an era when traditional sex values are also undergoing reexamination and change. As in any transitional period, varying reactions will occur. Some will view this period as a time for sexual license and exploitative sex; others will react defensively and retreat to the most conservative of sexual concepts. The majority will probably move to more moderate views than those expressed by the extremes. This is a period when more wholesome and firmer foundations are sought upon which to base sex values. We are moving away from repressive attitudes about sex toward a growing recognition that sexuality can have positive contributions to make. It is a move from the head-in-the-sand, "let's act as though sex does not exist" attitude to the conclusion that "sex is here to stay—let's examine its positive potentials!"

Six major conflicting value systems of sex that currently exist in this period of transition follow:

1. *Traditional repressive asceticism*—which is still embodied in most of our official codes and laws—prescribes any kind of sexual activity outside of the marriage relationship and accepts sex in marriage grudgingly, insisting upon the linkage of sex with procreation. This value system is intolerant of all deviations from restrictive patterns of heterosexual behavior, it places a taboo on public and scientific discussion and study of sex, and it conceives of sex morality solely in absolute terms of "Thou shalt" and "Thou shalt not."
2. *Enlightened asceticism*—as exemplified in views of such spokesmen as David Mace—begins with a basic acceptance of the ascetic point of view. Mace sees asceticism as a safeguard against the "softness" to which we so easily fall prey in an age when opportunities for self-indulgence are so abundant. He sees youth as the time when invaluable lessons of self-control and discipline must be learned, with sex as one of the supreme areas in which self-mastery may be demonstrated, and he opposes any slackening of the sexual code. However, he takes neither a negative nor a dogmatic attitude toward sex and has been an ardent exponent of the "open forum" in which issues can be stated and weighed.
3. *Humanistic liberalism*—has been best exemplified by the views of Lester Kirkendall. Kirkendall opposes inflexible absolutes and makes his prime concern the concept of interpersonal relationship. He sees the criterion of morality as not the commission or omission of a particular act, but the consequences of the act upon the interrelationships of people, not only the immediate people concerned but broader relationships. Kirkendall thus is searching for a value system which will help supply internalized controls for the individual in a period when older social and religious controls are collapsing.
4. *Humanistic radicalism*—is exemplified best by the views of Walter Stokes. He accepts the humanistic position of Kirkendall and goes further in proposing that society should make it possible for young people to have relatively complete sex freedom. He makes it clear that society must create certain preconditions

before this goal may be achieved. He envisions a cultural engineering project which may take generations to achieve.

5. *Fun morality*—has as its most consistent spokesman Albert Ellis. Without compromise, he upholds the viewpoint that sex is fun and that the more sex fun a human being has, the better and psychologically sounder he or she is likely to be. He believes that, despite the risk of pregnancy, premarital intercourse should be freely permitted, and at times encouraged, for well-informed and reasonably well-adjusted persons.
6. *Sexual anarchy*—has as its philosopher the late French jurist René Guyon. Guyon attacks chastity, virginity, and monogamy and calls for the suppression of all antisexual taboos and the disappearance of the notions of sexual immorality and shame. The only restriction he would apply is the general social principle that no one may injure or do violence to his fellows.[10]

Also emerging during this period has been the *Playboy* philosophy. *Playboy* has done well in exposing the hypocrisy of our society's sex attitudes and the inappropriateness of prudery. It also rejects sex behavior that is "irresponsible, exploitive, coercive or in some way hurts one of the individuals involved."[11] However, the impression that *Playboy* leaves the reader with implies that sex can be a casual way of saying hello and that it can be indulged in simply for the pleasure, devoid of any emotional involvement. The potential of sexual intimacy for psychological trauma, particularly where an insensitive partner is involved, is never alluded to. *Playboy* depicts the well-equipped male with a sports car, stereo, a bachelor's apartment, and a smiling robot-like girl prepared to serve his every whim and pleasure. It leaves one with the impression that technology has taken over and created an unemotional complying, thing of a woman—*a computerization of femininity!* The preceding value systems represent a great diversity of thought. What is simple, instinctive behavior for the animal is the basis of wide-ranging philosophy for man.

A feminist reaction to *Playboy* was of course predictable. An issue of *Cosmopolitan* magazine, effected an instant playback to *Playboy* by including in one of their publications the figure of a nude male in their centerfold. The point is clear. A person's integrity starts with one's personality and not with one's physiology.

Increasingly, religious leaders are recognizing that the rigid absolutes "thou shalt" or "thou shalt not" are not always appropriate bases for behavior and that the subjective morality of the individual must more often be called upon. With each period of liberation come the carpetbaggers selling their wares peculiar to the new found freedom accompanied by its inevitable naïveté. This implies careful preparation of the individual to make those most important decisions, lest we unshackle ourselves from the rigidities of the past to fall precipitously off the nearest cliff of licentiousness.

[10] Isadore Rubin, "Transition in Sex Values—Implications for the Education of Adolescents," *The Journal of Marriage and the Family*, Vol. XXVII, No. 2 (May 1965). Used by permission of the author.

[11] Hugh Hefner, *The Playboy Philosophy* (Chicago: H. M. H. Publishing Co., 1962–1965), Part 19.

Some Negative Bases of Sexual Involvement

It is important to note that a sexual relationship is a kind of social relationship. The motivations of the person in this type of relationship will not vary to any extent from those carried into other social interactions. The level of maturity and healthy-mindedness are also reflected in sex as well as other social relationships. Let us first consider some of the negative bases for this kind of involvement.

Sex—a thing. A person may view sex as a kind of commodity that is bought, sold, and paid for. The man with this point of view spends money on the girl he dates and regards it as an investment. He expects repayment in the form of physical pleasures that the female can provide. A girl who understands the rules of this game complies. This is but one form of sex commercialization that we see in our culture. A deep-rooted person-to-person relationship is not an outcome to be expected in such a situation. The focus in this case is not on persons relating to each other, but on services bought and paid for. Dr. Coffin, the chaplain at Yale University, has been prompted by this kind of sex-motivated activity to point out, "A society that places people in the category of things and values ability to purchase above the ability to relate is a society whose young people will grow up confused as to behavior and values."[12] It must be added that if a young person is confused with regard to sex values here, it is not the young person who introduced either the confusion or the value—but a society that does not recognize the bounds of propriety with regard to commercialism.

Exploitation. While the previously mentioned situation involved a type of reciprocal trade agreement, exploitation is based on the principle of getting something for nothing. The Don Juan needs to exploit others as a means of alleviating his fears with regard to his masculinity. It may be the nature of the individual to seek pleasure in the successful manipulation of others. Some people contend that we foster an exploitative male attitude in our society. They cite as evidence our concern with the problem of the unwed mother and the all-but-oblivious attitude toward the unwed father (the only one who seems concerned with the unwed father is the father of the unwed mother!). The idea is fostered that pregnancy is the girl's responsibility. Any girl that engages in sexual activity is no good, but—boys will be boys! It is contended that we equate male sexual irresponsibility with masculinity rather than with immaturity. The male who accepts the exploitative attitude, it is charged, betrays the "wholesomeness" of his activities when he reacts with all kinds of indignation if the girl in a like situation is his sister or later on his daughter.

This societal attitude is also apparently fed by the parents who view soaring illegitimacy rates with, "I don't have to worry, I have sons!" A recent study of unwed fathers indicates that perhaps there is cause for concern here. It presents evidence that the experience is also damaging to the unwed father. He is first of all denied identification with his own

[12] Mary S. Calderone, op. cit., p. 501.

creation and is further emasculated by his inability to see, much less take pride in, his offspring. Feelings of guilt that he may have are often heightened by the lack of punishment. The girl in the case usually is unwilling to identify him and in essence protects him. This serves to have a further distressing effect on the male who has been reared in a society where it is the masculine role to protect, rather than to be protected by, the female.

A salve for insecurity. The woman who places undue importance on her physical attractiveness needs constant assurance of its presence. She often becomes involved in a "Mirror, mirror on the wall" kind of game, seeking assurance from every male of the species that she is still "the fairest in the land." While it is quite natural and normal for a woman to want to be attractive to the opposite sex, preoccupation with the thought reflects a neurotic rather than a healthy need. When promiscuity is a result, the activity has hardly anything to do with sex, even though sex may be the distorted basis for attempting to satisfy security needs.

That biological urge. Satisfying the biological nature of the sex urge may be the sole motivation in some sexual involvements. Some find difficulty in acknowledging the existence of this aspect of their nature. They often attribute qualities of this kind of relationship that do not exist. Self-deluding attempts are made to believe that love was a motivating part of the experience. Marriages that result from a lustful relationship cannot be well based. A common cause of failure of early marriages is that they are often predominantly based on a sexual relationship. The young couple never learn to communicate on a higher level, preventing the fulfillment of each other's personality needs and the development of a more mature personal relationship. Unless the couple can find a more meaningful basis for a marital relationship, they quickly develop a feeling that they have turned into a dead-end road. Their relationship has already gone as far as it can go. An erroneous conclusion that is drawn when such a marriage goes sour (as it inevitably must) is that each made a poor choice of a marital partner.

There is an erotic element in man-woman relationships—even in one as casual as a verbal exchange. Those who recognize the potential of this powerful erotic force deal with it appropriately so they can control it rather than have it control them. They seek to avoid situations and behavior that would stimulate and unleash these forces with inappropriate partners. *There is nothing quite so ashen as meeting the gray light of dawn with the throbbing realization of overinvolvement with a person one cannot love.*

On Sex and Love: A Positive Basis for Sexual Involvement

Much has been written and said about the relationship of sex and love. It is rather basically agreed that they mutually benefit each other. Some feel strongly that sex without love is a barren experience, being equated to speech without thought. It lacks meaning. As expressed by Schwarz in referring to sexual activity, ". . . if we meekly submit to the physical impulse, we incur guilt. Because it fails the essentially spiritual nature of man, a purely physical intercourse is essentially immoral."[13]

The relationship of sex and love is often more casually viewed by the male as compared with the female. The male is more erotic in nature and his sex drive is more physiologically based. The male produces seminal fluids whose pressures create a sexual urgency not found in the female. His sex drive can serve as the motivating factor leading to intimacy, even with women he would otherwise have no regard for. Love, then, does not alway fit into the sexual pattern of things, particularly for the immature or exploitative male. The male in our society, often as a result of social conditioning, regards nonmarital sexual relations as more desirable than masturbation or nocturnal emissions. A common concurrent attitude is that "You don't touch the one you love." In such cases, the male learns more readily to equate sex with lust rather than with love.

Women, on the other hand, are not so strongly motivated by sex drive as by romantic influences. They view love and sex in closer context and in that order. The girl is more prone to view sex as part of a long-term relationship. Premarital sex is therefore stimulated in the female more commonly by the idea of not losing someone than by sexual urges. Where a girl's romantic notions are mixed with some naïveté, she may be coerced by the exploitative male to "prove her love." In recent years, however, with the biological protection of the contraceptive pill there has been a greater tendency for young women to accept sex activity on a more casual basis paralleling those of men. The further possibility of an abortion, should there be a "pill failure," serves as an added support for this attitude.

If love is viewed as the indispensable aspect of an ideal interpersonal relationship, one's interpretation of what is love becomes basic. Dr. Popenoe has reacted to the false values spewed out via the mass media by stating:

> The mass media picture love as a mysterious visitation that comes out of the nowhere and grabs hold of you like measles. Once it has you, the rest of your life should be an effortless ecstasy. If it turns out later that some effort is involved, it proves that you were mistaken in thinking this was your predestined soul-mate and there is nothing to do but throw him or her out and try again. . . . The net result has been to produce a culture that is based far more than is tolerable, on sex without love and marriage without responsibility.[14]

The nature of love is often overidealized with the emphasis on a sacrificial and an unrealistic selflessness. This interpretation gives it a saccharine flavor that could in time nauseate even the most romantic. The ability to give love is unquestionably an essential quality for the lover. The person's ability to receive love is equally important. It should be recognized that some of the person's own needs are being met by the relationship. The love relationship is

[13] Oswald Schwarz, *The Psychology of Sex* (Baltimore: Penguin, 1962), p. 22.

[14] Paul Popenoe, "Sex Education," *Family Life*, Vol. XXII, No. 8 (Los Angeles: The American Institute of Family Relations, August 1962). Used by permission of the author.

characterized by a couple's feeling of warmth, pride, and identity with one another. There is also the mutual satisfaction of security needs. A oneness emerges from the interaction of the two people involved. There develops a related emotional dependence and an ability to communicate, not only in terms of words, but in attitudes, feelings, and thoughts. In a new or developing relationship each person tries to put his best foot forward as a means of impressing the partner. In a mature love relationship, this kind of thought and action is not necessary. A man and woman can stand before each other and bare their complete psychological and physical selves with all inherent strengths and weaknesses. The commitment is complete. Sexual expression in this context then becomes a physical enactment of an existing mental, emotional, and social state of unity. In a love relationship, sex plays the secondary role of expressing and complementing the emotion. A mature love relationship is not one that all people are capable of attaining. Nor is it a state that once reached is forever propelled under its own power. It is a relationship that requires consistent attention or it dies of neglect like the unwatered plant.

Sexual Outlets

Masturbation is the self-stimulation of the genitals to effect sexual arousal and often orgasm. For the young male, masturbation is the most common sexual outlet until marriage. Over 90 per cent of the males have masturbated by the time they reach their sixteenth birthday. It is estimated that over half of the females have also masturbated. The frequency of the practice is usually much lower in the girl.

There were at one time many misconceived ideas about masturbation. It was erroneously related to just about everything from club feet to poor vision. Because uninhibited mental patients were observed to masturbate openly, it was even considered a cause of mental illness. The fear that it may later on affect sexual potency is equally unjustified. Clinicians now view it as a harmless practice physically. Masturbation as a physical excess is considered impossible because the body sets its own limits with regard to fatigue and endurance. At a given point it will no longer respond erotically.

Concern with regard to masturbation revolves around its psychologically caused misuse. When masturbation is not used in its sexual context, but in reaction to failure or rejection, there may be cause for concern. Its use as a source of solace and a retreat from problems reflects unwholesome attitudes. Those who have been taught that masturbation is evil or sinful will often develop guilt feelings when they participate in this activity. Masturbation may also serve as a source of marital problems. The male or female with a well-established habit of masturbation may find that it is not easily discarded. The heterosexual relationship found in marriage may not displace the practice of masturbation. Not recognizing this, the partner reacts with feelings of rejection; if for no other reason, the individual will find it wise to exert some control over this activity.

Views with regard to masturbation in our society

are becoming more objective. It is no longer regarded as often with alarm, but increasingly with the knowledge that it is a part of psychosexual development.

Nocturnal Emissions occur as a result of dreams of a sexual nature. An orgasm occurs during sleep and in the male semen is ejaculated, hence the term "wet dream." Females may have similar dreams, but of course ejaculation is not associated with them. The individual has no control over these experiences; they just happen.

Athletes are sometimes troubled by nocturnal emissions because they feel that they are weakened by them. It is believed that a decline in performance following a "wet dream" is psychologically induced by the thought that it may have this effect rather than by any actual physical changes that have occurred.

Occasionally, sexual dreams may involve a person the individual would not consciously consider as a sex partner. This could result in the development of guilt feelings. These feelings will be reduced if the person does not attach too much importance to the dream and places it in proper perspective. To attach moral meanings to nocturnal emissions is inappropriate because they are beyond one's control.

Petting can include a wide range of activity from kissing to the stimulation of the partner's genitals to orgasm. There are varied motivations for petting. It may serve as a means of expressing love and affection or it may be stimulated by a curiosity with regard to the opposite sex. It may be used by the wily and unscrupulous as a means of exciting the partner for seductive purposes. In other instances, the person may be seeking to establish that he or she is attractive to the opposite sex. It becomes important to give definition to a petting situation. Does one indulge for the pleasure of the moment, or does it mean the development of a more serious relationship between two people? If one person gives the activity one meaning while the partner gives it another definition, difficulty will inevitably be an outcome. Petting tends to be progressive with greater intimacies developing on a given occasion or with succeeding dates. Understanding one's motivations and those of the partner becomes increasingly important. It is also important to understand one's physiological reactions as well as those of the partner. A girl's slower sexual response may lead her into underestimating the male's level of excitation. The young man, conversely, may misjudge the girl's response by his more rapid reactions. Petting leads so naturally to sexual intercourse that a couple may reach the point of no return before they realize it. When intimacy goes beyond the level desired by those involved, strong feelings of guilt and degradation may follow. If the intent is to keep petting under control, its limits should be decided beforehand as a guard against impulsive behavior that one will later deeply regret.

Studies show that petting to orgasm is becoming more common as a solution to sexual tensions short of intercourse. As stated by Hettlinger:

> It is of course, possible to be a "promiscuous virgin" and to engage in petting to orgasm with a variety of casual partners and without any serious commitment. In such cases, the technical preservation of virginity is purely

superficial, and the level of sexual maturity is less than that of the person who has intercourse with one partner in the context of a loving relationship.[15]

Sexual Intercourse can serve to enhance a love relationship, particularly when the relationship is protected by the sanctity of marriage. Whether to participate in premarital intercourse is often a difficult question for a couple to resolve. "Premarital" would in this case be defined to mean that the couple have made commitments for marriage to each other. Intercourse without such commitments would be considered "nonmarital" in nature. Some couples have reported that as a result of premarital sex activity they felt they had developed a closer relationship. Others report negative reactions. Where sex activity is undertaken accompanied with fear of discovery, pregnancy, and guilt, more may be done to tarnish the feelings the couple have for one another, than to strengthen their relationship. Good sexual adjustment after marriage may also be negatively affected by hurried, fearful, and guilt-tinged premarital attempts. Because it may take a period of time for a couple to adjust to each other sexually, early premarital relations often give false indices as to the kind of sexual adjustment they will ultimately be capable of. Careful consideration must be given to the decision of premarital sex to determine if the couple will be helped or hurt by the experience, particularly in view of the circumstances and attitudes that often surround such practices. What effect an unexpected pregnancy will have on the relationship must also be taken into account. It has also been noted that when a couple engages in premarital relations, feelings of jealousy and greater possessiveness often develop. Should one of the partners decide to break off the relationship, it becomes more difficult to do so. A more unstable personality in this circumstance may threaten to expose the couple's premarital relationship. In a few cases, one of the partners may even threaten suicide. These latter actions usually do no more than demonstrate instability and confirm the individual's unsuitability for marriage.

The question of nonmarital sexual relations has also been raised. There are those who advocate complete sexual freedom in reaction to past sexual repression. Most people see both these points of view as creating their own sets of problems, with neither being a solution for the other. Reducing sex to the fun-and-games level with indiscriminate premarital intimacy appears to bear the same seeds of destruction as would the indiscriminate use of just about anything else. The difference, if any, is that here we are dealing with a sensitive part of life, requiring sensitive considerations. Equating sex that is based on sadism, masochism, exploitation, or self-indulgence with sex based on sincerity, love, and understanding cannot be justified by stating that sexual activity is "natural." There are mushrooms and there are mushrooms; there are berries and berries. Some will sustain the person; others will poison him. The skill comes in distinguishing between the two.

[15] Richard F. Hettlinger, *Sexual Maturity*, Basic Concepts in Health Science Series (Belmont, Calif.: Wadsworth, 1970), p. 47.

Homosexuality

Homosexuality and heterosexuality are often viewed in terms of absolutes. Actually, there are various gradations of sexuality from one polarity to the other. Many psychiatrists view homosexuality in terms of those persons who seek sexual gratification predominantly with members of their own sex. There is apparently a rather large percentage of the population who may be erotically aroused by members of both sexes. Research shows that approximately 37 per cent of all males have had some overt homosexual experience to the point of orgasm. However, studies show that only 4 per cent of white males are exclusively homosexual all of their lives.

There are various theories to explain the possible causation of homosexuality. Increasingly, researchers in this field are finding agreement that psychological, social, and cultural factors are more important than genetic or glandular ones. A number of studies indicate that identification with the parent of the opposite sex can be a strong contributing factor. This is particularly so where the parents have reversed roles, with the mother serving as the dominant partner and the husband playing a more passive role in the family. There is general agreement that multiple factors probably play a part in the development of the homosexual state. Some of these include disturbed parent-child relationships, arrested psychosexual development at an immature stage, and cultural overemphasis on "masculinity" resulting in feelings of inadequacy in males.

There is a question of whether homosexuality is an illness. Some feel that emotional personality problems found in homosexuals are often the result of punitive cultural attitudes leveled at this group, rather than an inherent part of the homosexual state. More research in this area, however, is needed before definitive answers can be given to the question. Psychoanalysts have in some instances been able to convert the homosexual individual to a completely heterosexual state. In most cases, however, therapy is considered successful if the person can learn to become somewhat more heterosexual than homosexual.

In 1969 the Gay Liberation movement had its birth in the form of a riot at a gay bar in Greenwich Village, New York. The movement represents a revolt against social persecution and seeks to assist the rights of the homosexual. The North American Conference of Homophile Organizations put forth the following formal statement.

> In our pluralistic society the homosexual has a moral right to be a homosexual, and being a homosexual, has a moral right to live his homosexuality fully, freely and openly, free of arrogant and insolent pressures to convert to the prevailing heterosexuality, and free of penalities, disabilities or disadvantages of any kind, public or private, official or unofficial, for his nonconformity.[16]

The Gay Liberation movement has also taken the stand that homosexuality is not pathological and does not belong in the realm of the psychiatrist and psychologist but view it instead as a sociological

[16]Joseph A. McCaffrey, ed., *The Homosexual Dialectic* (Englewood Cliffs, N.J.: Prentice-Hall, 1972).

problem in which prejudice and discrimination are directed against a minority in much the same way that other minorities are recipients of such treatment. "It is society that is defective and at fault and needs our attention, not the homosexual."[17] The emotionalized attitudes toward homosexuality in our culture are found to inhibit research in this area and add the problem of social rejection and persecution to the difficulties of the homosexual.

In Conclusion

The individual, as well as society, is challenged to develop sex values that may be useful as guiding principles in the determination of sex attitudes and behavior. We are moving from the point of view that sex per se is dirty and inherently evil to the recognition that sex can be a dynamic, powerful, and creative force. This change, in itself like a breath of fresh air, should prepare the groundwork for more enlightened objective discussion of the issues and problems previously mentioned.

Review Questions

1. "Sex is not something we do but something that we are." Explain.
2. What are the influences of the culture on concepts related to masculinity and femininity?
3. What changes have taken place with regard to the role of women in our society? What are the implications of these changes for the men and their concepts of masculinity?
4. What are the six major conflicting value systems related to sex that were identified by Dr. Rubin? Why are they particularly significant in a society whose sex values appear to be undergoing change?
5. What constitute some of the negative bases for sexual involvement? Why do they fail to serve the individual properly?
6. Why do many consider sex to be in the most desirable context when it is part of a love relationship?
7. What will probably be some of the outcomes of the feminist movement?
8. Why have the feminists reacted negatively to the Playboy philosophy?
9. How have societal attitudes toward masturbation been changing? What kinds of concerns are *now* expressed with regard to this practice?
10. What can be the varied motivations for petting? Why is it important to recognize the nature of these motivations in oneself as well as one's partner?
11. Distinguish between premarital and nonmarital sexual intercourse.
12. How do premarital relations encumber the breaking off of a relationship, should this decision be reached?
13. The terms *homosexuality* and *heterosexuality* should not be viewed as absolutes. Explain.
14. What are believed to be some of the causations of homosexuality?

[17] Ibid., p. 188.

Chapter 5
Preparation for Marriage

Preparation for marriage does not start at the time that one begins to give consideration to marital possibilities. To be quite precise about it, since one's genetic makeup represents an initial contribution in this area, preparation for marriage starts at the time of conception. Because the individual has no control over his inherited characteristics, he must accept it all gleefully or philosophically, as the case may be. Regardless of genetic endowments, the kind of marital partner a person *will be* is determined to a greater extent by the kind of person he *has become*. Marriage is essentially a close, intimate, social relationship between two people. The most important thing a person brings to this union is himself.

The prerequisite to a successful marriage is maturity. The complexities and responsibilities of marriage are not for the immature. Because the term "maturity" is subject to interpretation, it would seem appropriate to give some indices of its presence.

The mature person can accept responsibility for his own acts. This means that he is not trying to blame others for his failures or to exaggerate his accomplishments. He also does not take offense easily in reaction to what others may say or do. The immature often feel that people are picking on them. This kind of oversensitivity will hardly prove to be an asset in marriage, or in any interpersonal relationship, for that matter.

Maturity also means the ability to endure present deprivation in order to effect more meaningful future gain. A college student may accept some financial setbacks in order to complete professional education. He does this in the knowledge that the temporary setback is compensated for by his ultimate ability to earn a better income and do more meaningful work. The person whose wants and urges need immediate gratification has not outgrown a childlike mode of behavior. This also implies a nonexploitative attitude toward others. The immature regard other people as things to manipulate and use for their own purposes.

The mature person is also socially responsible. His natural regard for others and his sense of responsibility make him one who has a concern for other individuals as well as for his community. He participates in community activity without the expectation of personal reward other than the satisfaction of contributing to a better-functioning society.

The selflessness characteristic of the mature makes them better prepared to live in close association with others and to contribute positively to their lives. The close interpersonal relationships that exist in successful marriage require acceptable levels of maturity as prerequisites.

Motivations for Marriage

The reasons why people marry are many and varied. The wholesomeness and unwholesomeness of the reasons may run an equally wide range. Positive motivations for marriage revolve about the desire to develop a close interpersonal relationship with another. This is usually described as a love relationship. The marriage serves to give this union religious sanction and legal protection. Thus protected by marriage, the relationship is provided an environment in which it can best grow. It is thus also regarded as a favorable environment in which to bring the products of this relationship—namely children. Many people see in marriage a stable structure within which love relationships and families are best developed.

There are also some negative motivations for marriage. Many times a girl has been indoctrinated with the unfortunate notion that her major function in life is to "get her man." In this case, the focus is not the development of a meaningful relationship with someone, but how to get him to the marriage ceremony. The wedding then becomes a day of triumph and a celebration of accomplishment. The groom in such an unfortunate circumstance is not loved, but is a piece of property that represents some temporary social status. With the next day often dawns the realization that she is committed to share a lifetime with a symbol of success. Unless her attitude toward marriage is changed, there will be other days of celebration with equally short-lived "triumphs."

An individual may use marriage as a way of removing himself from an unhappy home situation. Where the predominant motive to marry is one of escape, the basis for another unhappy marriage may be in the making.

People who have been thwarted in a love relationship may decide to salve their bruised egos by impulsively marrying "on the rebound." The business of marrying the next eligible person to come along is an emotional reaction aimed to prove that the person *can* find someone to marry him or her. It also is designed to show that the rejecting party was not really needed, anyhow. Generally, such marriages are as likely to be successful as a series of shots in the dark. The element of emotional immaturity that leads to precipitous actions of this type is also one that does not lend stability to a marriage.

Sometimes wealth may serve as a prime motivator for marriage. People who would use marriage for this purpose usually feel unloved and unsuccessful and strive to marry profitably as a means of compensating for both. The most that can be hoped for under the circumstances is misery in comfort. The close personal relationship necessary to a marriage cannot be based on a bank account. The price for fraud in marriage can be brutally high for both the victim and the perpetrator.

The unexpected pregnancy sometimes serves to initiate marriage. However, the biological father may not be emotionally mature enough to be a husband, much less a meaningful father—to say nothing of the readiness of the girl for motherhood and marriage. The compatibility of the couple may in other instances leave much to be desired. When all these things are considered, perhaps other means should be sought to resolve a difficult situation, rather than to aggravate it further by forcing an unsuitable marriage.

Social pressure cannot be overlooked as a motivating factor in marriage. The person who does not succeed in marrying is often viewed with a degree of suspicion or regarded as a kind of failure. Mothers often develop a good deal of the social pressure when they act as "coaches" and regard their daughters as "players." According to the rules of the game, the idea is to see how soon and how well the daughters can marry. How well the daughters can marry is usually measured in terms of nabbing someone's son a little higher on the social ladder.

In recent years some young people have been appalled at some of the poor marriages they have observed or have been the products of. They have seen people with the poorest of relationships who have entombed themselves in the concrete of marriage, thereby sentencing themselves to a lifetime of incompatability and unhappiness. Their reaction has been to reject marriage and indict *it* as the perpetrator of the crime. Others see those who inappropriately enter marriage as the precipitators of their own misfortunes. Relationships that are ill founded should not seek the religious sanction and legal protection of marriage. Perhaps it is time to stop viewing marriage as an end in itself and to recognize that not all people are suited for lifelong relationships. Despite the contrivances that may exist, our society generally expects people to marry and many of our laws and customs are based on this expectation.

Love

Most people, when asked why they married, will aver that they were in love. The meanings given to the word "love" are many. The word is used in innumerable contexts such as love of country, parents, siblings, animals, clothes, fishing, and so forth. However, its meaning even in regard to one's intended spouse varies widely. Some people feel that they "fell in love" or that they experienced "love at first sight." Both of these experiences imply a sudden happening, something on the order of a chemical reaction. It could easily be rationalized that one no longer has control over a situation where "love has taken over." ("It's bigger than both of us!"). All that is left to say where such thinking prevails is "lover—beware!"

Closely akin to this kind of thinking is the concept of the "one and only." The thought is that there is only one person in the whole wide world with whom one could possibly fall in love. The fact that a large percentage of people marry individuals who live but a few miles from their homes represents a rather extraordinary level of coincidence that is blithely overlooked.

"Love conquers all" is a concept that leads a person to believe that love is an impenetrable shield against all problems. Such thinking is either a rationalization devised to ignore problems or potential problems a person does not choose to own up to, or an unfortunate naïveté. The thought that love will solve problems related to finances, education, children, parents, and religion by a magical waving of its wand cannot be equated with a realistic approach to life and living.

The decision of whether one is in love is an obviously important one. The rest of one's lifetime will be affected by it. A person about to abandon himself to love, needs as criteria for judgment more than wishful thinking or a hunch. As indicated in the previous chapter, love is based on rather complete understanding, communication, and commitment between two people. The bases of understanding, communication, and commitment are not established by a sly glance across the room. The criteria listed here for the evolution of love probably do not rate very high with the romantic. However, without these basics the most violent of infatuations is nothing more than a blazing star.

Physical attraction and infatuation are usually pleasant, exhilarating factors in the initial stages of many love relationships. Love, however, probably starts when the *I* becomes *We*. It does not *happen* so much as it *develops*, and it is not as exciting as it is comforting. Love is like an oasis; it serves as a kind of solid spot—a piece of rationality in an irrational world. It is a constant in an era of kaleidoscopic change. It gives a person purpose and direction as the North Pole does a compass. Fickleness and self-centeredness are immiscible with it. Love is tough, durable, and unshakable because it is a kind of personality fusion, welded by time and understanding.

Values

No two people have identical values. Marriage involves some adjustments to the values of the partner that are divergent from the person's own. These differences need, however, to be within the range of negotiability. Divergent attitudes toward money and how to use it, for instance, can be, and usually are, basic concerns in marriage. One partner may be quite frugal, desiring to set up as soon as possible a savings account and family insurance plans. The other partner may see immediate needs in terms of a new car or a fur coat. A man may judge his success by his professional contributions, a wife by how much money he makes.

Some people would not think of marrying and moving any distance away from their parents. Others abhor the idea of living near parents or in-laws, fearing possible marital interference from such sources. The thought of living in the country is incomprehensible to those who feel that the only place to live is in a large city. Conversely, others view cities as nice places to visit, but would not possibly think of living there.

It becomes apparent that one needs to look beyond those qualities that initially attract a person to another, as desirable as those attention-getting qualities may be. In choosing a partner for life, one needs to look past the more superficial and become acquainted with those values the prospective partner considers important, if not essential. The identification of those essential and important values in oneself and the prospective partner is necessary if one is to make some intelligent judgment with regard to compatibility.

Personality Characteristics

It has been found that good personal adjustment is a vital prerequisite for successful marriage. The person who can assume responsibility and is capable of making decisions is a desirable candidate. Conversely, the individual who needs to rely heavily on parents and other authority figures to make decisions is probably not quite ready to assume marital responsibilities.

Persons who can control their emotions and are not chronically subject to fits of anger or changing moods are easier to live with. The person who is capable of staying angry and sullen for days demonstrates an inability to overcome a basic emotion. His ability to function in a close relationship with another is accordingly limited. To be able to express affection comfortably and to possess a sense of humor can be invaluable assets. The ability of a couple to express affection and see the humor (even the bitter humor) in a situation can become important when things get rough—as they invariably will at times. The person who is basically optimistic will seek solutions to problems and will generally find them. The pessimist will view problems with cynicism and be content to wallow in its negative outcomes.

The person who is basically a considerate individual and can relate to others without being domineering or self-centered can readily make the transition from *I* to *we*. The factors we have discussed can serve as barometers for the measurement of a personal level of maturity.

Background

Where couples have similar backgrounds, areas of agreement are expanded and possibilities for conflict minimized. Couples whose levels of education are similar also find it easier to communicate with each other. If the levels of education significantly differ, then the levels of native intelligence should be comparable. When there are incompatibilities in this area, a couple may find it difficult socially as well as interpersonally. Friends that one partner may seek out are of no interest to the other and vice versa. Marital partners with dissimilar educational or intelligence levels will ultimately find many of their interests to be different and develop a tendency to drift away from each other.

Those people who come from happy marriages and childhoods have increased prospects for a happy marriage of their own. The adoption of those values and patterns of behavior that led to the successful marriage of the parents usually follows. Those coming from less happy homes need to develop insights into the failures of their parents' relationships and learn how to avoid similar mistakes. A happy home is usually synonymous with well-adjusted offspring who are in turn better able to interact positively with other people.

Economic Status

In early marriages, when both partners are still in college and not working full time, the factor of economics can rear its ugly head. The thesis that "two can live as cheaply as one" is largely fallacious, particularly if the two should become three or four. A couple needs to assess carefully their living costs for rent, food, clothing, utilities, tuition, and so forth, against what current income exists. In some instances parental help is available and can work out if it is offered with no strings attached and graciously

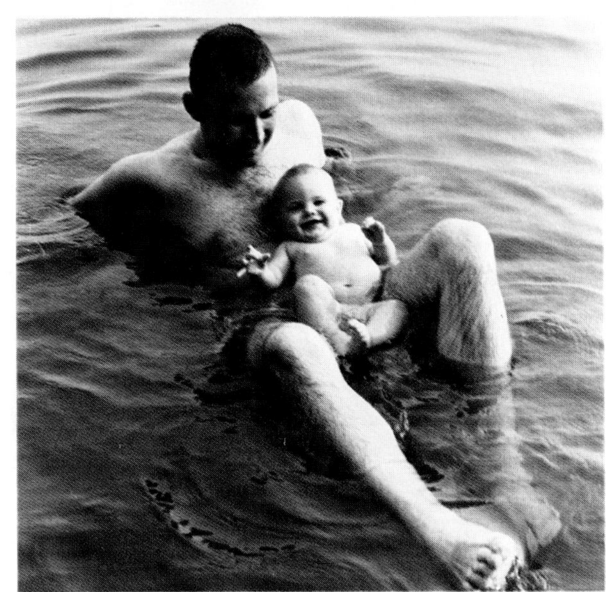

Fig. 5-1. *The father's role in the family should be more than an economic one. (Susan Johns)*

accepted. Student loans can also be a source of assistance. In most cases the situation will call for some belt tightening and the giving up of some "luxuries" to make the marriage solvent. When couples are mature enough to work through a more arduous situation they may even be better off for having done it. Many couples in their later years speak nostagically of the early "rough" days that caused them to live under more adverse conditions but which apparently drew them closer together as a result. Overcoming a challenge is always satisfying. The more challenging the situation overome, the more satisfying the experience, and the greater the risk.

A marriage that is economically stable has many advantages. The complex economic system we live in requires a steady and adequate income. What is adequate will depend to a great extent on what a person judges it to be. A person coming from a high-income family may have drastically different concepts of income adequacy as compared with those of one whose origins are in the lower-income groups. This is particularly a factor when the male who views himself as the breadwinner is in the lower economic echelon. The female in the case may suddenly find that things that she routinely purchased are now luxuries. Willingness to accept this change is important. Parents with money will place more value on the "happiness" of the daughter and be perhaps too eager to help. The male in the situation may feel threatened and inadequate, and the marital relationship possibly undermined.

In recent years greater numbers of people have reacted negatively to materialism as the primary goal in life. Many have sought simple ways of living in country settings in vain attempts to escape materialism and a highly technological society that overshadows the quality of human relationships. Others question if materialism should not be rejected as a value and if control over technology cannot be learned. The latter is a more realistic approach.

Marriages in which both partners were gainfully employed prior to the marriage usually have a high degree of success. This is particularly so when the woman was employed in a professional or skilled office position. The woman who brings to a marriage a potential for a second income affords it several advantages. This potential income can be used when desired to help set up a home or later on by helping to finance college costs for the children. It also gives the family a measure of security should there, for any reason, occur the loss of the breadwinner. The woman who has had work experience is also in a better position to discuss and share with her husband his professional work and related experiences.

The question of whether a mother should work while her children are quite young or living at home is a common issue. Ideally, children should have a great deal of contact with *both* parents. In an agrarian economy this was easily accomplished with both parents working at home. As our economy became industrialized, it was the father who went off to work leaving the child-rearing responsibilities largely to the mother. The family role of the father has heretofore been minimized. Studies are beginning to show, however, that the absence of the father contributes in his children (particularly sons) a low

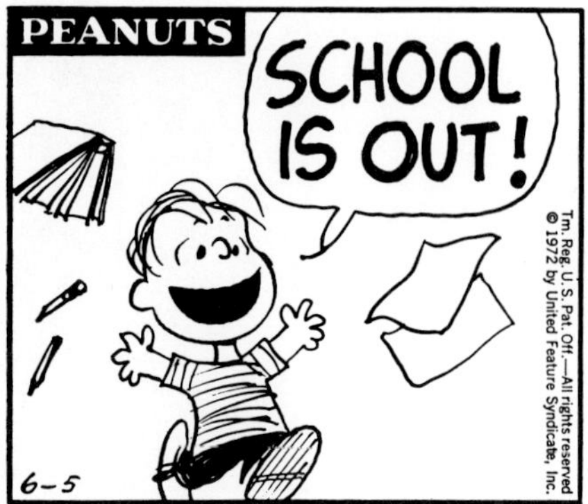

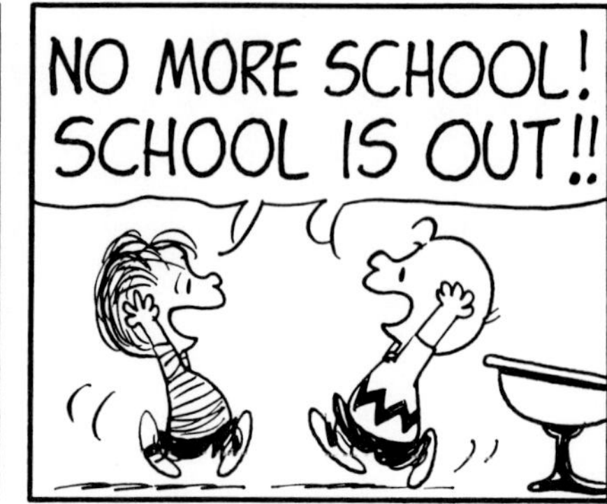

motivation for achievement, the need for immediate gratification of needs at the expense of long-range benefits, low self-esteem, and an unusual susceptibility to peer group influence. It is being realized that prolonged absence of either parent can be potentially damaging to the child. The issue of how children will fare with one or both parents working will largely depend on how much time the parents spend with their children daily and the quality of these parent-child relationships. The level of security of the children and the worth of their self-concepts will be thus determined.

The many social changes that have taken place in this country during the last twenty years warrants our reevaluating the role of the family as it concerns bringing up one's children. A number of factors have diminished the opportunities for adults to come in contact with children. The nuclear family no longer has access to grandparents, aunts and uncles. The working mother rationalizes that a child is better off in a "professional" child care situation. Gone is the apprentice system where a father taught a son his trade. We have followed this up within the home by relegating the children to the "playroom" and leaving them with babysitters while parents "get away from it all." As described by Dr. Urie Bronfenbrenner we are experiencing an age segregation and must make every effort to "bring adults back into the lives of children and children back into the lives of adults lest we complete the breakdown in the process of making human beings human."[1]

[1] *Today's Health,* June 1972, p. 37.

Sexual Considerations

Those who are comfortable and at ease with their sexuality are of course the best marital candidates. This would include men who like being men and women who like being women. They are not inhibited by shyness or feelings of guilt where sex is concerned. The woman who does not fear pregnancy and who desires children is positively prepared to fulfill her function in childbirth and motherhood. The woman who views childbirth and motherhood as personal sacrifices for which she must be forever reimbursed by husband and child alike is not prepared for either.

Relative interest in sex can be a factor in the success or failure of some marriages. Usually the sex interests of the male exceed those of the female. If these differences are not emotionalized and if each person is reasonable in his or her sexual demands or refusals, adjustments in interests can easily be worked out.

It is generally found that most sex difficulties in marriage are really reflections of difficulties in the personal relationships of the couple. When a couple enjoys each other's company as people, this compatibility carries over into all their interactions, including a sexual one.

Religious Matters

Even people of the same religion may view religious matters and responsibilities quite differently. Some measure religious obligation by attendance at the

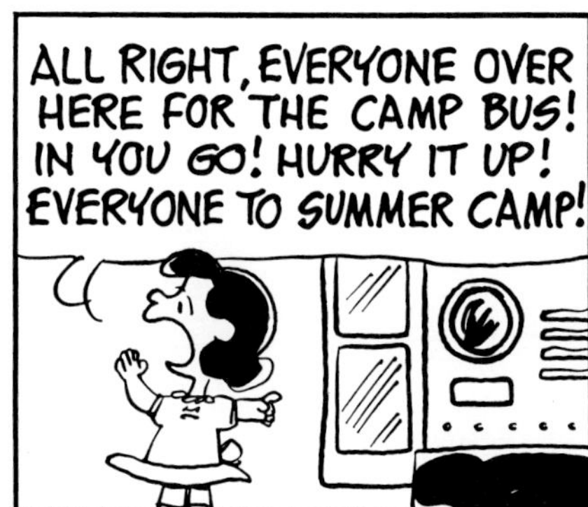

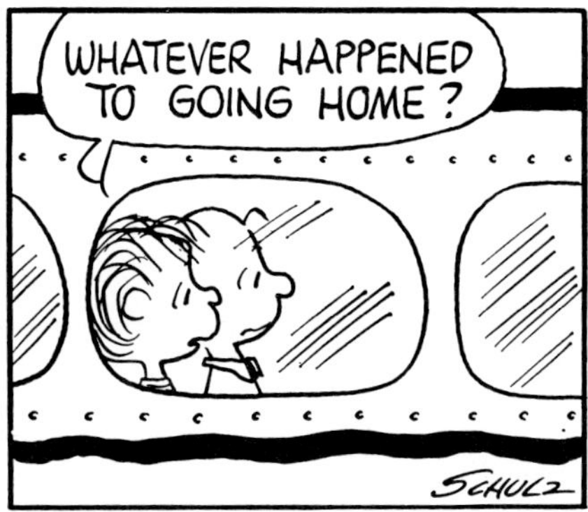

Fig. 5-2. "Whatever happened to going home?" Peanuts cartoon by Charles M. Schulz. (© 1972 by United Feature Syndicate, Inc.)

place of worship. Others may see greater importance in the application of religious principles in their interactions with others. The greater willingness of people to discuss religious issues brings to light variances in thinking that were previously undetected. While it is important to discuss issues within a religion, the discussion of religious variance in anticipated interfaith marriages becomes necessary. The number of such marriages is large and increasing. It is important to understand differences in religious philosophy so that the marriage may be served rather than hindered by them. It is of equal value to take stock of how one feels about one's own religion. The person who considers his religion to be the only true one or superior to others is probably a poor candidate for an interfaith marriage. It is important for a couple of varying religious backgrounds to discuss the topic objectively, rationally, and without emotion. The couple who postpone discussion here because they seek to avoid emotional scenes are developing a kind of time bomb. Many couples have worked out satisfactory arrangements with regard to religious differences. What is usually required is that one or both of the partners make concessions in this area. In some instances, a person may convert to the other religion to help resolve these differences. When this is done, it should not be regarded as a mechanical function or a procedure of convenience, but should be based on religious conviction. Where both decide to retain their religious affiliations, the question is raised of the religious affiliation of the children the marriage may produce. Deciding to let a child grow up to make his own decision on which religion he will choose may not always produce satisfactory results. A child growing up without religious training may, when he becomes of age, decide to be just that—irreligious. An alternate situation that could develop would be one in which both parents would compete for the child's religious preference. This kind of competition would hardly make for a happy home life. Decisions of this type are best made before marriage. Studies show that where the children are raised to follow the religion of the mother there is a greater degree of success. Because the mother assumes greater responsibility in the rearing of the child, her assumption of the religious training is more natural. Although there have been equally successful situations with the children reared in the father's religion, the percentage of trouble-free situations here is not as high.

Role Expectations

How do a man and woman view their prospective roles in marriage? Compatibility of the role concepts each is to play in a marital situation is important to the success of a forth-coming marriage.

Traditionally, we have held patriarchal ideas in our society, where the father has been the authoritarian in the family. The Old and New Testaments have indicated that the husband is the head of the household and the wife follows and obeys him. In recent years there has been a definite trend away from this thinking. More democratic views have developed with the wife assuming rights in marriages

Fig. 5-3. "Berry's World" by Jim Berry. (©1972 by NEA, Inc.)

BERRY'S WORLD

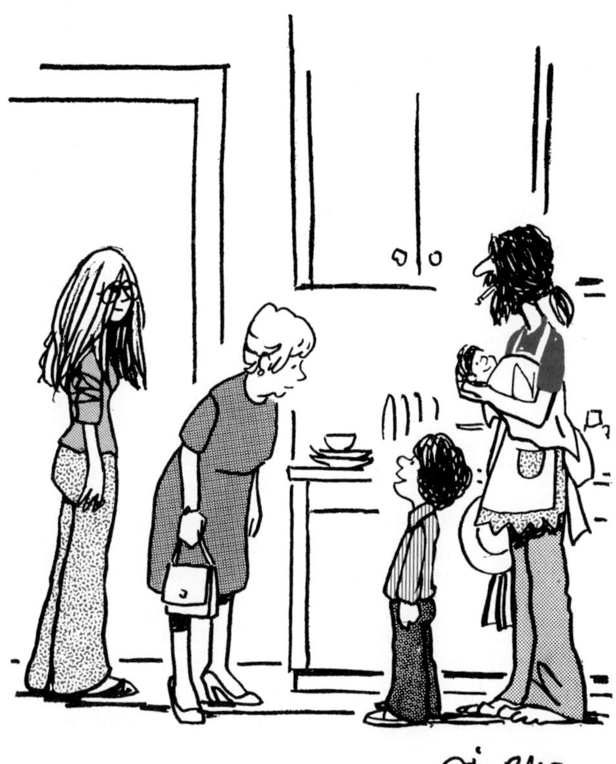

"When I grow up, I want to be a good mother, like Dad!"

equal to those of the husband. Transitions in thinking that have taken place in this area are by no means complete. We find people with various gradations of thinking from the patriarchal concepts to the equalitarian ones. It becomes important for a couple contemplating marriage to find out where each stands on this issue. In most instances, the strongest influence on how a person views his role in marriage is his family. Learning in this area takes place so gradually and subtly over the years that there is often little realization of the extent of this influence.

Traditionally, masculinity has been measured by the individual's ability to achieve economic success. The man who is not a good provider is considered a failure in his primary role. The man who is a successful breadwinner may find that the job can take him away from his family for long periods of time. He may then have his delinquencies as a father pointed out to him. The demands of his occupation on his time tend also to undermine any authority or guidance roles he plays at home. The conflict between job and home is a significant one for the male even though this kind of conflict is generally thought of solely in terms of the working woman.

In the past, the household roles of the husband and wife were well defined. How much housekeeping a man will do now depends on the amount of time he has available for the tasks as compared with the wife, and on attitudes toward particular household chores. These decisions are best resolved by the individual couple in accordance with their particular situation, their personalities, abilities, and values involved.

Nena and George O'Neill, in their book *Open Marriage,* introduced some new ground rules for marriage they consider to be essential changes if marriage is to survive as a viable institution. Open marriage is based on an honest and trusting relationship and on equal freedom and identity for both partners. A given partner is not dominant or submissive. The roles of the partners is not caste by predetermined rules. Domestic chores may be shared, and the woman may pursue her personal or professional interests as does the man. In essence the nature of the marital relationship is determined by the particular couple rather than by preset societal concepts of marriage.

Equality and role flexibility are two basics in the open marriage. In reaching out for equality the O'Neills feel that marriage should not be a 50-50 deal with compromises or where giving up certain things takes place—that is, the wife gives up a career and the husband going out with the boys. Rather it is viewed more as a 100-100 equation where each permits the other to pursue his or her individual interests. Role flexibility in open marriage, they feel, can be tested by a couple exchanging roles on occasion, with the husband cooking the meals and the wife fixing the screen door (provided each has the capabilities). The objectives of the open marriage thus aim at greater self-development with both partners growing in a compatible relationship. It seeks to avoid the stifling effects of more traditionally based marriages.

The Engagement

The engagement period affords the couple a period of time for the development of a closer relationship prior to marriage. This period of belonging to each other tests the relationship of the two people in a manner that casual dating cannot. It is assumed that engagement follows a period during which the couple have had the opportunity to become well acquainted. Some people establish an informal or pre-engagement period before making the more formal and public commitment of marriage. The informal engagement period gives the couple the opportunity to get to know each other better without the public commitment to marry. If the relationship does not work out, it is socially more comfortable to ease out of the situation.

The commitment of a couple to each other for marriage can have sobering effects. Girls may become less interested in expensive dating and begin to think of saving for the marriage. The realization of the forthcoming responsibilities of setting up a home and possibly having children lends a tone of seriousness to the relationship.

The formal engagement is usually sealed with a ring, more often than not a diamond ring. The size of the diamond is not necessarily indicative of the intensity of the love. It probably more nearly reflects the size of the bank account. Those who "splurge" on a ring will soon find that there are other things with less ceremonial value but greater practical value for which they could have saved the money.

The engagement period serves as a last trial run

to test compatibility before marriage. When a couple have come to know each other well, new incompatibilities rarely show up at this time. There may occasionally be a gnawing doubt about the whole thing, but this is not unusual. There are, however, a number of engagements which for one reason or another do not make it to the altar. Studies show that anywhere from one-fourth to one-third of engagements are broken. A number of relationships run into difficulty because they were not well founded in the first place. In other instances, incompatibilities did not become evident until this late date. When it is apparent that an engagement should be terminated, it is best to face this reality squarely. There are some who have managed to avoid the issue until after marriage, with resultant divorce. It is better to break an engagement than become involved in the more complex business of disassembling a marriage. When one partner desires to break off the relationship and the other does not, the situation becomes a more difficult one. The same principles, however, still apply. With tact and firmness it is best to make a clean break of it. This approach ultimately proves to be the most merciful. Being ambivalent and dragging out the agony with feelings of guilt and indecisiveness on one hand and rejection on the other is not the "easy" way out. When one is the rejected in such a situation, it proves bruising to the ego. It must be kept in mind, however, that one's capacity to love another has not been reduced. In looking back on the experience, it seems not as serious as it first appeared. The philosophic thought, that an engagement broken is a divorce prevented, helps.

A basic purpose of the engagement period is to prepare for the marriage ceremony. Increasingly clergy are permitting young couples to plan their own wedding ceremony with their selection of the music, readings, and even the format of the ceremony. Planning the wedding can be a complex affair if preparations are not started months in advance. Even with an early start the wedding day can take on some semblance of a Keystone Cops farce. Basic attitudes that people have toward weddings in terms of how they should be conducted, who should be invited, who pays the bills, and so on, must be contended with. Where both families decide to plan the wedding jointly, the project needs to be approached carefully, lest the negotiations become chilled with the inevitable areas of disagreement. Early planning permits rational discussion without the panicking pressures of time. Planning the wedding day is often the first important project that a couple embarks upon together. It often reveals aspects of the partners' personality not seen before. This should not come as any great surprise; one can expect these kinds of "discoveries" to continue many years into the marriage.

Engagement should be synonymous with a deepened relationship and a comfortable feeling of belonging to each other. There is a security that is not found in other kinds of relationships in being able to share life's experiences with another. The feelings of elation at having "found" each other is generally present in engaged couples. In good relationships, this feeling remains as the couple continue to complement each other throughout life.

Fig. 5-4. *In a good relationship love is not a sometime thing, but continues throughout life.* (*Susan Johns*)

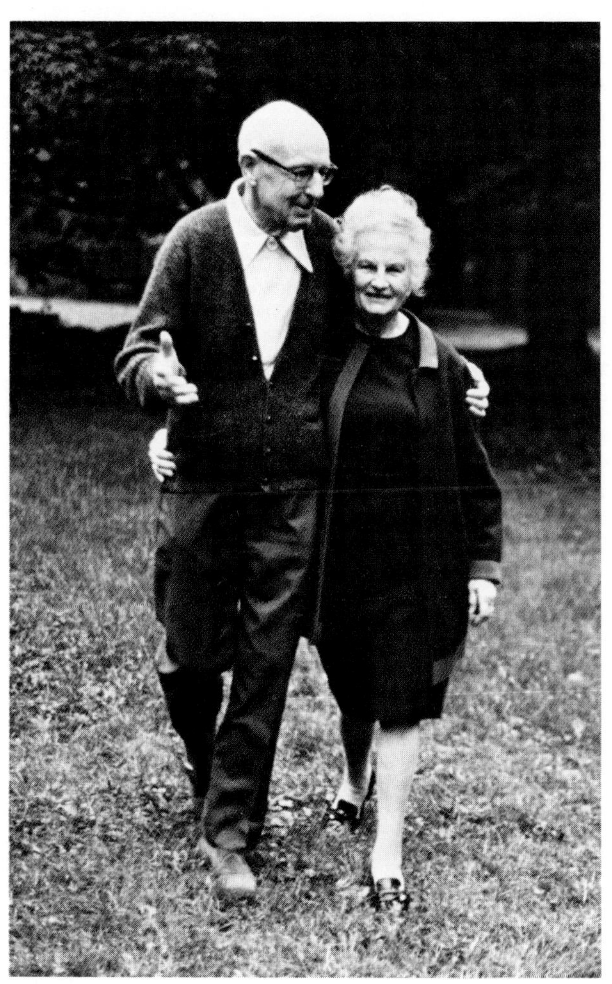

The Premarital Physical Examination

A complete physical examination is appropriate before marriage. Those defects that may be found are in the vast majority of instances remediable. In some few cases, the examination may reveal that a partner is sterile and that the couple would be incapable of having children. This kind of information could at times alter the marriage plans. In other instances, the couple might decide to adopt children or be willing to try artificial insemination, should the man be the sterile one. Another alternative would be to proceed with the wedding and accept the childless state. Genetic counseling has created the possibility of avoiding or preventing birth defects. It is the couple's responsibility to seek out such advice, to determine the prospects of their possibly producing children with such avoidable conditions as sickle-cell anemia, Tay-Sachs disease, hemophilia, cystic fibrosis, among others (see Chapter 6).

The premarital physical examination will occasionally reveal minor infections in the genital area that are common in women. In a pelvic examination the physician can also detect whether the hymen will prove to be a problem after marriage. It is sometimes necessary to perform minor surgery to cut the particularly tough fibrous tissue of the hymen. The opportunity to receive from a physician information about contraception and sexual intercourse also presents itself during the premarital examination. The couple may want to discuss these matters jointly with the doctor.

Occasionally a visit to a physician before marriage reveals an emotional problem that needs correction. Heeding the wise advice of the doctor, be it in terms of seeking psychological help or postponing the wedding, can go a long way in preventing difficulty or premature marriage.

Increasingly, physicians are using the premarital examination as an opportunity to give the Papanicolaou (Pap) test, a means of detecting cervical cancer. The greatest value from this procedure does not come from the comparatively rare incidence of cervical cancer in the young age group tested. Rather it can serve as a means of initiating a routine yearly "Pap test" habit. Fatalities from cancer of the reproductive organs would be eliminated if all women were to have this test administered yearly. In addition, most states in the United States require that a blood test be performed on prospective marital partners as a precautionary measure against syphilis.

Physical examinations should be routine procedures in preparation for marriage as well as throughout life. The person owes it to himself, to the prospective marital partner, and to the marriage they are establishing to assure as completely as possible full preparation for a lifelong partnership.

On Having Children

The question of whether to have children and how many is a matter that should be discussed by the intended. *What* is said is not the only important thing here, but also *why* it is said. The motivations of people who desire or do not desire children can be more involved than at first appears. In primitive societies, a great premium was placed on having children to perpetuate the race, and establish a large work force. At that time the infant mortality rate was high, so that if a woman had nine children she was fortunate if four or five reached adulthood. It was also recognized that the children would later care for the parents in their declining years. The child became an almost necessary form of old age insurance. In our more sophisticated society, which boasts medicare and varied retirement income plans, the child no longer serves this function. Our concerns for the perpetuation of the race need not be directed toward increasing the number of live births; infant mortality rates have been significantly reduced by advances in modern medicine. Our concerns for survival are now directed toward preventing a nuclear holocaust and controlling threatening broad-scale environmental health problems which are partially based on *over*population. The alarm has been sounded by some scientists that if we do not stabilize our population growth, we will exceed the resources of the planet Earth to sustain a desirable quality of life. Therefore the decision to have children is being influenced by societal concerns now related to overpopulation, as compared with primitive man's concern with underpopulation or the survival of the species. The decision therefore to have children can to a greater extent be based on a couple's desire to have them or not.

The bases of such a decision could include religious beliefs and whether or not the parents feel physically, psychologically, and financially capable of taking care of a child. They should have enough love and energy to share not only with each other but with a new baby as well. An interesting point was made in a study done at the University of Pennsylvania, where sociologists found that children raised in large families very rarely followed that pattern. In fact they tended to have small families—smaller than average. Therefore the size of the family from which the individual comes may be the determining factor in the projected size of his family.

A complicating factor in deciding to have children is that many people grow up with the idea that they *must* have children, or that they are not very wholesome people if they avoid parenthood. The influence of religion can be felt on this issue. Some religious organizations strongly encourage parenthood. In those cases where religious belief delimits birth control methods, choice as to parenthood is also delimited, as well as the size of one's family. How effectively *any* birth control measure is used is another factor. (This matter will be discussed in greater detail in Chapter 6, "Human Reproduction.") When people genuinely do not desire to have children and are forced by a vague sense of morality or obligation into a childbearing situation, we have the basis for a problem. While babies coo and are cute, they are also demanding. They want to be fed, changed, and loved. When these needs are not fulfilled, they cry at all hours of the day or night. The parent who does not really want the child in the first place feels put upon and becomes indignant. The end result is not only a disturbed parent but also an inevitably emotionally disturbed child. If only those people who genuinely *desired* children were to have them, the incidence of emotional disturbance could be significantly reduced on this basis alone.

At the risk of sounding ambivalent, we must also emphasize that determining whether one genuinely *desires* children is a difficult assessment to make. In essence, the person is asked to make a judgment in an area where he has no experience. Many a couple initially cool to the idea of parenthood become ecstatic over their firstborn. The creation of another human being in one's own image can obviously have profound effects on the individual. The miracle of birth can bring with it an unmatched humility and a sense of awe that accompanies only human creation.

How completely a person can understand all his motivations in any area is open to question. Unconscious motivations cannot be accounted for by the individual. The unconscious desire to prove manhood or womanhood may, for instance, be the prime mover in parenthood. Although self-understanding is never complete, discussion can lead to greater insight into one's own motivations and those of one's partner.

Review Questions

1. Why is maturity an essential quality for a successful marriage?
2. What are some of the negative motivations for marriage? Why are they poorly based?

3. Love has been defined in many ways. How do you interpret the term?
4. What are the traditional concepts regarding the roles of the man and woman in marriage?
5. How has the greater equality of the sexes in our society created some conflicts in the marital roles of the husband and wife?
6. Identify those values and personal characteristics that are conducive to successful marriages.
7. Discuss the importance of an economically stable marriage.
8. Why should religious viewpoints be discussed before marriage even if both parties are members of the same religion?
9. What are the potential problems that need careful discussion by a couple contemplating an interfaith marriage?
10. What are the advantages of an informal engagement period before the declaration of a formal engagement?
11. What are the purposes served by the engagement period?
12. Describe the functions served by the premarital physical examination.
13. How have changes in our society affected the necessity of producing offspring?
14. What factors must a couple consider in deciding upon parenthood?
15. How significant is the role of the father in successful child rearing?

Chapter 6
Human Reproduction

In his earlier days, man viewed his ability to reproduce with a certain amount of anxiety as he struggled against the elements to assure the survival of the human species. He suffered, at that time, losses from high rates of maternal mortality and even higher rates of infant mortality. If a child survived his first year of life, he was then challenged to weather a variety of childhood infections. As child and adult he was exposed to the plague and other epidemic diseases. Living in the shadow of the specter of mortality, man recognized the fragility of life and was preoccupied with the struggle for his survival.

With the advent of modern medicine, there has been a significant recession of the epidemic diseases, with their virtual disappearance in more highly developed communities of the world. It is now possible to immunize against many of the childhood diseases. The advances in pediatrics and obstetrics have reduced to all-time lows the infant and maternal mortality rates. Gradually man is becoming preoccupied with problems related to overpopulation. In this context, the tendency to view the creation of life with a disdainful casualness becomes possible. An appreciation of this phenomenon may be enhanced by the realization that man can initiate life, but he cannot create it. Man's role in this process is really no different from that of lower animals. We serve perhaps more as abject participants. As stated by Kahlil Gibran:

Your children are not your children.
They are the sons and daughters of Life's longing for itself.
They come through you but not from you,
And though they are with you yet they belong not to you.
You may give them your love but not your thoughts.
For they have their own thoughts.
You may house their bodies but not their souls,
For their souls dwell in the house of tomorrow, which you cannot visit, not even in your dreams.
You may strive to be like them, but seek not to make them like you.
For life goes not backward nor tarries with yesterday.
You are the bows from which your children as living arrows are sent forth.
The archer sees the mark upon the path of the infinite, and He bends you with His might that His arrows may go swift and far.
Let your bending in the archer's hand be for gladness;
For even as he loves the arrow that flies, so he loves also the bow that is stable.[1]

The Male Reproductive System

The basic purpose of the male reproductive system is to produce and deliver the male reproductive cells to the female genital tract to effect the fertilization of an egg cell. The male apparatus consists of the penis, the prostate and Cowper's glands, the testes, the vas deferens, and the seminal vesicles.

The testes, the two male reproductive glands, are suspended in a musculomembranous pouch called the scrotum that hangs from the groin. A short time before the birth of the human male (around the 7th

[1]Kahlil Gibran, "On Children," from *The Prophet* (New York: Knopf, 1945), p. 18. Reprinted by permission of the publisher.

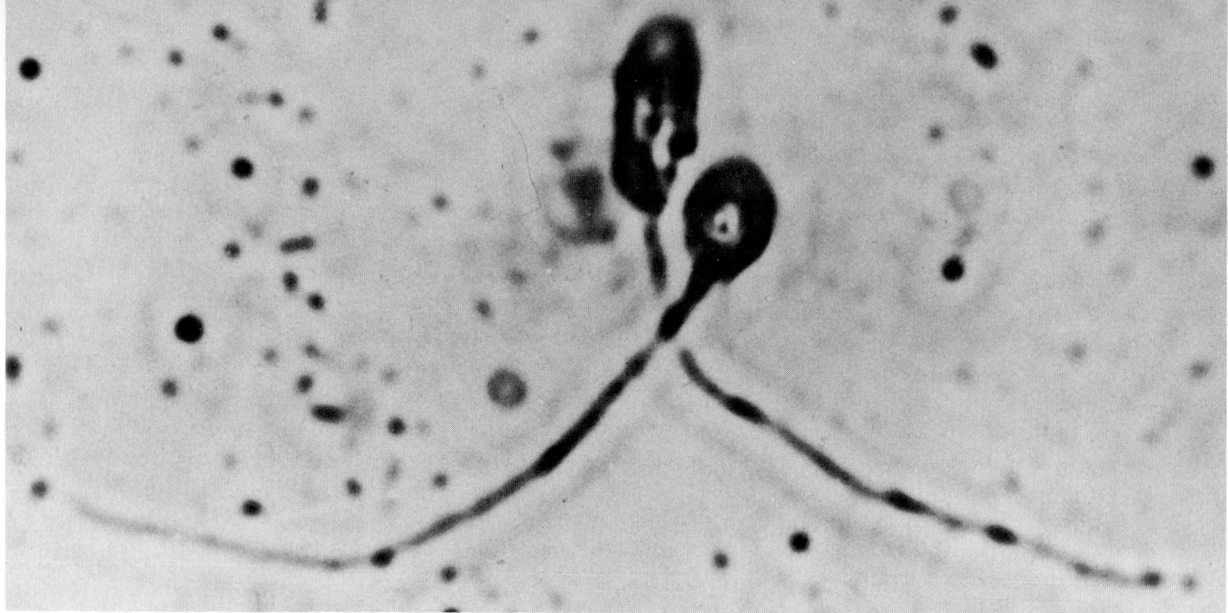

month), the testes descend into the scrotum. A major function of these glands is to produce male reproductive cells (sperm cells) following puberty. These cells are produced in the seminiferous tubules called the epididymis that lie on top of the testis. A reason for the location of the testes in the scrotum outside the body is related to the sensitivity of sperm cells to body temperature. The cooler temperature of the scrotum (about 3 or 4 degrees below body temperature) is more conducive to the production of sperm cells and their continued life. In addition to producing reproductive cells, the testes also produce the male sex hormone testosterone. The hormone influences the development of secondary sexual characteristics that occur at puberty involving the growth of a beard, a deeper voice, pubic hair, a masculine type of musculature, and the development of the male sex organs. The testosterone is produced by the cells found in between the seminiferous tubules of the testes.

The vas deferens conducts the sperm cells from the epididymis. The duct of the seminal vesicles joins the vas deferens just before the prostate gland. The secretions of the seminal vesicles, prostate gland, and Cowper's glands make up a thick, whitish, alkaline seminal fluid in which the sperm cells float. Semen, then, is composed of the secretions of these three glands, plus sperm cells. In ejaculation (or orgasm), the semen is propelled through the urethra of the penis to the outside. Ejaculation occurs as the result of the rhythmic contraction of smooth muscle tissue. (This muscle reaction is due to the stimulation of the head of the penis.) The reaction may also be effected by an erotic dream and result in a nocturnal seminal emission, or by masturbation. The semen ejaculated contains approximately a half billion sperm cells. Since only one will fertilize an egg cell, the oversupply reflects nature's way of guaranteeing the continuation of the species.

Sperm cells are microscopic in size. They consist of a head, neck, and a whiplike tail for locomotion. The sperm cell becomes self-propelled when it is deposited in the female reproductive tract and moves to the location of the egg cell. The head of the sperm cell is made up mostly of nuclear material containing paternal genetic characteristics. The responsibility for the determination of sex remains solely with the father. If the fertilizing sperm carries an X chromosome, the baby will be a girl, whereas if the sperm carries a Y chromosome, the baby will be a boy. Recently Dr. Landrum Shettles discovered that the size and shape of the heads of sperm cells varied. This variation corresponded with the X or Y chromosome the sperm carried. Oval shaped, larger sperm carried the X chromosome while round, smaller heads of sperm cells indicated they were carrying a Y chromosome.[2]

The function of the penis in the reproductive process is to conduct semen into the female genital tract. In order to perform this function, the usually flaccid penis becomes enlarged and erect as a result of sexual excitement and stimulation. This erection takes place because the erectile tissue of the penis

[2]David Rorvik, with Landrum Shettles, M.D., *Your Baby's Sex: Now You Can Choose* (New York: Dodd, Mead, 1970).

Fig. 6-1. *The oval-shaped, larger sperm carries the X chromosome. The round, smaller sperm cell carries the Y chromosome.* (*Landrum B. Shettles, M.D.; Columbia Presbyterian Medical Center*)

Fig. 6-2. *Male reproductive system.* (*Adapted from "Male Sex Parts," Family Life Publications Inc., Saluda, N.C.*)

Male Sex Parts

1	Rectum
2	Seminal vesicles
3	Bladder
4	Vas deferens
5	Prostate gland
6	Cowper's gland
7	Anus
8	Urethra
9	Epididymis
10	Testicle
11	Penis
12	Glans penis
13	Foreskin
14	Scrotum

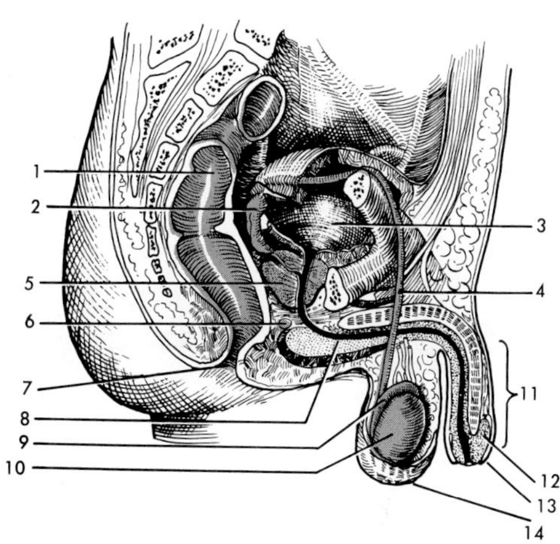

becomes engorged with blood. In this state, the organ can be introduced into the female vagina.

The penis is covered by a loose sheathing of skin, with that portion covering the head of the penis called the prepuce or foreskin. The foreskin is often removed shortly after birth in an operation called circumcision. Among Mohammedans, Jews, and some other religious groups, circumcision is part of religious ritual that dates back many centuries. It is now performed not only for religious reasons, but because it serves as a sanitary measure as well. In some cases, the foreskin is too tight and is removed because it will interfere with the copulatory function of the penis.

The Female Reproductive System

The female reproductive system consists of the two ovaries that produce ova (eggs) and give off hormonal secretions, two fallopian tubes, the uterus, vagina, the external genitals, with the breasts sometimes being considered a part of this system. Most of the structures of the more complex female reproductive system are located within the body where they can best carry on the function of nourishing and sustaining the unborn child.

The ovaries are two almond-shaped glands that are located on either side of the midline of the body. They are attached to the uterus by means of a short ligament and reside by the openings of the fallopian tubes that emanate from the uterus. The basic functions of the ovaries are to produce ova (eggs) and secrete hormones. One of the ovaries will produce an ovum every 28 to 30 days. Although the ovaries have a potential for the production of many thousands of ova, only about 300 to 500 mature egg cells are produced during the reproductive life of a woman. When the ovum erupts from the ovary (ovulation), it finds its way into the broadened end of the fallopian tube.

The hormones released by the ovaries help to control the monthly rhythm of ovulation and menstruation. They also influence the development of the secondary sexual characteristics, such as breast development, pubic hair, and the development of the typically female contours of the body.

The two fallopian tubes are about four inches long and extend outward from the uterus. Their main function is to collect ova released by the ovaries with the slender processes on the ends of these tubes. The ciliated lining of the fallopian tubes conducts the egg to the uterus.

The uterus is a hollow, pear-shaped, muscular organ about the size of a closed fist. It has an enormous capacity to enlarge and become many times its normal size during pregnancy. During this period of time, it expands upward into the abdominal cavity. The uterus is suspended in the pelvic cavity by ligaments with the top or fundus tilted forward and the cervix (mouth) of the uterus extending into the upper portion of the vagina. Its basic function is to receive ova from the fallopian tubes and if they have been fertilized to retain and nourish them until they have developed to a full-term fetus. The environment within the uterus is generally alkaline.

The vagina is a highly elastic musculo-

Female Sex Parts

15	Ovary
16	Fallopian tube
17	Rectum
18	Uterus or womb
19	Cervix
20	Bladder
21	Vagina
22	Urethra
23	Anus
24	Clitoris
25	Hymen
26	Labia

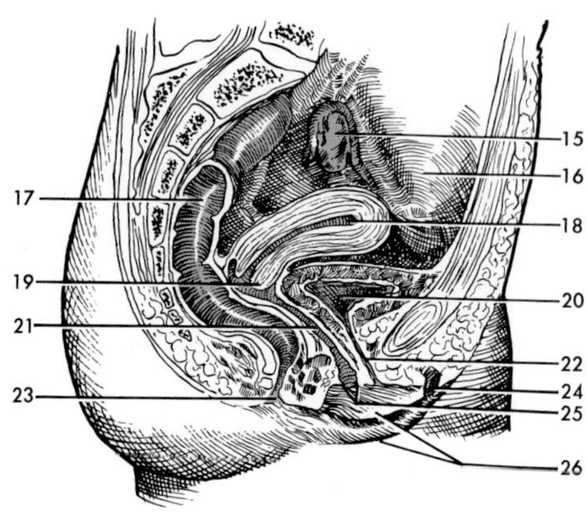

Fig. 6-3. Female reproductive system. (Adapted from "Female Sex Parts," Family Life Publications Inc., Saluda, N.C.)

membranous canal that extends downward and forward from the uterus. It serves as the female organ during intercourse and as the birth canal for the newborn during the birth process. The mucus membrane of the vagina is lined with mucus glands called Bartholin's glands. These serve to secrete a viscous fluid when stimulated into activity by sexual excitation. This fluid acts as a lubricant for the sex act and is generally acidic in nature. As the woman approaches the moment of ovulation the environment near the cervix becomes more alkaline. These changes in the pH of this environment are said to be a factor in the sex determination of a fetus. During the climax of the sex act (orgasm), there are rhythmical contractions of the vagina along with diffuse pleasurable sensations.

The external female genitalia are composed of the vulva, which covers the opening to the vagina, and the clitoris. The vulva is made up of the labia majora and the labia minora. The majora consists of two longitudinal folds of skin covered with pubic hair in the adult. Situated between the labia majora are two smaller longitudinal folds called the labia minora. At the anterior junction of the labia minora is the clitoris. This small body is made up of erectile tissue and corresponds to the penis in man. It contains many sensory nerve endings and responds to tactile stimulation. The hymen is a thin fold of perforated mucus membrane that covers the opening to the vagina. This structure is peculiar to the human species and its biological function is unknown. It is made up of material that is quite elastic and much like the tissue of the eyelid.

Ovulation, Hormones, and the Menstrual Cycle

From the earliest of times there have been many superstitions related to menstruation. It was once thought that a menstruating woman was possessed of the evil spirits. In some cultures, she was considered as being unclean and had to live in separate quarters. A number of old wives' tales and admonitions still persist today, as, for example: loss of menstrual blood weakens you; do not bathe; a permanent wave will not take during this period of time; stay in bed a day or two; do not exercise; cold drinks will cause menstrual cramps, and so forth. The woman who feels comfortable about herself and her menstruation is not affected by weird, exaggerated, or emotionalized notions. It is now recognized that the individual's routine should not vary markedly during the menstrual period. Reasonable exercise and bathing or showering should be part of the daily activity. Any blood loss that occurs during this period of time is in terms of a few ounces and should not affect the person. The more casual the attitude toward menstruation by the woman, the better she will take the process of daily living in her stride.

The ability of the ovaries to produce eggs is stimulated by the follicle-stimulating hormone (FSH) of the pituitary gland. Without this hormone, an egg cell (ovum) would never be formed. In conjunction with FSH, the pituitary gland secretes the luteining hormone (LH). This hormone helps FSH to ripen the follicle and cause ovulation (the release of the egg from the ovary). LH then stimulates the develop-

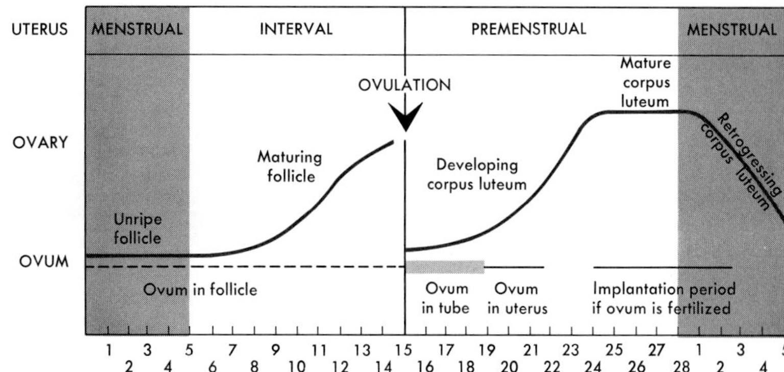

Fig. 6-4. The menstrual cycle.

ment of a corpus luteum from the ruptured follicle. It further stimulates the corpus luteum to secrete two ovarian hormones, estrogen and progesterone. These hormones prepare the lining within the body of the uterus (the endometrium) for the reception of the egg. Further interaction of these hormones causes the uterine lining to disintegrate if the egg is not fertilized. This results in the beginning of the menstrual flow. The cycle is then ready to start over again.

The menstrual cycle is usually approximately 28 days long, with the menstrual flow lasting an average of five days. The length of the cycle can vary from one woman to another as well as within the same person. Tension or emotional trauma among other factors, have been known to disrupt this process. Some women have highly predictable cycles; in others quite the opposite is true. Ovulation occurs at about the 14th day in the cycle, when the egg enters the fallopian tube. If the egg is fertilized by a sperm cell in the fallopian tube, it will progress to the lining of the uterus and implant itself.

The attitudes developed toward menstruation are often reflective of the woman's adjustment to her sexuality. There are those who accept this as a normal and natural process, while others regard menstruation as a "curse" or a period of illness. Where negative attitudes are present, even slight cramps can become causes of incapacitation.

A few days before the menstrual flow starts the woman often has a feeling of fullness in the lower abdomen. This is due to the engorgement of the lining of the uterus and the woman may as a result feel some discomfort. There is in some women a tendency to retain fluids at this time, resulting in a puffy feeling. Actual weight gain due to increased fluid retention is sometimes noted. A let-down or "blues" feeling may also be present. This can be attributed to a cessation of secretion of those hormones that stimulated the formation of the endometrium. They are known to give a feeling of well-being and their absence sometimes causes an opposite mood reaction.

Occasionally, menstruation is accompanied by cramps and pain beyond normal discomfort (dysmenorrhea). The pain is usually related to the efforts of the uterus to contract in order to expel its lining. Hormone imbalance and a deficient blood supply are among many possible reasons for the symptoms.

The cessation of menstrual periods or their failure to appear in the adolescent girl is referred to as *amenorrhea.* This condition can be caused by a wide variety of factors such as malnutrition, various diseases, sedentary living, and underdeveloped uterus or ovaries. Where unusual conditions related to menstruation appear, the individual should consult with a physician, preferably a gynecologist.

Menopause

The cessation of the menstrual cycle begins in the middle to late forties. Menstrual periods become irregular with longer time intervals between, until the period of cessation is reached. The ovarian func-

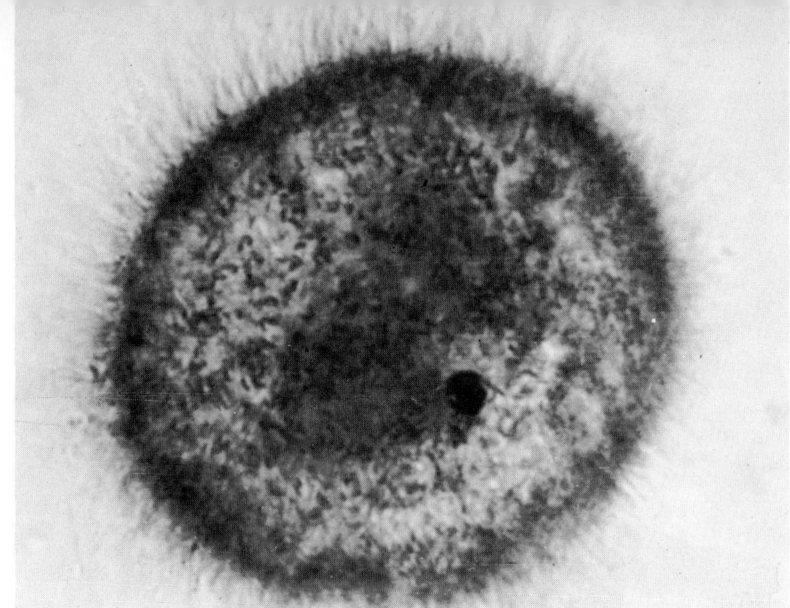

Fig. 6-5. An egg cell surrounded by many sperm cells that seek to fertilize it. (Dr. L. B. Shettles, Ovum Humanum, *Hafner Publishing Co., N.Y.)*

tion of producing eggs is over. The ovaries continue, however, to produce those hormones not related to ovulation. This period in a woman's life is the menopause, often referred to as "change of life." Because childbearing is a basic function of the woman, a number of women reach menopause feeling that their most important purpose in life has come to an end. Others become preoccupied with the idea that they are now aged. Periods of depression and other disorders can thus be associated with this period. Actually, negative attitudes related to menopause often reflect a narrowed perspective toward life. A woman may view motherhood as her only role in life, to the exclusion of "wifehood" and "womanhood." At about this time the children may marry, further aggravating her loss and her developing sense of uselessness. A woman whose interests are broadly based, who has achieved a status of good emotional health and who prepares herself to assume varied roles in life, sees nothing tragic in menopause. In fact, she may now be relieved of a fear of pregnancy and see opportunity to do things that were inhibited by previous family commitments.

During menopause, hormonal secretions undergo change, with the result that a number of physical symptoms may appear. These include hot flashes, palpitations of the heart, sweating, and periods of general discomfort. Physicians now prescribe hormone therapy to help a woman through this transitional period. Hormone therapy has been so successful that at a recent meeting of the American College of Obstetricians and Gynecologists it was agreed that women should receive doses of estrogen hormone not only during menopause, but thereafter. During postmenopausal aging, it has been noted that skin loses its tone, bones their hardness, and that fatty deposits begin to accumulate in the arteries, increasing the woman's vulnerability to heart disease. The administration of estrogen delays the onset of these changes and keeps the woman younger for a longer time. This represents a major step forward in the area of hormone therapy.

The Reproductive Process

During sexual intercourse, the male ejaculate is deposited in the female vaginal tract. Sperm cells from the semen will swim into the uterus and fertilize the egg cell, if one is present, in the fallopian tube. In the process of fertilization, the nucleus of the sperm cell unites with the nucleus of the egg cell. Each cell brings to this union 23 chromosomes, and the resultant fertilized egg contains 23 *pairs* of chromosomes. There is evidence that more than one sperm cell penetrates the egg cell. However, the egg cell will be fertilized by only one sperm cell. It is at this precise moment of conception that the sex of the new individual is determined. Dr. Shettles has indicated that the timing of intercourse is the critical factor in the sex determination of children. Male-producing sperm (or androsperm) are more sensitive to an acid environment and do not survive as long as the female-producing sperm (gynosperm). However, in a more alkaline environment the androsperm have the distinct advantage of speed and agility and are able to reach a waiting ovum far ahead of the gynosperm. If intercourse takes place very close to the time of ovulation in the female, when the cervical secretions become more alkaline, chances are the child will be a boy. If, however, intercourse takes place two or three days before ovulation, when the acidic environment of the vagina still persists, chances are the baby will be a girl.

It usually takes three to four days for the fertilized egg to tumble its way through the fallopian tube and become imbedded in the lining of the uterine wall. During this time, the fertilized egg has already begun cell division. The one cell divides into 2 cells, then to 4, 8, 16, and so on. The embryo grows and is suspended within a structure called the amniotic sac. The fluid in this sac serves to cushion and protect the developing embryo. The embryo is attached to the placenta by means of an umbilical cord. The placenta is a special disclike organ that develops shortly after the implantation of the egg in the wall of the uterus. Projections (villi) from the placenta extend into the uterine wall to facilitate the nutritional function of this structure. Nutrient material and oxygen from the maternal blood, by the process of osmosis, enter the villi of the placenta. The small blood vessels in the villi conduct these materials through the umbilical cord to the embryo. Waste products from the embryo are removed by the reversal of this process. The gestation period for humans is approximately 280 days or a little more than nine months.

Signs of Pregnancy

The cessation of menstruation can be one of the first signs of pregnancy. This is not always a reliable indication because a number of factors (such as emotional upset or illness) can result in a missed menstrual period. In other cases, a woman's menstrual cycle may be so irregular that the skipping of menstrual periods is not unusual. Morning sickness in either mild or severe form occurs in approximately two-thirds of pregnant women. The nausea that accompanies this condition usually disappears after the third month. Medication is available to relieve the symptoms that occur at this stage. A number of changes also take place in the breasts. They become fuller, with darkening and an enlargement of the nipples. The increased blood supply to the breasts may become evident by the increased visibility of the enlarged blood vessels. The foregoing signs may or may not be apparent in early pregnancy. Given enough time, of course, even a five-year-old could make an accurate diagnosis. For more positive indications of early pregnancy there are several laboratory tests that can be employed. In response to pregnancy, the body produces large amounts of hormones that spill over into the urine. Two commonly used tests for pregnancy are the Pregnosticon and Gravindex. A urine sample is put through an agglutination test and the results are read in three minutes. The tests are extremely accurate even 7 days after a missed menstrual period and virtually 100 per cent accurate 14 days after a missed period. Pregnancy tests may be ordered by the physician, who should

Fig. 6-6. A 44-day-old embryo about ½-inch long in a "weightless" state within its fluid-filled amniotic sac. Its umbilical cord carries food and oxygen from the placenta. Note the lidless eyes and the first joints of the fingers and toes. (Carnegie Institution of Washington)

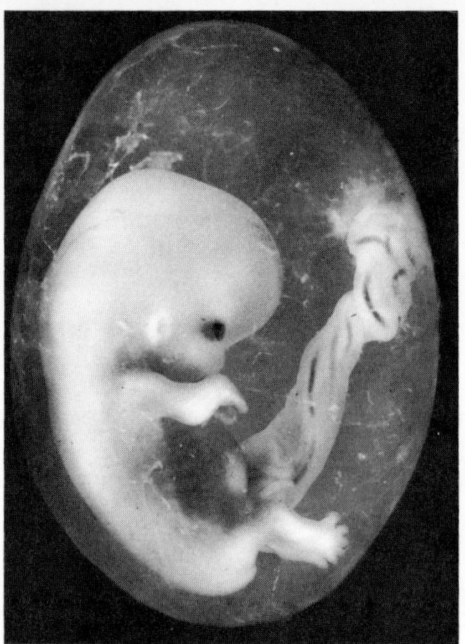

Fig. 6-7. A 16-week-old fetus which now has all of the essential organs. It is only about 4 inches in length at this time. (Carnegie Institution of Washington)

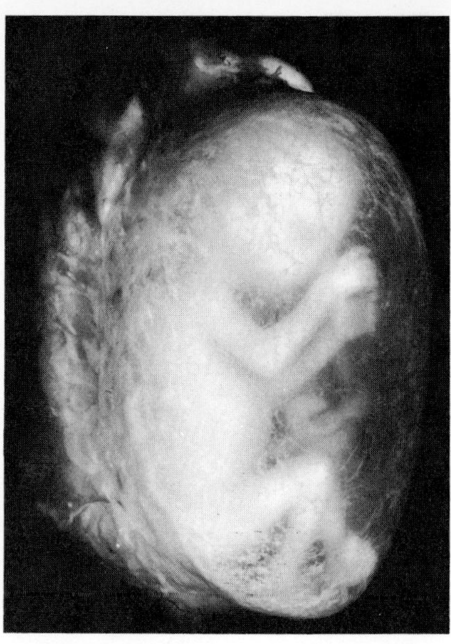

be visited when the person has missed two menstrual periods in a row.

Prenatal Development

The First Trimester starts, of course, at conception in the form of a single fertilized egg. The embryo at the end of the second month is referred to as the fetus. By the end of the third month, the fetus is three inches long and has arms, legs, hands, fingers, toes, and ears. It has a definite human appearance. Even the teeth have begun their development in the jawbones. At the end of the three-month period, the fetus weighs in at about one ounce.

During this period the expectant mother may experience the early signs of pregnancy, namely, morning sickness and breast development. The woman may also find that the feeling of fatigue occurs more easily at this time. A more frequent need for urination is caused by the compressing of the bladder by the enlarging uterus. A craving for unusual foods or those out of season may occur. Researchers have had difficulty substantiating why particular cravings should come about. There are those dastardly enough to suggest that this is a woman's way of getting some small luxuries normally not available to her. However, when a pregnant woman living on the Canadian border desires watermelon in January . . . who is to deny her? Certainly not her husband!

The Second Trimester results in a growth in length of the fetus to about 14 inches and in weight to about two pounds. The heartbeat of the fetus is now audible and its movements felt. If the child were born at this stage of development, it would have only a slight chance for survival. The mother during this period shows definite signs of abdominal enlargement and usually begins to wear maternity clothes at about the fifth month.

The Third Trimester is a period during which the child grows bigger and stronger and becomes ready for the outside world. The weight usually reaches seven to eight pounds, with the length ranging around twenty inches. The fetus gains about 50 per cent of its weight during the last two months. It will have periods of activity and periods of rest—periods of wakefulness and sleep. A child born during the seventh month of pregnancy has a fair chance of survival. Its chances of sustaining life increase rapidly from this point on as it approaches full term. During this period, the child can develop the ability to kick rather vigorously. These movements usually slow down during the ninth month. The mother's need for frequent urination reoccurs during this trimester as the enlarged uterus exerts pressure on the bladder. The pressures created by the added weight and fluids of the pregnancy may result in enlarged veins in the legs. During the last two weeks, the fetus moves gradually downward toward the pelvis in preparation for the eventual birth.

Prenatal Care

Modern medicine has made childbirth much safer for both mother and child. A major contribution to this accomplishment has been better prenatal care. While pregnancy is a natural process, hazards related

Fig. 6-8. A 24-week-old fetus within the muscular wall of the uterus. The umbilical cord connects the fetus to the placenta implanted on the inner wall of the uterus. (*Carnegie Institution of Washington*)

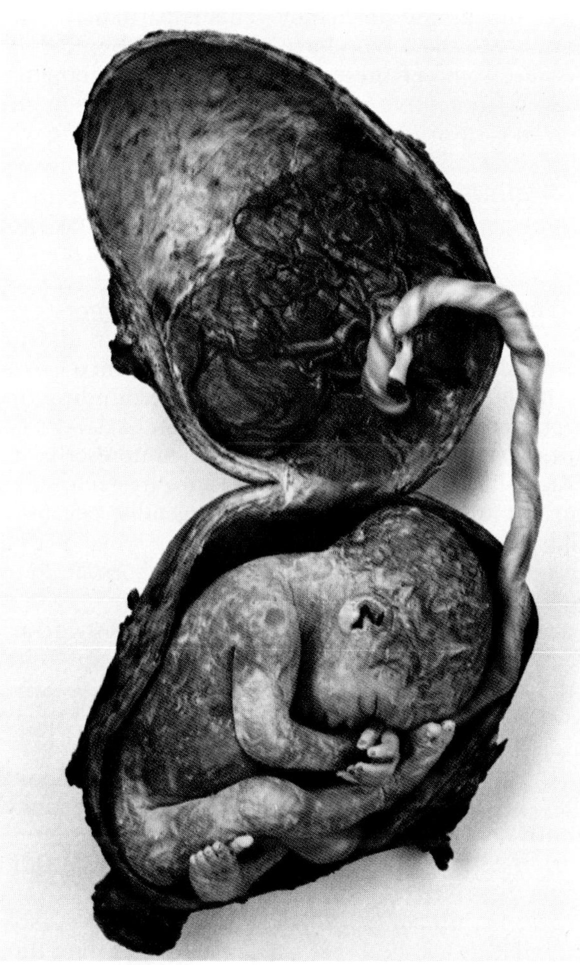

to it are minimized when this period is supervised by the obstetrician. The expectant mother will usually see the physician once a month during the early months of pregnancy. The visits are increased to every two weeks in the latter stages. The physician will take a medical history to evaluate the woman's capability to handle the stresses and strains of pregnancy. He will also give a complete physical examination including the pelvic region. He checks the size of the pelvis to make sure it will permit the passage of a normal-sized child at birth. The physician will routinely check the weight of the expectant mother as well as chart the rate of growth of the fetus. Weight control during pregnancy is a real concern to the doctor. A weight gain of not more than twenty pounds is desirable. Excessive fat formation during the prenatal period can be a source of difficulty at the time of childbirth. The common old wives' tale that a pregnant woman needs to eat for two can serve as a bit of misleading information resulting in undesirable, if not dangerous, weight gain. It is important to note that it is not the size of the child that will be affected by the amount of food intake, but of the expectant mother. The child's weight is determined basically by heredity, the development of the placenta, and the length of pregnancy.

The need for a well-balanced, nutritious diet is important to the expectant mother. The child will draw from the tissues of the mother for its growth. Where inadequate diets are followed, it is the mother who will suffer the deficiency, not the unborn child.

Fig. 6-9. A quiet moment for mother and child. (Ken Heyman)

Urinalyses serve to check that the pregnancy is progressing routinely. During this period, the kidneys are under the double strain of excreting wastes for both the mother and child.

There are few organisms that can pass from the mother's body through the placenta to the child. However, a few disease-producing bacteria and a number of viruses can. Rubella (German measles, or three-day measles), while not dangerous to the adult, can cause harmful effects to the fetus in its first trimester. Fetal death, mental retardation, cataracts, and deafness are among its varied effects. Since a vaccine for rubella has been developed (see Chapter 9) it is hoped that routine vaccination of children will eradicate this disease. The mumps and other viral diseases can also affect the fetus. When expectant mothers are exposed to viral diseases to which they may not be immune the physician may recommend injections of gamma globulin. Gamma globulin is a derivative of human blood that contains antibodies and will give the person a temporary immunity that serves to protect the fetus. It is wise for the expectant mother to avoid people with various infections as a precautionary measure. Because we know that several diseases can affect the unborn, particularly during the first trimester of pregnancy, it is best to err on the side of caution. We cannot discount the fact that our information in this area is incomplete. The number of diseases that are capable of affecting the early pregnancy is not known at this time.

Part of the prenatal care involves informing the mother about the various changes that will take place during the pregnancy. This is particularly important for those who have not had children before. Because some of these changes are rather dramatic, they do not serve as sources of anxiety when the person is informed about them. The obstetrician will also advise the woman to inform him of any unusual happenings, such as vaginal staining or bleeding, cramps, or backaches. These signs may or may not be serious. However, the doctor should make the judgment and act accordingly.

The use of drugs needs to be handled more cautiously at this time. The thalidomide drug disaster resulted in the birth of thousands of deformed babies in Europe. This demonstrated with resounding impact that a normally harmless drug can be dangerous during pregnancy. Even the use of nonprescription drugs should be checked with the physician. The current injudicious use of sleeping pills, pep pills, alkalines, tonics, and alcohol singly or, worse yet, in combination, can be threats to the unborn child as well as the prospective mother.

It has also been noted that those children who are X-rayed in utero have a higher incidence of leukemia later in life. For this reason it is wise for a woman to inform a physician other than her obstetrician of her pregnancy.

Tooth decay is another possible source of difficulty that should be corrected preferably before pregnancy. Tooth decay is in essence an infection and its elimination deletes any possible toxic effects on the child from this source.

The maintenance of good muscle tone is always desirable, but it becomes particularly important dur-

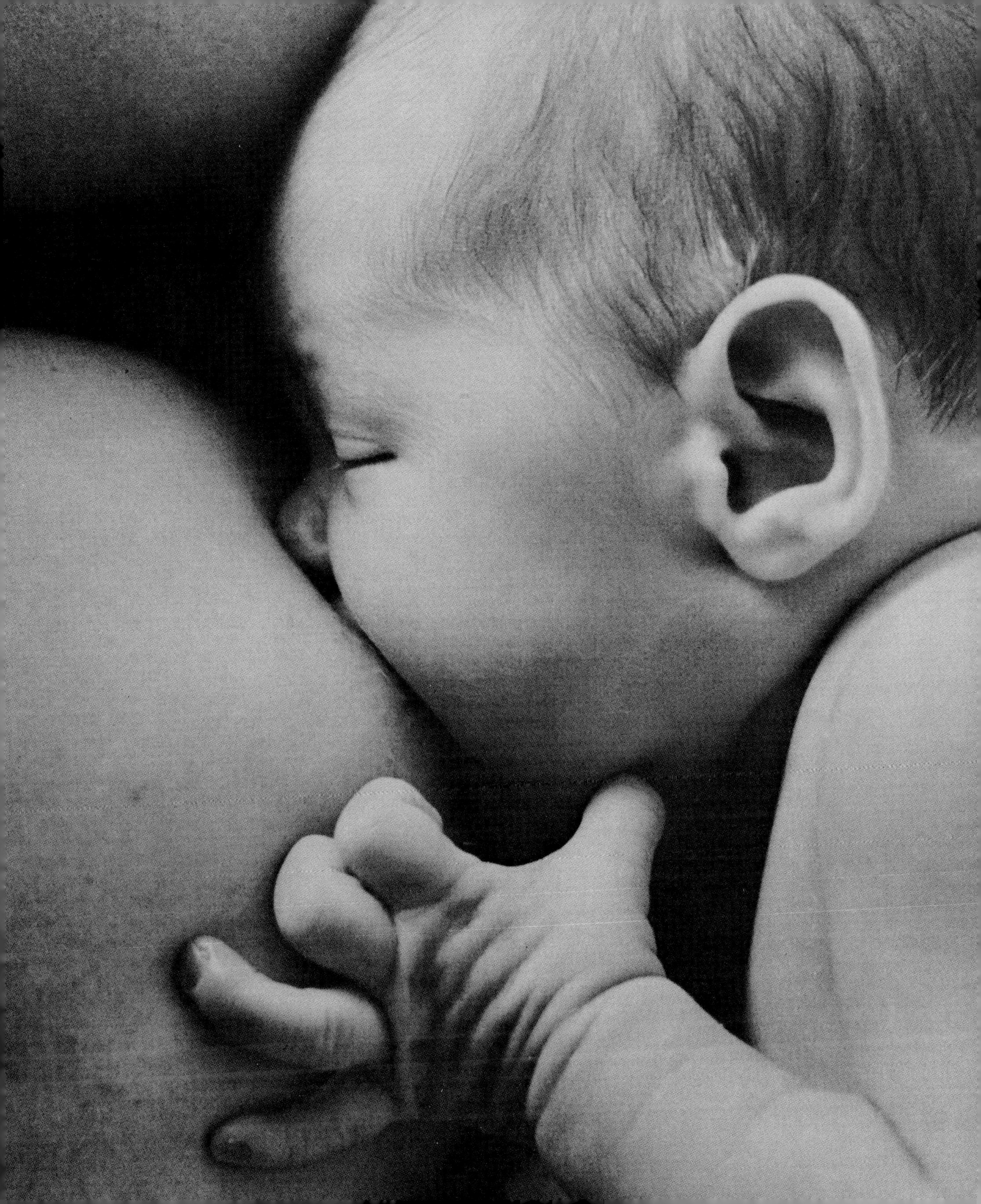

ing childbirth. Strong abdominal and back muscles will not only make a pregnancy more comfortable for the expectant mother but will also play a significant role in the birth process itself. The woman who has always exercised regularly is better prepared for the function of childbirth.

Breast Feeding

The question of whether or not to breast-feed the newborn is a decision each mother must make. Attitudes toward breast feeding are often consciously or unconsciously developed fairly early in life. The woman is often faced with the decision without having given it much prior thought. Some advantages of breast feeding are found in the development of a closer child-parent relationship. Mother's milk is also rarely one that does not agree with the baby. Allergy and other feeding problems have greater incidence with formula-fed babies. Some women prefer this method of feeding because it does away with a lot of paraphenalia in the form of nipples, bottles, sterilizers, and so forth. It is also cheaper, which is a factor in some families. Several studies have also shown that the incidence of breast cancer is lower among women who breast-feed their young. There has, however, been a growing tendency away from the breast-fed child in our society. Some mothers are repelled by the whole idea and see only animal-like qualities in the process. There is also the fact that where babies are bottle-fed the father can give the 2 A.M. feeding as well as the mother. The decision as to how to feed the newborn is dependent to a great extent on the psychological preparation of the mother for this function and what are perceived to be the advantages and disadvantages of either method.

The Rh Factor

This factor is an inherited protein substance found in the red blood cells. Approximately 85 per cent of white people have this protein material and are therefore designated as being Rh+. The other 15 per cent are described as being Rh−. Approximately 93 per cent of blacks are Rh+, and the factor is even higher among Asians. The Rh symbol was given to this blood protein because it was first detected in the rhesus monkey.

The Rh factor has caused some concern because under certain circumstances it can be responsible for such conditions as mental retardation, cerebral palsy, and spontaneous abortion. These developments are possible only when the mother is Rh− and the father is Rh+, and the fetus is Rh+. Not every pregnancy of this type is necessarily affected. In order for there to be a reaction, some of the Rh+ blood of the fetus must leak through the placenta to the mother's bloodstream. The mother's blood in reaction to the blood of the fetus will develop antibodies. The quantity of antibodies developed is in proportion to the amount of fetus blood that leaks into the mother's bloodstream. In large enough quantities, these antibodies could begin to destroy

Fig. 6-10. As diagrammed, some of the RH+ blood of the child leaks through the placenta to the Rh− blood of the mother. The mother's blood reacts by developing antibodies that return to the baby's bloodstream and destroy some of his red blood cells. If enough antibodies reach the child, anemia of varying severity will result. (Adapted from René Dubos, Health and Disease, *Life Science Library, 1965)*

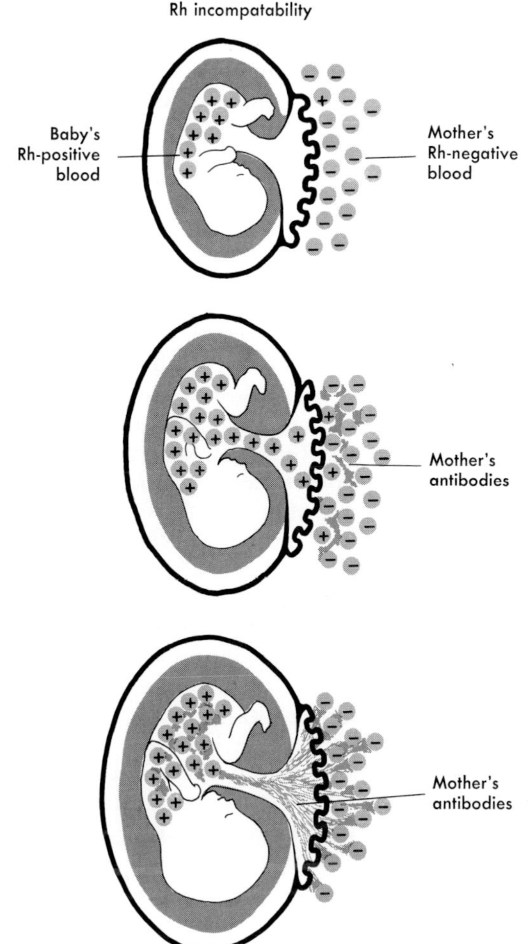

the red blood cells of the fetus, resulting in anemia, a jaundiced condition, or even death. The first such pregnancy will probably produce no reactions. It may take several pregnancies before the mother's blood has been sensitized enough to produce sufficient antibodies to affect the child. Up until now, when the obstetrician had a case with an Rh− mother and an Rh+ father, he would periodically check the mother's blood for antibody level. If necessary, the child's blood was replaced by an exchange transfusion immediately after birth, or the child was delivered prematurely in order to save its life. Newer medical techniques now enable the physician to give the baby a blood transfusion while it is still in the womb. Early in 1968 a new *preventive* treatment was developed. A vaccine, called anti-Rh immune globulin, is administered to an Rh− mother within three days after the delivery of an Rh+ baby. In the mother, this blocks the development of a sensitization against the baby's Rh+ red blood cells that entered her circulation. This protection lasts long enough for the baby's blood cells circulating in her body to wear out and disappear. The mother whose blood has already been sensitized against the Rh factor by previous pregnancies or blood transfusions may not benefit from this new preventive measure. It is therefore important for the girl with Rh− blood never to receive blood transfusions with Rh+ blood and for her to receive anti-Rh immune globulin within the first three days following the delivery of an Rh+ baby or miscarriage. This process will be repeated after each pregnancy involving an Rh+ baby. Since the use of the vaccine has been so nearly

100 per cent effective, parents with an Rh incompatability can look forward to having additional children safely.

Childbirth

Childbirth starts with the onset of labor, the somewhat rhythmic contractions of the uterus. During the pregnancy, the muscle cells of the uterus increase in number and size in preparation for the birth process. Labor can be subdivided into three stages. The first and longest stage starts with the first uterine contraction and ends with the complete dilation of the cervix of the uterus. The second stage starts at this point and terminates with the birth of the child. The third stage extends from the birth of the child to the expulsion of the afterbirth (placenta) and the final contraction of the uterus. Generally, labor will last for about 7 hours for the first birth and 4 hours for subsequent births. There can, of course, be great variance in the duration from one woman to another and in the same woman from one birth to another. The figures cited cannot be viewed by any means as absolutes.

The uterus, as a means of maintaining its muscle tone, undergoes gentle rhythmic contractions even when it is in a nonpregnant state. During pregnancy, contractions continue and become more noticeable, particularly during its latter stages. These contractions are referred to as false labor. They have caused many an unneccessary trip to the hospital at odd hours of the night and early morning.

Uterine contractions are at first about fifteen to twenty minutes apart, and fairly mild. Succeeding contractions become more intense, closer together, and last longer. Initial contractions may last about thirty seconds; later on they may last a minute or more.

The amniotic sac ("bag of waters") which surrounds the child in the uterus and is filled with fluid will often break during the first or second stage of labor. This occurs in response to the increased pressures created by the contracting uterus. The breaking of this sac is usually a signal for the expectant mother to get to the hospital if she is not already there. The amount of fluid released is anywhere from a cupful to a quart. Increased uterine contractions usually follow the "breaking of the water." Obstetricians will sometimes break the amniotic sac in order to induce greater uterine activity.

When an expectant mother arrives at the hospital during this first stage of labor, a number of routine procedures are performed. Her contractions are timed, the baby's heartbeat is recorded, and body temperature is taken. Preparation is then made for delivery. For hygienic reasons, the pubic hair is shaved and an enema containing antiseptic fluid is given to clean out the lower bowel.

The obstetrician can then check the progress by a vaginal examination to determine the extent of dilation of the cervix. When the cervix is completely dilated, the second stage has begun. Contractions become quite strong and are assisted by abdominal muscles when the mother bears down with each contraction. She is guided in this process by nurses

Fig. 6-11. ***A.*** *The first stage of labor: Uterine contractions have started and the cervix of the uterus has begun to dilate.*

B. *The second stage of labor: The uterine contractions force the child through the birth canal (vagina) with the head making its appearance at the vaginal opening.*

C. *The second stage of labor will soon end. After the head of the child has cleared the vaginal orifice the body will quickly follow.*

D. *The third stage of labor: The child has been born and its umbilical cord cut and tied. The placenta has detached itself from the wall of the uterus and will soon be expelled. The uterus begins its return back to its normal size.*

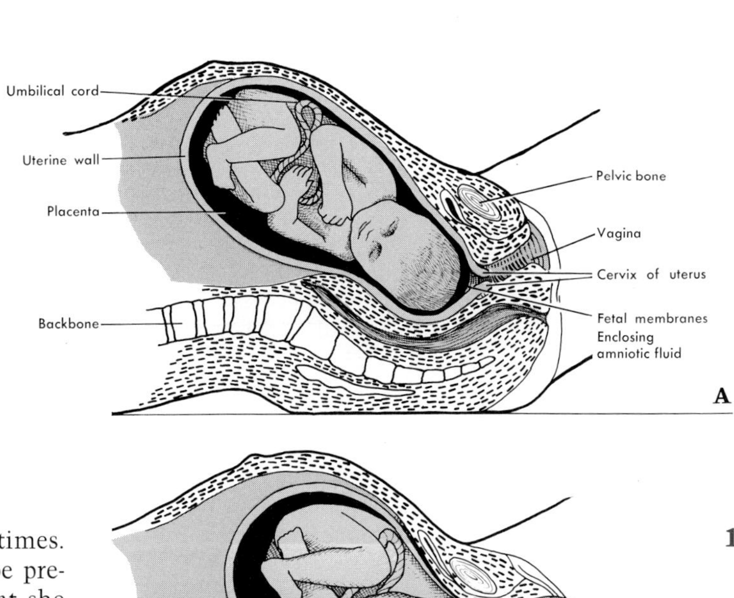

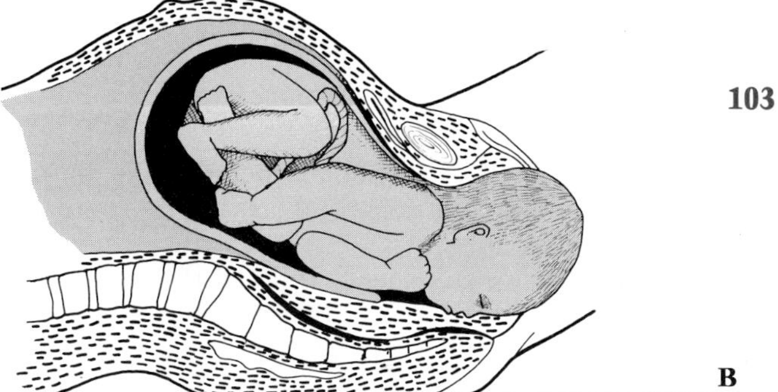

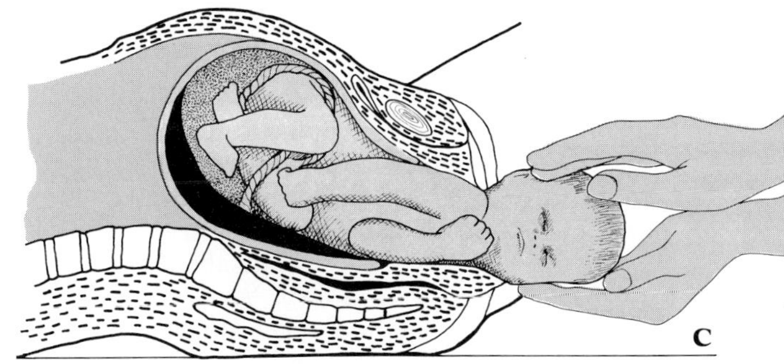

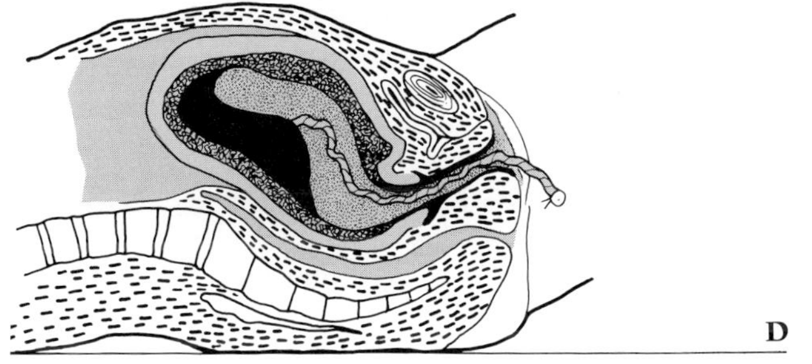

encouraging her to bear down at the proper times. It is particularly important that the mother be prepared for this part of the birth process so that she knows what to expect and what is expected of her. The most difficult time comes when the baby's head reaches the muscles surrounding the vaginal opening. If the physician deems it necessary, in order to prevent the tearing of these tissues, he may perform an episiotomy. This is a small incision made at the bottom of the vaginal wall, usually at an angle to the side rather than straight down. This type of incision heals fairly quickly and functions to facilitate the birth. Once the head of the child is cleared, the body follows rather quickly. The baby at this point is still attached by its umbilical cord to the placenta (afterbirth) in the mother. Two clamps are placed on the umbilical cord and the cord is then cut between them. Upon being born, the child is held by its heels to help drain out any fluids that it may have in its mouth and throat. The child usually cries and inflates its lungs for the first time and begins to take care of its respiratory needs. The stump of the umbilical cord that remains ultimately dries up and drops off, leaving the navel or umbilicus as its mark of birth. The baby is cleaned and an identification bracelet is usually placed on it. It will also have a 1 per cent solution of silver nitrate placed in its eyes to avoid possible infection.

In the third stage of labor there is the expulsion of the placenta from the uterus. This takes place within fifteen or twenty minutes after the birth by contractions of the uterus or at times by pressure applied by the physician.

Caesarean Section

Birth by Caesarean section is the surgical removal of the baby from the uterus. This is not the preferred manner of birth and is used when, for one reason or another, normal delivery through the birth canal is not possible or advisable. This method is employed when the child is too large to pass through the pelvic opening of the mother. In other cases, the mother with a heart, lung, or kidney condition may be a poor candidate for the vigorous second stage of labor, which is physically demanding.

The frivolous and uninformed sometimes think that a Caesarean section is a good way to avoid the discomfort of a normal birth. It still represents major surgery, and though it can be skillfully done by the capable surgeon in a well-equipped hospital, it remains a good *second choice* for delivery. The usual procedure is to perform the section about two weeks before the expected date of birth. After a woman has had a child by this method, succeeding children are almost always delivered the same way. There is some fear on the part of physicians that the uterine scar left by the operation may weaken and rupture during labor. There have, however, recently been some obstetrical centers that have succeeded in having normal births follow Caesarean sections. The number of births that a woman can have via Caesarean section has also been a concern. Many physicians recommend that sections should not be performed more than three times. In some rare cases, women have had as many as nine sections successfully performed.

The Breech Birth

Normally, the child in the birth process moves down the birth canal head first. In about 4 per cent of the cases, there is a breech presentation with the baby's buttocks, shoulders, or feet appearing first. These deliveries are invariably more difficult and sometimes more hazardous to the child. The experienced obstetrician, however, can effectively deal with the situation.

Natural Childbirth

In recent years, there has been a great deal of discussion about natural childbirth. The aim of this method is to effect the birth of the child without the use of drugs. The woman is prepared for this event by following a regimen of exercise, good health practices, and by psychologically preparing herself. The latter is accomplished by increasing her understanding and acceptance of childbirth, thereby eliminating tension and fear.

There is great variation in the way drugs may be used in childbirth, ranging from general anesthesia to the injection of drugs to make specific parts of the body insensitive. Some advocates of natural childbirth have displayed a missionary zeal and feel that all childbirth should be drug-free. Obstetricians generally feel that this is an irresponsible attitude. The decision of whether to use a drug, when, what kind, and how, should be that of the trained obstetrician. Many women suited for natural childbirth physically and psychologically report great exultation

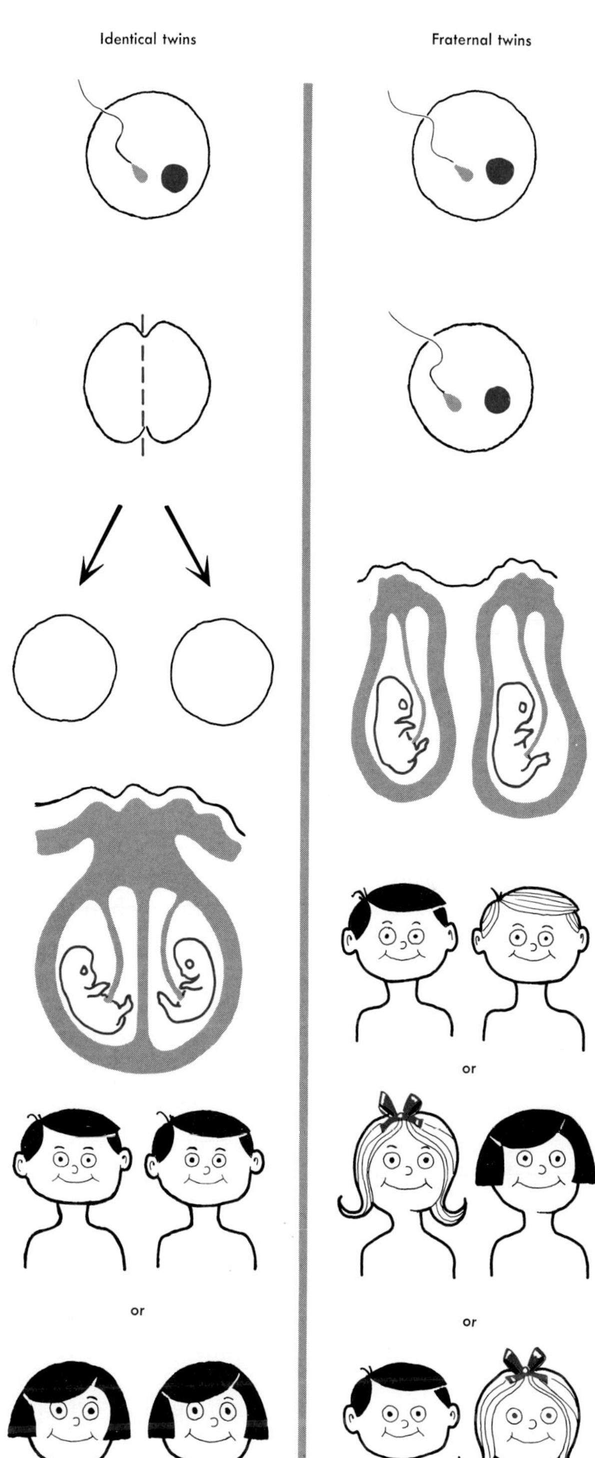

Fig. 6-12. Twinning. (Adapted from World Health, *Aug.–Sept. 1966)*

in experiencing childbirth. Herein lies the contribution made by this method and its advocates. It has tended to blunt the stories of horror about childbirth told by those who would enshrine themselves in martyrdom. Somewhere in between these two extreme sweeps of the pendulum lies the average woman's thinking. She is inviting neither unwholesome fear of childbirth nor adolescent enthusiasm. When a woman feels that the fewer drugs used the better, an obstetrician can be found to be guided by the principle. A competent physician, however, does not want his actions dictated before the fact. When circumstances demand that drugs or other actions be taken to save child and/or mother, he does not want to have his hands tied by misplaced enthusiasms.

Multiple Births

The incidence of twinning in the United States (where at least one child is born alive) is one set of twins for every 99 births. A set of triplets is delivered for every 10,200 deliveries and a set of quadruplets for every 900,000 deliveries. It is interesting to note that the chances of a multiple birth are over twice as high in mothers between the ages of 35 and 39 as compared with mothers in the 15- to 19-age group. The reason for the increased multiple birthrate with higher age groups is not clear.

Twins that develop from the same fertilized egg are identical twins. It is believed that the fertilized egg splits resulting in the development of two babies who have identical genetic makeup, and will therefore be of the same sex and of very similar appearance.

Fraternal twins occur as a result of the mother's producing two eggs at the same time. The eggs are then fertilized by different sperm cells. The genetic makeup of fraternal twins is as different as in children born in separate births. About two-thirds of all twins born are fraternal, with the remaining third being identical.

It appears that there is a hereditary factor associated with twinning, as evidenced by the higher number of twin births in some families. The pattern that it follows is not too well understood.

The Premature Child

A child that is born before 36 weeks after conception is regarded to be premature, 40 weeks being considered full term (slightly more than 9 months). Another criterion for determining prematurity is that of weight. Any child born weighing less than 5 lbs. 8 oz. is classified as premature. The closer to full term the fetus is, the bigger and more highly developed will be its organs and body systems. Its chances for survival, therefore, are proportionately increased.

Those born within the 32- to 36-week period will usually weigh from 3½ to 4 pounds. The infant will be weak, but can manage to cry for its food when hungry. Careful supervision and nursing care are needed if the baby is to live. When birth occurs 28 to 32 weeks after conception the fetal infant will weigh about two pounds. An infant of this size and maturity would require constant medical supervision for survival, because it cannot nurse and has particular difficulty maintaining a constant body temperature. A fetal infant born sooner than 28 weeks after conception is not given any chance for survival.

One of the several handicaps that the premature child must overcome is the difficulty of regulating body temperature. This difficulty results from the large body surface in proportion to its weight, a lack of insulating subcutaneous fat, and an incompletely developed sweating mechanism. The nutritional needs of a normally rapid growing fetus are high. Yet its sucking and swallowing reflexes are weak or absent, and the ability of its digestive tract to handle and absorb foods is often lacking. The premature are also more vulnerable to infectious diseases.

The greatest problem the premature baby will encounter, however, is the respiratory difficulty caused by hyaline membrane disease (HMD). When babies are born, the inner surface of the lungs contain a surfactant which lubricates these surfaces. After one breath is forced out, this surfactant allows the lungs to expand again to let the next breath in. Premature babies born with hyaline membrane disease are born *without* this surfactant or lubricating device. Their lungs do not inflate enough, and a struggle for oxygen develops. If the baby lives for three days, he will usually begin to produce surfactant and may survive. The problem, then, has been to prevent brain damage from oxygen deprivation in those first critical days. Three medical approaches are being used to produce a higher survival rate for the baby with hyaline membrane disease. The first involves the mechanical technique of artificially inflating the infant's collapsed lungs by forcing air through a tube inserted into the baby's lungs. This method has achieved an unprecedented 80 to 90 per cent survival rate.[3] A second method concentrates on preventing the disease by determining prenatally through amniocentesis whether the baby's lungs are ready for their first breath. By examining the levels of certain substances in the amniotic fluid (lecithin and sphingomyelin), Dr. Gluck,[4] of the University of California at San Diego, has been able to foretell whether the infant is producing surfactant. More recently, Dr. John A. Clemente and colleagues at the University of California at San Francisco, have come up with a "foam test"[5] of the amniotic fluid which determines the presence of pulmonary surfactant.[6] Since HMD is especially prevalent in babies born prematurely by induced labor or Caesarean section, if the Gluck test or "foam test" is administered and indicates that the baby is *not* producing surfactant in many cases the Caesarean section may be postponed and labor not induced. Finally some research with animals in Canada indicates that surfactant production can be stimulated by administering steroids at birth. Ultimately, it is hoped, the treatment could begin prenatally for humans too.

[3]Dr. George Gregory, University of California, *New England Journal of Medicine*, June 1971.

[4]*Medical World News*, December 11, 1970, p. 4.

[5]"foam test"—Equal amounts of amniotic fluid and ethyl alcohol are shaken vigorously until bubbles and froth appear. If the froth lasts for 15 minutes, the baby's respiratory development has progressed sufficiently so that there will be no respiratory distress. If no bubbles or froth develop from the shaking, or if the bubbles do not last, then there is not enough pulmonary surfactant, and this baby may well experience respiratory distress.

[6]*Today's Health*, September 1972, p. 7.

Causes and Prevention of Prematurity

More than half of the neonatal deaths (within a month after birth) are due to prematurity. Some of the causes of prematurity revolve around the mother, with injury, malnutrition, infectious disease (tuberculosis, syphilis), cardiac or diabetic disorders, and toxemia with multiple pregnancy as the most common. Those causes that are related more closely to the child include malformation of the fetus, premature separation of the placenta, Rh factor difficulties, as well as a large group of undiagnosed causes. It must be noted that a number of the factors causing premature births are also related to the incidence of stillbirth (birth of a dead child).

Prevention of prematurity is considered the basic aim rather than focus on the improvements of the scrambling efforts to save the fetal infant who has made a precipitous entry into the world. Research efforts are focusing on toxemia and the premature separation of the placenta as well as other related factors. In the meantime, good prenatal care properly utilizing medical information already known is the best guarantee of a healthy child.

Abortion

Man has struggled for centuries with the complex multifaceted social, medical, legal, and moral problems related to abortion. In recent years there has been a great deal of public discussion centered on these issues. The more recent discussions do not differ to any great extent from the following discussion that took place between two physicians in another century. "About the terminating of a pregnancy, I want your opinion. The father was syphilitic. The mother tuberculous. Of the four children born, the first was blind, the second died, the third was deaf and dumb, the fourth also tuberculous. What would you have done?" "I would have ended the pregnancy." "Then you would have murdered Beethoven."[7]

Abortion refers to the separation of the fetus from the uterus during its first twenty-eight weeks of prenatal life. After the twenty-eighth week it is termed a premature birth. When this occurrence is precipitated by natural causes, it is referred to as a *spontaneous abortion.* The term "miscarriage" is often used in referring to this kind of abortion. It is believed that the improper implantation of the fertilized egg, hormonal imbalance, or imperfections in the fetus are the primary causes of the occurrence. In the 1940's and early 50's, obstetricians in an attempt to correct the hormonal imbalance administered estrogenic hormones to women with histories of spontaneous abortion. Recently, however, a warning to discontinue the use of synthetic estrogens during pregnancy has been circulated because of the possible link to vaginal cancer in the female offspring born to women so treated. The mother often relates the spontaneous abortion to a fall, a bumpy ride, or similar incident. However, these are considered to be at most secondary causes. Most spontaneous abortions occur in the first three months of pregnancy.

A *therapeutic abortion* is one that is induced by a physician. There are several methods that have been widely used by physicians because of their practicality and safeness. The criterion for the choice of method is usually the length of the pregnancy. Prior to twelve weeks of pregnancy a dilatation and curettage (more commonly known as a D & C) is the preferred method. Under local anesthesia the cervix of the uterus is dilated, and with the use of an instrument called a curette the lining of the uterus is scraped free of all embryonic material. A variation on the D & C is the vacuum aspiration technique. The cervix is dilated and a small tube that is attached to a vacuum pump is inserted into the uterus. The fetal matter is drawn off in this manner. It has been determined from initial studies in New York with therapeutic abortions, that 77 per cent were done either by a D & C or a suction curette. The injection of prostaglandins intravenously or directly into the uterus were first used experimentally in 1970 to induce therapeutic abortions.

If the pregnancy has continued to the 16th through 24th week the preferred method is saline induction. The amniotic fluid is drawn from the amniotic sac and a saline solution is substituted for it. This foreign solution kills the fetus. Within 24 to 72 hours a miniature labor begins until the fetus is expelled. In New York 20 per cent of the thera-

[7]Norman St. John Stevas, *The Right to Life* (New York: Holt, Rinehart & Winston, 1964), p. 16.

peutic abortions were done in this way. When sterilization of the mother is indicated in addition to a therapeutic abortion, physicians may remove the pregnancy by hysterectomy, which is the removal of the entire uterus. This is rarely done and accounted for only 3 per cent of all therapeutic abortions done in New York.[8]

The Legality of Abortion

The legislative developments relative to abortion laws in the United States during recent years have been nothing short of revolutionary. Although women have sought and found abortion since the beginning of time, it is only now in this period of rapid social change that we have shed the Victorian cloak of silence to witness the pendulum swinging full arc to "abortion-on-demand!"

The new abortion laws that began to make their appearance in 1967 varied somewhat in their provisions. Basically, however, three kinds of modernized abortion laws emerged at that time. Those that stated abortion was not a crime when performed by a licensed physician because the pregnancy would impair the physical or mental health of the woman or that the child would be born with a grave physical or mental defect, or in cases of pregnancy resulting from rape or incest. Colorado, in 1967, became the first state to liberalize its law in this fashion. The second type law expanded the provisions of the first to include an evaluation of the mother's actual or foreseeable total environment. This is sometimes thought of as abortion on social grounds where the family size, level of income, and marital status may be taken into consideration. The third kind of law was the most permissive, for it removed all criminal penalties for abortion, provided the abortion was done early in pregnancy and by a licensed physician. This more permissive law has been adopted by the states of Hawaii, Alaska, Washington, and New York.

[8]Center for Disease Control, Report to New York City Health Dept., August 1970.

The variations to the basic laws were many. While *all* states required that abortion be done by a licensed physician, some states insisted it be done in a hospital, whereas others merely stated it could be done in another place designated by law. Age limits of the mother were set in some states and pregnancy time limits established in others. Approval by hospital therapeutic abortion committees, consultants, or hospital boards may be required to justify an abortion, and finally some states have established residency requirements. In addition to the individual state variations, it has been determined that the actual practice of abortion may vary from the provisions established by state law.

In 1973 the United States Supreme Court handed down a precedent-setting decision on abortion. The decision in effect legalized abortions desired by the mother and recommended by a physician during the first trimester of pregnancy. The state may regulate abortion procedures after the first trimester to the extent that the procedures relate to the preservation and protection of maternal health. The court saw the state interest in potential life during the last ten weeks of pregnancy when the fetus could survive

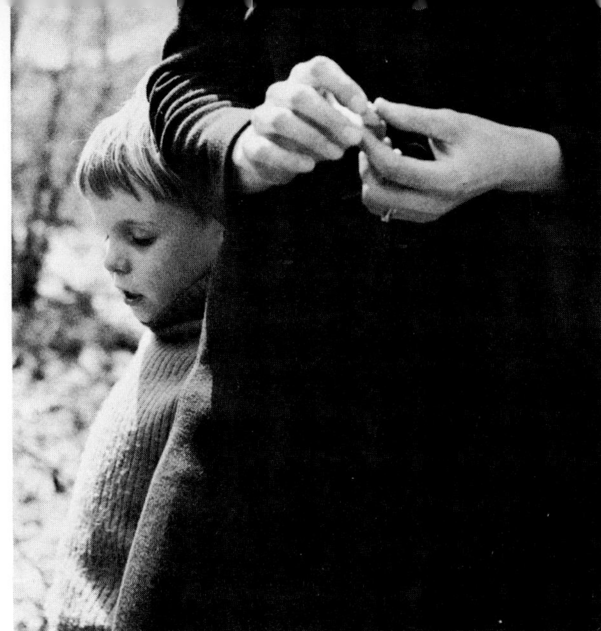

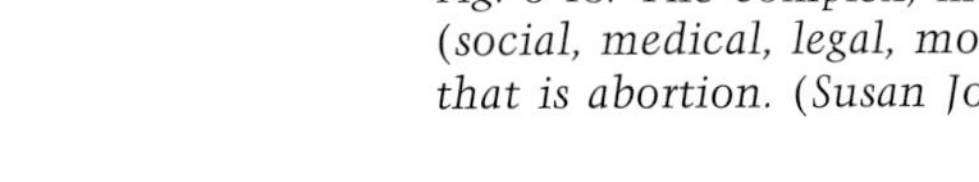

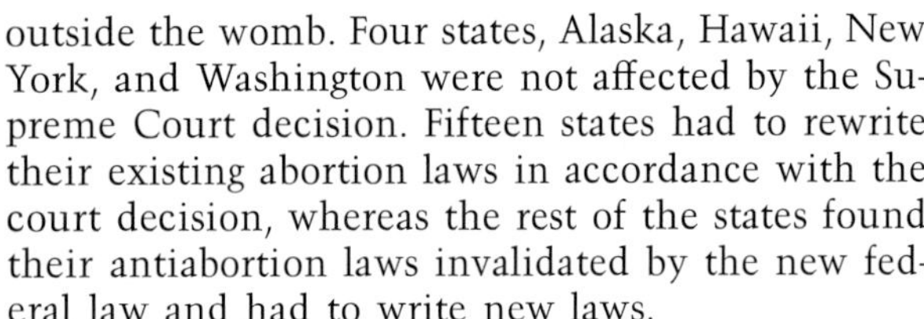

Fig. 6-13. The complex, multifaceted (social, medical, legal, moral) problem that is abortion. (Susan Johns)

outside the womb. Four states, Alaska, Hawaii, New York, and Washington were not affected by the Supreme Court decision. Fifteen states had to rewrite their existing abortion laws in accordance with the court decision, whereas the rest of the states found their antiabortion laws invalidated by the new federal law and had to write new laws.

The Morality of Abortion

The liberalization of the abortion laws is not a complete answer to this dilemma. There are those who feel that an abortion results in the destruction of a human life. A very real moral issue needs, then, to be dealt with. There is also a difference of opinion at what point the destruction of the unborn is morally right or wrong. Some feel abortions can be permitted before the fetus resembles a child and others feel it is permissible before the mother feels movement of the fetus (quickening). Another point of view is that the abortion should not take place after the time when the child would live if it were born at that moment. This usually refers to a seven-month-old fetus or older. Others feel that life begins at birth and the destruction of the unborn child at any time before that is capable of moral justification. Then there are those who state that a woman cannot be half pregnant. She is either pregnant or she is not. If she is pregnant, then she is bearing a life. The destruction of that life, this group feels, is as morally wrong as the murder of an older person. Birth is only the separation of one phase of development of a human being from another. Each individual, then, needs to develop values upon which to base his thinking on this issue.

The reasons why abortions may be sought must be considered in this decision. A pregnancy that results from rape or incest is a case in point. Should a woman who has been violated suffer the further indignity of bearing the child? There are responses to this query to the effect that you cannot correct one crime by performing another. Yet, is it not criminal to expect a woman to bear a child she cannot love? It is not the intent of the author to confuse the reader, but merely to indicate the complexities involved in the issues. The woman who contracted German measles during her first trimester of pregnancy has a similar decision to make. This unfortunate occurrence means that her unborn child has a significantly increased chance of being born with a deformity. Many women would seek an abortion on these grounds. Yet, there is a chance that the abortion would result in the destruction of a normal child. The decisions here do not come easily.

Many public health experts point out that we have exerted great efforts to reduce infant mortality. There have been the development of vaccines for diphtheria, tetanus, poliomyelitis, whooping cough, measles, and improvements in nutrition, prenatal care, obstetrics, and other areas. At the same time, estimates indicate that over a million fetal lives are lost in abortions. The two facts stand in contradiction to each other. The more effective use of known birth control methods, it is felt, could make a preventive contribution to this problem.

Many a hospital nurse who has been trained morally and professionally to preserve life is revolted at having to discard a human being in development like so much refuse. On the other hand, there are those who accept abortion with a disdainful casualness, and a callousness inconsistent with humaneness. At best, abortion should be regarded as a distasteful correction for a situation that in most instances should not have occurred in the first place. Several European countries have had liberal abortion laws for a good number of years. Sweden and Denmark started liberalizing their abortion statutes in the 1930's. Hungary and Czechoslovakia in the 1950's. In Hungary the increase in legal abortions has risen to the point where they exceed the number of births. As the abortion rate in that country has gone up, there has been a corresponding decline in the birthrate. This suggests that abortion is being used as a birth control measure. Because liberalized abortion laws caused a significant drop in the birthrate, two countries of Eastern Europe, Romania and Bulgaria, developed more restrictive statutes to reverse the trend. If abortion is accepted as a primary birth control method, or an unqualified adult right, some fear that it may serve as the basis of a greater problem than those it is seeking to correct. Abortion should therefore be used as a reluctant last resort.

Contraception and Family Planning

The concept of family planning and contraception too often is interpreted solely as a means of keeping families small. There are many indications for use of contraception within marriage. These include some medical reasons such as advanced diabetes or cancer. Kidney disease, neurological diseases, and some inherited conditions might require strict use of contraception or even sterilization. For many, the basic purpose *is* to regulate family size and to effect a more judicious spacing of children, particularly since it has been shown that repeated closely spaced pregnancies have a higher incidence of stillbirths and premature births. It is recommended that two years elapse between pregnancies.

Contraception outside of marriage has become a current issue which is being dealt with in several ways. Social agencies concerned with birth control and illegitimacy will advise and prescribe contraceptives to anyone seeking them. Their theme is if you are going to be sexually active, then you must be responsible for the prevention of any births outside of marriage.

There are various devices and methods related to contraception. They can take the form of mechanical devices, chemical substances, or natural methods. No contraceptive method is foolproof, but each helps in producing the desired results. Ideally a contraceptive should be harmless, reliable, free of objectionable side effects, inexpensive, readily reversible, simple to use, and should not interfere with the sexual satisfaction of either partner. The following birth control methods will be listed in order of effectiveness with sterilization and the contraceptive pill being virtually 100 per cent effective and ending with the vaginal douche which is only 69 per cent effective.

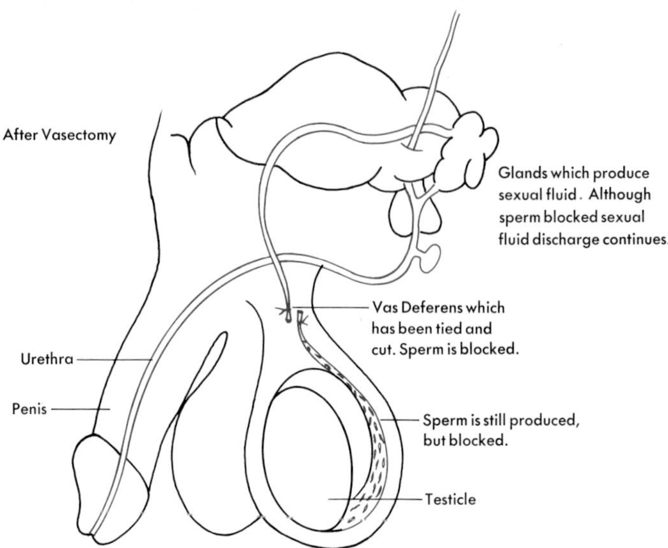

Fig. 6-14. Diagram of vasectomy.

Sterilization

Sterilization of the man or woman is a permanent means of preventing conception. In the man, a *vasectomy* involves simple surgery with a local anesthetic to cut and tie the vas deferens (tube leading from the testes) thus preventing the passage of the sperm cells. After the operation, sperm continue to be produced by the testes but, since their pathway is blocked, they simply disintegrate and are reabsorbed by the body. A vasectomy in no way alters sexual desire or performance. In the woman, a *tubal ligation* is more involved and requires major abdominal surgery to cut and tie the fallopian tubes. An alternate procedure would be a salpingectomy, which is the removal of the Fallopian tubes. Very often this is done shortly after childbirth. It can, however, be done at any time. A newer technique called a *laparoscopy* is being more widely used because the surgical procedures are simpler and allow the patient to leave the hospital the same day. In a laparoscopy, two tiny incisions are made in the abdomen to separate the organs and a laparoscope is used to locate the Fallopian tubes. Through the second incision the physician inserts the electric cautery and a tiny surgical knife that cuts and cauterizes the tubes. Sterilization is legal in the United States, and there is evidence that increasing numbers of older couples who feel their families are complete are being sterilized.

The religious positions on sterilization vary and must be one of the factors a couple must consider in making this decision. Orthodox Judaism is strongly opposed to sterilization except for an urgent medical reason. Likewise the Catholic doctrine prohibits sterilization when the sole purpose is to render the person sterile. In cases where the organs must be removed because of disease entities, surgery can be performed morally, and the sterility becomes a secondary outcome. Physicians will very often consult with the husband and wife to establish clearly the motivations for their decision, and to confirm that their patient understands that for all intents and purposes this procedure is irreversible. The couple should also be warned that sperm reappearance may occur temporarily in a small number of cases.

Oral Contraceptives (The Pill)

Several kinds of oral contraceptives are now available and all must be prescribed by a physician. Reexaminations are usually performed at 6- to 12-month intervals. The hormones contained in these pills prevent the ovaries from releasing an ovum, thus inhibiting ovulation. Basically there are two methods of pill use. The most commonly prescribed pill is the "combination" or "balanced progestin-estrogen" method. Each pill contains a combination of both synthetic estrogen and progestin. One begins to take the pill on the 5th day after the start of menstruation and continues to take a pill for 21 days. No pills are taken for the next 7 days, thereupon the entire procedure is repeated. A variation of this procedure is to take pills for 28 days. The last 7 pills in this regimen are placebos containing no hormones. For the woman who is prone to forgetfullness, the 28-day-pill routine is probably easier for her because

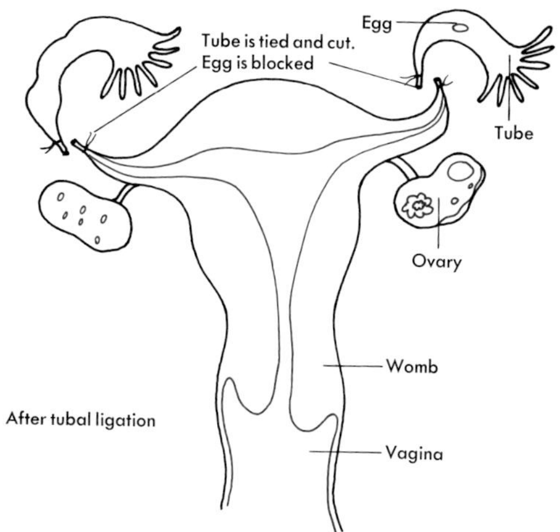

Fig. 6-15. Diagram of tubal ligation.

her pill-taking routine is not interrupted. She merely takes one pill a day month after month.

The second method of pill use is the sequential method. For the first 14–16 days a pill containing *only* estrogen is taken, thus preventing ovulation. For the next 4 to 6 days a pill containing a combination of estrogen and progestin is taken to assure orderly bleeding within 3 to 5 days after the last pill is taken. Most studies show a slightly higher failure rate for patients on the sequential method who forget to take one or two pills as compared to women who forget to take their combined pills.

Some minor side effects are sometimes described by a few patients who begin using the oral contraceptive. These include nausea, breast tenderness, skin pigmentation, headaches, and weight gain. There have also been some positive side effects reported such as the regularity of menses in heretofore irregular women and the elimination of dysmenorrhea (painful menstruation) and premenstrual tension. A curious relationship has also been drawn between users of the oral contraceptive and venereal disease. It seems that changes in the vaginal tissues resulting from pill use render one more susceptible to venereal disease. When one has contact with a person infected with venereal disease there is a 50 per cent chance of contracting the disease. However, for the woman using the pill, the chances of her contracting the disease are greatly increased.

The question of safety has arisen time and again since the introduction of the oral contraceptive in May 1960. At that time recommended use was limited to two years. This was later extended to four years and finally in 1966 all restrictions on length of use were removed. The FDA's appointed Obstetrical and Gynecological Advisory Committee have the problem of pill safety under constant surveillance. Two studies from England in 1967 and 1968 have indicated that there is a very small but real danger from using the pill. Many scientists who support the oral contraceptive will quickly point out that the incidence of thromboembolic (clotting in a blood vessel) disorders in pregnant or recently delivered women is almost three times greater than for those nonpregnant women taking the pill. They also state that the death rate per 100,000 women involved in automobile accidents is much greater, and finally that the lives claimed from smoking resulting in lung cancer and heart disease is also much greater than the threat posed by oral contraceptives. The FDA has indicated on the labeling of all contraceptives that use of the drug is associated with potential danger.

More than a decade has elapsed since the oral contraceptive became a household word. It has been blamed for the changes in social mores and for the increase in venereal disease. The scientific studies are finally gathering the great numbers needed to develop any study with validity and the next few years should be rich in statistical yields concerning the Pill.

Intrauterine Devices

Intrauterine devices are made of plastic or stainless steel and come in a variety of shapes. They are placed in the uterus by a physician and serve as a

95 per cent effective means of birth control. The device does not interfere with the menstrual period and requires little attention from the physician after it is in place. It can be removed at a later date when pregnancy is desired. How the device works is not completely understood by the scientists. Unlike the oral contraceptive, ovulation does occur; however, the egg does not implant itself in the uterine lining while the foreign body is within the uterus. Heretofore, the intrauterine device was least satisfactory in young women who have never had children, since insertion was more difficult and spontaneous expulsion of the device more common. Specially designed IUD's have now been made available for women who have never borne children. Other problems associated with the IUD are infection and perforation of the uterus. Pregnancy can occur with the device in place and usually remains in the uterus to be expelled with the afterbirth following childbirth. Intrauterine devices are used by about 7 per cent of obstetrician's contraceptive users.

The Diaphragm and Cervical Cap

The diaphragm is a hemispherical rubber dome which women insert into the vagina to cover the cervix. It is usually used with a cream or jelly that contains a spermicide. It must be left in place at least 6 hours after intercourse and must be properly fitted and prescribed by a physician. It is about 88 per cent effective as a birth control measure, since it can become dislodged during intercourse. Many women use the diaphragm, while others dislike the entire procedure.

The cervical cap is a smaller plastic or metal cup that fits securely over the cervix. Physicians carefully fit the cap, very much like a thimble is placed on a finger. Sometimes women insert the cap after menstruation and leave it there until a few days before the onset of the next menses. The drawback of this method is that the placement technique is more difficult than the diaphragm, since the cervix is so deep within the vagina.

The Condom

The condom is one of the more popular methods of contraception. It is simple to use, can be purchased without a prescription in any drugstore, does not require fitting or consultation with a physician and, properly and consistently used, is 86 per cent effective. The condom, "rubber," or "prophylactic," is a strong sheath of rubber that fits over the man's erected penis before sexual intercourse. It catches the man's ejaculation thus preventing it from entering the vagina. In addition to its contraceptive qualities, it is also considered a good preventive for venereal disease because contact with infected tissues is limited.

Chemical Contraceptives

Chemical contraceptives include vaginal foams, jellies, creams, suppositories, and tablets. They are available without prescription and are generally less effective when used alone as compared to use with a diaphragm or condom. They are more effective than the following contraceptive methods, and some women find them acceptable primarily because they are available to them without a prescription.

Withdrawal

Dr. Guttmacher, President of Planned Parenthood—World Population, describes withdrawal or coitus interruptus as probably the oldest technique used to avoid having children. Some in fact would not even consider it as a contraceptive method at all. In this method of contraception the penis is withdrawn from the woman's vagina just prior to ejaculation so that the semen is deposited outside the genital tract. Very often this is not a successful method of birth control, since it becomes difficult for the man to withdraw in time and since there are enough sperm in the preclimax lubricating fluid to cause pregnancy.

Rhythm, or "Safe Period"

The rhythm, or "safe period," method of contraception is based on the principle of avoiding intercourse during that period when an egg cell is present in the woman's fallopian tube. In a 28-day menstrual cycle, the woman is expected to ovulate on the 14th day. A four-day period before and a four-day period after the 14th day make up the "unsafe" period. The greatest difficulty with this method is attempting to ascertain when ovulation takes place. Menstrual cycles are often not very regular, or are disturbed by illness, emotional upset, and other causes. For this reason, the rhythm method is an unreliable means of contraception. The method can be made more accurate if the woman keeps a daily record of her temperature upon awakening each morning. When ovulation occurs, the body temperature will go up one-half to one degree and remain at that level for the rest of the cycle. A further disadvantage is that the couple's sex life may be controlled to an uncomfortable extent by the calendar and temperature readings rather than by love and desire. At best most couples will require assistance from a doctor or rhythm clinic if the effectiveness of the method is to be increased. Both must also be willing to accept long periods of abstinence each month.

Douches

The vaginal douche following sexual relations is probably the least effective birth control measure. The sperm enter the uterus within seconds after the male climax so that the woman would literally have to jump out of bed and race to the bathroom in order to flush out the vagina with a douche. There is also some question that the douche itself may help push the sperm farther into the uterus. Many physicians feel douching too frequently can be harmful because it destroys the protective bacteria in a woman's vagina and renders her more susceptible to vaginitis.

The Contraceptive Promise of the Prostaglandins

Prostaglandins are fatty acid compounds that occur naturally in the body. They were first identified in 1930 and finally produced synthetically in 1966. They have remarkable effects on the female reproductive system, as well as other systems. Some scientists are saying that these substances hold a new promise as a "morning after" method of fertility control. For some time it has been known that they stimulate contractions of the uterus and therefore play an important part in inducing childbirth within a few hours after its administration. Injection of prostaglandins to induce therapeutic abortions was first used in 1970. Laboratories are endeavoring to develop a pill that would be the first "post conception contraceptive."

In addition to their possible use as a birth control measure this versatile family of substances seems to hold promise for the prevention of peptic ulcers, regulating blood pressure, opening airways to the lungs of asthmatics by relaxing the smooth muscles of the bronchi, and regulating metabolism.

Some Aspects of Infertility

While many young married couples are preoccupied with keeping the size of their families small, there are about 15 to 20 per cent of married couples who are faced with the aspects of never having children born to them. The reasons for infertility vary and are equally shared by either the husband or the wife. In the male the numbers of sperm produced may not be sufficient, the amount of seminal fluid may be scant, there may be an obstruction somewhere in the pathway from the testes to the end of the penis, or there may be some difficulty in maintaining an erection. In the female the infertility may arise from the ovaries not producing mature ova, or a malformed uterus that is not responding to the hormones in the bloodstream. There sometimes occurs, as a result of infection or disease, a blockage of the fallopian tube so that the egg cannot pass through. In addition, the vaginal environment may sometimes be overly hostile to the sperm. Through medical detection once the problem is identified in either or both partners, therapy can begin. It is estimated that $\frac{1}{3}$ to $\frac{1}{2}$ of infertile or subfertile couples can be helped to have children by either surgical or medical means.

The rash of multibirths that we are beginning to accept as commonplace are usually due to fertility drugs. Some hormones have the undesirable side effect of promoting maturation of more than one egg, hence the birth of quintuplets and even octuplets.

The therapy most people are aware of is artificial insemination (AI). This is the process of transferring sperm-filled seminal fluid from the male to the female by artificial means. If the male whose sperm is used is the husband, then the process is called AIH (Artificial Insemination–Husband). If a donor other than the husband is used, as in cases where the husband is irreversibly sterile or carrying an undesirable genetic trait, then the process is termed AID

(Artificial Insemination–Donor). Couples may choose artificial insemination as a more desirable alternative to a childless marriage or to the adoption of a child. A couple needs to be thoroughly familiar with all the facets of this procedure. In some cases, the husband finds it difficult to accept his own infertility, let alone accept a child born of such an arrangement. Women who have been artificially inseminated without the husband's written consent have been accused of adultery. Some men who have given written consent for this procedure reverse themselves years later, suing for divorce and attempting to deny paternal responsibility for child support because the child is not "biologically" his. Questions of legitimacy have also arisen. The legal ramifications of artificial insemination at times have become most complicated, and for these reasons couples should not take donor insemination lightly. The State of Oklahoma in 1967 developed legislation to confer legality on the use of artificial insemination and to spell out the rights of children conceived in this way. Hopefully other states will follow this pattern for legislation.

Needless to say, a majority of the couples resorting to AID or AIH are delighted with their decision and as Dr. Guttmacher claims, "Once an AID procedure has been accomplished, I advise the couple to forget the whole business. Ideally, by the time the infant is delivered, the husband, the wife, and the doctor are no longer thinking about the fact that donor impregnation was involved."[9] Again it is important for those couples contemplating artificial insemination to seek out religious counsel on this issue, for some religions accept the procedure as moral, but others do not.

[9] Alan Guttmacher, M.D., *Birth Control and Love* (New York: Bantam, 1970), p. 239.

Genetic Counseling

There was a time when being a "carrier" meant that a person was harboring a dread communicable disease. In these days of greater sophistication, the term can now mean that the person is a carrier of a defective gene. Such a person could have offspring with a genetic disease (see Chapter 11).

The worst genetic mistakes are usually aborted early during pregnancy, sometimes before the mother even knows she is pregnant. Nature's correction of its own mistakes, however, is not foolproof, and genetic mishaps do occur. Many persons are unaware that they are carrying defective genes until they have a child born to them with a genetic disease. Where there is such a family history, genetic counseling can offer a couple some hope for the future. Through genetic examinations of both parents, physicians can indicate what the risks are of having an abnormal baby. Some alternatives available to a couple running a high risk of producing a defective child may well be to remain childless, adoption, artificial insemination, or perhaps, in the near future, inovulation (the prenatal adoption of someone else's fertilized egg).

As a result of a medical technique called *amniocentesis*, physicians can now for a number of diseases accurately predict whether the fetus is the

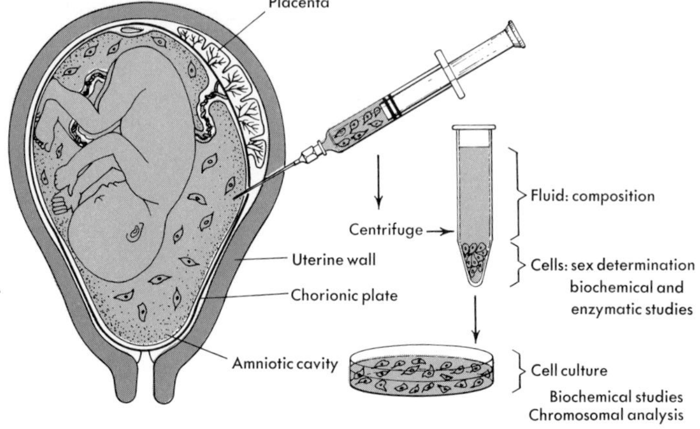

Fig. 6-16. Diagram of amniocentesis. (From "Prenatal Diagnosis of Genetic Disease" by Theodore Friedmann. Copyright © 1973 by Scientific American, Inc. All rights reserved.)

victim of a genetic disease. This involves microscopic examination of the chemical composition of the amniotic fluid or the cells found in the amniotic fluid surrounding the fetus. Ideally the fluid sample is drawn during the 14th to 18th week of pregnancy and will clearly detect over 70 inborn errors of metabolism or other genetic faults. A family alerted through an amniocentesis that they will bear a hopelessly defective child may either seek an abortion or carry the child to full term and care for it as best they can. In some instances, techniques have been developed to aid the fetus in spite of his genetic weakness. The physician thus alerted to the problem may act to correct it or minimize its effects. In counseling parents, only information is given. All decisions on planning or terminating a pregnancy are left to them.

One problem in developing genetic disease prevention programs is the difficulty in identifying high-risk pregnancies. For example, if amniocentesis would be performed in all women over 35 years of age who became pregnant, the estimates are that the rate of occurrence of Down's syndrome would be cut in half. When a woman has already borne a child with a genetic disease, we have a second justification for amniocentesis in future pregnancies.

It has been suggested that if prenatal diagnosis and selective abortions were coupled with screening programs to find carriers of genetic diseases, very significant reductions could be effected in these diseases. If the screening program discovered those families where *both* parents were carriers, the monitoring of all their pregnancies would result in the detection of many cases of genetic disease. It would then be possible to offer selective abortion for those fetuses affected. Since it is estimated that it costs $250,000 to care for each infant born with Down's syndrome, it would be *economically* feasible to conduct such a program of detection and prevention. The greater issue that surfaces here goes well beyond the economics of things. Man is entering an era where he can control the quality of life born to him. It is time to review the ethics upon which such profound determinations are to be made.

Review Questions

1. "Man can initiate life, but he cannot create it." Explain.
2. Describe the functions of the testes, the male reproductive glands, and the ovaries, their female counterparts.
3. Abortion should not serve as a birth control measure. Explain.
4. Describe the menstrual cycle with regard to hormone secretion and ovulation.
5. How do a woman's reactions to menstruation sometimes reflect her adjustment to her sexuality?
6. Describe the emotional and physiological difficulties that may occur at the onset of menopause.
7. What are the early signs of pregnancy? Which tests may a physician employ to confirm the condition?

8. Describe the significant developments during each trimester of pregnancy.
9. How has good prenatal care made childbirth safer for mother and child?
10. What are the major factors to be considered in determining if the baby will be breast-fed or bottle-fed?
11. Describe the three stages of labor in childbirth.
12. Define: (1) Caesarean section, (2) breech birth, (3) natural childbirth, (4) premature child, (5) abortion.
13. What are some of the measures that can be taken to prevent the birth of the premature child?
14. What are the medical, social, and moral issues in the discussion about liberalizing abortion laws in the country?
15. What are the emotional and legal considerations related to pregnancies via artificial insemination?
16. How do you view some of the research implications related to human reproduction?
17. How can amniocentesis prove helpful in the area of genetic counseling?

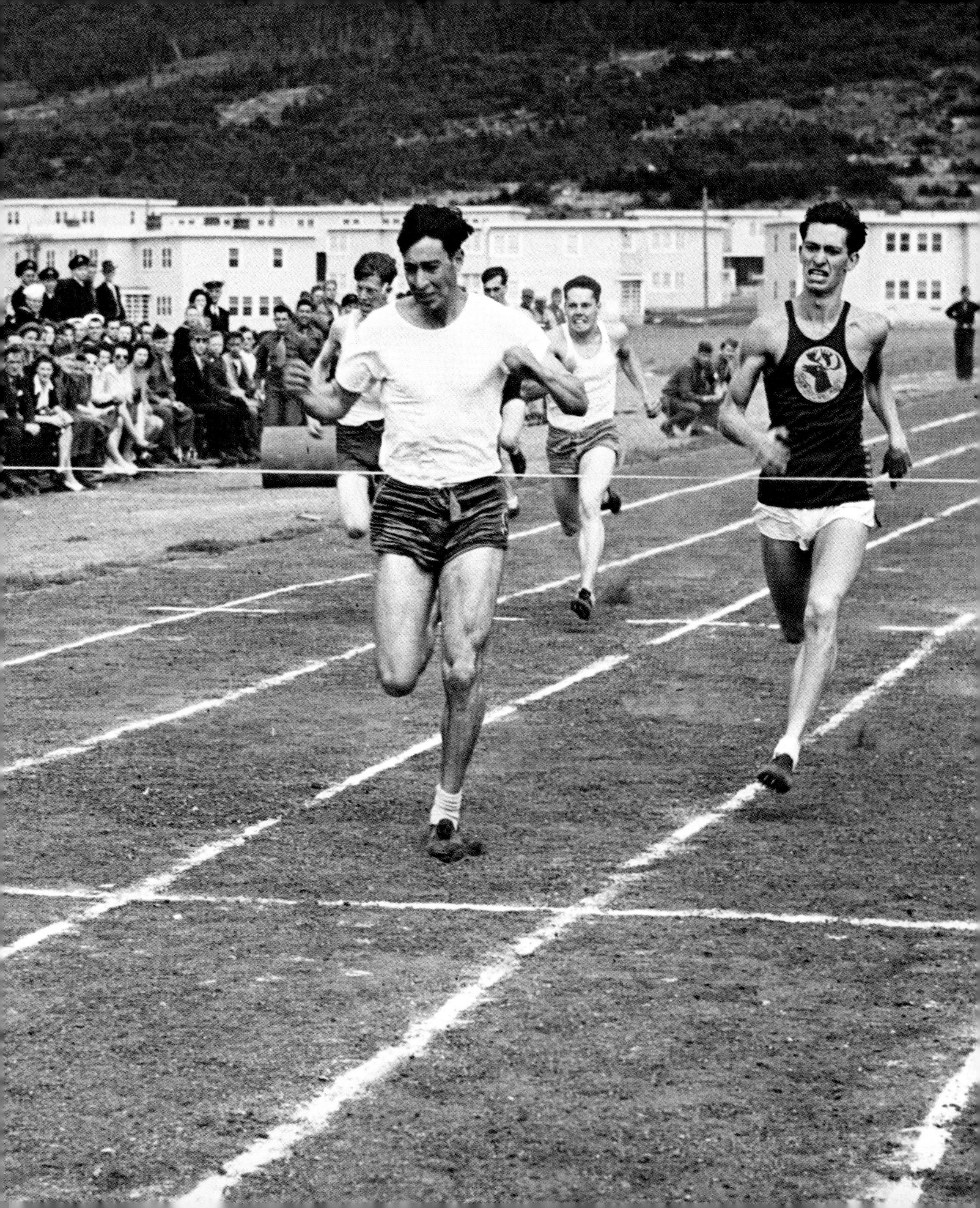

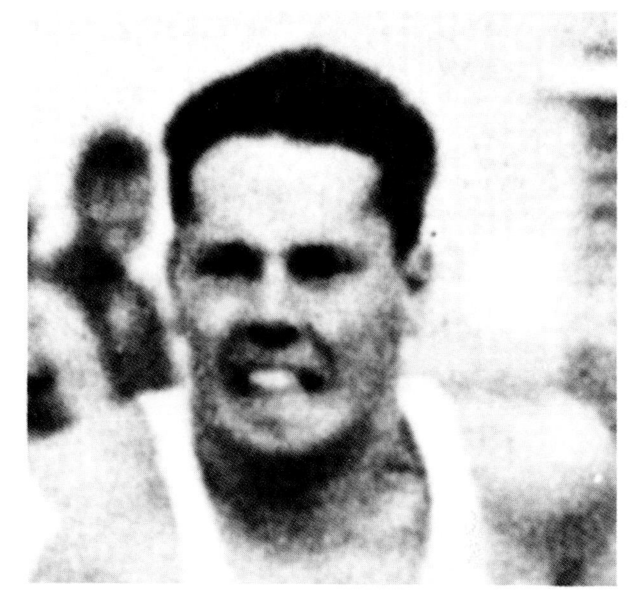

Part Four
Maintaining Health Status

Chapter 7
Personal Health

Physical Fitness

The human body is a mechanical structure unique in that its continued use results in greater efficiency. We know from the training of athletes that if we gradually increase the work load, the body adapts to meet the increased demands by anatomical and physiological changes of its organ systems, with the result that it functions more efficiently. For example, in a trained runner, the heart beats more slowly, yet with greater force, and thereby provides more blood per unit time than the heart of the sedentary person. Oxygen delivery and transport systems become more efficient in reaction to endurance exercises, and programs that are planned for the improvement of muscular strength result in the toughening and strengthening of muscular tissue. The human body was made to be used and therefore thrives on being active.

In our highly mechanized and specialized society, work is often *not* a source of activity. The many appliances used in the home have reduced the level of activity for the housewife. The man at work is often reduced to watching the dials on a machine performing the task that formerly required his physical effort. Some industries have gone so far as to give their employees exercise breaks to encourage activity. In West Germany, industrial concerns have made some efforts to develop broad-scale physical reconditioning programs for thousands of their sedentary workers. The question that physiologists are now faced with is, What happens to an organism that thrives on activity when it is placed in an environment that strongly discourages it? At what level of lowered activity will disfunctions appear in the human mechanism? What form will they take? As expressed by Morehouse, "If man lies too quietly, bones dissolve, pressure reduces circulation causing death of tissues, muscles atrophy, fascia contracts, and neuromuscular and vasomotor coordinations are forgotten. Habitual quiet sitting produces similar, but lesser effects."[1] A great deal of evidence points to inactivity as at least one factor related to cardiovascular disease. The fat American is no doubt one whose caloric intake exceeds caloric output. Overweight is invariably accompanied by a greater susceptibility to a number of diseases and a shortened life-span. In recent years, the increases in mortality from cardiovascular disease among relatively young men have caused particular concern. Numerous studies have indicated a higher incidence of cardiovascular disorder among those in occupations requiring little activity. This factor in combination with emotional stress, cigarette smoking, and overweight often proves to be lethal. The need to reverse this trend relates not only to the desirability of increasing longevity of life but to a higher quality of living as well. When young women lack proper muscle tone and strength for such natural functions as childbirth, we begin to realize how basic fitness can be. The vigorous, successful, professional often needs the physical mechanism as well as the mental abili-

[1]Laurence E. Morehouse, "American Living—A Threat to Fitness," *The Journal of Health, Physical Education and Recreation* (September 1956). Reprinted with permission.

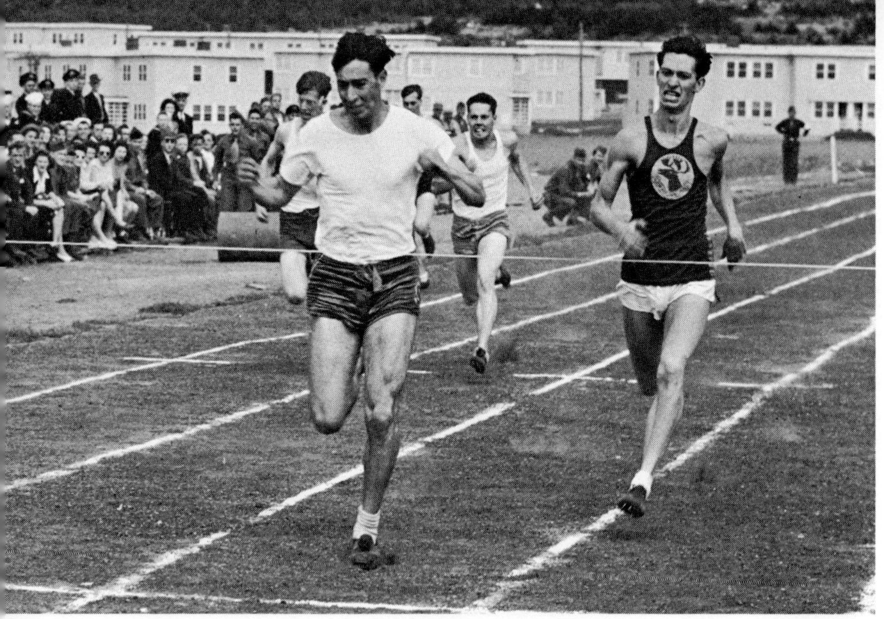

Fig. 7-1. Activities such as track or swimming can produce high levels of physical conditioning. They must, however, be continued in some modified form as the person grows older in order for a reasonable level of fitness to be maintained.

ties to carry on a strenuous schedule of professional activity. While the "tired old man" can be related to the aging process, the "tired young man" can be more closely associated with inactivity and its erosion of youth.

> Suffice it to conclude here that the development of obesity (and of heart disease as well as a number of other pathologic conditions) is to a large extent the result of the lack of foresight of a civilization which spends tens of billions annually on cars, but is unwilling to include a swimming pool and tennis courts in the plans of every high school.[2]

It is a rather fundamental conclusion that the activity once demanded by people's work must now be provided as part of their leisure time activity. There are those who would compound the error by following a leisure time regimen of being among the thousands in the stands or among the millions of home viewers watching the athletes perform. The person who would become a chronic watcher of an activity rather than a participant has developed a disease of civilization known as "spectatoritis."[3] The man who worked in order to support his family and the woman who worked to maintain a home were understandably strongly motivated to do so. Is it possible to have motivations of equal strength related to leisure time activities? The question no doubt presents a challenge to the professionals in the areas of physical education and recreation. The answer appears to lie in those activities that one has developed enough skill and interest in to enjoy. The person who becomes a golf bug hardly needs to be motivated to get out to the golf course. If anything, the problem may be one of getting him home! We are witnessing for example, the largest wave of bicycle popularity in its 154-year history. Greater numbers of people are riding bikes for physical fitness reasons, or in other cases the bike is being used by environmentalists as a partial solution to our pollution problems. It makes little difference whether the motivations stem from wanting to strengthen one's internal environment or to cleanse our external environment—the results are laudatory.

Those, on the other hand, who participate in activities because "it's good for me" are placing exercise in the category of a pill. Perhaps this is reflective of a society that is leaning toward attitudes encouraging self-doting and that is overemphasizing its "illnesses" and "unbearable stresses." In the "it's good for me" group are those who exercise on the living room floor to the count of a shoulder-padded television personality. The interest in this "game" is usually short-lived. There are also those who visit "health" clubs for a dosage of fitness. Fitness cannot be prescribed. It is often best attained as the side effect of one's intense interest in one or preferably several kinds of physical activity. Many of our present-day gropings for exercise and fitness appear to be inappropriate, with "commercialized exercise" being packaged and sold. The result is the loss of those satisfactions that should be derived from phys-

[2]Jean Mayer, *Overweight* (Englewood Cliffs, N.J.: Prentice-Hall, 1968), p. 83.
[3]A term coined by Dr. Jay B. Nash.

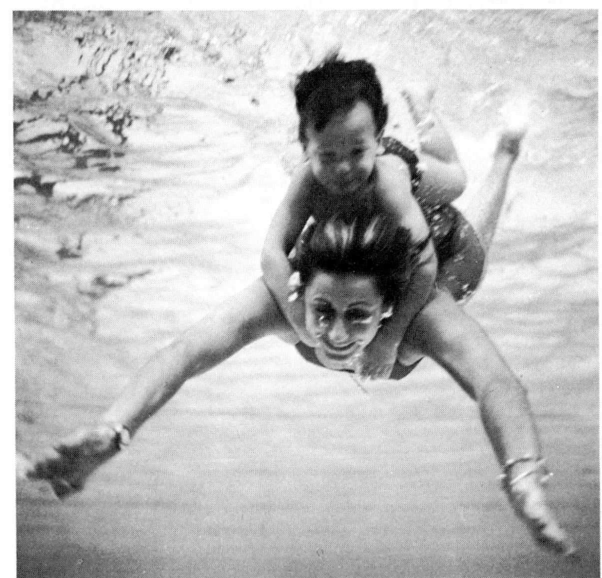

Fig. 7-2. Some activities can be pursued all of one's life. A key to success is learning skills early. (WHO Photo—Paul Almasy)

ical accomplishment. The skill of the fencer, the persistence of the runner, the tenaciousness of the mountain climber, the freedom of the camper are lost to those who would buy fitness by the dollar. Lost also are the exhilarations of the baseball well hit, the bowling ball well delivered, the swimming stroke executed with power and grace. These results lead one to question the misguided motivations and depths of interest of those who would "purchase" exercise.

Physical Education Needs

Physical education programs aimed at developing those skills that can be used after the age of 30 can make a major contribution to the present and future fitness of its participants. While big-muscle sports, like basketball, baseball, and football, are fine they do not represent lifelong kinds of activity. We are all too familiar with the college varsity athlete who graduates and suddenly finds himself divorced from the source of intense activity that once occupied major portions of his time. If his work requires that he function from behind a desk, his life could become a very sedentary one with the usual weight gain and deconditioning of muscles.

Physical education and recreation programs should include activities such as swimming, tennis, badminton, volleyball, handball, as well as other activities that can be used for most if not all of one's life. The success of such programs may be measured not only by proficiency of performance in a formal class but the degree to which the individual uses these activities as part of his pattern of living.

As part of the space program, a mechanism is being developed to keep the heart muscles of astronauts in good condition during long voyages in the gravity-free atmosphere of space. The lower portion of the body is placed in the mechanism. Air forced out by the device creates a partial vacuum around the lower body and limbs. This results in the drawing of blood into the lower portion of the body by the higher air pressure on the upper torso. The heart thus has to work to pump the blood to the upper parts of the body. This results in a work load comparable to that created by the earth's gravity. Without such a mechanism an astronaut's heart might become so deconditioned after a long space voyage that his return to the earth's atmosphere would create too great a work load for his heart.

In the absence of meaningful motivations for activity, is there the possibility that such devices, when perfected, might be used for men on earth? There has also been developed and patented a device which enables the person to "exercise" while reading a book or watching television. The mechanism electrically stimulates the skeletal muscles and is claimed to increase their tone. Those inclined toward ease and comfort may view automated exercise with some delight. The ever-ingenious athletic coach may see possibilities for such mechanisms in producing finer conditioned athletes. Some observers of the American scene have hopes that the advanced technology that created our "soft" living and its ensuing problems will also provide the devices of automated exer-

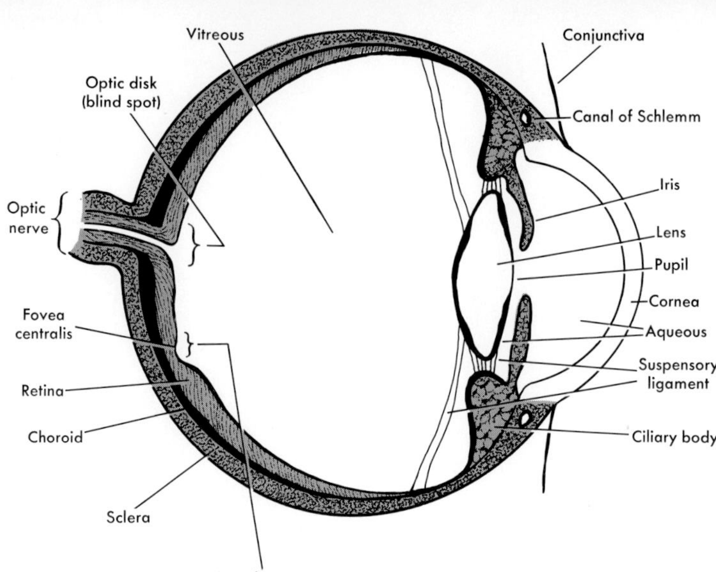

Fig. 7-3. Horizontal section of right eyeball.
(The American Optometric Association)

cise that will correct them. Others feel that the best advice that can be followed in our present state of knowledge is, "Run, for your life!"

Vision

The eye is essentially a mechanical structure that can record images and pass them on to the brain for interpretation. What we see is therefore not solely dependent on the eyes. This is exemplified by the old saying, "There are none so blind as those who will not see." The wide range of interpretation that can be given to what is seen is influenced by emotions, position in life, sociological factors, and so on. One need only observe the opposite "interpretations" of a ball player and an umpire after both have watched the same sphere travel a distance of 60 feet. The interpretations given to the flight of that ball may differ widely enough to start a violent argument. Granting that the vision passed on to the brain is subject to varied judgments, let us first study the eye as the exacting, marvelous structure that it is. We can then leave for later conjecture the colorations that man gives to precise images and the kind of care he is capable of giving to structures he has limited ability to repair and can never replace.

The Structure of the Eye

The eye is an optical instrument often compared with a camera. Its walls are made up of three layers. The outer protective layer is the sclera, referred to as the "white" of the eye. In the front of the eye the sclera is transparent and is called the cornea. The middle coat is the choroid, which contains blood vessels, pigment, muscles, and nerve tissue. In front, the choroid forms the iris, the colored part of the eye which controls the amount of light entering it. This control is accomplished by two sets of muscles that enlarge or make smaller the opening in the iris. The third layer is the retina. Receptors known as rod cells and cone cells make up the retina. The rod cells perceive light while the cone cells perceive color and detail. The cone cells occur in greater numbers in the center of the eye. One effect of this arrangement is that a person needs to look more directly at an object in order to perceive its color. The rod cells are found in greater concentration on the outer parts of the retina. The macula is located in the very center of the retina and is the area of greatest visual acuity because the light rays are generally focused onto it by the lens. The image picked up by the retina is transmitted by the optic nerve to the visual centers of the brain.

The point where the optic nerve enters the eye is called the blind spot. There are no rods and cones in this area, so vision in this spot is not possible. In a two-eyed person the blind spot of each eye is not significant, because the fields of vision of the two eyes overlap. In a one-eyed person, however, the blind spot could mean not seeing a child at a distance of 30 feet. At twice that distance it could blot out something as large as a car. To demonstrate the presence of the blind spot, close the left eye and stare at the square below with your right eye. Bring the book slowly closer to your eye. At a distance of about

Fig. 7-4. Test for blindspot.

9 inches, the circle will disappear from view. You may repeat this by gazing at the circle with the left eye and closing the right eye.

The aqueous humor, found in the forward chamber of the eye, is a clear fluid which carries nutrient material to the tissues of the lens and cornea. It also helps the cornea to maintain its proper curvature. The vitreous humor, found in the chamber behind the lens is a jelly-like material that gives the eye its shape.

The lens of the eye is a double convex, transparent structure that focuses on near and far objects by changing its shape. This ability is referred to as *accommodation.* The ability of the eye lens to accommodate is greatest in childhood and diminishes with age. This is why five-year-olds can sit so close to a television set without visual distress. The distress is with the parents who have diminished power of accommodation and cannot understand how a child can perform such a feat without eyestrain. Change in the shape of the lens is effected by the action of the ciliary muscles. Contraction of the ciliary muscles results in a relaxation of the ligament surrounding the lens, thus causing the lens to thicken. This permits the eye to focus on nearby objects. When the ciliary muscles relax, the reverse occurs and the eye can focus on distant objects.

Refractive Errors

In *myopia* (or *nearsightedness*), the light rays come to focus in front of the retina, making it difficult to see distant objects distinctly. This condition tends to develop some time after the fourth year of life. As the eye grows in size, myopia will develop if the focusing apparatus of the eye is not equipped to bring light rays to a focus over this greater distance. As the size of the eye continues to grow with the development of the child, the myopia becomes progressive until growth levels off at approximately eighteen to twenty years of age. Though the exact cause of myopia is unknown, it is generally considered to be related to structural development and part of the growth process. A strong hereditary tendency is involved in this condition. When one parent is myopic, 60 per cent of the children can be expected to be myopic. One study has shown a relationship between the incidence of myopia in children and diets deficient in animal protein.

Two main types of professional men specialize in matters concerning the eye, the optometrist and the ophthalmologist. The *optometrist* is a graduate of a school of optometry. He is licensed in all fifty states to measure visual acuity, to prescribe glasses, and to perform other nonmedical measures. He is not a medical doctor and is therefore not trained to treat diseases of the eye.

The *ophthalmologist* (oculist) is a medical doctor who has specialized in ophthalmology. He is qualified to treat all conditions of the eye. He is licensed not only to measure for visual acuity, but to treat diseases of the eye and to perform eye surgery.

The relationship of eye exercises and myopia has been an issue between some optometrists, who claim that eye exercises can significantly correct myopic conditions, and ophthalmologists who see no evi-

Fig. 7-5. ***A.*** *The Normal Eye;* ***B.*** *The Myopic Eye;* ***C.*** *The Hyperopic Eye;* ***D.*** *The Hyperopic Eye—Accommodating.*

The Normal Eye

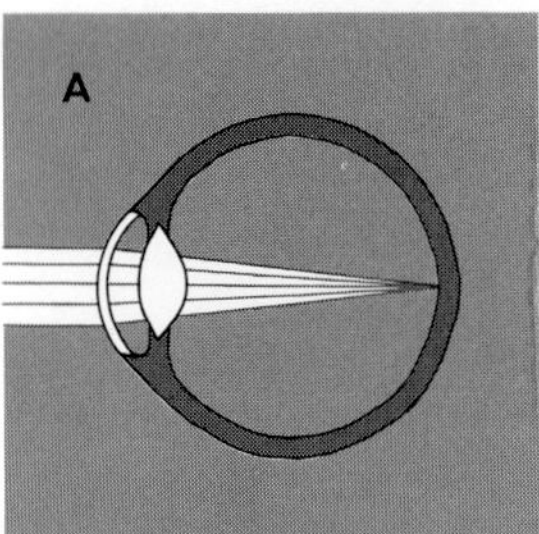

Parallel rays of light (from a distant object) are focused on the retina

The Myopic Eye — (Elongated Eye)

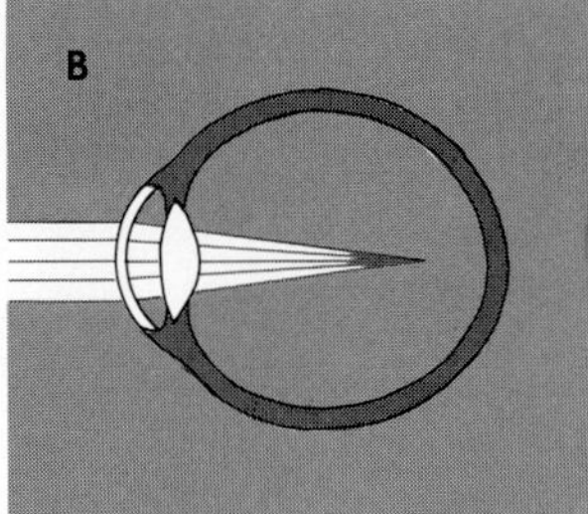

Parallel rays of light focus in front of the retina (distant objects are not in sharp focus)

The Hyperopic Eye (Short Eye)

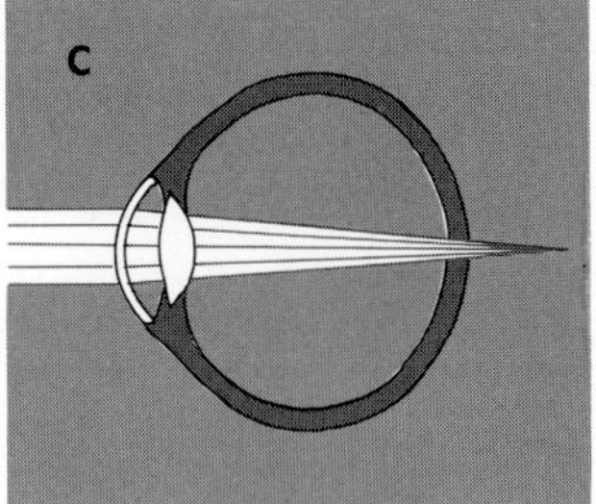

Parallel rays of light come to a focus behind retina

The Hyperopic Eye — Accommodating

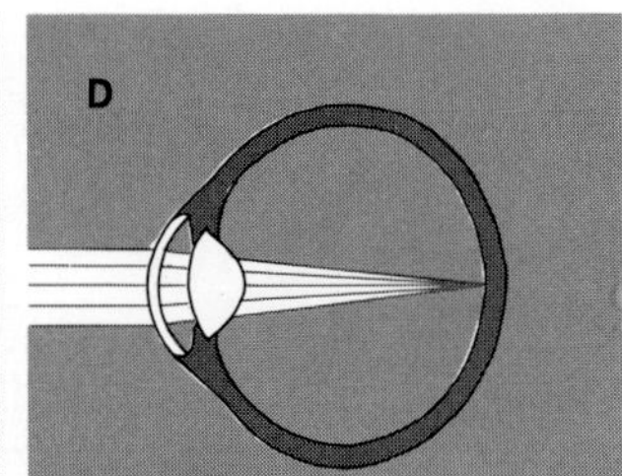

Parallel rays of light are brought to a focus on the retina by accommodation (lens becomes thicker, thus increasing its refractive power)

dence for such a claim. Recently a group of ophthalmologists, with the cooperation of optometrists, undertook research in an effort to determine the value of such visual training. The results indicated that 20 per cent of the cases showed some improvement in reading ability but no change in the degree of myopia. A conclusion reached was that one could learn through experience to interpret and fill in the incomplete or blurred images when the myopic correction by glasses was discontinued. The ophthalmologists in the study therefore decided that visual training (eye exercises) had no value in the treatment of myopia. The condition, however, can be corrected by eyeglasses with concave lenses.

Another factor related to myopia is the greater tendency of myopes to develop detached retinas. For this reason they sometimes are advised by ophthalmologists to avoid contact sports.

In *hyperopia* (or *farsightedness*), the light rays tend to come to a focus behind the retina. This occurs when the eyeball is too short for the focusing mechanism of the eye. Though children are usually born hyperopic, they are generally not bothered by the condition because of their great ability to accommodate. The need for glasses in hyperopia would therefore depend on whether the continuous use of accommodation is causing discomfort and fatigue. Dislike of close work, complaints of dizziness, headache, and nausea are some of the symptoms that might appear. Where correction is necessary, eyeglasses with convex lenses are used. In most cases, as the child grows, the eyeball lengthens and the focal point in the eye returns to the retina.

In *presbyopia,* the lens loses some of its elasticity and thereby its ability to focus, particularly on near objects. This condition is often associated with middle age. The person usually finds that he has to hold the newspaper or phone book farther and farther away in order to read it. The inflexibility of the eye lens and its resultant inability to focus on objects is thereby compensated for by the bifocal eyeglasses. Bifocal lenses are used to correct the condition with the upper lenses in these eyeglasses used for viewing distant objects and the lower lenses used for reading or other close work.

Astigmatism results in the blurring of vision because of an improper curvature of the cornea or the lens, and represents the most common type of refractive error. The improperly shaped cornea or lens creates visual distortions, such as those seen in wavy panes of glass. Astigmatism can occur in combination with hyperopia or myopia, although its causes are not related to these conditions. It can be corrected by specially ground lenses that will eliminate the distortions arising from this structure defect.

Vision Testing

The most common screening test used is the *Snellen Visual Acuity Test.* 20/20 vision on this test indicates normal vision and the ability to read letters of a given size at 20 feet. 20/40 vision refers to the ability to read letters of a larger size at 20 feet that the normal eye can read at 40 feet. Therefore, 20/200 vision represents the ability to read a letter of an even larger size at 20 feet when the normal eye can

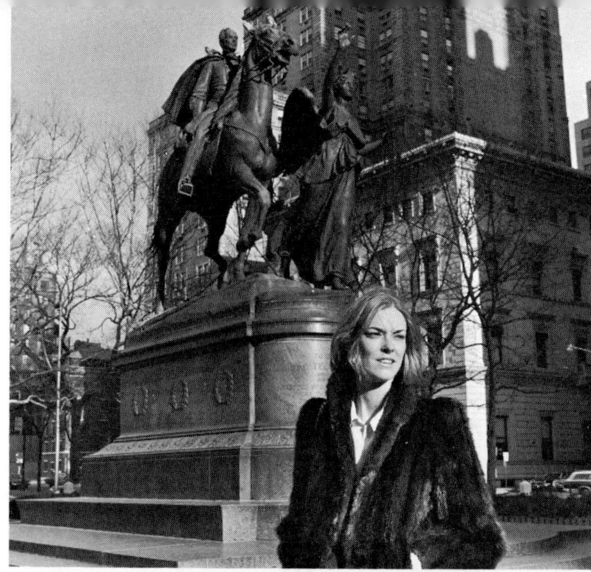

Fig. 7-6. *Normal vision. Both near and far objects are in focus. (N.Y. Eye and Ear Infirmary by J. P. Goeller)*

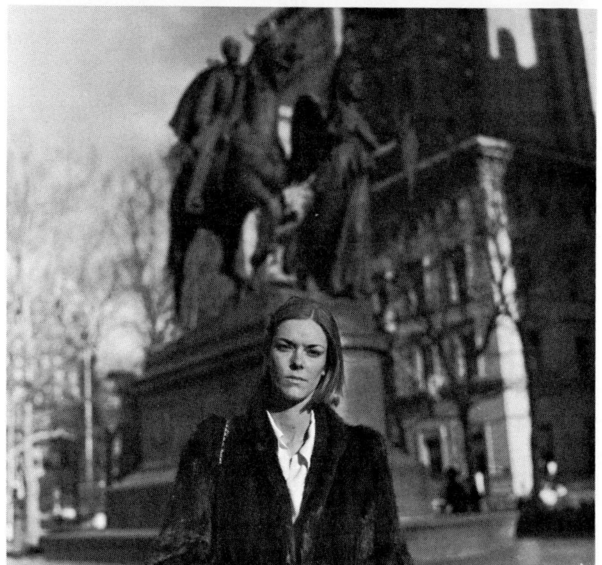

Fig. 7-7. *Myopia (nearsightedness). Near object is in focus, far objects are not. (N.Y. Eye and Ear Infirmary by J. P. Goeller)*

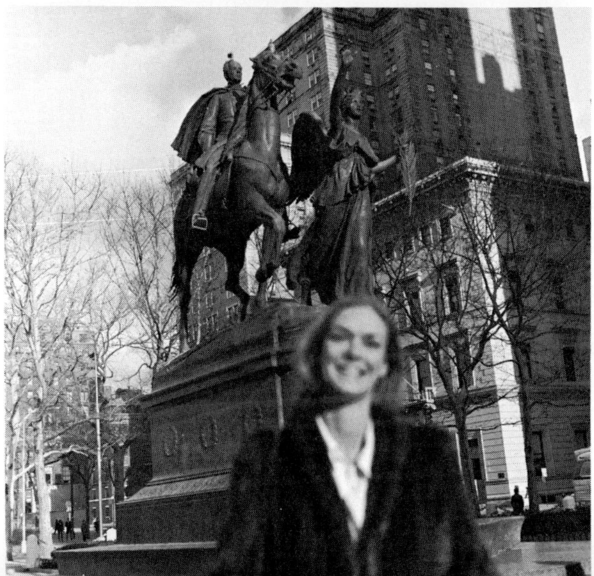

Fig. 7-8. *Hyperopia (farsightedness). Far objects are in focus, near object is not. (N.Y. Eye and Ear Infirmary by J. P. Goeller)*

read it at 200 feet. This test can identify myopia when the individual's vision indicates visual acuity of 20/40 or more.

Hyperopia can be tested for by having the individual look at the Snellen Chart through a plus lens. If the person can read the 20-foot line while looking through a plus lens, he is hyperopic. The 20-foot line would look blurred to the normal eye when this type of testing lens is utilized.

A significant difference in the visual acuity of one eye as compared with that of the other could be an indication of strabismus (crossed eye). It must be

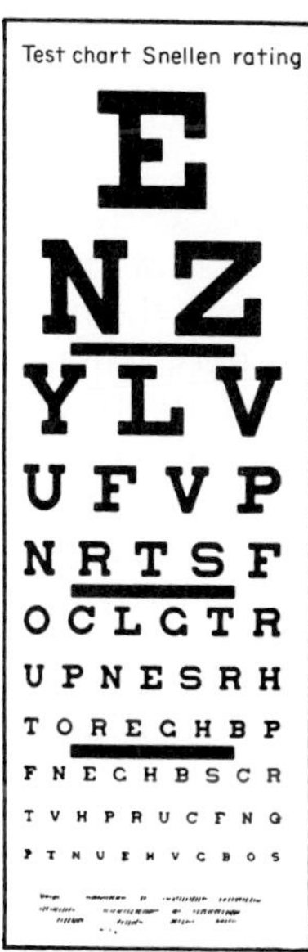

Fig. 7-9. *A Snellen chart. (Bausch and Lomb Optical Co.)*

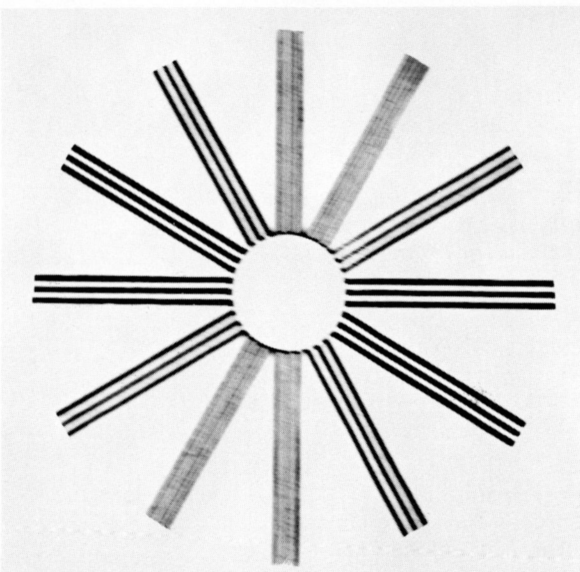

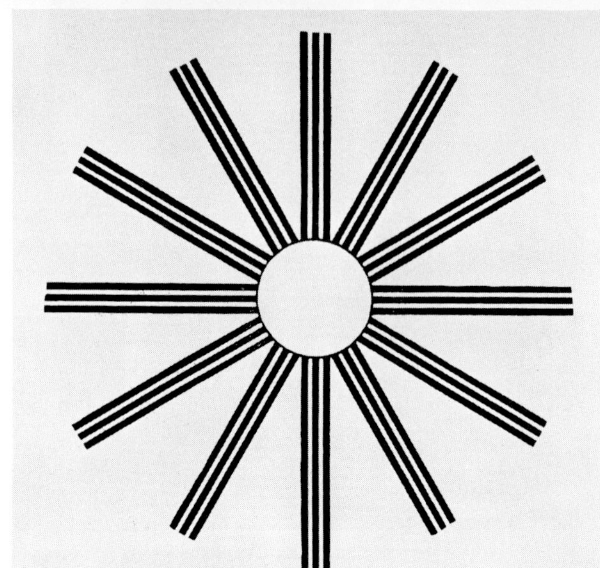

emphasized that the Snellen Visual Acuity Test is merely a screening device. For a complete eye examination one should see one's ophthalmologist (oculist).

The test for astigmatism is positive if the spokes of a wheel are not straight or look gray. If the spokes are straight and all of the same black intensity, the person is not astigmatic.

Eyeglasses

Eyeglasses compensate wholly or in part for refractive errors of the eye. Their function is corrective, and not therapeutic. A person who does not wear his glasses will not ruin his eyes any more than a person wearing them will cure his refractive error. Eyeglasses correct refractive errors to varying degrees while they are worn. This seems to be reason enough to wear them.

Safety lenses are eyeglass lenses that have been heat-hardened by being exposed to a temperature of 1300 degrees F. The result is that the lenses will not break as easily, and should they be broken the edges of the broken lens will not be as sharp.

In 1970 the Food and Drug Administration announced its new regulation that all eyeglasses be made of either heat-tempered glass, laminated glass, or plastic lenses. This regulation removed from the market lenses made of crown glass that shatter upon impact into potentially blinding slivers. The thousands of cases of eye injury or blindness because of such lenses is well documented.

A further safety need that still remains is the production of flame-resistant eyeglass frames. While American manufacturers produce flame-resistant frames, foreign-made frames often are made of cellulose nitrate, a highly flammable material. Eyeglass frames made of this material can explode into flames by the person lighting a cigarette or merely leaning over a gas stove burner or barbecue.

An *optician* is the craftsman skilled in the grinding of lenses according to the prescription of the ophthalmologist (oculist) or optometrist and in setting these lenses properly in frames.

Contact Lenses

The concept of the contact lens dates back to 1887, when an artificial eye manufacturer made a simple glass shell to fit over an eye whose lid had been removed. It was later discovered that a phenomenon known as surface tension could hold a properly shaped, moistened glass disk against the surface of the eye. Early experimentation with contacts was directed primarily to the scleral lenses. This larger type of contact lens covers not only the cornea, but most of the sclera (white of the eye). Scleral lenses are used by some individuals whose occupations might lend to the easy dislodging of the smaller corneal lenses. The corneal type contact lens covers the cornea and the iris that lies behind it (covering only the colored portion of the eye). Though the scleral lens has been greatly improved, the corneal lens is by far the more popular. These lenses have

Figs. 7-10 and 7-11. This is a test for astigmatism. The faded and blurred lines in Fig. 7-10 are indicative of astigmatism. Fig. 7-11 should appear dark and clear. If it does not, see your eye doctor! (N.Y. Eye and Ear Infirmary by J. P. Goeller)

also been reduced in thickness to 4/1000 of an inch. With the advent of plastics in the early 1950's, and the concept of an individualized curved lens, comfort has increased and the popularity of contact lenses has soared. Today it is estimated that 7 million Americans own contact lenses.

The motivation for the use of contact lenses is usually cosmetic in nature (improved appearance). Contact lenses also offer advantages in certain occupations and activities. Surgeons, actors, musicians, policemen, and other outdoor workers may find them advantageous because they do not fog up or get wet in the rain or reflect stage lights. Contact lenses can also provide a better correction for severe myopia than regular eyeglasses. They also correct corneal astigmatism more effectively because they replace the distorted surface of the cornea with a properly shaped one.

Research conducted by the Food and Drug Administration in 1964 and several independent studies published in medical journals have noted that numerous eye injuries result from the use of contact lenses. The difficulties are caused basically by improper fitting of lenses, unsanitary practices by the wearer resulting in infections, and wearing of the lenses for too long a time. A moment of forgetfulness, as in going to sleep without removing the lenses, can result in permanent damage to the eyes. In a study conducted by Dr. William Stone, almost 50,000 lens users were surveyed. He found that six eyes were removed because of infections caused by the lenses, seven had vision permanently reduced to less than 20/200, and another required a corneal transplant. A few hundred suffered less serious injuries that were corrected with the discontinued use of the contact lenses.

Because properly fitting lenses are of utmost importance if eye injury is to be avoided, identifying the skilled practitioners in this field is essential. The two kinds of professionals qualified to prescribe contact lenses are those selected ophthalmologists or optometrists who do a good deal of work in this area. These should be individuals who have had specific training in the fitting of contact lenses. When in doubt, a person may write to the Contact Lens Association of Ophthalmologists, 40 West 77th Street New York, New York 10024, or the American Optometric Association, 7000 Chippewa Street, St. Louis, Missouri 63119, for the name of an experienced practitioner in his locale.

Regardless of how well a person may be fitted with contact lenses, not all people can wear them. People with chronic infection or inflammation of the eyes or eyelids are poor candidates. People with allergies or other disorders that make the eyes water would also do well to avoid them. There is a period of discomfort and adjustment that the wearer must go through in being fitted for these lenses. Contact lenses are, after all, foreign bodies that are placed in the eyes and they take some getting used to. It is during this initial period of use that close professional supervision is necessary. Pain that the wearer may experience can be normal reaction to the lenses or may be indicative of a poor fit, damage to the cornea, or a given person's inability to wear such lenses.

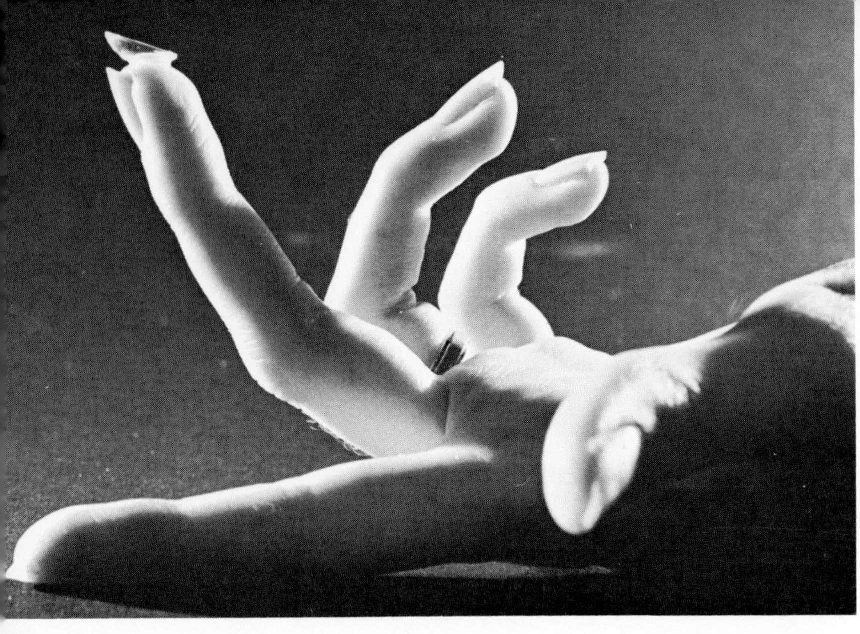

Fig. 7-12. A soft contact lens. (Consumers Union)

Sanitary handling of contact lenses is essential to avoid infection. Before each insertion, the wearer should wash his hands carefully and wash the lenses in a wetting agent and under tap water. After each removal, the lenses need to be stored in a special case.

Some practitioners contend that contact lenses have a therapeutic effect on refractive errors of the eye. To date, this contention is without substantive evidence.

> The small, but real, danger of eye damage from wearing contacts, the expense and inconvenience of getting properly fitted, the discomfort of adjusting, the need for regular checkups, the care required in use, and the strong possibility of losing lenses are all major disadvantages the potential wearer should consider carefully before buying.[4]

In fact, it has been determined that of the Americans who purchase hard contact lenses, half of them give up the battle and go back to eyeglasses.

The appearance of the *soft* contact lens in 1971 promised new hope.[5] The soft lens is made from a water-absorbing plastic that is soft and pliable when moist and hard and brittle when dry. They are slightly larger than the hard contact lenses (soft lenses range in diameter 12.3–15.5 millimeters; hard lenses range in diameter 8–10.2 millimeters) and are invisible on the eye. The soft lenses are more comfortable to use, particularly at the beginning. They adhere better to the eye and do not fall out as easily as the hard contact lenses and they allow the individual to switch back to regular eyeglasses with little or no blurring of vision. They have been highly effective in treating diseases of the eye, either in using them as "bandages" for the cornea or by impregnating them with medication for the treatment of glaucoma. They have also been successfully used on infants and young children who underwent cataract surgery and heretofore could not tolerate the hard contact lenses.

The soft lenses now available to the public correct for myopia only. Experimental lenses for hyperopia and aphakia (removal of the lens resulting from cataract surgery) are being tested. Soft lenses are not as effective in treating astigmatism as the hard lens, since the soft lens takes the shape of the cornea and becomes almost as irregular as the cornea it covers. For those individuals with a combined myopia-astigmatism, they will have success correcting the myopia, but will continue to be astigmatic.

The cost of the soft lens is about $100 more than the hard contact lens and up to $300 more than for regular eyeglasses. A major drawback with the current soft lenses is the nightly 15-minute sterilization procedure to keep the lenses free of bacteria. Another concern is the possibility that soft lenses might absorb harmful vapors or fumes from paint sprays, tear gas, smoke, hair spray, or industrial chemicals. If an individual without glasses came in contact with

[4] "Contact Lenses—Can You Buy Them Safely?" *Consumer Reports* (Mount Vernon, N.Y.: Consumers Union, March 1967).

[5] The following discussion of soft contact lenses has been adapted from "Soft Contact Lenses: They Have Their Limitations," *Consumer Reports* (Mount Vernon, N.Y.: Consumers Union, May 1972), pp. 272–278. Copyright © 1972 by Consumers Union.

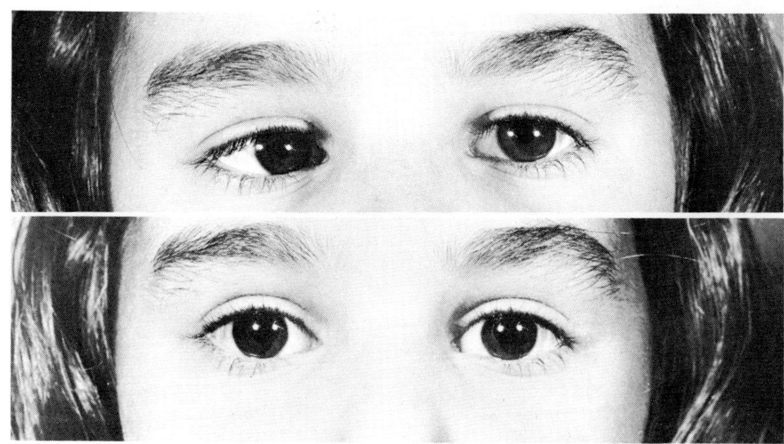

Figs. 7-13 and 7-14. A child with strabismus (crossed-eye) before and after treatment. (Today's Health)

Fig. 7-15. Double vision as it would appear to a person with a crossed eye. (N.Y. Eye and Ear Infirmary by J. P. Goeller)

these harmful substances normally the flow of tears would quickly wash them away. However, with the soft contact lens, chemicals may be absorbed and held against the eye until the lens was removed.

Strabismus (Cross-Eyed)

The eyeballs are coordinated in their movements by a set of six muscles for each eye. When a muscle of the eye is not of balanced strength with its counterpart, it will cause a cross-eyed condition (strabismus). There is a hereditary factor associated with the condition. Strabismus occurs in varying degrees of intensity. In some instances, the condition is noted only when the eyes are tired, resulting in a slight wandering of one eye out of position. In the more severe forms, an eye is in a fixed misaligned position. The crossed-eye is usually turned inward or outward, although there are other possibilities. Double vision is an effect of this condition. As a result, the individual suppresses the vision of the crossed eye as a way of eliminating the double image. Eventually, this will result in the loss of sight in this eye. Experience has shown that children do not outgrow this condition and that it should be treated early. If it is ignored until after eight years of age, considerable, if not complete, visual loss can be expected in the crossed eye. Strabismus can be corrected by prescribing special glasses, by exercising eye muscles, by placing a patch over the good eye (forcing the crossed eye to straighten), or by performing surgery on the eye muscles. In the latter cases, the shortening of the weaker muscle through

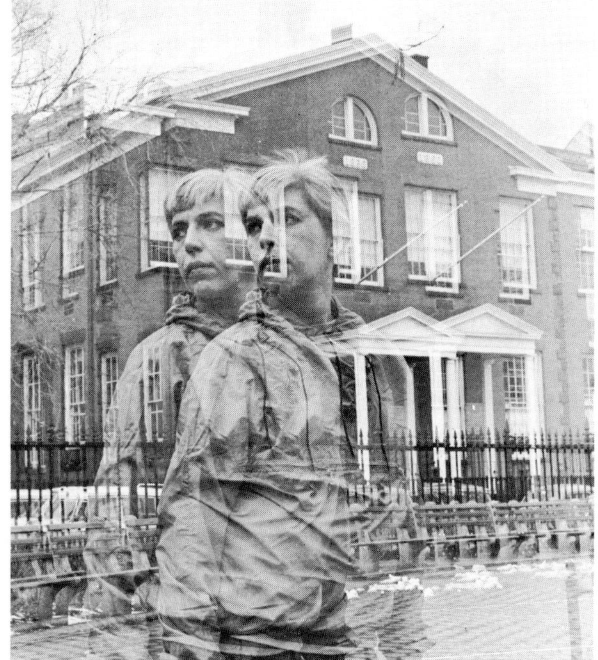

surgery will straighten the eye. When the child fails to receive early medical attention for strabismus, the resultant loss of vision in one eye handicaps the individual in several ways. He will have a narrowed field of vision, a blind spot in the good eye that cannot be compensated for, and the inability to perceive depth accurately (that is, to judge the distance of objects from oneself). Our depth perception is the

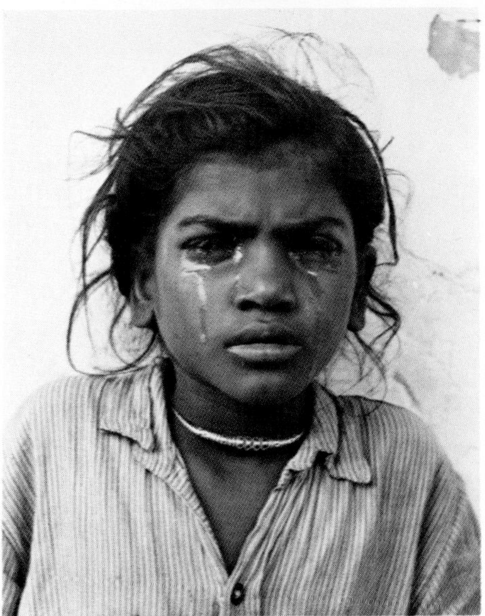

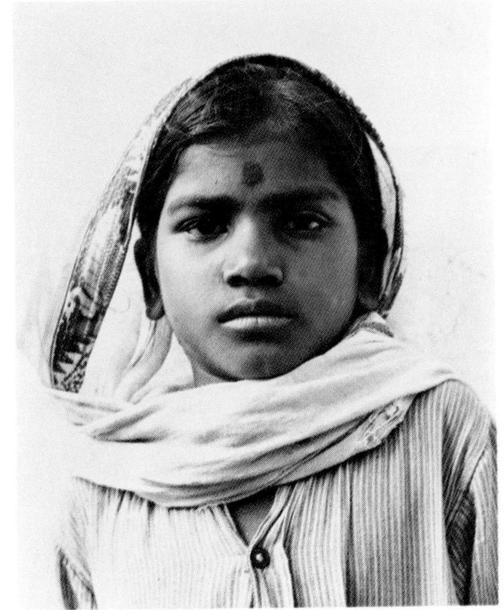

result of our binocular vision. To demonstrate this, one need only place a book on its side. Closing one eye, attempt to bring the forefinger down on the front edge of the book. You will find that you can perform this task more accurately with both eyes open. In the late teens, some people have crossed eyes straightened for cosmetic reasons. This does not, however, correct the visual loss, which is usually considerable by this time, if not complete.

Detachment of the Retina

A conservative estimate is that one person in 20,000 suffers from a detachment of the retina. Two out of three cases occur in persons with a high degree of myopia. Blows to the head are also recognized as contributing factors.

In the past, a detached retina meant blindness in the eye or eyes affected. At the present time there are several methods of treatment available. So called "shallow" detachments may be treated by using the xenon arc or the laser beam. In more extensive detachments a variety of surgical techniques may be used. Critical to the success of any treatment procedure is the length of time that elapses from when the detachment occurs to when treatment is sought. The retina is basically made up of nerve tissue and constantly needs a source of nourishment if it is not to degenerate further.

Recent research indicates that about 6 per cent of the population of the United States show certain degeneration or holes in the retina. Many of these include apparently healthy people. It seems likely that a prevention measure that will be increasingly used in the future is that of photocoagulation involving the use of the xenon arc or laser beam. This procedure will strengthen the retinal attachments around these weakened areas. Such preventive treatment would only take place after careful clinical examination by the eye specialist.

Diseases of the Eye

Trachoma is a chronic infection of the lids caused by a filterable virus. This is the most widespread infection of the eye and the leading cause of blindness in the world. It is not prevalent in the United States, but can be found in countries with low standards of living and unsatisfactory sanitary conditions. It responds readily to sulfonamides and antibiotics. In the absence of treatment, the virus attacks the conjunctiva and cornea of the eye. The World Health Organization has been active in combating this disease by establishing community clinics, dispensing antibiotics, and educating the people in the endemic areas.

"Pink-Eye" is an infection or inflammation of the conjunctiva. It is an acute, highly contagious infection. It readily responds to treatment and can be cleared in two days or linger for two weeks if untreated, thereby remaining a source of infection for an extended period of time. Dust, smoke, and powders can also cause the inflammation of the conjunctiva. Because of its highly contagious nature, the use of a separate face towel is recommended.

Styes are caused by bacterial (staphylococcal) in-

Figs. 7-16 and 7-17. *A case of trachoma showing some of the effects of the infection and the change as a result of treatment with antibiotics. (World Health Organization Photo by Homer Page)*

fections of the small glands on the margin of the eyelid. Repeated styes reflect a poor state of general health. Medical attention should be sought in such repetitive cases or when the stye becomes quite painful.

Cataract is the development of an opacity of the eye lens or the capsule in which it is enclosed. It is *not* a growth. The disease often progresses slowly, and when the lens can no longer be seen through, vision is restored by the surgical removal of the lens. Eyeglasses are then used to replace the removed eye lens. In Europe, some experimentation has sought to replace the eye lens with a plastic lens inserted in the aqueous humor in front of the iris. Cataracts may be caused by injury or by diseases such as glaucoma, diabetes, and prenatal exposure to German measles. Two-thirds of occurring cataract conditions, however, are from unknown causes.

Glaucoma. There are two types of glaucoma: the acute type and the chronic. The acute type is characterized by sudden onset and extreme pain, with the eyeballs becoming stony hard. Surgery for this type of the disease must be performed promptly, usually within 24 to 48 hours in order to prevent blindness. The chronic or insidious version of the condition is the more common type. Symptoms include headaches, nausea, and the seeing of colored halos around lights. The symptoms are frequently vague and go unnoticed until irreversible damage to the retina has occurred. In glaucoma, increased fluid develops pressure within the eyeball which can cause the destruction of the retina and the optic nerve. This disease is a leading cause of blindness in the United States, despite the fact that we know how to detect the condition, treat it, and prevent the ensuing blindness. Early detection of glaucoma is important, because the progress of the disease can be arrested through treatment with drugs or surgery. It is estimated that 2 per cent of the population over 40 years of age has developing glaucoma. The incidence tends to rise sharply in the 50- to sixty-year-old age groups. Periodic examination of the eyes by an ophthalmologist should include the testing of fluid pressure with a tonometer. This is recommended as a preventive measure, particularly for people over 40.

Color Vision

Varying wave lengths of light give us color. This was demonstrated by Sir Isaac Newton, when he passed a colorless beam of light through a prism and split it into seven colors or wavelengths, (red, orange, yellow, green, blue, indigo, and violet). Our ability to perceive these varying wavelengths of light depends upon the cones which are located almost exclusively in the macula of the retina. Defective color vision (color blindness) results from the inability of the cones of the retina to perceive all colors. The degree of this inability varies from complete color blindness to difficulty distinguishing one shade of color from another. The defect is hereditary, with 1 male out of every 25 and 1 female out of every 200 affected. There is no way of correcting the defect. Color perception tests are usually administered in schools to determine if defective color vision is present and to what degree. The most common color vision defect found is the inability to distinguish red from green; blue-yellow defective perception is the next most common. Defective color vision can be an inhibiting factor where employment is concerned. Occupations in which the ability to identify color accurately is important are best avoided by people with this defect.

Sunglasses

Sunglasses may be worn to diminish discomfort from sunlight of high intensity. They should not be worn to eliminate headlight glare, because when they are worn at twilight or in darkness they can blot out enough vision to constitute a safety hazard. The constant use of sunglasses can limit one's ability to tolerate light. Should a person develop the symptoms of photophobia (the inability to tolerate light), it is an indication that medical attention is needed, not sunglasses. Looking directly into the sun even with sunglasses can result in serious damage to the eyes. In spite of warnings via the mass media before each eclipse of the sun, a number of persons do damage to their eyes by looking at the sun through sunglasses or smoked glass. The safest way to watch an eclipse of the sun is via the television set. The use of neutral sunglasses as opposed to colored sunglasses is recommended, because they do not affect color perception.

Night Vision

The ability to see in dimly lighted areas is dependent upon the production of the pigment in the retina called visual purple. Visual purple is bleached by bright lights. Entrance into a dimly illuminated room results in a temporary loss of vision until this pigment is produced in sufficient quantities. The production of visual purple is dependent on an adequate amount of vitamin A in the body. Inadequate amounts of vitamin A can cause night blindness. Vitamin A in excess of that recommended in a satisfactory general diet, however, will not make night vision keener. As indicated in the chapter on nutrition, this kind of deficiency may be more closely related to a bodily inability to absorb vitamin A than to a dietary deficiency. A physician should be consulted in cases of suspected night blindness to determine if the condition exists, and if so, why.

Lighting

Proper lighting for study should be at least 20 footcandles of illumination at the top of the desk. An unshaded 75-watt bulb will provide 9 footcandles of illumination at a distance of 3 feet. The colors of the walls and ceilings of a room will have an influence on lighting because light colors reflect light, and dark colors absorb it. Glare from glossy paper or highly polished furniture can cause a good deal of unnecessary eye strain. Good lighting does not refer merely to an adequate amount of illumination on one's work. It also refers to the avoidance of sharp contrasts in light, such as that produced by a well-lighted desk in a dark room. Contrasts in lighting cause eye fatigue and thereby lessen the effectiveness of one's work and shorten his work period.

PERMISSION TO DONATE EYES*

I ______________________ OF ______________________
(RELATIONSHIP) (DONOR)

DO HEREBY GIVE PERMISSION TO HAVE HIS OR HER EYES DONATED TO THE EYE-BANK FOR SIGHT RESTORATION, INC.
AND/OR ______________________ HOSPITAL
(LEAVE BLANK)

AT THE TIME OF DEMISE.

____
SIGNATURE

TEL. __________ ______________________
ADDRESS

DATE __________ ______________________
WITNESS

*TO BE GIVEN BY NEXT-OF-KIN OR WHOEVER LEGALLY RESPONSIBLE
IDENTIFICATION ON BACK OF CARD

Fig. 7-18. An authorization card to donate one's eyes. (The Eye Bank, New York)

Watching television in a darkened room is a comparable situation that could lead to eye discomfort after a period of time.

Eye Banks

Eye banks have significantly contributed to the reduction of blindness due to damaged corneas. People wishing to contribute their corneas to a blind person need to register with an eye bank sometime during their lives. After the death of a donor, the cornea is removed and within a matter of a few days transplanted to the person in need. Not all transplant operations are successful. A bodily response to injury is to grow small blood vessels in the area to heal the wound. When the "wound" is corneal surgery, the small blood vessels that occasionally grow into the area will cover the new cornea, thus blocking the vision once more. This reaction is called vascularization.

A corneal transplant whereby a clear, healthy cornea replaces a damaged one will restore vision to an affected person. This act literally becomes the gift of sight. Donating one's eyes in a will is not recommended because by the time the will is read, tissues of the cornea are beyond use. Registration with an eye bank is the recommended procedure.

The Visually Handicapped

A person whose vision is 20/70 or less in the good eye after correction (i.e., with eyeglasses) is considered to be visually handicapped. Children whose visual acuity falls into this category are often placed in special classes. They are provided with books with larger print, are taught to use a typewriter early, and in all ways provided a setting that will best facilitate learning.

Blindness is often regarded as the complete loss of sight. *Legal blindness,* however, is commonly defined as 20/200 vision in the good eye after correction, or loss of 80 per cent or more of his visual field. The latter condition is often referred to as tunnel vision. Though a person with tunnel vision may have 20/20 vision in his narrowed visual field, he is considered to be blind. Decisions concerning the giving of financial aid to individuals who are visually handicapped are often based on these definitions.

The adjustments of the blind to their handicap can be extremely difficult. They must learn to read Braille; traveling requires assistance from a seeing eye dog or other people. Even everyday tasks such as preparing meals and moving about one's home require learning. Though a great deal has been written and said about the blind and their adjustment to their handicap, little has been said about the poor adjustment made by seeing people to the blind. A blind person who attempted to be a comedian would be severely handicapped by his lack of vision even though it had nothing to do with his ability to tell jokes. People often seem to be so overwhelmed with the handicap that they become blind themselves to the personality before them. The greatest loss of the blind is often not their vision, but normal interrelationships with "normal" people.

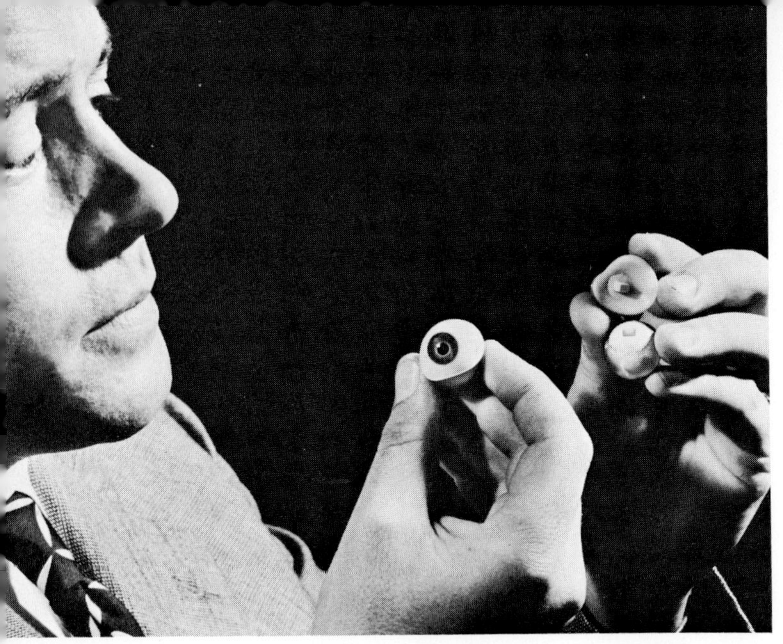

Figs. 7-19 and 7-20. When a person has lost an eye due to accident or disease a helping hand is offered in restoring the person's cosmetic appearance, with a plastic artificial eye. The man in Fig. 7-20 demonstrates how the artificial eye can move with the natural one. This is accomplished by suturing the eye muscles to the mesh surface of the prosthesis. (*American Optical Company*)

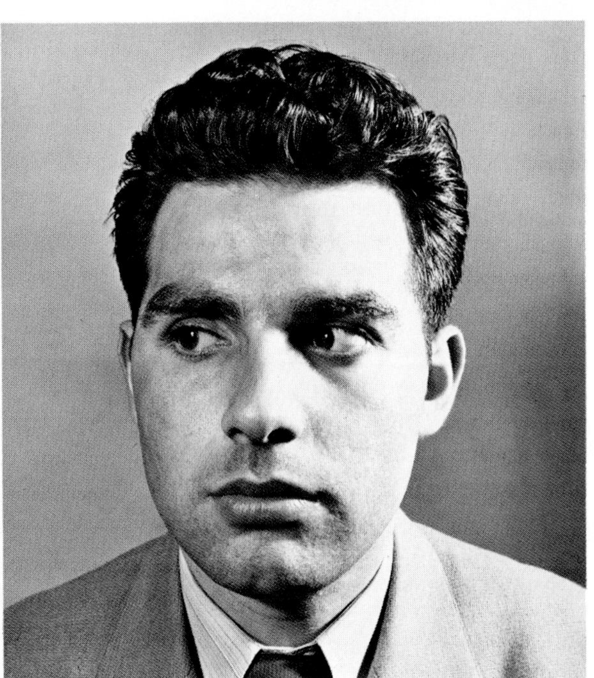

The Artificial Eye

There has been real progress made in the development of artificial eyes for those who lose one of these sense organs. These artificial devices, developed to maintain the cosmetic appearance of the person, can now be made to match the color and size of the person's other eye. In addition, they can be made to move in unison with the real eye.

Hearing

The sense of hearing, though obviously valued by people, is probably underrated in its importance. Our ability to communicate with others depends on it more than on any other of our senses. The loss of hearing immediately transforms the world around us into one of silence and isolates the individual. If one were to sit quietly and listen to all the background noises in the environment (whether in an office of a busy city or sitting on a stump in a wooded area), one would become aware of the many noises one hears but is often not conscious of. We live in a world of sound—sound that is not only a means of communication, but may be a warning of danger, a gauge of emotions, or a spark of humor. The familiar sounds often envelop us in a cloak of security. The ear is the mechanism that serves as the vehicle for this major means of communication. Let us examine its care and functioning.

The Outer Ear

The Pinna, the external part of the outer ear, serves to catch sound and send it into the auditory canal. Because the muscles that control the movement of the pinna in animals are vestigial in man, we do not have the ability to turn the pinna in the direction of sound as do horses or dogs. Instead, we need to turn our head so an ear points in the direction of the sound. A simple experiment to demonstrate this is to have a person close his eyes and point in the direction from which he hears sound. An-

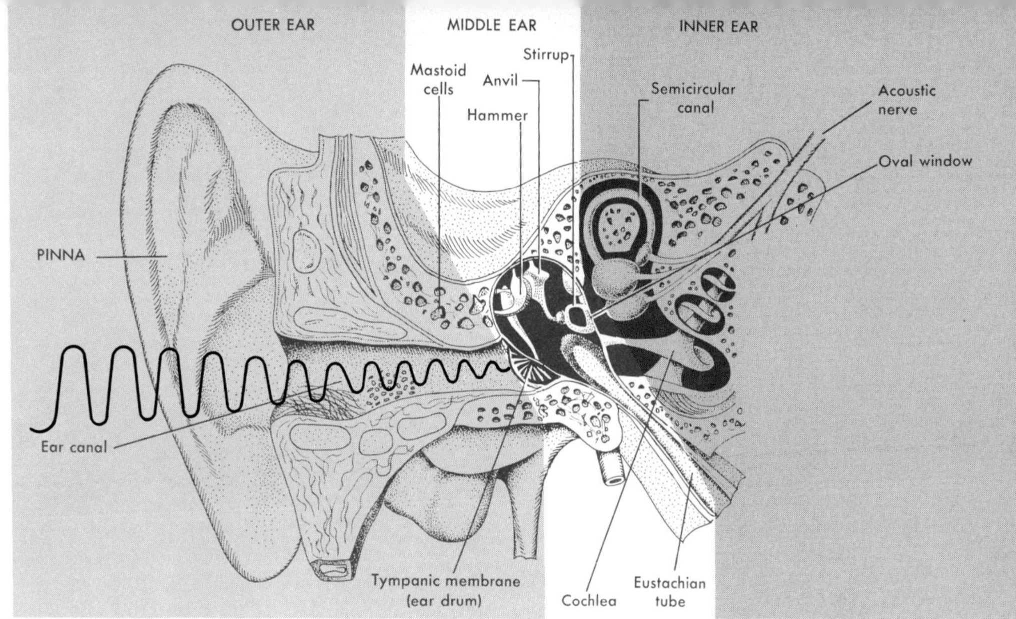

Fig. 7-21. The human ear. (Maico Electronics, Inc.)

other person clicks coins along the person's medial line between the ears, starting at the forehead and ending at the back of the head. The person will make a number of errors in identifying the direction from which these sounds come, though he will have little difficulty with those made to the left or right of the head.

Inside the auditory canals are the glands that produce cerumen, or ear wax. The cerumen not only helps to keep inquisitive insects out of the ears but also has an antiseptic action (with respect to bacteria), thus performing a further protective function. In some instances, an oversecretion of cerumen may block the auditory canal thus affecting the hearing acuity of the individual. In such cases, the cerumen should be removed by a physician. Attempts to remove excess cerumen with hairpins or match sticks may not only push the wax further back into the canal, but may result in damage to the walls of the auditory canal and possible perforation of the eardrum.

The Middle Ear

The Middle Ear is made up of the eardrum (tympanic membrane), the three ear ossicles, hammer (malleus), anvil, (incus), stirrup (stapes), and the eustachian tube. Its function is to conduct sound waves received from the auditory canal to the inner ear. The eustachian tube connects the middle ear to the back of the throat and keeps the air pressure on the inside of the eardrum equal to that on the outside. This permits the eardrum to vibrate properly when sound waves strike it. Anything inhibiting the vibration of the eardrum will affect hearing. Because of the position of the eustachian tube, throat infections can migrate up through it to the middle ear. Blowing of the nose too vigorously when one has a cold can force infectious material into the middle ear, with resulting fuzzy sensation in the ears. Blow gently with both nostrils open! *Middle ear infection* (otitis media) is a leading cause of hearing

Fig. 7-22. Diagram of outer ear. (Maico Electronics, Inc.)

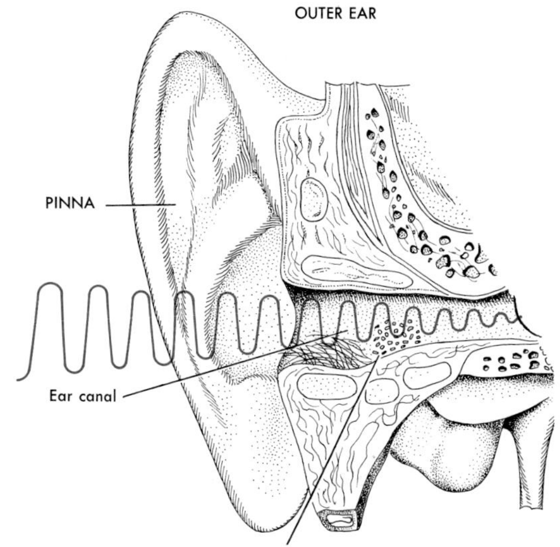

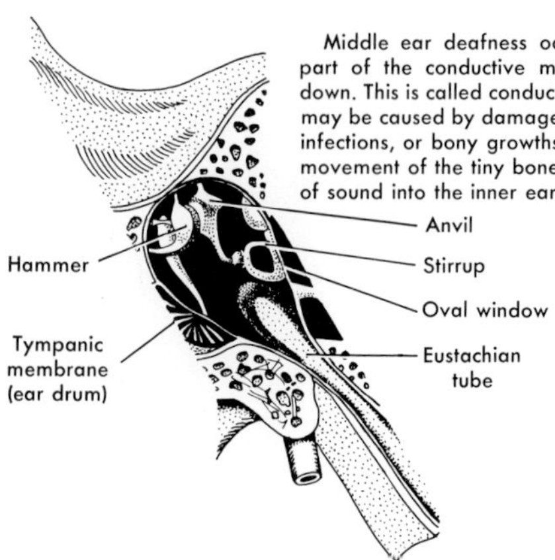

Fig. 7 23. Diagram of middle ear. (Maico Electronics, Inc.)

loss in young people. Infection can damage the ear ossicles, and in some cases completely destroy them. Infectious fluid can also build up in the middle ear cavity. If this is not relieved by medical attention, it may break through the eardrum and result in a draining or "running" ear. Whether hearing is affected by a perforation of the eardrum, or the extent to which it is impaired depends on how badly the eardrum is damaged. A good rule to follow is to have all earaches checked by a physician. The self-medicating use of heat, oils, or other things may relieve the pain but not the infection, and does not prevent ensuing damage.

Damaged eardrums can now be replaced surgically. A surgeon may use the eardrum of a donor as well as the ear bones if necessary and replace the damaged parts of the middle ear. This procedure has been highly successful in restoring hearing to the normal range.

Otosclerosis is a disease or disorder in which calcium deposits cause a fixation of the stapes (stirrup) so that it cannot efficiently conduct vibrations to the inner ear, with a resultant hearing loss. Although this hardening tendency is hereditary and is present at birth, it often does not produce a noticeable hearing impairment until later in life (usually between the ages of 20 and 40 years). It is twice as common in females as in males, and pregnancy may accelerate the process. Both ears are usually affected. The cause of otosclerosis is unknown.

The symptoms of clinical otosclerosis include impaired hearing, tinnitus (head noise), brittle bones, a family history of progressive deafness, a tendency for the hearing loss to increase during pregnancy, and papacusis willisiana, which is the hearing of speech better in a noisy environment than in a quiet one. Diagnosis of otosclerosis may be made with relative certainty in the typical case by history, hearing tests, and otoscopic examinations. The hardening process of otosclerosis may cease at any time and the hearing may remain on a stationary level throughout life. Fortunately, few persons with otosclerosis advance to total deafness. However, in some cases, as this bony hardening continues, it may involve the inner ear mechanism and result in deterioration of the hearing nerve.

As a result of many years of research, two operations have been developed to overcome the obstruction caused by the bony fixation of the stapes. These are known as *stapes mobilization* and the *fenestration* operation. Both operations were done before the turn of the century by European surgeons, but because of the lack of adequate illumination, magnification, and modern drugs to combat infection, these operations were abandoned as being unsatisfactory procedures. Modern instruments and new drugs have reinstated surgery as a corrective measure.

The fenestration operation does not attempt to treat or cure the underlying otosclerotic bone disease. It merely bypasses the obstructed oval window by creating a new window. Done under general anesthesia, the new opening (window) is made in the bone over the inner ear in such a way as to allow the sound vibrations to bypass the fixed stapes area and stimulate the nerve directly through the new window. In approximately 80 per cent of the cases

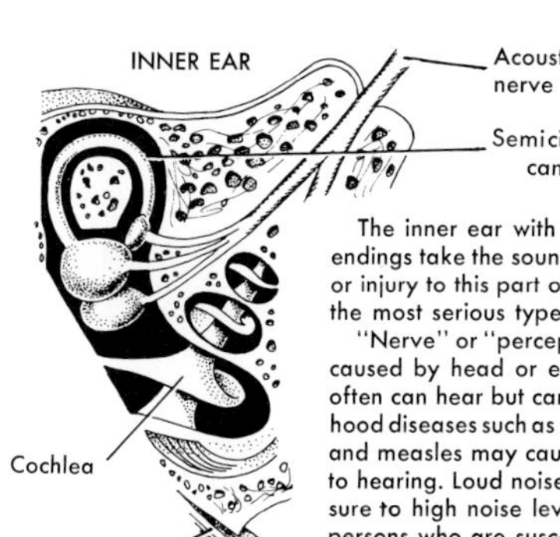

Figure. 7-24. Diagram of inner ear. (Maico Electronics, Inc.)

the patient with otosclerosis who is suitable for fenestration surgery will have his hearing permanently restored to a practical level.

The stapes mobilization operation is done under a local anesthetic so that hearing tests can be done during the course of the operation. The eardrum is carefully elevated to expose the fixed stapes, and a small instrument is placed gently on this bone. The stapes is delicately manipulated until it is loosened and again becomes movable. The eardrum is then replaced in its normal position. If there is no immediate improvement in hearing, the operation has been unsuccessful, and a fenestration operation may be later performed in the same ear. The stapes mobilization operation is successful in improving the hearing to the serviceable range in approximately 60 per cent of the patients operated on.

The Inner Ear

The Inner Ear is made up of the semicircular canals and the cochlea. The semicircular canals do not have a hearing function, but serve to give us our sense of balance. They can be troublesome when overstimulated by plane, car, or boat travel causing motion sickness. Drugs such as dramamine are available for the control of this ailment. Their effectiveness is generally greatest when taken sometime prior to travel. Because of the possibility of side effects in certain individuals, the use of these drugs should be medically supervised.

The second structure of the inner ear, the cochlea, is a snail-shaped structure that is filled with fluid into which project nerve endings. Vibrations received from the stapes (stirrup) of the middle ear set this fluid into motion which in turn stimulates the nerve endings. Some nerve endings pick up high-pitched sounds, while others are sensitive to low-pitched sounds. These thousands of nerve endings come together to form the auditory nerve carrying the sound to the brain for interpretation. Damage to the auditory (eighth) nerve is sometimes due to the side effects of drugs such as salicylates, quinine, and streptomycin. Physicians are, of course, aware of these drug side effects and prescribe them judiciously.

Hearing loss due to inner ear malfunction can be precipitated by a number of causes. Diseases such as measles, scarlet fever, and syphilis (congenital or acquired) can damage the inner ear, as well as circulatory disturbances and loud noises.

Noise and Hearing Loss

Noise pollution is best described as unwanted sound. Besides being annoying, loud noise over a period of time can cause permanent and irreversible damage to the auditory nerve. Federal and state health and safety codes have set 90 decibels as the maximum level of noise that workers should be exposed to without wearing ear protection. To maintain a lower noise level, industry has in many instances redesigned machinery or modified manufacturing processes. When noise levels exceed 90 decibels, ear protection in the form of earplugs or earmuffs are worn.

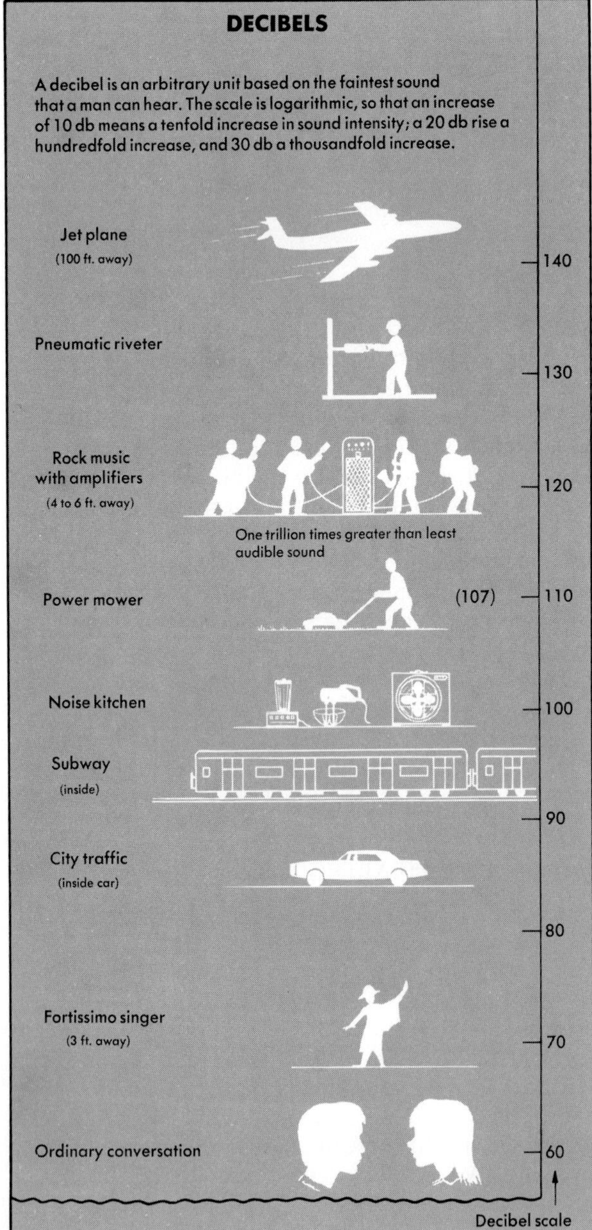

Fig. 7-25. Human hearing: schematic representation of intensity and frequency characteristics of the human ear and loudness of sounds. (*V. Puglisi,* Time *Magazine, August 9, 1968*)

Concern in recent years has been expressed by hearing specialists with regard to hearing loss caused by electronically amplified music. Rock music groups can produce sound at the level of 120 decibels if you are 4 to 6 feet from them. This is well above what is considered a safe level of sound. It is estimated that 10 per cent of those who expose themselves to music of that loudness will not have their hearing effected. Ninety per cent will suffer from significant hearing loss at least temporarily. Permanent hearing loss will occur for some listening to loud music for a week or two. For others it may take a year of exposure before permanent damage is effected. Tests show that hearing losses occur in the high frequency speech range. This is similar to the hearing losses experienced by older people who urge others to stop mumbling and to speak up!

The Nature of Hearing Loss

The usual concept is that people either have the ability to hear or are deaf. The gradations and types of hearing loss are generally overlooked.

Sound is measured in terms of two basic qualities: its loudness, measured in terms of *decibels* of sound; and its pitch, measured in terms of sound wave *frequencies.* In measuring one's hearing acuity, an instrument called an audiometer is used. Its function is to detect a person's ability to hear sounds of various frequencies (pitches). When a sound of a given pitch cannot be heard at normal decibel (loudness) level, then the audiometer measures how much louder that sound must be before it is heard. In

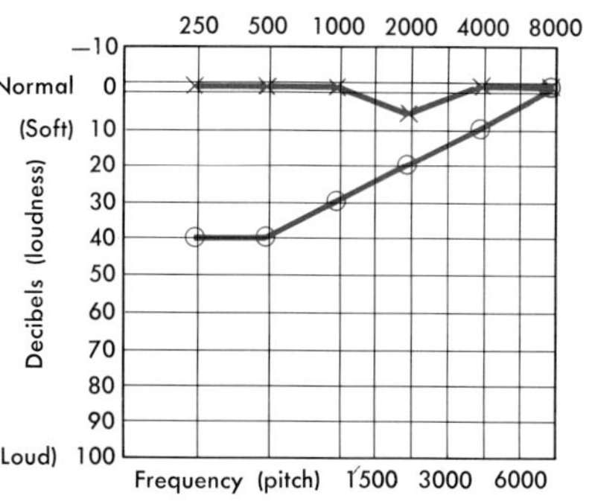

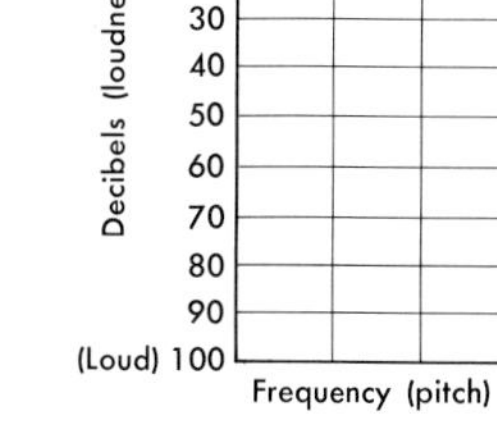

Fig. 7-26. (left) Audiogram of a person with a low frequency loss due to a middle ear infection. (right) Audiogram depicting high frequency or nerve loss due to inner ear involvement.

effect, the person's hearing can be measured and then charted in a diagram known as an audiogram. Specific types of hearing loss are thus identified.

A *conductive hearing loss* is due to a malfunction of one of the conductive parts of the ear (outer or middle ear). It usually results in the person's having difficulty hearing the low-pitched sounds (vowel sounds).

In the *neural (nerve) type of hearing loss,* the nerve endings in the inner ear are damaged, and the person usually has difficulty hearing the high-pitched sounds (consonant sounds).

There are instances of a *mixed hearing loss,* where both a conductive and a neural loss are present, with the result that the person has difficulty with both high- and low-pitched sounds.

When emotional problems affect a person's hearing, it is said that the individual is suffering from a *psychogenic hearing loss.* This would be part of a neurotic behavior pattern and is not to be confused with inattentiveness. Although there is nothing organically wrong with the ear, the person does not hear. Distinguishing a psychogenic hearing loss from a loss faked by a malingerer seeking disability compensation poses problems for specialists who measure hearing. A number of effective tests, however, have been developed for this purpose.

Hearing Specialists

An Otologist is a medical doctor who specializes in the care and treatment of disorders of the ear and hearing.

The Audiologist is a highly specialized technician trained to measure hearing acuity with the use of such instruments as audiometers and is usually certified by the American Speech and Hearing Association (ASHA).

The Otorhinolaryngologist is a medical doctor who specializes in the care and treatment of disorders of the ear, nose, and throat.

When hearing loss is suspected, competent professional help should be sought. One should start with the family physician or seek out an otologist. Speech and hearing centers are available in some larger communities. The audiologist will many times be called in by the physician for additional diagnostic help. Some confusion arises between the ASHA (American Speech and Hearing Association) Certified Audiologist and the Hearing Aid Audiologist. The latter is either a hearing aid salesman or works for one and does not have the in-depth training and education that the ASHA Certified Audiologist has. Only after careful examination and testing can an accurate diagnosis and possible course of treatment be prescribed. Treatment may include a wide variety of possibilities: medication to clear up an infection; a stapes mobilization operation; speech reading (lip reading); speech therapy (particularly where hearing loss has affected the speech development of young children); or the use of a hearing aid.

Hearing Aids

Hearing aids should be purchased on prescription very much the way eyeglasses are. They should be

Fig. 7-27. (left) Dentition of the child. (right) Dentition of the adult. (Copyright by the American Dental Association. Reprinted by permission.)

 prescribed by an otologist with the possible consultation of an audiologist. The type, cause, and severity of the hearing loss will help determine the nature of the hearing aid prescribed. A person with a high-frequency loss who hears low-frequency sounds normally would be further handicapped by a hearing aid that amplified low-frequency sounds rather than the needed high-frequencies. It would be comparable to a nearsighted person's wearing the eyeglasses of a farsighted person. Those hearing aid salesmen (or Hearing Aid Audiologists, as they sometimes refer to themselves) who attempt to diagnose the nature and cause of a hearing loss and subsequently prescribe and sell hearing aids (worth hundreds of dollars) are perpetrating a fraud either in ignorance or by design. Legislation is needed to help correct this unfortunate practice. Many such instruments wind up as permanent fixtures in the bureau drawer because they are not suitable for the particular person's condition or because the person was not trained in its use. Hearing aids are of two basic types and work on the principle of air conduction or bone conduction. *Air conduction* hearing aids send sound through its normal route via the auditory canal. *Bone conduction* hearing aids send sound directly into the inner ear usually via the mastoid bone located behind the ear. They are used when the conductive parts of the ear are not functional. Hearing aids also vary with regard to their power. Small hearing aids, such as the type that can fit into the ear canal, are usually adequate for moderate hearing losses. They are not powerful enough, however, for the more severe losses. Some people are inclined to shout at those who wear aids, overlooking the obvious fact that the hearing aid is already amplifying their voices.

A major objection to the use of hearing aids used to be their size and weight. With the introduction of transistors, these instruments can now be placed in eyeglass frames, or even be worn as a barrette in a woman's hair. The tendency is still to hide the hearing aid. We have, to very great extent, overcome this negativism with regard to the use of eyeglasses, and it is to be hoped the acceptance of hearing aids will soon follow. It is recommended that a hearing aid be purchased on a trial basis. After the dealer shows one how to use and care for the aid, the otologist or audiologist should check to see if it is working properly. Chances are there will be a free postevaluation of the mechanism included in the purchase price. If within a month an individual cannot adjust to the hearing aid, perhaps there is a need for more rehabilitative help.[6]

The Psychological Aspects of Hearing Loss

Those who have severe hearing loss or deafness have more than just an auditory loss to deal with. Their relations with others can be seriously affected. While blindness evokes a sympathetic reaction, deafness many times stimulates an opposite kind of response in people. Severe hearing loss or deafness tends to

[6]The Buying Guide Issue, *Consumer Reports,* 1972. Published by Consumers Union, Mount Vernon, N.Y. 10550.

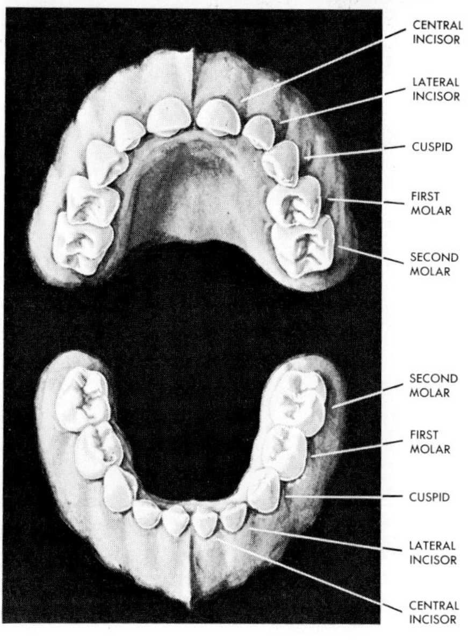

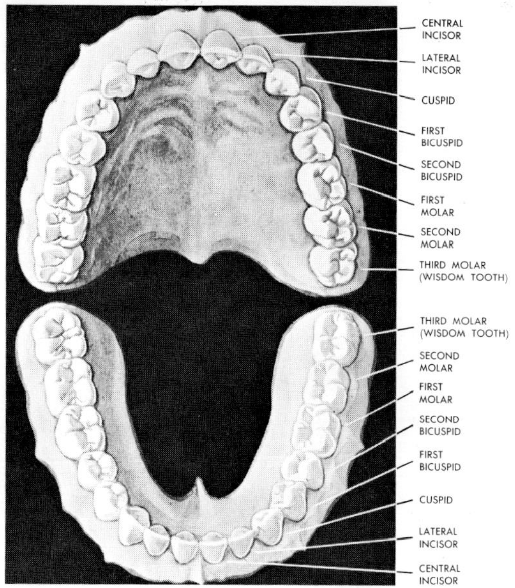

cut off the major means of communication and serves to isolate the individual. The person sometimes becomes suspicious of the motives of others, with ensuing effects on personality and sociability. The person who does not hear cannot use his ears for cues to danger in the environment, such as a siren, a whistle, or a car horn. He uses his eyes for this purpose and must be ever alert to changes in light and movement. We have a responsibility to help those with hearing losses to make a good adjustment to their handicap by contributing when possible to the emotional security of these individuals.

Dental and Oral Health

The almost universal prevalence of dental and oral disease combined with a lack of appropriate attention to them has resulted in a health problem of almost monumental proportions. By the age of 16, the average youth has seven to eight decayed, filled, or missing teeth. By 45 years of age, the average adult has lost half of his teeth. The American Dental Association has reported surveys estimating that there is a backlog of 700 million unfilled cavities among Americans. There are over 100 million people who have suffered tooth loss because of diseases of the gum or supporting structures.

Primary Factors in Tooth Decay

Susceptibility to tooth decay seems to involve a number of factors. "It has been found that genetic factors in various oral conditions ranging from tooth decay to cleft palate contribute a small but significant variable to resistance and susceptibility to caries."[7] In addition, tooth decay has been related to the presence of oral bacteria which react with carbohydrates (particularly refined sugars and starches). This interaction results in the production of organic acids that will dissolve the enamel of the tooth and thus initiate dental caries. Dental plaques, a gelatinlike film that adheres to the teeth, can act as protective mediums for oral bacteria. Proper cleaning of the teeth will help temporarily to remove dental plaques. Controlling the intake and frequency of refined carbohydrates is particularly important if tooth decay is to be minimized among young children. Children's teeth seem to be particularly susceptible to the development of caries. Tooth brushing or rinsing of the mouth with water immediately after eating refined sugars and starches helps prevent dental caries.

Fluorides and Tooth Decay

Minute amounts of fluorides used in various ways have been found to be remarkably effective in preventing tooth decay. When one part fluoride is added to every million parts of drinking water, dental caries experience is reduced by about 65 per cent in children who drink fluoridated water from birth. Several fluoridation programs have been in effect for

[7] "NIDR Reports on Dental Research." (Bethesda, Md.: National Institute of Dental Research, National Institutes of Health, January 1964), p. 5.

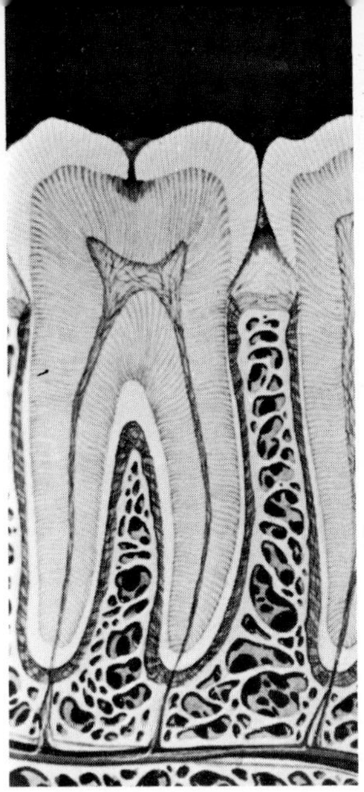
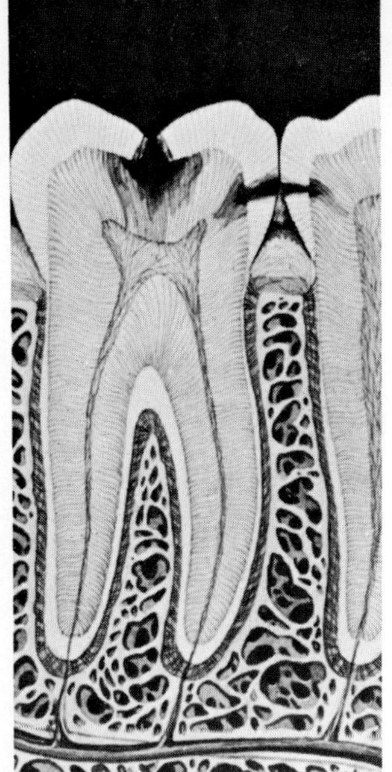
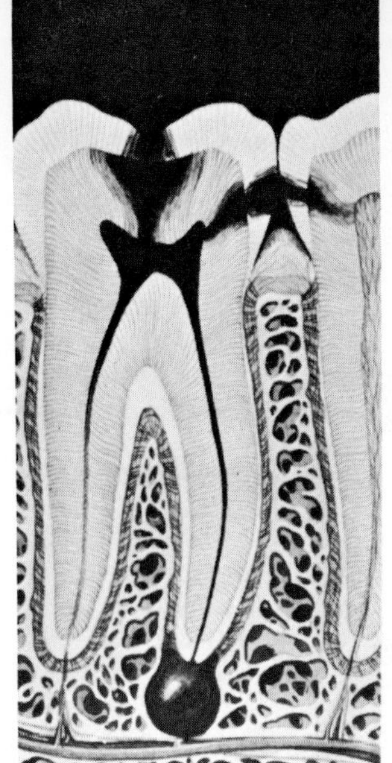
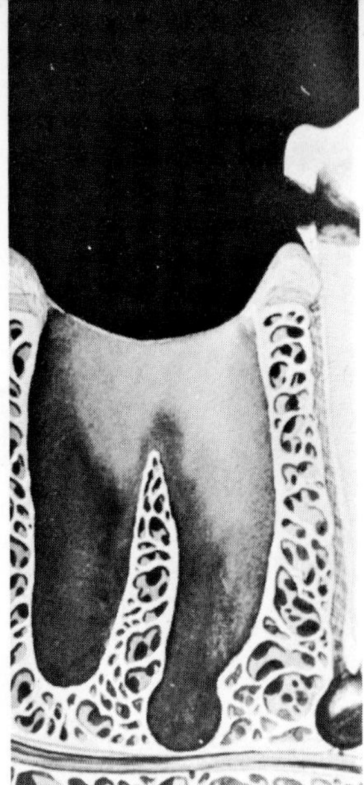

more than twenty years, consistently substantiating their contributions to dental health. Over 1300 communities in the United States have now had programs of this type for over ten years.

The manner in which fluorides work is not completely understood. It is generally believed that they combine with the tooth enamel to make it harder and more resistant to decay.

Where communities do not yet fluoridate their drinking water, other means may be utilized to give children the benefits of fluorides. The dentist can give topical applications of a fluoride solution. Tablets that contain appropriate amounts of fluoride can also be given to children from birth up to completion of the development of the second molars. A fluoridated dentifrice can also be used. Although these methods of fluoride use are helpful, they do not decrease the amount of tooth decay as effectively as fluoridation of the water supply. In addition, research has shown a beneficial supplemental effect of fluorides when added to those obtained in the water supply.

Almost all of our major cities use fluoridated drinking water. This public health measure is strongly endorsed by the major health organizations in the United States. In spite of this, there is still opposition by sincere, but misinformed people to proposals for the fluoridation of drinking water. Those in the community who are uninformed with regard to the safety and effectiveness of fluorides are often confused by the opposition. The result is usually a delay in the implementation of a much-needed public health program.

Periodontal Diseases

These diseases of the gums represent the major cause of tooth loss in adults over 35. More than 70 per cent of all Americans suffer from these disorders by the age of 50, with almost all being affected by the age of 75. A number of factors can contribute to disease of the gum; among them are malocclusion, bacteria and their products, dental plaque, and vitamin C deficiency. Its major cause is usually tartar (calculus) that accumulates on the teeth. Tartar is a crusty deposit that can irritate the gums. The chronic irritation of the gum tissues leaves them prone to infection which attacks the periodontal membrane and bone which support the tooth. The tooth is then without support. Some people who have had little or no tooth decay lose their teeth to periodontal disease.

Through early diagnosis by the dentist, and *proper,* daily brushing of teeth, periodontal disease is minimized. It is important to brush away from the gums with the stroke beginning on the gum tissue. In addition, it is advised to have a dentist or dental hygienist remove tartar that may form on the teeth. This cleaning or prophylaxis should take place at the interval suggested by the dentist. Gums that become inflamed or swollen or have a tendency to bleed should be checked by a dentist.

Malocclusion (irregularly positioned teeth) can often precipitate periodontal disease by causing undue pressure on some teeth, entrapping food debris, and creating a chronic gum irritation.

If periodontal disease has developed, the dentist

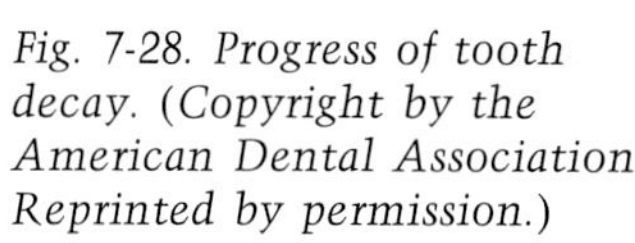

Fig. 7-28. *Progress of tooth decay. (Copyright by the American Dental Association. Reprinted by permission.)*

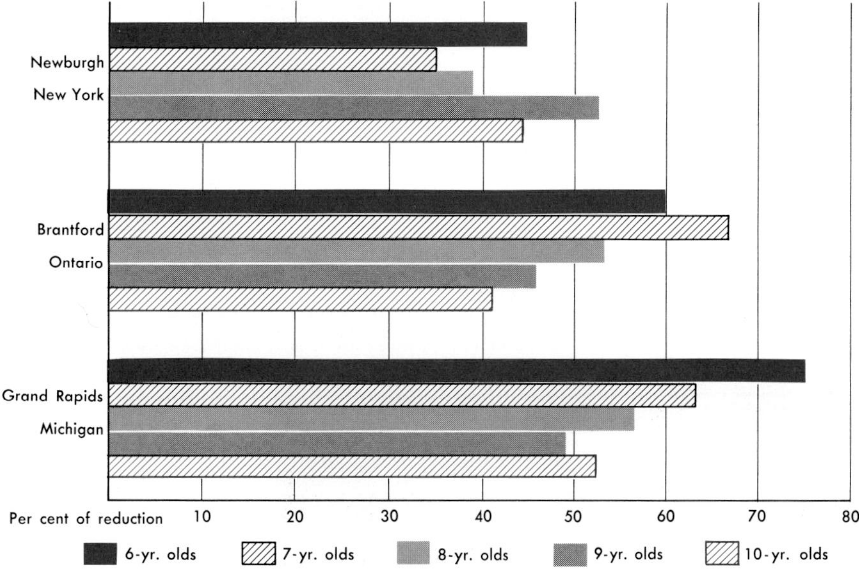

Fig. 7-29. *Reduction of dental caries in permanent teeth of children in continuous residence in three areas after ten years of fluoridation. (Copyright by the American Dental Association. Reprinted by permission.)*

may refer the patient to a periodontist. The periodontist will treat the infected gum tissue and recommend home care. He may utilize gingivectomy (surgical removal of gum tissue) as a treatment.

Malocclusion

The irregularity of tooth position or a "poor bite" (improper fitting together of teeth when the jaw is closed) is malocclusion. There are two general types of causes for this condition, namely those that are hereditary in nature and those that are acquired.

Hereditary factors include dental arches of inadequate size and primary teeth that are shed too early or retained too long. Acquired malocclusion may result from thumb-sucking or the early loss of primary or permanent teeth with the resultant drifting of some teeth out of position. The prevention of early tooth loss can prevent malocclusion and subsequent periodontal disease. Early dental care is therefore important to long-term dental health.

The *orthodontist* is the dental specialist who treats malocclusion. Through a variety of treatment methods, he brings teeth and jaws into proper relationship. Malocclusion can be corrected even in adults, although there are advantages to early attention to this problem.

Cleft Palate

Cleft palate is a congenital condition wherein an opening or furrow exists through the roof of the mouth. It occurs about once in every 700 live births in this country. Cleft palate occurs during early uterine life, when the two sides of the palate do not grow together and meet in the middle. This condition may be mild, involving only the soft palate and resulting in a double uvula. A more extensive cleft may involve both the hard and soft palates, and in more extreme cases the cleft may also involve the jaw and lip. The more severe cases of cleft palate are serious for the infant because he is unable to suck nourishment from a bottle or breast. Specially designed feeding tubes are used which utilize the force of gravity and prevent food from going up into the nose. Surgical repair provides a roof for the mouth, thus preventing food from spilling into the nasal cavity. In some severe cases, a special plate which attaches to the teeth is fashioned by the dentist and surgeon to cover the cleft. Surgery also corrects the obvious facial disfigurement. Correction of faulty speech is usually facilitated with the help of a speech therapist.

When there is a fissure or opening of the upper lip, the condition is sometimes called harelip. In simple conditions of harelip, there is no interference with feeding or tooth structure and the cosmetic effects of surgery are most successful. Correction of the cleft palate usually involves the combined services of a plastic surgeon and dental specialists.

Problems of the Foot

The layman's concept of foot problems usually starts with corns and callouses and ends with bunions and ingrowing nails. However, problems related to feet

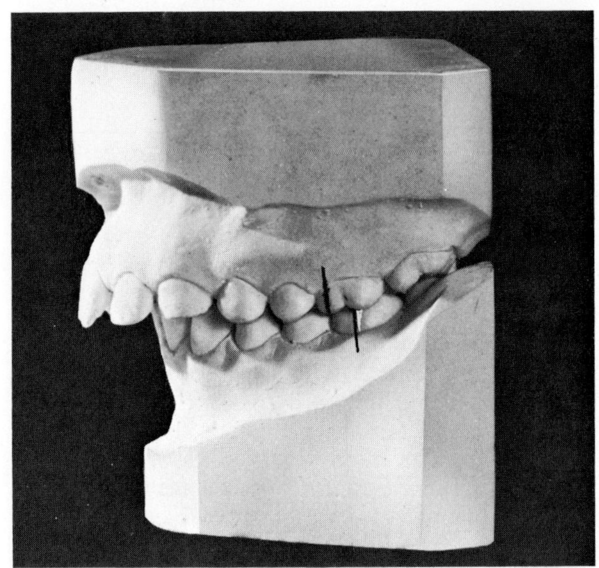

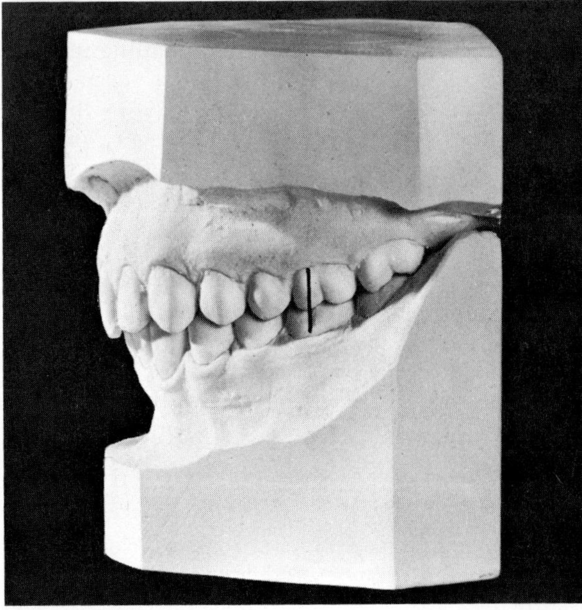

Fig. 7-30. Malocclusion before and after treatment. (Copyright by the American Dental Association. Reprinted by permission.)

stem from many and varied causes. They can be congenital, hereditary or neurogenic in nature, as well as metabolic, infectious, traumatic, or environmental.

Foot Care for Youth

It seems ironic that about 99 per cent of us are born with perfect feet, but all too soon develop foot problems. It is documented that well over three-fourths of our schoolchildren already are plagued with foot ailments. During childhood the foot is a pliable structure reacting to many stresses and strains. As the child grows, the foot becomes sturdier. It is during this period that the child's feet must be carefully observed and protected, for they can be distorted, made weak, and deformed. Very often these deformities are imposed by well-meaning, but uninformed mothers and shoe salesmen. Some babies spend their entire infancy in stretch suits that could serve as a toe-curling device if the size of the garment is not checked periodically. Booties and socks on infants should be loose and floppy. Some physicians are convinced that crooked shoes are being put on straight feet. In one instance a toddler toed in when walking in his "high, sturdily built, good supporting, expensive shoe." When the shoe was removed the child walked straight. The shoe's structure was such that although it looked straight, the forefoot pointed inward. The physician's advice was for the child to walk barefoot where there was no danger of injury to his feet, but if protection was needed, for the child to wear a soft shoe or sneaker. The misconception

Fig. 7-31. *Happiness is feet that don't ache.* (Popular Science)

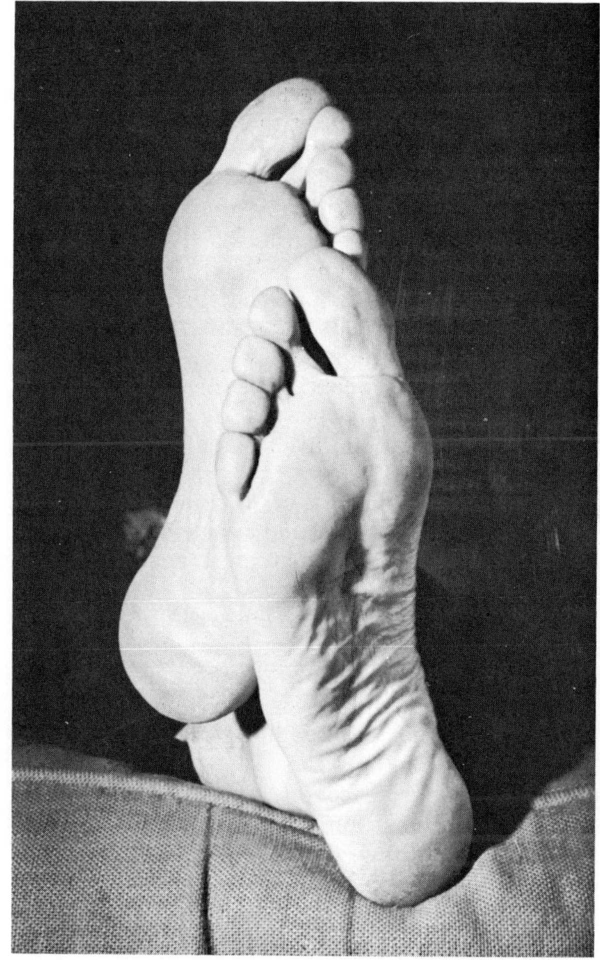

that the lace-up oxford-type shoe will prevent foot deformities still persists, even though most physicians feel that if the foot is normal there is no need for rigid special supports.

Clubfoot is a congenital malformation in which the tendons of the foot are misplaced and turn in at an awkward angle. Years ago, a person born with this affliction went through life with an ungainly shuffle. Today, when the condition is recognized at birth a plaster cast is applied to the foot soon thereafter. The casts are changed frequently as the foot assumes a more normal position. In some cases where the foot does not respond, surgery may be performed by an orthopedist to correct the condition. An orthopedist may also treat pigeon toes (or metatarsus adductus) early in a child's life when the bones are still soft and pliable. Here again casts are used to urge a more correct position of the foot.

Those Environmental Factors

Foot troubles can also arise from *environmental factors* such as overweight, overwork, ill-fitting shoes, tight hosiery, and abuse or neglect of the foot. A great offender of these environmental factors seems to be ill-fitting shoes. Since 80 per cent of podiatry patients are women, one would suspect that women are driven by the dictates of fashion into shoes that are incorrectly shaped for their feet. The habitual use of high-heeled shoes shifts the body weight forward to the metatarsal heads, almost completely eliminating the heel as one of the weight-bearing

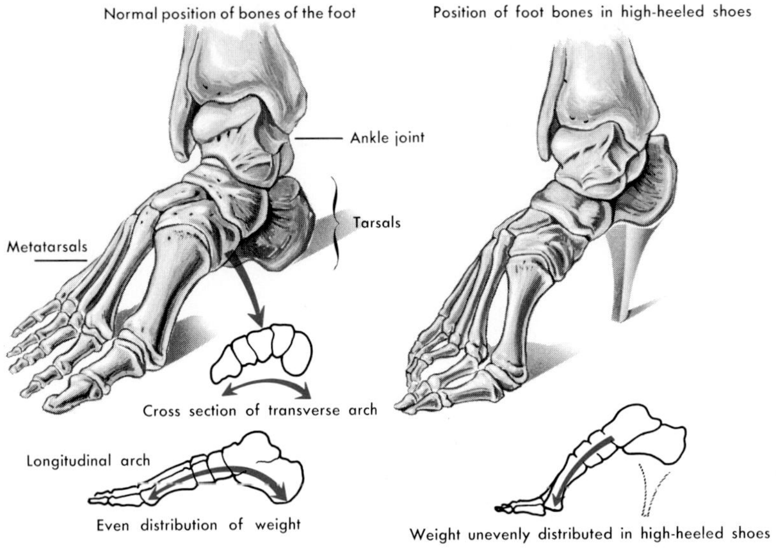

Fig. 7-32. *What high heels do to your feet.* (*Courtesy* Today's Health)

points. The foot is also pushed forward so that the toes are shoved into the narrow toe area. An additional result of the constant wearing of high heels is that the calf muscles will shorten and decrease the range of dorsiflexion of the foot.

Sneakers have finally been redeemed. The idea that sneakers caused flat feet has been a part of our culture for too long. Likewise the idea that arch supports will *correct* flat feet has flourished from generation to generation. Actually very little is known as to the causes of a flattened longitudinal arch (officially known as pes planus). Many people with flat feet suffer no foot pain and have full range of use. After many years of treating flat feet with steel arch supports (now plastic) some physicians are beginning to question this form of treatment for fallen arches.

The rule of thumb on shoes is comfort, not price. A soft shoe with low heel and a wide space in front for uncramped toes is what most podiatrists and physicians are recommending.

The new phenomenon of not wearing any shoes among our teenagers and young adults has stirred some mixed feelings. Some shopkeepers feel compelled to publicly display signs prohibiting the entrance of bare-footed individuals for "sanitary" reasons. The barefoot ones themselves see and feel the disadvantages of bare feet on city streets. The pounding of the pavements on an unprotected sole is very tiring to say nothing of the fungus infections, the cut toes, and the burning from hot pavements. Many physicians contend, however, that "walking barefoot on softer surfaces—sand and earth—is still considered the best of foot exercises for young and *old.*"[8] With some reservations, physicians welcome the barefoot trend as the end of years of foot constrictions that led to bunions, hammer toes, corns, and aching feet.

Serving the Aged and Infirm

Medical advances by extending the life-span, paradoxically increase the proportion of aged and disabled persons. A good percentage of podiatrists' patients are in their senior years. Frequently, complaints are symptoms of serious general medical problems. If the podiatrist recognizes systemic diseases from early signs in the feet, he refers the patient to his physician while he keeps the patient ambulatory by alleviating foot disorders. Many times, the physician refers his patients with arthritis and circulation problems to the podiatrist to facilitate proper foot care. Amputation of limbs was once not uncommon among people with circulatory and diabetic problems. But modern medical techniques are now saving the entire limb or limiting amputations to only a portion of the foot. Orthopedic and podiatric care in rehabilitation often reveals that people who can move about are more likely to accept other rehabilitative measures. Podiatry departments in mental institutions provide examination and treatment on a regular basis. Here again, recovery need not be impeded by aching or diseased feet.

[8] "Shooting Out Myths About Footwear," *Today's Health* (May 1971), p. 34.

Review Questions

1. How does "commercialized exercise" fall short of the physical and emotional satisfactions that can be derived from physical activity?
2. What appear to be the answers to our declining levels of physical fitness?
3. Why is hyperopia in children a lesser problem than myopia?
4. Eyeglasses are corrective, but *not* therapeutic. Explain.
5. What are some of the dangers involved in the use of contact lenses? How may these difficulties be minimized?
6. What kinds of visual problems are associated with strabismus? How can this condition be corrected?
7. Why is glaucoma an unnecessary cause of blindness?
8. What are some of the limitations that should be observed in the use of sunglasses? Under what circumstances can sunglasses be harmful?
9. Describe the operation of an eye bank. What kind of blindness does it serve to correct?
10. What are the adjustments that blind people need to make? How does the sighted person at times further handicap the blind?
11. What are the common causes of hearing loss in the middle ear?
12. How do various types of hearing loss differ? What implications do these differences have for hearing aids used to correct them?
13. Define: (1) otologist, (2) audiologist, (3) otorhinolaryngologist.
14. What are the sociopsychological implications of hearing loss?
15. What have been the contributions of fluorides to the prevention of tooth decay?
16. What are the relationships of malocclusion to periodontal disease?
17. Describe a cleft palate condition. How can this condition and its effects be corrected?
18. What are some of the environmental factors that contribute to foot problems?

Chapter 8

Our Shifting Nutritional Problems

It appears to be a rather common human tendency to solve problems by sometimes overcorrecting them. At one time, there was concern for the incidence of vitamin deficiency diseases in this country, such as rickets, beriberi, and pellagra. With the discovery of vitamins, we have seen the development of food enrichment programs, vitamin tablets in almost every food and drug store, vitamin-loaded tonics, and a rising incidence of *hyper*vitaminosis—vitamin poisoning! Most of us have replaced a struggle for an adequate amount of food with weight problems from overindulgence at the dinner table. In our efforts to make food more plentiful, thousands of chemicals are used in the form of food additives and pesticides. Checking the safety of food additives and what constitutes safe amounts of pesticide residue on fruits and vegetables has already become a routine public health procedure. The nutritional status of the American people has obviously improved, as indicated by the relative absence of nutritional or related diseases and a taller, presumably healthier generation of youth, but a plentiful food supply does not insure adequate nutrition for all. While significant progress has been made in nutrition, it would be worthwhile to consider the shifting personal and public health concerns in this area and their implications.

Poverty, Hunger, and Malnutrition

The Citizens' Board of Inquiry . . . found across this country what some public officials suspected, but which too many ignored or denied: that in the wealthiest nation in the history of the world, millions of men, women and children are slowly starving.

They found that American babies die in infancy, because their mothers cannot nurse them, and cannot buy the milk to keep them alive.

They found that thousands of American children are anemic and listless, their physical growth stunted because they lack adequate protein.

They found that scurvy and rickets, surely diseases of an alien past, cripple American children who never drink citrus juice, and who rarely drink milk.

They found that American children in large number suffer from hookworms and roundworms, parasitic infections that drain what strength these children have.

They found that hundreds of thousands of school children cannot learn their lessons, because they go to school without breakfast, have no money for lunch, and return to a supper without meat or green vegetable.

And they found that countless old people in America exist almost entirely on liquids, because they cannot buy or find a decent meal.[1]

In the last several years, the problems of hunger and malnutrition associated with poverty have come to the forefront of the nation's social and political conscience. In 1967 and 1968, several reports documented the existence of hunger and malnutrition among poor people in the United States. In 1967

[1] *Hunger, USA,* A Report by the Citizens' Board of Inquiry, with an introductory comment by Robert F. Kennedy (Boston: Beacon Press, 1969), p. 7.

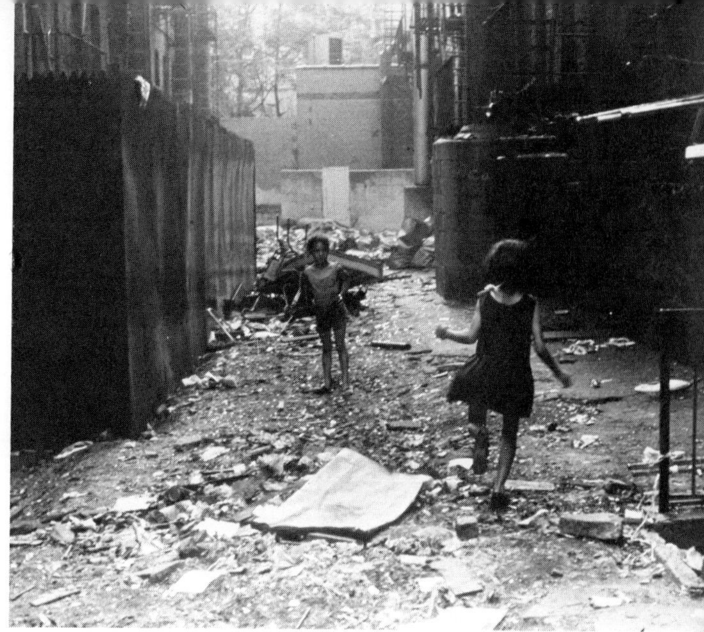

Fig. 8-1. *Poverty, hunger, and malnutrition are often found to be highly related.* (*Susan Johns*)

Senators Robert Kennedy and Joseph Clark made a trip to rural Mississippi to report on poverty programs, and came back dismayed at the overt hunger they had seen. The Field Foundation also sent a team of physicians to Mississippi. The team reported to a Senate Sub-Committee on Manpower, Employment, and Poverty, that they had found a surprising amount of hunger and malnutrition among poor people in the areas they had visited. In 1968 the Citizens' Board Of Inquiry, a private group, published a document entitled, *Hunger, USA.*[2] At about the same time (May 1968) CBS broadcast its documentary *Hunger in America.* Both of these served to spark debate in public and private forums as a result of documenting the extent to which hunger existed in our "land of plenty."

In December 1967 Congress authorized the U.S. Public Health Service to conduct a study of the nutritional status of poor people in the United States. Termed the National Nutrition Survey, this study began in 1968 in ten states and New York City. Field work was completed in 1970 and the data are still being analyzed. The survey focused on those areas of the ten states that contained the highest percentage of families with low incomes. The age groups most vulnerable to malnutrition seemed to be children through the age of 16 and the elderly, especially black and Spanish-speaking individuals over 60 years of age. In all areas surveyed, income showed a positive correlation with overall nutritional status, with the poorest of the poor having the least adequate diets and the greatest vulnerability to malnutrition. Impaired growth of children, low hemoglobin levels (reflecting low iron intakes), low plasma vitamin A levels especially in children, and poor dental health were major problems.

[2]Ibid.

Several governmental programs have been developed to combat hunger and malnutrition among the poor. One of these government food assistance programs for families and individuals is the Donated Commodities Program. This program was initially established to help the needy and provide a market for agricultural commodities in surplus. The theory was that by supplying some food for free, more of the family's limited money would be available for other kinds of food and other necessities. About 3 million people now participate in the commodity program. The government provides food bought on the open market, not necessarily in surplus, including staples such as flour, cornmeal, and dry milk, but also including canned meat, canned chicken and turkey, canned vegetables, and fruit juice.

The Food Stamp program was the result of food stamp legislation initially introduced in 1964 by President Kennedy. The Food Stamp Act went into effect in 1967. A family pays a limited amount per month (from nothing up to more than $100, depending on the family's income and the number of people in the family) and receives food stamps worth much more which may be spent in any supermarket or grocery store that accepts them. Food stamps allow freedom of choice to the family with the exception that they cannot be used for nonfood items and household supplies, alcoholic beverages, and imported items (with the exception of coffee, tea, bananas, cocoa). More than 10 million people are currently participating in the Food Stamp Program.

Government-subsidized School Feeding Programs include lunches in schools which participate in the National School Lunch Act, breakfast, and special feeding programs. In order to participate in the National School Lunch Act, schools must serve lunches that meet the "Type A" standard, which is planned to provide at least one-third of the Recommended Dietary Allowances for a child. Since 1968 schools must make lunches available free or at reduced prices to children unable to pay the full price. The system for determining which children get free or reduced prices is determined by the local school board, but must be a matter of public record and must not discriminate in any way against children receiving free or reduced-price lunches.

Weight Control

In spite of the fact that some individuals do not get enough to eat, a far larger number have the problem of obesity resulting from an excess of food intake and/or a lack of exercise. Obesity is by far the most common nutritional problem in the United States today.

Problems related to weight control are often considered to be synonymous with those of overeating and gluttony. Increasingly, evidence is being gathered to indicate that this is not necessarily so. There are studies which show that some overweight people eat less than individuals of normal weight. Current

Fig. 8-2. A recommended method of measuring obesity is with skinfold calipers. If the fold is more than an inch thick, the person is considered to be "fat". (Dan Bernstein)

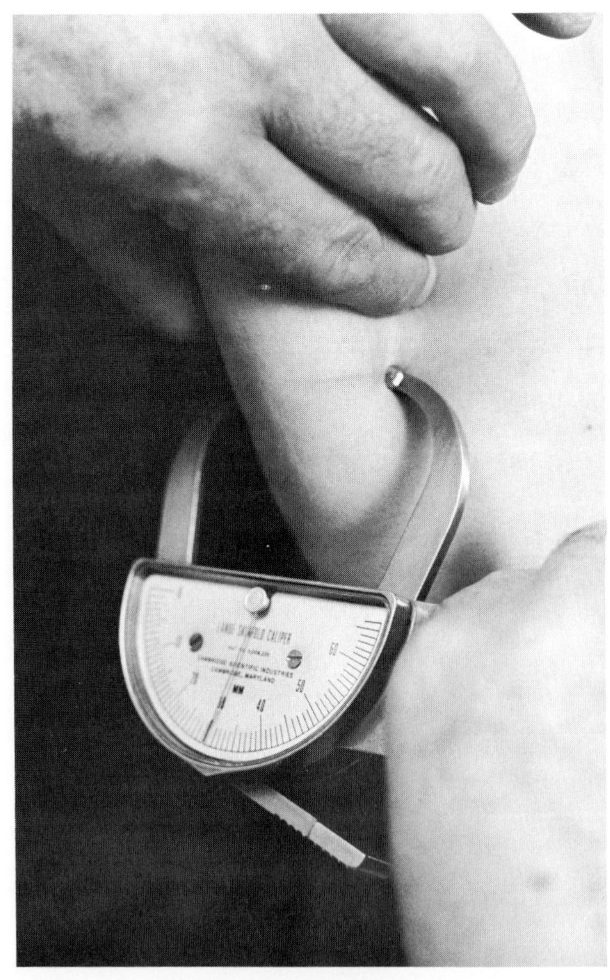

information indicates that fat metabolism in some obese subjects may differ from that found in subjects of normal weight. If this is so, a purely dietary approach to the correction of metabolic obesity would prove inadequate. It is becoming increasingly apparent that there are a number of factors involved in weight control.

One of these factors is that of exercise. Weight control is based on achieving a balance between caloric intake and caloric output. To concentrate solely on diet (caloric intake) is to focus on only one-half of the problem. It has many times been found that weight control can be adequately achieved by increasing the level of exercise alone. Studies have shown that overweight people are, in many instances, not as active as they might be. Observations of overweight children in physical education classes have indicated that these children are frequently much less active than individuals of normal weight. One reason for the neglect of exercise as a factor in weight control is the misconceived idea that exercise consumes very little energy. Examples indicating that one must walk 36 miles within a few hours to lose one pound of fat, present the problem in a negative and discouraging manner. It sounds much more positive and encouraging to indicate that a pound of fat may be lost by a person who walks one mile daily for 36 days. Should the person continue this practice throughout a year, he would achieve a weight loss of ten pounds. It has further been estimated that one-half hour of fairly vigorous exercise daily, will result in a loss of approximately sixteen pounds in one year. Another misconception that results in the underestimating of the value of exercise is that increased exercise invariably means increased appetite. Another factor generally ignored here is that exercise will raise the metabolic rate, not only during the exercise period but sometimes for hours after the individual has ceased activity.

Increasingly, the relationship between heredity and obesity is being explored. One study has demonstrated[3] that only 10 per cent of the children whose parents were of normal weight are obese, and that the proportion will rise to 40 per cent if one parent is obese. Where both parents are obese, the percentage of overweight children in the family rises to 80 per cent. Additional studies in this area indicate that where obesity runs in families, genetic as well as environmental factors may be involved. "Comparative lifetime studies of identical and fraternal twins have strongly pointed toward possible hereditary factors in their obesity. Food habits are not the only or even the main factor in their obesity."[4] Obesity, like any other problem, deserves early attention. Pediatricians become increasingly concerned where this kind of problem is ignored in childhood, when corrective measures can best be undertaken.

Emotional and psychological factors also have a role to play here. Such factors as grief, lack of affection, success, or popularity are involved as motivators of abnormal eating patterns. Many people will

[3] "Obesity in Adolescents," *Consultant.* A monthly publication of Smith, Kline and French Laboratories.

[4] *Obesity and Health* (Washington, D.C.: U.S. Dept. of Health, Education and Welfare, U.S. Public Health Service Publication No. 1485), p. 42.

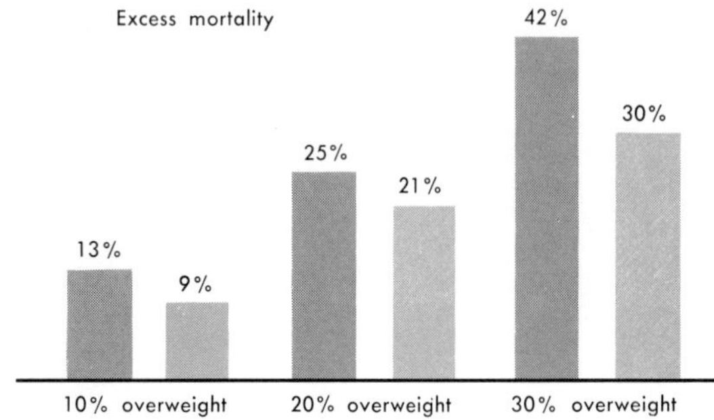

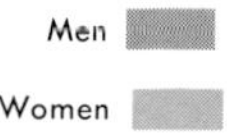

Fig. 8-3. Overweight shortens life. (Metropolitan Life Insurance Company)

eat out of just plain nervousness. Tensions before an examination or any situation contributing to stress might precipitate an evening-long session of "nervous eating." It has been found in those cases where emotional or psychological factors are involved that restriction of food is not necessarily the best solution to the problem. We may be sometimes superimposing an additional difficulty for the individual. If the person can be induced to increase his energy output by some kind of activity, the problem is more easily resolved.

Lack of information with regard to basic nutrition is an additional factor that might complicate the management of obesity. People are too often unaware of which foods are of high caloric value and which ones are not. Basic information in this area alone could prevent much obesity.

It is an established fact that the overweight do not live as long as those of normal weight. Cardiovascular disease, high blood pressure, diabetes, arthritis, cerebral hemorrhage, and nephritis are some of the conditions that occur more often in the overweight. In a study reported by the Metropolitan Life Insurance Company, it was found that excess mortality rose rapidly with an increased degree of overweight. A 13 per cent excess mortality rate was found for those 10 per cent overweight, 25 per cent for those 20 per cent overweight, and 40 per cent for those 30 per cent overweight.[5]

Cardiovascular disease is the leading cause of death in the United States (see Chapter 11). Many risk factors have been identified which may predispose an individual to atherosclerosis and to heart attacks. Among these are age, sex, heredity, stress, smoking, obesity, hypertension, and high levels of serum lipids. A general picture of the coronary-prone individual may be painted as an overweight, middle-aged male with a sedentary but highly stressful job, who has had high blood pressure for some time, smokes heavily, and has high serum cholesterol and serum triglyceride levels.

Since several of the risk factors (obesity, serum lipids, and possibly hypertension) may be related to diet, nutrition is one means of attacking the problem. Certainly the most important nutritional prevention that can be undertaken is the attaining and maintaining of normal weight by the individual. Aside from this, epidemiological data indicate that a lower fat intake, including less-saturated fat (primarily that from animal sources such as in butter, whole milk, meat, and lard), and a lower intake of refined sugar *might* be beneficial in lowering the rate of overt cardiovascular disease in the population as a whole.

Dieting

It has been found that only 10 per cent of people who see a physician about dieting are successful in losing weight and maintaining that reduced weight. One of the problems involved is that many physicians, like many lay persons, regard obesity as a

[5] "Overweight—Its Prevention and Significance." A series of articles in *Statistical Bulletin* (New York: Metropolitan Life Insurance Company, 1960).

moral issue rather than a complex medical problem not as yet completely understood. Those who have punitive attitudes toward their overweight patients are reinforcing feelings of guilt that have already been induced by family and friends. Physicians who use this approach are usually those not well trained to handle problems of this type and are acting out of frustration rather than in the context of medical know-how or technique.

In considering diets, the first concern should be with nutritional adequacy and balance. Often people establish a diet pattern that is unbalanced with regard to one or more nutrients. The result is the addition of a deficiency problem to the overweight problem they already have. Dieting patterns are also found too often to be temporary and emotional in nature. Individuals will attempt to modify their diet for one or two weeks when what is really needed is a change of eating patterns that will last for that individual's lifetime. The emotional nature with which some people approach dieting is exemplified by the woman who felt that she needed to have a banana split smothered with whipped cream and nuts in order to "reinforce" herself before undertaking the "ordeal" of dieting for the next two weeks. This approach immediately condemns the attempt at weight control to obvious failure. Diets that also exclude exercise as indicated earlier are narrow and shortsighted in scope; it must be remembered that some individuals who do not exercise extensively, in order to maintain their weight, go through life feeling constantly hungry. Some aids have been utilized in helping the individual to suppress appetite. They are at best, however, crutches and ultimately the individual must learn to "go it alone" on a restricted dietary pattern.

Quackery and Special Diets

Quackery in the area of nutrition, and particularly with regard to weight control, is literally running rampant in the United States. Wherever we run across a problem that is difficult to control, invariably people of questionable ethics will move in to sell quick cures. The market at the present time is flooded with publications that give what appear to be easy solutions to the problem. These books come under varying titles intimating that you can eat all you want and lose weight, provided you include some magic ingredient. These ingredients include vegetable oils, special dietary supplements, and homespun but unscientific dietary regimens. We have seen the increased sale of vibrating couches, belts, and other gadgets of this type. The federal government, after extensive testing, has indicated that there is no evidence to support the thesis that these vibrating gadgets will be helpful in weight reduction. For some, the most that can be said for them is that they can be relaxing; however, for others, the possibility for harm is present. The Relax-A-cizer, which promises to reduce girth by electrically stimulating muscles, is one such device.

In April 1970 a permanent injunction against the distribution of the *Relax-A-cizer* was issued by a U.S. district court. After a trial which heard the testimony of thirty-one medical authorities, the device was declared to be dangerous to health, having the potential effect of damaging the heart and other vital organs, and disseminating preexisting cancer cells throughout the body.[6]

Before-meal candies are often sold as a means of suppressing appetite. The person is supposed to eat two candies with the idea of raising the blood sugar level, which in turn is supposed to kill the appetite. The difficulty with this approach is that the caloric content of the candy is much too low to have any effect on the blood sugar level.

Some people are misled into believing that steam baths are a means of losing weight. The unhappy fact is that temporary loss in body fluids is regained with the first intakes of water and other fluid material, but the dollars and time invested are not.

Nutritional Misinformation

One problem area in nutrition against which little progress has been made is food faddism. The only thing that has changed here is the scene of the crime. The old food faddist sold his wares from the back of a covered wagon. Now he has the facilities of television and book publishers who have national distribution. Charlatans using twentieth-century methods are deluding the American public who have in very many cases nineteenth-century nutritional information. It is estimated that almost one billion dollars a year is spent in the United States in the area of food quackery. The range of activity here is a broad one, including the sale of food supplements, books, health foods, weight control plans, and "cures" for a wide range of ailments that even medical science cannot completely control.

The Appearance of Another Foolproof Diet?

Some books (see *Calories Don't Count* and *Dr. Atkins' Diet Revolution*) persist on best-seller lists in spite of condemnation by the American Medical Association and leading nutritionists. In 1962 the best-selling book in the nation was *Calories Don't Count*, by Herman Taller, M.D., with an estimated sales of 2 million copies. The author was later convicted of conspiracy and violation of federal drug laws because of a commercial tie-in of the book with safflower oil capsules. His license to practice medicine was revoked for three years in addition to being fined.

In 1973 a diet book called *Dr. Atkins' Diet Revolution*, by Robert C. Atkins, M.D., suddenly became a best seller. It told its readers what they apparently wanted to hear—that they could eat large amounts of food and still lose weight. What the author advocated was a high protein and fat diet and one low in carbohydrates. Nutritionists immediately labeled it as another rehashing of the "DuPont diet," the "Drinking Man's Diet," "The Mayo Diet" (not related in any way to the renowned Mayo Clinic) *Calories Don't Count*, and "The Air Force Diet." Nothing is new—at least not in this context.

[6] *The Medicine Show* (Mount Vernon, N.Y.: Consumers Union, 1971), p. 114.

Fig. 8-4. Some books (see Calories Don't Count *and* Dr. Atkins' Diet Revolution) *persist on best-seller lists in spite of condemnation by the American Medical Association and leading nutritionists. This is a classic example of a communication failure eroding the effectiveness of the country's health authorities. (© 1973, 1962 by The New York Times Company. Reprinted by permission.)*

Best Seller List

An analysis based on reports from leading booksellers in 38 cities showing the sales rating of 16 leading fiction and general titles over the last 3 weeks. Sales through the book clubs are not included. Figures in the right-hand column do not necessarily represent consecutive weeks and do not indicate week-to-week shifts on the chart.

April 8	April 15	April 22	This Week		Weeks on List
				Fiction	
	11	5	1	Ship of Fools. *Porter*	3
1	1	1	2	Franny and Zooey. *Salinger*	32
2	3	3	3	The Fox in the Attic. *Hughes*	10
3	4	4	4	The Agony and the Ecstasy. *Stone*	57
5	2	2	5	The Bull From the Sea. *Renault*	9
6	5	6	6	Six Crises. *Nixon*	7
4	6	7	7	A Prologue to Love. *Caldwell*	22
7	8	8	8	To Kill a Mockingbird. *Lee*	91
	16	12	9	Island. *Huxley*	3
9	7	9	10	Captain Newman, M.D. *Rosten*	14
8	10	10	11	Chairman of the Bored. *Streeter*	30
				General	
1	1	1	1	Calories Don't Count. *Taller*	21
2	2	2	2	My Life in Court. *Nizer*	22
4	3	3	3	The Rothschilds. *Morton*	8
3	4	4	4	The Guns of August. *Tuchman*	11
14	6	5	5	A Bridge for Passing. *Buck*	4
	10	7	6	In the Clearing. *Frost*	3
11	9	9	7	Scott Fitzgerald. *Turnbull*	5
5	5	6	8	The Making of the President 1960. *White*	42
7	8	8	9	The Last Plantagenets. *Costain*	11
9	12	11	10	The New English Bible: New Testament.	57
6	7	10	11	CIA: The Inside Story. *Tully*	12

Best Seller List

This Week		Last Week	Weeks on List
	FICTION		
1	JONATHAN LIVINGSTON SEAGULL. Bach	1	45
2	THE ODESSA FILE. Forsyth	2	18
3	SEMI-TOUGH. Jenkins	3	21
4	GREEN DARKNESS. Seton	5	11
5	THE CAMERONS. Crichton	6	15
6	THE PERSIAN BOY. Renault	8	15
7	AUGUST 1914. Solzhenitsyn	4	24
8	THE SUNLIGHT DIALOGUES. Gardner	9	4
9	ELEPHANTS CAN REMEMBER. Christie	7	6
10	THE EIGER SANCTION. Trevanian		9
	GENERAL		
1	DR. ATKINS' DIET REVOLUTION. Atkins	1	14
2	THE BEST AND THE BRIGHTEST. Halberstam	2	14
3	HARRY S. TRUMAN. Truman	3	11
4	I'M O.K. - YOU'RE O.K. Harris	4	46
5	"JOHNNY, WE HARDLY KNEW YE." O'Donnell & Powers	5	12
6	THE JOY OF SEX. Comfort	6	11
7	ALL CREATURES GREAT AND SMALL. Herriot	8	7
8	SUPERMONEY. Smith	9	21
9	JOURNEY TO IXTLAN. Castaneda	7	14
10	SOLDIER. Herbert with Wooten		1

This analysis is based on reports obtained from more than 125 bookstores in 64 communities of the United States. The figures in the right-hand column do not necessarily represent consecutive appearances.

Table 8-1. ***Desirable Weights of Persons 20 to 30 Years Old***

Height (without shoes)	Weight (without clothing)		
	Low	*Average*	*High*
Men	**Pounds**	**Pounds**	**Pounds**
5 feet 3 inches	118	129	141
5 feet 4 inches	122	133	145
5 feet 5 inches	126	137	149
5 feet 6 inches	130	142	155
5 feet 7 inches	134	147	161
5 feet 8 inches	139	151	166
5 feet 9 inches	143	155	170
5 feet 10 inches	147	159	174
5 feet 11 inches	150	163	178
6 feet	154	167	183
6 feet 1 inch	158	171	188
6 feet 2 inches	162	175	192
6 feet 3 inches	165	178	195
Women			
5 feet	100	109	118
5 feet 1 inch	104	112	121
5 feet 2 inches	107	115	125
5 feet 3 inches	110	118	128
5 feet 4 inches	113	122	132
5 feet 5 inches	116	125	135
5 feet 6 inches	120	129	139
5 feet 7 inches	123	132	142
5 feet 8 inches	126	136	146
5 feet 9 inches	130	140	151
5 feet 10 inches	133	144	156
5 feet 11 inches	137	148	161
6 feet	141	152	166

*Source: U.S. Dept. of Agriculture.

The AMA Council on Foods and Nutrition reviewed not only the Atkins' publication, but the history of similar diets that have been presented to the public in glowing and highly promissory terms. Within short periods of time they faded into obscurity with no nationwide decrease in obesity being effected. The Council described the diet as unscientific and potentially dangerous for these reasons:

1. A high-fat diet would pose greater risk for the development of heart disease, particularly in susceptible individuals.
2. A feeling of fatigue was a common complaint of individuals on this diet. The fatigue promptly disappeared following addition of carbohydrates to the diet.
3. The Atkins' diet would increase the blood uric acid level aggravating gout conditions or inducing a gout condition.
4. The Council felt it was unfortunate that no reliable mechanism exists to help the public evaluate and put into proper perspective the great volume of nutritional information and misinformation with which it is constantly being bombarded. Bizarre concepts of nutrition and dieting should not be promoted to the public as if they were established scientific principles.
5. Further, physicians were warned to counsel their patients as to the potentially harmful results that might occur because of adherence to the "ketogenic diet," and to report adverse effects from this diet in the medical literature just as in cases of an adverse drug reaction.

Ironically spokesmen for the AMA indicated that their criticisms would probably result in the publisher selling more books. In March 1973 an attorney filed a million dollar suit against Dr. Atkins and his publisher, David McKay Co., for more than 10,000 Ohioans who have bought the book. He asked that the book be banned in Ohio and that buyers of the book be reimbursed. He also asked that the author and publisher be required to pay for any medical problems caused by the diet.

These are classic examples of a communication failure eroding the effectiveness of the country's health authorities.

It is more than a bit ironic that the best-fed country in the world, one whose government pays its farmers not to overproduce, that enriches its bread with the vitamin B's and iron, adds vitamin D to its milk, iodizes its salt, and adds vitamin A to margarine, should also have such an enormous, useless sale of vitamin and mineral supplements. Why is it that books advocating the use of "miracle foods" or "health foods" persist on best seller lists in spite of condemnation by the American Medical Association and leading nutritionists? It is obvious that there is more at stake here than nutrition. The erosion of the effectiveness of authorities in any field spells trouble for a society. How does it happen that a country with a highly developed educational system and mass media second to none can be so badly deluded and uninformed in so basic an area? Let us look at some of the factors involved.

The motivations of the food faddists vary. Their actions are stimulated sometimes by ignorance, sometimes by the search for financial gain. Their false claims and methodical distortion of the truth have misled many. Some of their typical approaches follow:

Exaggerated and False Claims for Specific Foods

Honey is purported to be a preventive for many ills ranging from arthritis to bed wetting. Yogurt, which is the nutritional equivalent of milk, is often sold as a "miracle" food. Vinegar is claimed to help the body burn fats. These statements exemplify the many distorted and misleading claims made by food faddists. The source of miraculous and sweeping claims for specific foods should be carefully checked and should trigger a good deal of caution.

Myth of Soil Depletion

Faddists have been hard at work selling the idea that the soil in this country is depleted, resulting in food products lacking in minerals and vitamins. The United States Department of Agriculture, after a great deal of testing, has found that depleted soil, where it does exist, will result in a smaller yield. The food produced, however, will contain the same amount and quality of nutrients. Faddists will often claim that organic fertilizer is the answer to soil depletion, decrying the use of chemical fertilizers as dangerous. There is, of course, no evidence of this. Spreading such ideas usually results in the sale of unnecessary mineral and vitamin supplements by the food faddists. It also spurs the sale of organically grown "health" foods in "health food" stores at many times the normal price.

Myth of Overprocessing Foods

The claim is made that the canning and freezing of foods result in a significant loss of nutritive value. Although there may at times be some nutritive loss in processing food, it is an inconsequential one if it exists at all. The claim represents a gross exaggeration, the motivation for which is obvious.

Exaggerated Need for Vitamins

The discovery of vitamins was effective in significantly reducing the vitamin deficiency diseases. Enrichment and fortification programs followed, with vitamins being routinely added to foods, so that people could conveniently get adequate amounts of varied vitamins. However, as with many discoveries, an aura of exaggerated effectiveness and function has surrounded the use of vitamins. The faddist has exploited this. The food manufacturer who carefully prints vitamin content of his food, as if it were the only important nutrient it contained, contributes to this exaggerated concept. Pharmaceutical houses have also jumped on the bandwagon with advertisements implying the universal need for vitamin supplementation. Thousands of door-to-door salesmen daily canvas our neighborhoods making false claims for their products sold at ridiculously high prices. It is common for people to believe that vitamins will give them quick energy. Without their daily vitamin pill they expect to come apart at the seams. Many a college student has his or her suitcase packed for school with the inevitable bottle of vitamins. The idea that the only important nutrients in our foods are vitamins reflects a bit of nutritional misinformation.

Vitamin products have a recognized place as a part of preventive medicine when for some special reason the physician decides this kind of supplementation is needed. The indiscriminate use of vitamins is not only expensive but can in some instances be dangerous and represent a poor substitute for a physician when one does not feel well.

Subclinical Deficiency Claims

Faddists have sold the idea that fatigue and generalized aches and pains are symptoms of an underlying nutritional deficiency. Even something as common as feeling tired when one wakes up in the morning has been distorted to indicate the inevitable need for a food supplement. Millions of dollars worth of food supplements are sold by misleading people into making this type of erroneous *assumption*. This is followed by an equally misguided practice of self-treatment with the food supplement.

The Claim that All Diseases Are Due to Faulty Diet

Those diseases that the medical profession has difficulty in managing are the favorites of the faddists.

Heart disease, arthritis, anemia, even decreased sexual potency are given an airing. The usual food supplements are not the only items on sale here, but also the books that advocate a course of action.

One product which the Food and Drug Administration managed to restrict the sale of contained alfalfa, watercress, and parsley. Its salesmen claimed it would cure fifty-seven different diseases. "Groucho Marx, on his radio program a few years ago, interviewed the inventor of Hadacol, Louisiana State Senator Dudley J. LeBlanc. When Groucho asked him what Hadacol was good for, LeBlanc gave an answer of startling honesty. 'It was good,' the senator said, 'for five and a half million for me last year.'"[7]

The Health Food–Organic Food Movement

In the last few years consumers rightly concerned over ecology and pollution of the environment have extended their concern to the food supply. This concern about excessive use of pesticides, additives, and chemical fertilizers has overlapped considerably with and been taken advantage of by promoters of various expensive "health foods" and "organic foods." Scientifically speaking, any food that comes from an animal or plant is organic. The popular use of the term usually refers to food that is grown with naturally produced (i.e., not chemically synthesized) fertilizers and without the use of pesticides. Foods grown in this manner are perfectly good foods but usually have no different nutrient content from other foods and often are much more expensive.

Much publicity has been given to the announcement that a majority of students preferred organically grown foods, when offered a choice in a campus restaurant on the Santa Cruz campus of the University of California. Either no one has told them, or they don't believe, that there is no such thing as organic plant nutrition. Plants utilize only inorganic forms of plant food. Compost and manure are broken down by bacteria to components, such as nitrate, potassium ion, and phosphate, before they are assimilated. Hydroponics, in which plants are grown inorganically without soil, leads to the production of vegetables and fruits with the same protein, carbohydrate, vitamin, and mineral content as when the same strains of plants are grown in the ground with lots of manure. An important difference is that organically grown vegetables are more likely to carry Salmonella, which leads to a common form of food poisoning. Salmonella has recently been reported to be present in vegetables in Holland, grown with the organic benefits of sewage effluent.*

*Presented at the joint meeting of the California and Nevada Dietetic Associations in Las Vegas on April 19, 1971.[8]

The added expense of organically grown foods was explained by an interesting study conducted at the Virginia Polytechnic Institute in 1971 and repeated

[7] Martin Gardner, *Fads and Fallacies* (New York: Dover, 1957), p. 229.

[8] Thomas H. Jukes, "Chemical Residues in Foods," *Journal of the American Dietetic Association*, Vol. 59, No. 3 (September 1971), p. 203.

again in 1972.[9] The vegetable yields from two garden plots were compared. In one garden the vegetables were grown organically and in the other, the vegetables were grown with the help of modern agricultural techniques. The chemically protected garden yielded 1,954 pounds of vegetables whereas the organic garden yielded 237 pounds.

	Organic Yield (lbs)	*Chemically Protected Yield* (lbs)
Tomatoes	141½	446
Cucumbers	28¾	205
White Squash	3	157
Eggplant	no yield due to flea beetles	154¾

Among some younger members of society, dietary restrictions including eating only so-called organic foods and in some cases vegetarianism have become part of the cultural framework. The "counter-culture" food ideology is harmless in most cases, but when carried to extreme can be dangerous. For instance, the "Zen Macrobiotic" diet based on the writings of George Oshawa[10] recommends that the diet will help the consumer attain a spiritual state not attainable in any other way. In its extreme form (most desirable, according to the author) nothing but brown rice is to be eaten. This diet could be, and has been on occasion, fatal. Brown rice alone does not supply the nutrients needed for survival, let alone health. There is evidence that macrobiotic children are not growing properly—their birth weight is less than normal, they develop slowly, and they lose their hair. These are termed as classic marasmus (a nutritional deficiency brought on by a severe shortage of proteins and calories) symptoms. Most vegetarian regimes, however, can provide adequate nutrition if a *variety* of foods including cereals, legumes, nuts, fruits, and vegetables are consumed. Although legumes (peas and beans), nuts, and soybeans contain some protein, it is difficult to consume the great amounts needed for proper nutrition. If milk and eggs are allowed, then the chances are better that proper nutrition can be achieved. The extreme reaction of some groups to avoid processed foods has been disastrous. In some communes babies have been fed raw milk, resulting in diseases, such as typhoid, which were all but unheard of in this country a few years ago. A physician at St. Mark's Hospital diagnosed a case of ascariasis (infestation of the intestine by a parasitic worm, ascaris) in a young woman who for the past six months had eaten large quantities of raw, organically grown vegetables.

As one renowned professor of nutrition has indicated, "We have enough problems as a nation—poverty, ignorance, pollution, racial prejudice, poor planning of our material and intellectual processes, cloudy ethics—without encouraging the creation of new totally unnecessary health hazards."[11]

[9]Robert C. Lambe, Extension Specialist and Associate Professor in Plant Pathology at Virginia Polytechnic Institute, Blacksburg, Va., 1971.

[10]George Oshawa, *Zen Macrobiotics: The Art of Rejuvenation and Longevity* (Los Angeles: Ignoramus Press, 1965).

[11]Jean Mayer, Professor of Nutrition, School of Public Health, Boston, Mass. *New York Times*, April 2, 1972.

Unfortunately many manufacturers of health foods and "organic" vitamin supplements (which are no different chemically from synthesized vitamins) have taken advantage of the youthful counterculture for economic gain. Especially disturbing is the fact that some "health food stores" have been noted recently to be accepting food stamps. Surely the low-income person can least afford to spend extra money for food that will give him no more nutrition than the food he can buy in the supermarket.

Food Additives

The old country store is with us no more. Its familiar food odors and cracker barrel are part of a nostalgic past. The crackers are now double-wrapped to maintain freshness and crispness for months. The bread on the open shelf is now carefully wrapped and calcium propionate added to prevent it from becoming moldy. The age of the supermarket is upon us. The frozen food sections, with their increasing variety of foods, and the canned and bottled goods departments are part of an era marked by advances in the packaging and preservation of food. In the supermarket are also found maraschino cherries containing a color additive; marshmallows that stay fresh longer, not only because of better packaging, but because an additive helps it to retain its moisture. The poultry and fish have antibiotics added to retard spoilage. An era that has seen rather revolutionary changes take place in food processing and packaging also heralds the coming of age of the food additive, for without them many packaged food products could not be produced.

A food additive is a substance added to food in a variety of ways to make our food better and more abundant. There are two general types of additives. Those that are called *intentional additives* are substances used to perform a specific function, such as nutrient supplements, preservatives, and coloring materials. The others are called *incidental additives* and serve no function in the finished product, but somehow become a part of the food through some production method, processing, or packaging. Examples of incidental additives might be pesticides or chemical fertilizers that are needed to protect our crops from being consumed by insects.

In 1924, iodine was the first food additive used. It was added to table salt to prevent goiter. Iodized salt has been responsible for the practical disappearance of simple goiter in this country. As of July 1972 all salt was required to carry a statement regarding iodine content on its label; for example, next to Iodized Salt the statement "This salt supplies iodine a necessary nutrient," whereas next to the name Salt, the statement "This salt does not supply iodine, a necessary nutrient."[12]

In the thirties, the fortification of milk with vitamin D was begun. This procedure was developed to prevent rickets in children. Milk is rich in calcium and phosphorus, those minerals that are needed for the proper development of bones. Because vitamin

[12] "Information on Ingredient Labeling of Standardized Foods," FDA, March 1972.

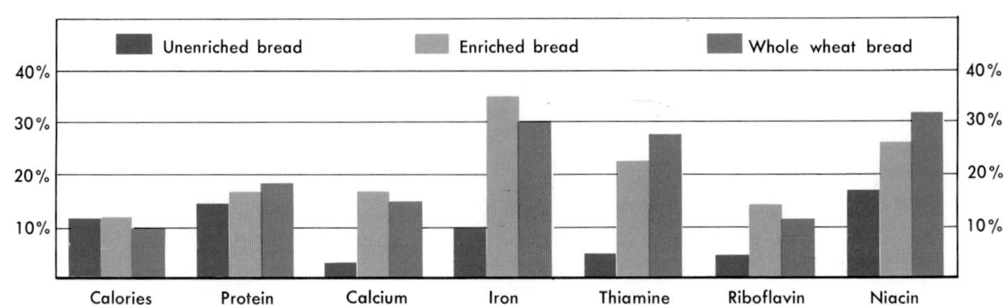

D helps the body to utilize calcium and phosphorus, it followed that milk should be the food selected for fortification with this vitamin. In the early forties, the enrichment of flour, bread, and cereal products with several B vitamins (thiamin, riboflavin, and niacin) and iron was begun. This program is believed to be a strong factor in the virtual elimination of pellagra in the southern part of this country. Vitamin A has since been added to margarine to make it the nutritional equivalent of butter. More recently the FDA has decided to increase the amount of iron and B vitamins in the grain products of American consumers. In this way the high prevalence of iron deficiency anemia found by the White House Conference on Food, Nutrition and Health and the Ten-State Nutrition Survey in 1969–1970 might be significantly reduced.

Though the early food additives were essentially *nutrient supplements,* those that followed were designed to preserve flavor or color, or maintain texture of processed food. Microorganism spoilage is controlled through the use of *antibiotics,* which inhibit the growth of molds and bacteria. *Sugar* is used as a preservative not only with jams and jellies but with canned and frozen fruits as well. *Antioxidants,* such as vitamin C, are used to prevent fruit from turning brown when being frozen. *Emulsifiers* are used so that substances that are normally immiscible will mix (such as oil and vinegar in a salad dressing). Emulsifiers are also used in bakery batters and ice cream to give these products a smoother texture. *Stabilizers and thickeners* will thicken and prevent chocolate from settling out of chocolate milk. Other examples of their uses are in cake mixes and gelatins, where they surround flavor oils and prevent their deterioration by oxidation. Acids, bases, buffers, and *neutralizing agents* control the degree of acidity or alkalinity in foods, which in turn affects their flavor and texture. *Sequestrants* are used to separate out certain substances in solutions, such as minerals from fats and oils, which act as catalysts to rancidity. They are also used as clarifying agents for beverages. *Humectants* are added to keep moisture in food, for example, shredded coconut and confections. *Anti-caking agents* are used to keep salts and powders free flowing. *Firming agents* maintain the texture of processed fruits and vegetables, and *coloring agents* are used in a variety of foods to improve their appearance. *Bleaching agents* bleach a number of foods, including flour, whose color after milling is yellow. It formerly required months of storage to bleach flour, which led to problems of insect and rodent infestation. (It was not uncommon to find insect fragments in flour and flour products at one time.) *Foaming agents* are used in pressure-packed products to facilitate the ejection of the material from the can as in the case of the many whipped toppings. *Foam inhibitors* are used in the canning of liquid foods (e.g., orange juice) where foaming interferes with the canning process. *Nonnutritive sweeteners* such as saccharin are used in dietetic foods and beverages.

These are a few of the types of additives currently being used. In terms of numbers there are literally thousands of food additives in use. The control and safety factors in the use of additives have been care-

Fig. 8-5. Most Americans consume five to six slices of bread a day. The chart compares nutrient contribution of six slices of enriched, unenriched and whole-wheat bread to the recommended dietary allowance for the normal man. (Today's Health)

fully worked out. When it is found that a chemical has use as a food additive, it is put through toxicity studies to determine if the substance is harmful to living things. These studies are conducted with laboratory animals, some being of a short-term nature while others are long-term studies. When it is determined that the chemical is safe for human consumption, the Food and Drug Administration is petitioned and the test data presented. When the scientists of the governmental agency are convinced of the safety of the chemical, they determine the safe amount and the foods it will be used in and how it will be labeled.

Federal Legislation Relating to Food in the United States

Federal Food and Drug Act of 1906

This legislation made illegal the adulteration of food entering into interstate commerce. In this law, adulteration was defined as:

1. The use of poisonous additives of any type.
2. The extraction of valuable constituents from the product. This was aimed at inhibiting manufacturers from utilizing cheaper and less nutritious ingredients in their products.
3. The attempt to conceal inferiority of the product in any way. This legislation was considered to be good for its time, but by 1938, needs for revision became apparent.

Federal Food, Drug, and Cosmetic Act of 1938

This law applied to imports and exports as well as interstate commerce. In it *food* was defined as articles used in food or drink for man or other animals. This legislation again prohibited the adulteration of food. In addition, it made truthful labeling mandatory. Weight and contents of a food package had to be accurately described and not in any way misleading. The name and place of the manufacturer, packer, or distributor needed to be listed on the food package. This legislation also set standards and definitions for foods. It enacted *standards of identity,* which described what the product was. For example, in the identification of fruit preserves, not less than 45 parts fruit or fruit juice needed to be present in the product, with the remaining 55 parts being sugar. If the proportion of fruit or fruit juice is less than 45 per cent, then the product must be labeled imitation. This legislation also set *standards of quality,* particularly for canned foods and vegetables, with regard to tenderness, color, and freedom from defects. If a product, for example, is excessively broken, it must be labeled "below standard in quality." The law also established *standards of fill* for a container. This was aimed at preventing deception of the buyer. It was at one time a practice for some manufacturers to place their products in a large container and then only half fill it. This misled the consumer into thinking that he was getting more of the product than he actually received.

Major amendments to the 1938 law have been

added. *The Miller Pesticide Amendment* was passed in 1954. The basic provision of this amendment was to set standards for safe amounts of pesticide residue that may be permitted to remain on fruits and vegetables. The *Food Additives Amendment* was passed in 1958. This amendment required proof of safety before a substance could be added to food. It also forbade the use of a substance which was found to produce cancer in man or animals. In 1960 the *Color Additive Amendment* came into being. This legislation placed under control the use of coal tar colors. It required that no coloring matter be approved if it was found to be carcinogenic to man or animal when used in any amounts. If a question arose as to whether a coloring material was carcinogenic, a scientific advisory committee would investigate the matter.

Protecting the Public from the Faddist

The question arises, how can we better protect the American public from health food faddists? Education with regard to the simple principles of nutrition would do much to handcuff quackery. In addition, however, some help is needed from the federal and state governments. Laws concerning food and drugs should be uniform throughout the states. What endangers the public health in Maine will surely be as hazardous in California! Many states take no interest in public health problems and very often these states become handy bases of operation for food quacks. Modernized drug, food, and advertising laws are needed so that the obvious loopholes of the old laws will no longer exist. Along with this modernization should go bigger budgets and larger staffs for the Food and Drug Administration and the Federal Trade Commission. Changes in our laws should permit the protecting agencies such as the Post Office, Food and Drug Administration, and the Federal Trade Commission to exchange information and permit court decisions won by one of the protecting agencies to be used by the others. Support from the nation's judges would also be invaluable. Quacks who are caught are usually lightly fined and set free to pick up where they left off.

Active, aggressive law enforcement is necessary to help control nutrition quackery. The Food and Drug Administration directs its activities against shippers and distributors whose food supplements and dietary preparations bear inaccurate or exaggerated claims on their labels. It has been active in running down the door-to-door salesmen of food supplements often referred to as "doorstep diagnosticians" who "prescribe" their products for a variety of ailments, including serious diseases. The Food and Drug Administration activity in this area also includes investigating "nutrition educators" and "health food lecturers" who rent halls to give pseudoscientific talks and misrepresent the products they sell.

The Federal Trade Commission has responsibility for checking promotional and advertising practices related to foods and cookware that are misleading. This federal agency works with one hand tied behind its back in that the burden of proof regarding any claim in dispute lies with the agency and not with the manufacturer or producer making the claim. Misleading advertising can go on until such time as the Federal Trade Commission, with its limited facilities, personnel, and budget, can prove it wrong. This issue will be further discussed in chapter 11, "Consumer Beware."

Law enforcement with regard to nutritional quackery, regardless of how effective it may be, is not a solution unto itself. Although it has a definite contribution to make, it is limited by personnel and facilities available. It can serve as a valuable adjunct to other measures.

The Need for Effective Nutrition Education

Education is a key to the prevention of food faddism and the practice of good nutrition. Nutrition education programs in our schools are not as well developed as they might be. They are often too narrow in their scope, concerning themselves only with the nutritional diseases or a recitation of nutrients and their functions. Many elementary teachers, poorly prepared in the area, are often sources of misinformation. In addition, they often use a fear approach and tend to preach instead of teach about nutrition. Secondary school programs are equally in need of review in terms of their content and student coverage. Certainly *all* high school seniors should have basic nutritional facts and be alerted to the public health problems and programs in this area. Public health organizations could then further educate a public that has been given a basis for additional information. The educational task of the public health agency is at present overwhelming. It is time for schools, colleges, and health agencies to coordinate their efforts to achieve adequate nutrition education in schools.

The White House Conference on Food, Nutrition, and Health held in December of 1969 recommended that a comprehensive and sequential program of nutrition education should be an integral part of the curriculum of all elementary and secondary schools in the United States and its territories. A few states have taken action toward implementing this recommendation, but at present far too many schools have made little or no effort in nutrition education or in coordinating school efforts with those of the community. The health education teacher trained as an educator and in the field of public health is in a unique position to coordinate efforts not only within schools, but with the community as well. The health teacher should coordinate existing programs, such as those which may exist in home economics, school feeding programs, and physical education in order to provide meaningful nutrition education for each child. The health educator can also tie his program in with community efforts such as the recent expanded Food and Nutrition Education Program, which is part of the Cooperative Extension Service. Under this program, indigenous nutrition aides are employed to carry out nutrition education programs in their own neighborhoods. As of 1971 about 9,000 aides were employed in the program throughout the country, reaching about 1.5 million individuals.

Until there are expanded efforts for meaningful

nutrition education programs for *all* age groups in the community, problems of nutrition can be expected to increase in scope and severity.

Problems Related to Food and Digestion

Food Poisoning

Common types of food poisoning involve *staphylococcal* and *salmonella* contamination. When contaminated foods are ingested, the symptoms of food poisoning appear 2 to 4 hours after eating in the form of nausea, diarrhea, and intestinal cramps, lasting a few hours and usually not more than a day. Improperly prepared foods, unpasteurized milk and dairy products, contamination of foods by roaches, rodent feces, or infected persons may be some of the ways this condition is transmitted. Some safeguards against food poisoning that can be taken are:

1. Wash raw foods thoroughly.
2. Wash hands *before* handling food, and after handling *raw* foods such as chickens, meats, eggs, and dairy products.
3. Refrigerate all dairy products and leftovers promptly.
4. Keep perishable foods chilled when going on trips or picnics.

In 1972 the American Public Health Association and six other organizations brought a public interest suit against the Secretary of Agriculture. These health organizations did this because of the consistent refusals of the U.S. Department of Agriculture to provide adequate labeling instructions on how to avoid food poisoning from disease-causing raw poultry and meat products. The APHA and its colleagues indicated that the label should warn the consumer of possible contamination and inform him of proper handling and cooking procedures. In explaining its action the APHA pointed out that:

> USDA warns in one of its own publications that "food poisoning ranks second only to the common cold as the most frequent cause of illness in this country" and that "food poisoning results most often from carelessness in the handling, preparation, and storage of food." Federal inspection procedures for raw meat and poultry products do not attempt to detect salmonella or similar bacteria causing food poisoning.
>
> The suit points out that the Center for Disease Control, an agency of the Public Health Service, knows of 20,000 reported cases of salmonella poisoning each year and estimates the total at 2 million. The Food and Drug Administration attributed approximately 100 deaths to food-borne salmonella poisoning in 1970. The National Academy of Sciences places the economic cost of this disease at $300 million annually, and has termed salmonellosis "one of the most important communicable disease problems in the United States. Between 15 per cent and 50 per cent of federally inspected meat and poultry has been found to be contaminated by salmonella. In a sworn affidavit filed with the court, Sussman cited these figures, and detailed one case of food poisoning.
>
> Two deaths resulted when 18 people at a Thanksgiving day dinner ate a USDA inspected turkey. Within 18 hours, 17 of the guests developed symptoms of gastroenteritis, including vomiting, diarrhea, fever, and abdominal pain. A 17-year-old boy and a 56-year-old woman died,

and the others were hospitalized for between four and twelve days, Sussman reported. Had proper food handling procedures been followed so that this turkey had not come into contact with other foods, and the cook's hands been washed immediately after handling the bird, this incident would never have happened, he said.

The suit seeks to have the court rule that USDA officials have violated their statutory duty, and that within 30 days USDA should propose new regulations, requiring that labels on inspected raw meat and poultry products contain instructions to the consumer on the proper storage, cooking, and handling precautions necessary to minimize the risk of salmonella and other bacterial food poisoning.[13]

Botulism is another form of food poisoning that is highly fatal. The early symptoms of botulism are characterized by double or blurred vision, slurred speech, and difficulty in swallowing. Death due to botulism is usually the result of respiratory and cardiac paralysis, since the poison primarily attacks the nervous system. This occurs in two-thirds of the patients and usually within 3 to 7 days. The symptoms develop in accordance with the amount ingested and appear within 18 hours. Most poisonings in the United States arise from the improper canning of vegetables at home. The botulism organism (Clostridium botulinum) is widely distributed in the soil and is normally harmless when surrounded by air. However, when the organism is in an airtight container, such as a can or a preserving jar, it grows and produces one of the most deadliest poisons known to man. When the homemaker is careless or unaware of proper sterilization methods in home-canning, some very serious consequences may be in store. There have been, however, cases of botulism caused by commercially canned products. In July 1971 a death was recorded as a result of botulism from a can of soup. In April 1970 there was a nationwide recall of 80,000 frozen pizzas believed to contain botulism-tainted mushrooms. During that year 13 people became ill from botulism and 5 died. In 1963, 14 Americans died from infected tuna and smoked fish from the Great Lakes.

Death from botulism need not occur at all since boiling the contents of a can vigorously for 3 to 5 minutes destroys the toxin. This would pertain to soups as well as vegetables—even those green or wax beans to be used for salads and are generally used straight from the can. Never buy cans that are swollen or misshapen and never taste-test a suspicious-smelling food, since only very small amounts of the toxin are extremely dangerous. The treatment for the condition consists of intramuscular injections of botulinus antitoxin only after certain diagnosis of botulism has been made.

Peptic Ulcers

Peptic ulcers can be described as an erosion of the mucus membrane of the stomach or small intestine. They are called *gastric ulcers* if they occur in the stomach and are referred to as *duodenal ulcers* when they appear in the upper part of the small intestine.

[13]*The Nation's Health,* April 1972. (The Official Newspaper of the American Public Health Association.)

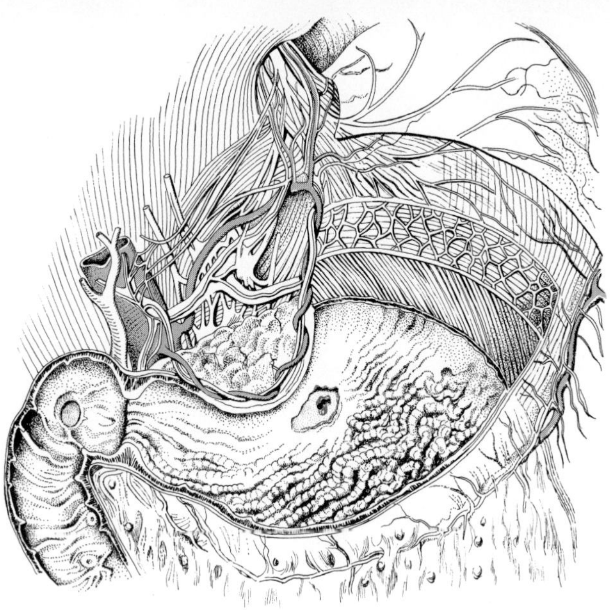

Fig. 8-6. Examples of gastric and duodenal ulcers. (Adapted from a drawing by Roche Laboratories, Nutley, N.J.)

The condition is often related to nervous and emotional states. It is believed that stress will many times cause in the stomach an increased flow of hydrochloric acid which will precipitate the development of ulcers. The condition can become complicated when erosion through the stomach wall strikes a blood vessel and bleeding results. This is referred to as a *bleeding ulcer* and can cause anemia or endanger life if the bleeding is profuse. When the erosion perforates the stomach, we have what is known as a *perforated ulcer* which can lead to rather serious complications.

Treatment for ulcers often consists of a bland diet, with many small meals recommended in place of the usual three. Drugs are occasionally prescribed in addition to the modification of diet. Where the ulcers are of a serious nature, surgery may be the recommended procedure. The surgery is usually designed to remove the ulcerated part of the stomach or to permit food to bypass this portion of the stomach.

A factor in ulcer incidence is the self-medicative use of alkalis to relieve symptoms of stomach discomfort. Alkalis will cause the stomach to increase its acid production, particularly if the alkalis are used habitually. This acid rebound can be a factor in ulcer production. It has further been found that alkalis interfere with nutrition by destroying vitamins such as vitamins C and B_2. It is interesting to note that the incidence of gastric ulcers increases as socioeconomic class is lowered. There are some sources of information in our society that try to contradict this basic fact. The incidence is also three times as high in the male as in the female. It has also been observed that ulcers in women tend to go into remission during pregnancy. However, attempts at hormone therapy to alleviate ulcers have been ineffective.

Gall Bladder Disease

The function of the gall bladder is to produce bile. The bile emulsifies fat, breaking down fat globules into smaller ones so that they may be more easily digested. It was once erroneously believed that this disease was more prevalent among women who tended to be overweight and of middle age. It therefore was considered to be the disease of the "fair, fat, and forty." Recent studies, however, have shown that these three factors do not necessarily apply to this condition. Gall bladder disease is often caused by infection that migrates from the intestine through the bile duct and into the gall bladder. Symptoms that generally appear as a result include nausea, heartburn, indigestion (particularly after eating fats), and pain on the right side under the ribs. The treatment usually consists of diet control (particularly the restricted use of fats in the diet) or the removal of the gall bladder. *Gallstones* represent another form of gall bladder malfunction. These stones or crystals precipitate out of the solution of bile and can be a cause of pain. The stones sometimes block the bile duct or cause pain by scratching their way through it. Because of the dangers of cancer due to chronic irritation, the gall bladder is often removed under these circumstances.

Constipation and Laxatives

"No organ of the body is so misunderstood and maltreated as the digestive tract. It has been purged, irrigated, lavaged, massaged, and pummelled, all in the name of that great American obsession, the daily bowel movement."[14] The idea that a daily bowel movement is synonymous with good health has caused a preoccupation with this function. Six out of ten Americans use laxatives, and there are 500 different brands of laxative products on the market. In most instances, the use of these products was completely unnecessary. Most cases of constipation can be relieved without the use of drugs. It must further be recognized that in the great majority of cases where laxative drugs are used, constipation is not even present. Constipation cannot be defined in terms of a daily bowel movement. What is normal functioning here will vary from one individual to another. This variance may be from one or more movements a day to an evacuation only once in two or three days without the slightest of ill effects. Physicians are many times concerned because people overlook the fact that any laxative is potentially harmful and that there is no such thing as a laxative that is natural and harmless in all instances. The theory that a laxative "cleans out" the digestive tract is quite a misleading one. Essentially, what the individual does is to introduce into the digestive tract a cathartic drug which can have a number of harmful effects including dehydration, irritation, and inflammation of the digestive tract. There is a relationship between the incidence of hemorrhoids and fissures of the anus and the habitual use of cathartics. Besides, the very cause of chronic constipation is often associated with the use of these types of drugs. In essence, they may be causing the very condition that they are supposed to be preventing. The best preventive measure against constipation would be for most people to resist taking self-medicative action in the form of laxatives, suppositories, and enemas. A very positive step that can be taken in combating constipation is to add to the diet such foods as fruits, vegetables, and whole wheat grain cereals. These will add roughage to the diet that will maintain proper functioning of the digestive tract. Probably the greatest problem that we have in this country in connection with constipation is the current hysteria related to its supposed existence.

[14] *The Medicine Show* (Mount Vernon, N.Y.: Consumers Union, 1971), p. 47.

Basic Nutritional Needs

There is nothing more basic to survival than food. The quality of that survival is strongly related to the quality of one's nutrition. What constitutes good nutrition, however, varies with the person, his age, sex, size, his rate of growth, physical activity, or the presence of stress such as disease or fever. Nutrition is thus a science. There are, however, few people who treat it as such. Health motives and knowledge of nutritional needs may play a part, but are hardly the only motives for the selection of foods. What a person eats will be influenced by the season of the

Fig. 8-7. *A guide to good eating. Used daily, these foods are the foundation of a good diet. Eat more of these and other foods as needed for growth, activity, and desirable weight. (National Dairy Council, Chicago, Ill.)*

year, the amount of money available to buy food, and his geographical location. Within that framework the person will make food choices strongly influenced by his cultural and personal background as well as his tastebuds. Add to this already complex situation misinformation deliberately disseminated by food faddists and some misleading advertisements and it becomes apparent that developing good nutritional practices is a complex process. Be that as it may, let us not shrink from adversity. On the following pages are tables and criteria that will assist you in measuring nutrition practices. Also see Appendix B for a comprehensive Table listing the nutritive values of foods. Perhaps with the assistance of your instructor, you may choose to measure your nutritional practices and those of your classmates, your family, or selected groups in your community. In the process you may gain some insights into the factors that lead to varying levels of nutritional status.

The Balanced Diet

An adequate diet is usually discussed, particularly in health texts, from the point of view of what constitutes adequate nutrition. This is probably as it should be. We cannot ignore the fact, however, that the reasons for food intake include other motivational factors besides health. There has been increasing recognition of the role of emotional factors as related to food intake. The insecure person may choose to eat food as an infant uses a pacifier. Food is frequently offered as a social grace. In many such instances, the person is made to feel awkward if he refuses the offering. Social pressure, therefore, becomes a reason for eating in this case, not nutrition. This may be particularly true when you are offered a piece of grandmother's favorite pie and are expected not only to eat the first piece, but enthusiastically ask for a second. Food tastes, the manner in which food is prepared, how much time we allow for a meal, and family eating patterns are other factors related to what and how much we eat. We could go on. The point is that through this maze of motivational factors and circumstances we must keep in mind the basic purposes of food intake. Those who live to eat die early. For those of us who eat to live, let us consider those combinations of foods and nutrients that can help us to do it best.

A varied diet is in itself insurance that we are getting the variety of nutrients needed to maintain health. Using a guide such as the basic four food groups is an easy, yet a fairly specific, check on the nature of our food intake. The basic four food groups include:

1. The Milk Group

Foods included in this grouping consist of milk and milk products, such as cheese and ice cream. The daily amounts recommended for foods in this group include the following: For whole milk, three to four cups for children; four cups or more for teenagers; two or more for adults; four or more for pregnant women; and six or more for nursing mothers. The milk in these cases may be in the form of skim milk, butter milk, evaporated milk, or dry milk. Cheese

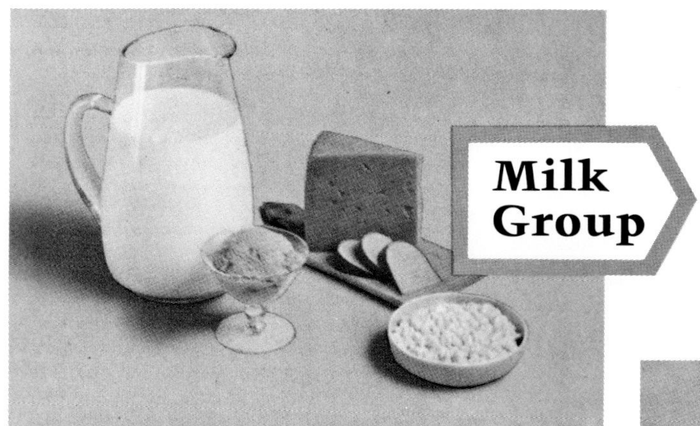

Milk Group

3 or more glasses milk—Children
smaller glasses for some children under 8

4 or more glasses—Teen-agers

2 or more glasses—Adults

Cheese, ice cream and other milk-made foods can supply part of the milk

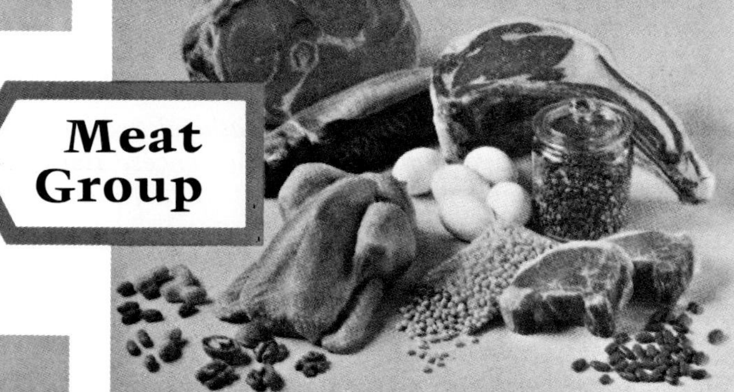

Meat Group

2 or more servings

Meats, fish, poultry, eggs, or cheese—with dry beans, peas, nuts as alternates

Vegetables and Fruits

4 or more servings

Include dark green or yellow vegetables; citrus fruit or tomatoes

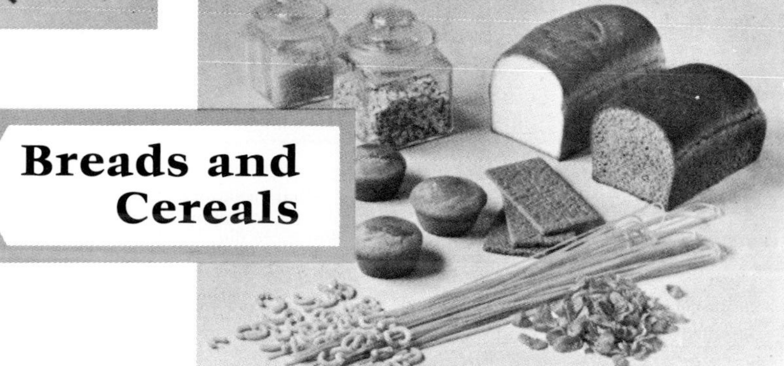

Breads and Cereals

4 or more servings

Enriched or whole grain
Added milk improves nutritional values

Table 8-2. ***Food and Nutrition Board, National Academy of Sciences-National Research Council Recommended Daily Dietary Allowances,[a] Revised 1974***
Designed for the maintenance of good nutrition of practically all healthy people in the U.S.A.

								Fat-Soluble Vitamins			
	Age (years)	*Weight*		*Height*		*Energy*	*Protein*	*Vitamin A Activity*		*Vitamin D*	*Vitamin E Activity[e]*
		(kg)	**(lbs)**	**(cm)**	**(in)**	**(kcal)[b]**	**(g)**	**(RE)[c]**	**(IU)**	**(IU)**	**(IU)**
Infants	0.0–0.5	6	14	60	24	kg × 117	kg × 2.2	420[d]	1,400	400	4
	0.5–1.0	9	20	71	28	kg × 108	kg × 2.0	400	2,000	400	5
Children	1–3	13	28	86	34	1300	23	400	2,000	400	7
	4–6	20	44	110	44	1800	30	500	2,500	400	9
	7–10	30	66	135	54	2400	36	700	3,300	400	10
Males	11–14	44	97	158	63	2800	44	1,000	5,000	400	12
	15–18	61	134	172	69	3000	54	1,000	5,000	400	15
	19–22	67	147	172	69	3000	54	1,000	5,000	400	15
	23–50	70	154	172	69	2700	56	1,000	5,000		15
	51+	70	154	172	69	2400	56	1,000	5,000		15
Females	11–14	44	97	155	62	2400	44	800	4,000	400	12
	15–18	54	119	162	65	2100	48	800	4,000	400	12
	19–22	58	128	162	65	2100	46	800	4,000	400	12
	23–50	58	128	162	65	2000	46	800	4,000		12
	51+	58	128	162	65	1800	46	800	4,000		12
Pregnant						+300	+30	1,000	5,000	400	15
Lactating						+500	+20	1,200	6,000	400	15

[a]The allowances are intended to provide for individual variations among most normal persons as they live in the United States under usual environmental stresses. Diets should be based on a variety of common foods in order to provide other nutrients for which human requirements have been less well defined. See text for more detailed discussion of allowances and of nutrients not tabulated.

[b]Kilojoules (kJ) = 4.2 × kcal

[c]Retinol equivalents

[d]Assumed to be all as retinol in milk during the first six months of life. All subsequent intakes are assumed to be half as retinol and half as β-carotene when calculated from international units. As retinol equivalents three fourths are as retinol and one fourth as β-carotene.

Water-Soluble Vitamins							Minerals					
Ascorbic Acid (mg)	*Folacin*[f] (μg)	*Niacin*[g] (mg)	*Riboflavin* (B_2) (mg)	*Thiamin* (B_1) (mg)	*Vitamin* B_6 (mg)	*Vitamin* B_{12} (μg)	*Calcium* (mg)	*Phosphorus* (mg)	*Iodine* (μg)	*Iron* (mg)	*Magnesium* (mg)	*Zinc* (mg)
35	50	5	0.4	0.3	0.3	0.3	360	240	35	10	60	3
35	50	8	0.6	0.5	0.4	0.3	540	400	45	15	70	5
40	100	9	0.8	0.7	0.6	1.0	800	800	60	15	150	10
40	200	12	1.1	0.9	0.9	1.5	800	800	80	10	200	10
40	300	16	1.2	1.2	1.2	2.0	800	800	110	10	250	10
45	400	18	1.5	1.4	1.6	3.0	1200	1200	130	18	350	15
45	400	20	1.8	1.5	2.0	3.0	1200	1200	150	18	400	15
45	400	20	1.8	1.5	2.0	3.0	800	800	140	10	350	15
45	400	18	1.6	1.4	2.0	3.0	800	800	130	10	350	15
45	400	16	1.5	1.2	2.0	3.0	800	800	110	10	350	15
45	400	16	1.3	1.2	1.6	3.0	1200	1200	115	18	300	15
45	400	14	1.4	1.1	2.0	3.0	1200	1200	115	18	300	15
45	400	14	1.4	1.1	2.0	3.0	800	800	100	18	300	15
45	400	13	1.2	1.0	2.0	3.0	800	800	100	18	300	15
45	400	12	1.1	1.0	2.0	3.0	800	800	80	10	300	15
60	800	+2	+0.3	+0.3	2.5	4.0	1200	1200	125	18+[h]	450	20
80	600	+4	+0.5	+0.3	2.5	4.0	1200	1200	150	18	450	25

[e]Total vitamin E activity, estimated to be 80 percent as α-tocopherol and 20 percent other tocopherols.

[f]The folacin allowances refer to dietary sources as determined by *Lactobacillus casei* assay. Pure forms of folacin may be effective in doses less than one fourth of the recommended dietary allowance.

[g]Although allowances are expressed as niacin, it is recognized that on the average 1 mg of niacin is derived from each 60 mg of dietary tryptophan.

[h]This increased requirement cannot be met by ordinary diets; therefore, the use of supplemental iron is recommended.

and ice cream would make adequate replacements for milk. The amounts it would take for either one of these items to replace milk needs to be estimated on the basis of calcium content. A good rule of thumb is that a one-inch cube of cheese will equal $\frac{2}{3}$ cup of milk; $\frac{1}{2}$ cup of cottage cheese is equal to $\frac{1}{3}$ of a cup of milk; $\frac{1}{2}$ cup of ice cream is equal to $\frac{1}{4}$ cup of milk.

The major contribution that these foods make to our diet is that they are good sources of calcium as well as protein, vitamin A, and riboflavin.

2. The Meat Group

This group would include a variety of meats such as beef, veal, lamb, pork, and organ meats. It would also include poultry, fish, eggs, and shellfish. When some of these foods cannot be obtained, alternatives in this group consist of dry beans, peas, lentils, nuts, and peanut butter. It is recommended that a person choose two or more servings each day from the foods found in this group. Each serving should consist of approximately two to three ounces of meat, poultry, or fish. Two eggs, one cup of beans, peas, or lentils, or four tablespoons of peanut butter would count as a serving. The foods in this group are important because they are sources of protein, iron, and the B vitamins (thiamin, riboflavin, and niacin).

3. The Vegetable/Fruit Group

All fruits and vegetables are included in this grouping. It is recommended that four servings each day be included in the individual's diet. Because foods in this group are generally good sources of vitamins C and A, it is recommended that one give consideration to those fruits and vegetables that are rich in these nutrients. Good sources of vitamin C would include the citrus fruits, as well as strawberries, broccoli, and green peppers. Good sources of vitamin A include the dark green or yellow vegetables. These are exemplified by such items as Swiss chard, apricots, broccoli, kale, spinach, pumpkin, sweet potatoes, and turnip greens, among others. Particular attention should be paid to the sources of vitamin C, because of the high incidence of borderline deficiency in this nutrient.

4. The Bread and Cereal Group

This group includes those foods made from grain, namely breads and cereals, cakes, crackers, and other baked products, as well as cornmeal, macaroni, oats, and rice. It is recommended that four servings be chosen daily from this grouping. A serving would be defined for this group as one slice of bread, one ounce of cereal or $\frac{1}{2}$ to $\frac{3}{4}$ of a cup of cooked cereal, cornmeal, macaroni, or rice. The foods in this group, in addition to serving as supplementary sources of protein and iron, are also rich in the vitamin B's and serve as sources of food energy.

Anyone selecting his foods on the basis of the recommendations of the basic four food groups should have a balanced diet. When an individual seeks to lose weight, the recommendation is that the amount of food be somewhat restricted. However, the variety of foods as listed in these four groups should remain consistent if one is to maintain an adequate level of health.

Review Questions

1. What changes have been taking place in the nature of our nutritional problems? To what extent are some of our new nutritional problems the result of overcorrecting for some of our former problems?
2. What are some of the typical approaches used by the modern-day food faddists?
3. What protection is provided the public from the food faddist? Evaluate the effectiveness of this protection.
4. What is the role of education as a means of combating food faddism?
5. Describe the dramatic changes that have been brought about by the introduction of food additives.
6. How did the purposes of the early food additives differ from those of the most recent ones?
7. In what way does the Federal Food, Drug and Cosmetic Act protect the health of the consumer? What are the provisions of the major amendments to this law?
8. What are the factors that make the problem of weight control difficult and complex?
9. Why do so many attempts at dieting fail?
10. Why has quackery in the area of weight control been so successful?
11. What particular nutritional problems do poor Americans face?
12. Evaluate the effectiveness of existing programs to improve the nutritional status of the low-income segment of our population.

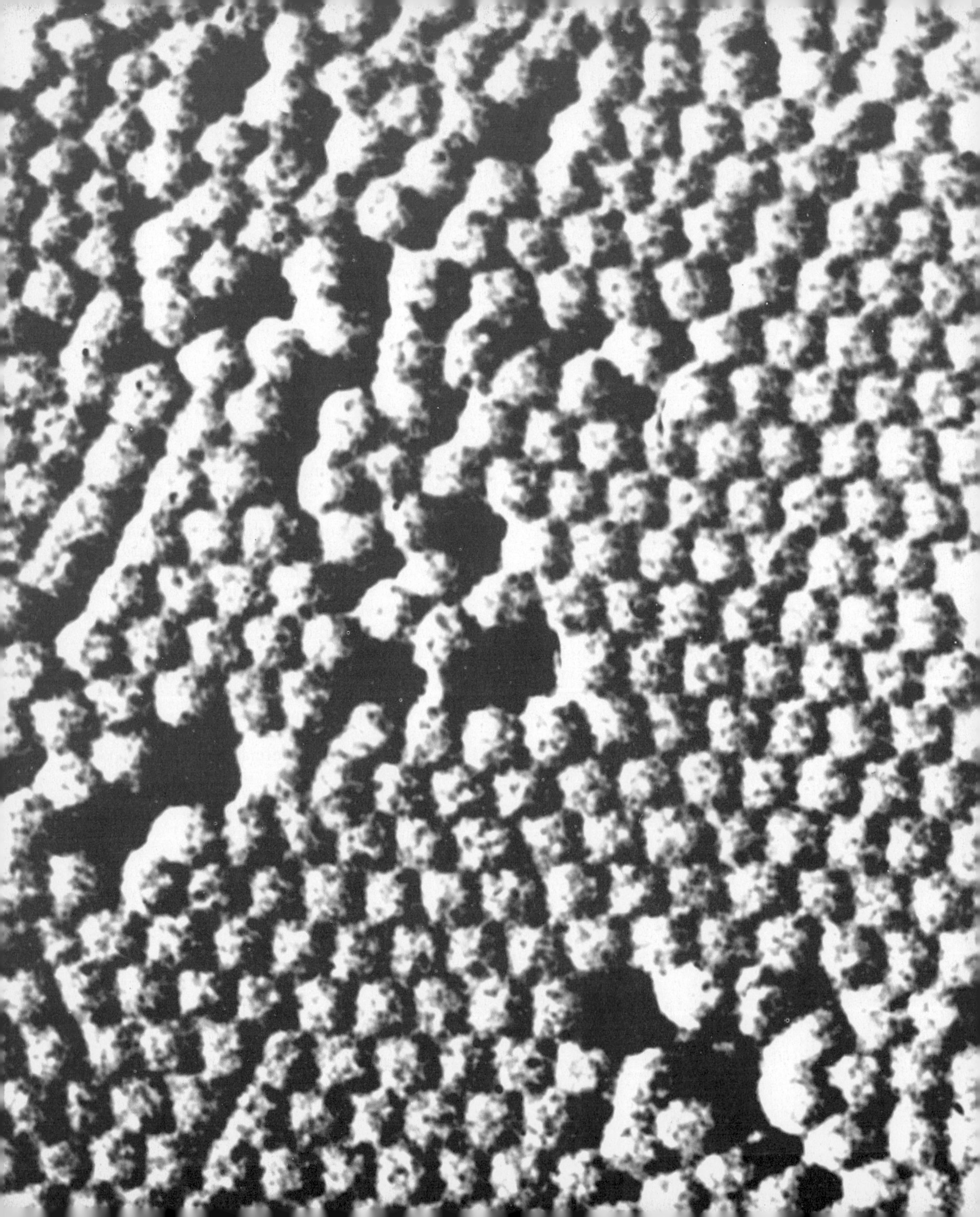

Part Five

Disease Prevention and Control

Chapter 9
Man's Control of Communicable Diseases

Through the centuries since prehistoric times, man has relentlessly and unremittingly struggled against the ravages of communicable disease. He has often enjoyed greater success in his efforts to control communicable disease than in any other health sphere. In spite of this success, he has failed to eradicate a single disease. Every communicable disease ever known to man still exists today in some part of the world. Though man's progress with this kind of health problem cannot be measured by his ability to eradicate disease, there are other means of measuring his success.

A comparison of long-term mortality rates from selected communicable diseases illustrates the dramatic downward trend in the number of deaths from these diseases. Similarly, a decreasing incidence of a particular illness suggests that a measure of control has been achieved. Fig. 9-1, for example, provides data indicating the extent to which smallpox caused illness and death in the United States during the period of 1921–1971. Smallpox is perhaps the most vivid example of a communicable disease that has been effectively controlled in our country. Widespread immunization programs and increased public awareness are undoubtedly the essential factors in the changing status of smallpox in the United States.

In 1972, the U.S. Public Health Service issued a historic recommendation that routine smallpox vaccinations be discontinued in this country. This decision was based on the fact that there had not been a case of smallpox in the United States since 1949 and the risk of complications from the vaccinations now outweigh the probability of the person contracting the disease. Six months after the United States suspension, there occurred an epidemic of the disease in Yugoslavia and an outbreak of it in West Germany. A number of health professionals have nervously suggested that the suspension of smallpox vaccination might be premature and could reexpose the nation to a deadly disease. Others have maintained that our national surveillance system to identify suspect cases and carry out emergency procedures can prevent the spread of the disease. In addition, smallpox vaccination *is* required for people who travel to countries where smallpox still occurs and for health professionals who may come in contact with patients.

To emphasize further the point that control of a disease does not imply eradication, one need only glance at the morbidity and mortality data relative to poliomyelitis over the past few years. In 1954 there were 38,476 cases of poliomyelitis reported and 1,368 deaths resulting from the disease. Following the development of the first successful vaccine in 1954–55, by Dr. Jonas Salk, and the perfecting of the first live-virus vaccine by Dr. Albert B. Sabin in 1961, an abrupt change in the poliomyelitis patterns became evident in this country. By 1963 the number of cases of this disease was reduced to 449, with only 27 deaths. A milestone was reached in 1969 when for the first time no fatalities due to polio were recorded and with only 21 cases of the disease reported in 1971. A surprise outbreak of polio occurred in 1972 at a school in Greenwich, Connecticut.

The private coeducational school—whose 129 pupils are

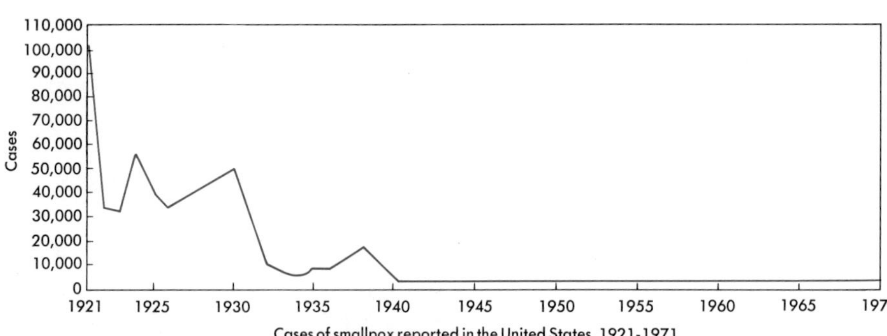

Fig. 9-1. Graph of smallpox cases. (*Center for Disease Control*)

for the most part Christian Scientists—was the scene of the most serious outbreak of paralytic polio in the United States in the last seven years. Eleven students are suffering the symptoms of the disease, and at least four have been partially paralyzed. And all the stricken youngsters—as well as most of the student body—had never been immunized against polio because of their parents' religious beliefs. . . . After parents agreed to have their children vaccinated in an emergency mass immunization session, the health officials decided not to quarantine the school, and classes continued in a relatively relaxed atmosphere.[1]

The American Academy of Pediatrics has warned that immunization efforts are lagging. They estimate that 50 per cent of inner city children have not been vaccinated against polio. Obviously, if we are to continue our remarkable control over poliomyelitis, efforts to encourage mass immunization of the public must be continued.

Despite these impressive achievements, a number of diseases such as hepatitis, influenza, and pneumonia are still taking their toll. Venereal disease incidence in recent years has become epidemic, rapidly climbing, even though effective treatment for these diseases was discovered over a quarter of a century ago.

If one broadens one's perspective of communicable diseases and considers their international significance, it becomes tragically apparent that in many regions of the world, smallpox, plague, cholera, and other diseases persist as leading causes of mortality and human misery. These diseases are most prevalent in areas where man has been deprived of the scientific and technological expertise that has enabled other men to understand, control, and modify their physical environment. Our discussion of World Health deals with the health problems of deprived countries and national and international efforts to eliminate these conditions. Our concerns here are primarily with those diseases of a communicable nature which appear to be most prevalent and/or problematical in our nation today. Attention will be directed toward that group of diseases that presents the most serious threat to the young adult.

Terminology of the Communicable Diseases

Familiarity with terminology frequently encountered in any formal discussion of diseases is essential if the student is to develop a depth of understanding of the subject. These terms may at first seem cumbersome, but will soon prove to be invaluable as your acquaintance with the subject broadens.

Communicable disease is illness "due to a specific infectious agent or its toxic products, arising through transmission of that agent or its products from reservoir to susceptible host, either directly as from an infected person or animal, or indirectly through the agency of an intermediate plant or animal host, a vector, or the inanimate environment."[2]

[1] "Polio: The Price Paid by Believers," *New York Times*, October 29, 1972.

[2] *Control of Communicable Diseases in Man*, 10th ed. (New York: American Public Health Association, 1965), p. 13.

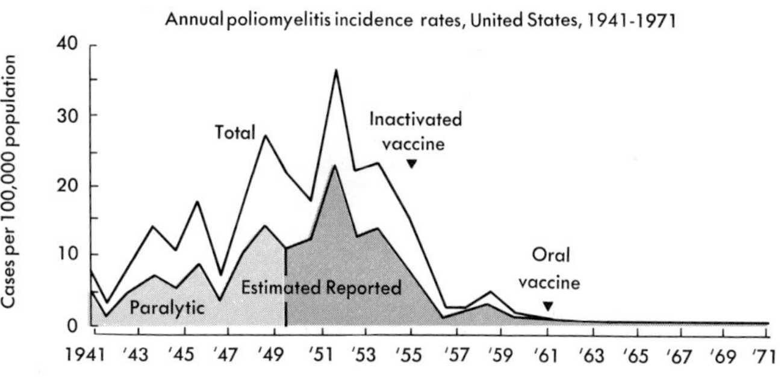

Fig. 9-2. Vaccines have nearly eliminated these major diseases in the United States. (Center for Disease Control)

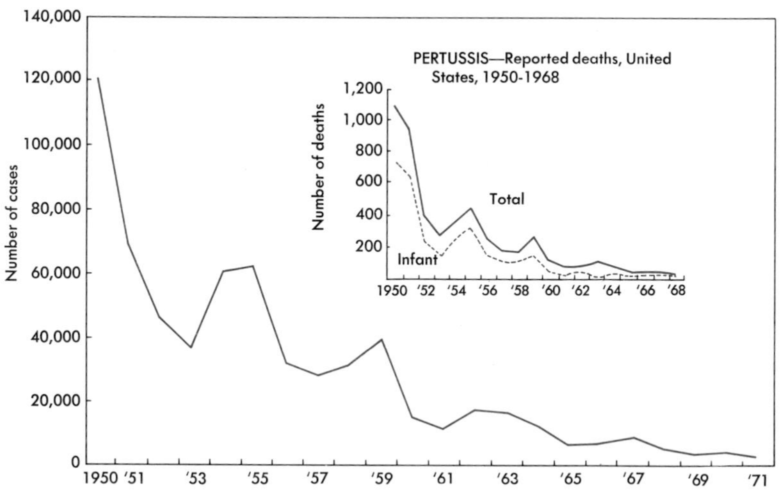

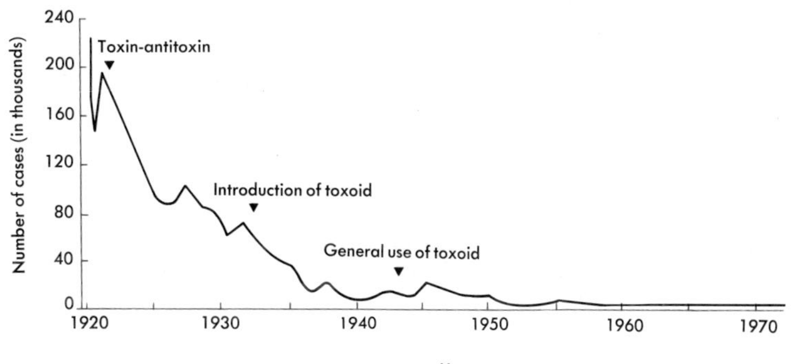

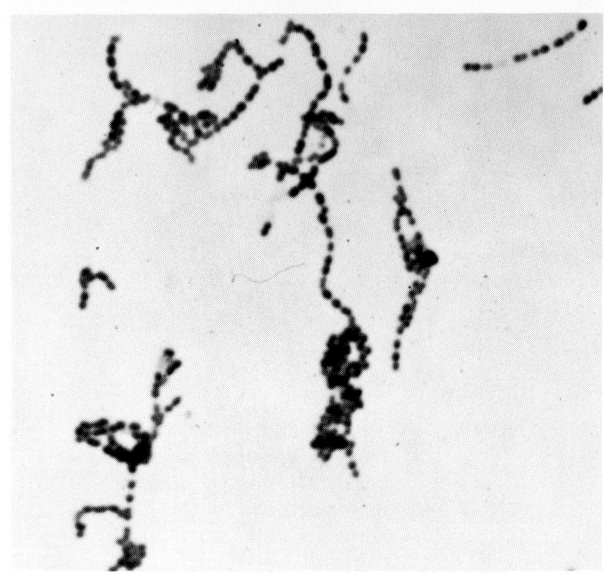

Use of the term *communicable disease* is favored by the health scientist; lay people frequently employ the term *contagious* when referring to the same group of diseases. Although these two designations may be used interchangeably, a distinction between these terms and "infectious" diseases is in order. *Infectious diseases* are those diseases of man and other animals resulting from infection. For example, tonsilitis is an infectious disease which is not transmissable. Serum hepatitis, on the other hand, is both infectious and communicable. While all communicable diseases are also infectious, it is clear that not all infectious diseases are communicable.

Morbidity statistics are used to indicate the number of cases of a disease in a given population. Generally, these data are expressed in terms of the case-rate per 100,000 population per year. The number of deaths attributed to a specific disease is often expressed in terms of the *mortality rate* for a given population. The size of the reported population may vary, depending largely on the nature of the disease and the characteristics of the group in question. Often, mortality rates are given for specific diseases, age-groups, sexes, and other significant differentials which may be appropriate in statistical reporting.

The American Public Health Association defines the *incidence* of a disease as "the number of cases of disease, of infection, or other event occurring during a prescribed time period, in relation to the unit of population in which they occur; thus the incidence of tuberculosis expressed as a rate is the number of new cases reported per 100,000 population per year." If one interprets this as a "dynamic" measurement, or one that involves a considerable span of time, it becomes a simple matter to distinguish between the incidence and the *prevalence* of a disease. Data which indicate the prevalence of a disease relate to the number of cases of a specific disease *at a particular time.* Thus, the prevalence of infectious hepatitis is a "static" measurement of the number of persons ill from hepatitis existing at a given time, per 100,000 population.

Disease-Producing or Pathogenic Organisms

Bacteria are one of the lowest forms of plants. While most of these microorganisms are helpful or harmless (decomposing organic matter, making cheese) some can cause disease. These organisms take three basic forms, being rod-shaped (bacilli), round (cocci), or spiral (spirochetes). They cause such diseases as tuberculosis, typhoid fever, whooping cough (pertussis), or "strep" throat, among others.

Viruses are the smallest of the disease-producing organisms and can be seen only under the electron microscope. They require living cells for their growth and reproduction. Poliomyelitis, the common cold, measles, mumps, and hepatitis exemplify diseases produced by them. Drugs that are effective against viral diseases are rare. The main means of combating these diseases are prevention via those vaccines that are available, or avoidance of the sources of infection.

Fig. 9-3. Chains of streptococci: bacteria as seen under a microscope. (Center for Disease Control)

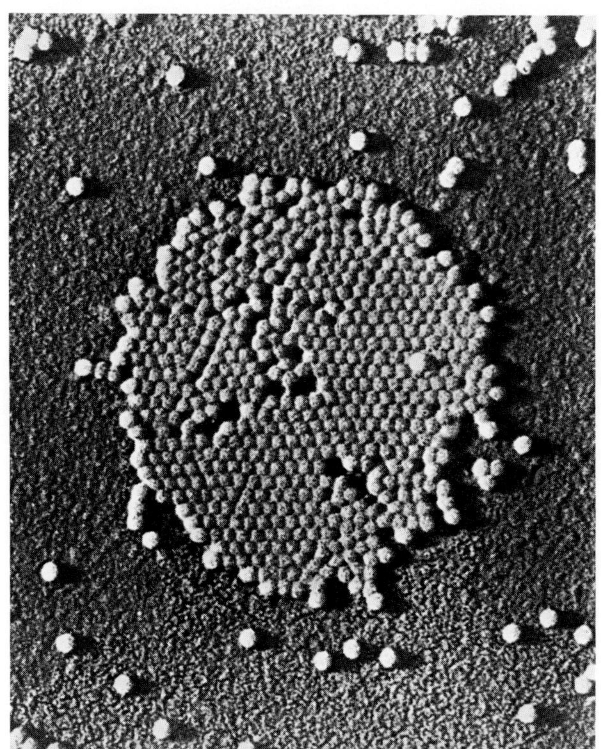

Fig. 9-4. Polio virus as seen through an electron microscope. (Center for Disease Control)

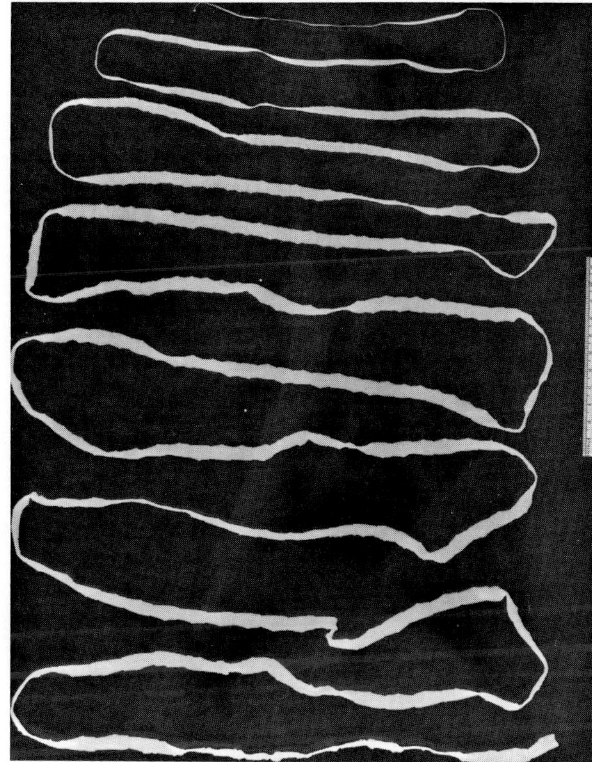

Fig. 9-5. Tapeworm—a parasitic worm found in the intestinal tract. (Center for Disease Control)

Fungi are plant forms that include yeast and molds. Infections that come under the category of "athlete's foot" or "ringworm" are caused by fungi. "Ringworm" gets its name from the ringlike appearance that the fungal growth often takes in scalp infections.

Protozoa are one-celled animals and represent the simplest form of animal life. Some protozoa are parasitic to man and can cause such disorders as malaria, amebic dysentery, and African sleeping sickness.

Parasitic Worms take varied forms and can produce a number of human diseases. These organisms can vary in size, with many being visible to the naked eye. Hookworm, tapeworm, and schistosome (the agent causing schistosomiasis) are examples.

Rickettsia are organisms smaller than bacteria and are barely visible under conventional microscopes. They are responsible for such conditions as Rocky Mountain Spotted Fever, typhus, and Q fever.

Transmission of Infectious Organisms

Modes of transmission of these organisms are the means whereby they are carried from a source of infection to a susceptible person. Transmission can be accomplished through *direct contact* with an infected person, as in touching, kissing, or sexual intercourse. Transmission of infectious agents can also take place through *indirect contact,* that is, through the touching of contaminated articles such as eating utensils, clothing, food, and so forth. *Droplet infection* takes place when the agents are carried

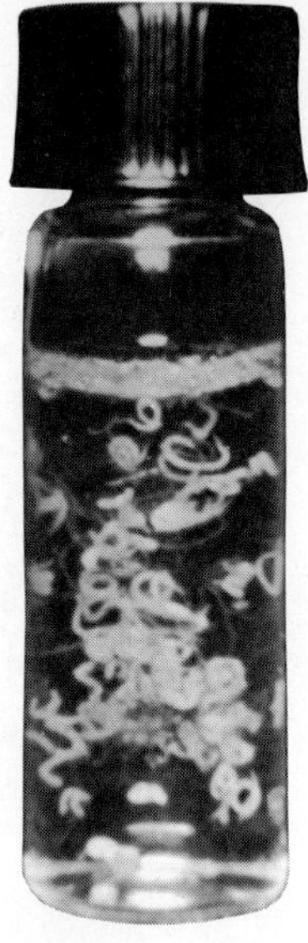

Fig. 9-6. Photograph of schistosomes filtered from the blood of an infected person. This was done by means of an experimental surgical approach to the treatment of schistosomiasis. (*B. H. Kean, M.D.,* Journal of the American Medical Association, *January 23, 1967.*)

by small droplets through the air, usually a matter of a few feet. This represents a type of contact infection because of the close proximity of the people involved. Coughing, sneezing, or talking can serve as means of facilitating droplet infections.

Vectors are insects or animals that serve to transmit disease. The mosquito that carries the protozoan that causes malaria from an infected person to the uninfected acts as a vector. Mosquitoes that carry the virus that causes encephalitis perform a similar function as do the ticks that carry the rickettsia that cause Rocky Mountain Spotted Fever. Vectors often serve as reservoirs of infection. Control of a given disease frequently depends on effectively diminishing the population of the vector.

Resistance and Immunity to Disease

What course of action can one take to protect oneself from communicable diseases? If your childhood learnings have carried over into early adulthood, your response to this question will probably reflect parental teachings relative to the "theory of disease resistance." Most young adults tend to support the concept that by following basic hygienic principles it is possible to maintain a reasonably high level of resistance to disease. The protection thus attained is general in nature and is not specific for any disease. On the other hand, any single element of a healthful regimen does not constitute a panacea of disease prevention. That is, healthful exercise does not guarantee protection from disease any more than either proper diet or recommended amounts of sleep can be expected, in themselves, to provide ultimate resistance. Yet, it is not uncommon for some individuals to engage in rigid dietary programs or weight-training plans designed principally to protect them from infectious disease. When an individual is obsessed by such health fads, practices, or beliefs, it is apparent that his concept of disease resistance is limited and that his efforts to maintain a desirable state of mind and body are misdirected.

Disease Immunity

Protection from specific communicable diseases is spoken of in terms of *immunity* to these illnesses, and is strikingly different from the ill-defined concept of resistance. Immune persons are believed to possess substances called *antibodies* which provide varying degrees of protection from different diseases. When certain foreign substances (almost always protein in nature) are introduced into a person's body, complex protective reactions may result. The foreign substance, perhaps a virus, is the *antigen* and its presence stimulates the production of substances (antibodies) having the capability of destroying the antigen. An important characteristic of antibodies is that each particular type is effective in destroying only one variety of organism. Thus, measles antibodies protect only against measles virus, and mumps antibodies are specific only for mumps.

These protective substances have been detected in the circulating blood and are believed to be formed by cells of the reticuloendothelial system (certain tissues in the spleen, lymph nodes, and bone marrow). When exposed to antigens, these antibody-forming tissues are so modified that they are capable of producing new antibody supplies on contact with the same antigen in the future. This explanation is a gross oversimplification of the complex process known as the antigen-antibody reaction. It is important to note that not all disease-producing organisms provoke this physiological response. Modifications of this defensive mechanism are apparent in diseases such as the common cold, where immunity, if at all present, is of short duration (probably a few days).

Immunity resulting from antigen-antibody reactions never provides total protection from the disease that originally triggered the reaction. Experience has demonstrated that antibody levels which have proven to be effective under normal living conditions may be overwhelmed by unusually high concentrations of antigenic material.

Clearly, the ultimate purpose of all varieties of antibodies is essentially the same—to destroy antigens. A closer examination of the manner in which they perform this function is fascinating. Some antibodies, classified as *agglutinins,* cause a clumping of bacteria. As a consequence of this agglutination, the mobility of the bacteria is reduced and they are more easily devoured by leukocytes (white blood cells). Other antibodies, the *bacteriolysins,* possess the peculiar ability to form a solution (lysis) of bacteria, thus destroying the organisms. *Opsonins* are yet another antibody type that cause bacteria and other antigens to be more attractive to white blood cells. They appear to act much as a catalyst in the reaction between certain antigens and antibodies.

Types of Immunity

An immunity is classified as being *active* when the body's own efforts are involved in the development of protective antibodies. This would occur when a person has a disease or when he receives a vaccine (antigens with weakened virulence). A *passive* immunity can be effected by injecting into the person ready-made antibodies produced in another person or animal. For example, the antibody for German measles can be isolated from the blood of those people who have had the disease. The injection of these antibodies (in the form of gamma globulin) will produce a temporary immunity. Because these antibodies were "borrowed," the immunity is considered passive. Whether artificially induced or the result of actually being ill with a disease, active immunity provides more lasting protection than passive immunity and in many instances is lifelong. Passive immunization may be advised in response to the need for protection after exposure, or in cases where one anticipates exposure to a disease. Such might be the case when an expectant mother, in her first few months of pregnancy, is exposed to German measles. In an effort to protect the fetus from harm, the physician may recommend the administration of immune serum in the form of gamma globulin. Such a procedure would of course be unnecessary for the expectant mother who had been vaccinated against German measles.

Fig. 9-7. A modern vaccine in the making. (World Health Organization)

Modern freeze-dried smallpox vaccine is prepared from virus grown on the skin of a living animal: calf, sheep, ass, buffalo-calf, etc., and is a purified virus suspension.

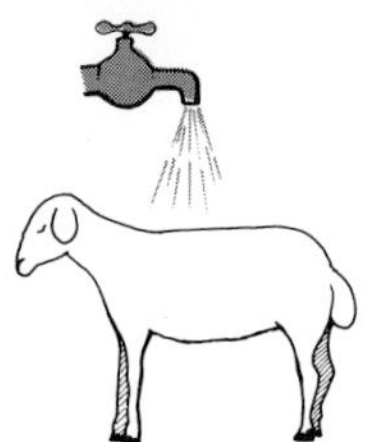

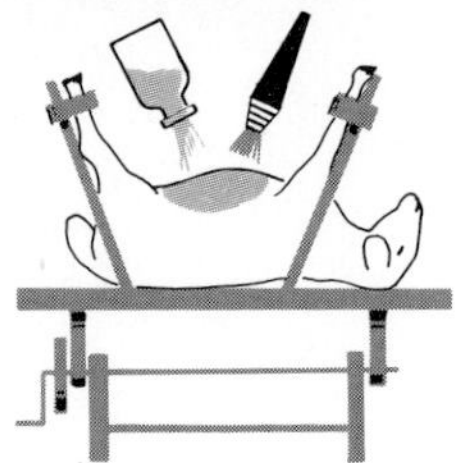

Shaving and cleaning of the vaccination area—the abdomen, for example—of an animal known to be free from any disease transmissible to man.

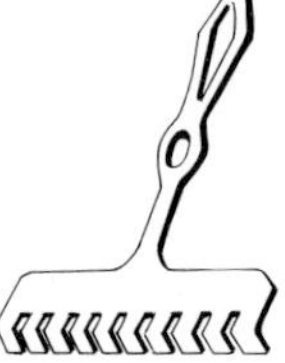

Scarification of the skin surface with a scraper which slightly draws blood

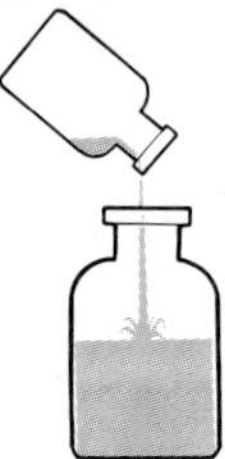

Storage of the harvest at +20° centigrade, for a few hours in a phenolic solution, to destroy the rest of the bacteria.

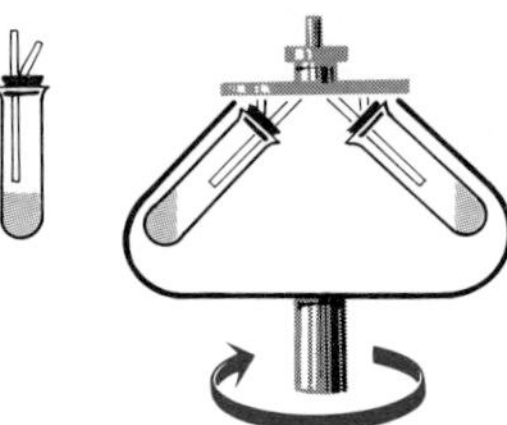

High-speed centrifugation to eliminate the phenol and other soluble substances.

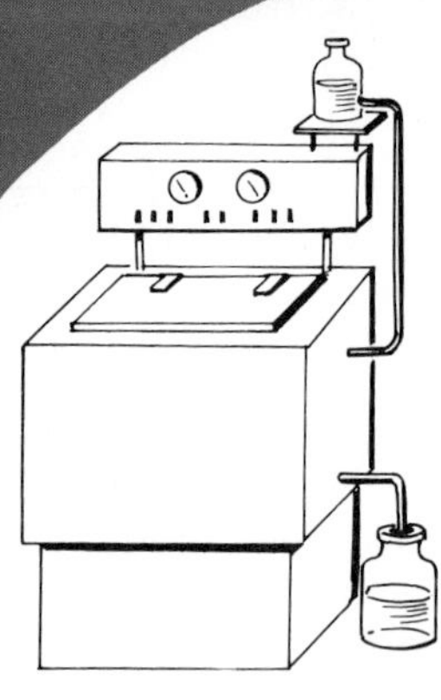

High speed centrifugal machine

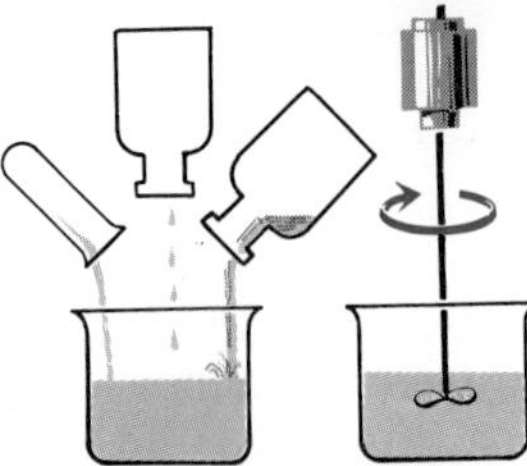

Resuspension of the vaccine virus thus obtained in a buffer solution with peptone to assure full preservation during drying process.

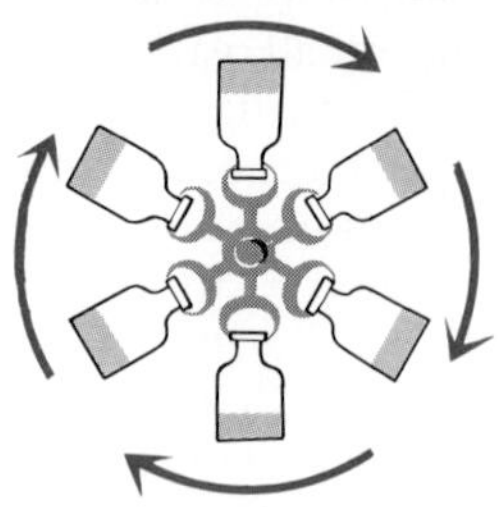

Low-speed centrifugation to eliminate conglomerates.

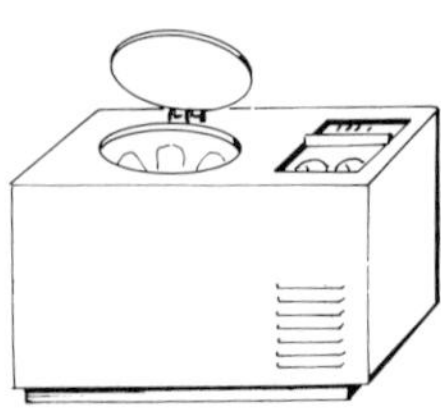

Low-speed centrifugal machine

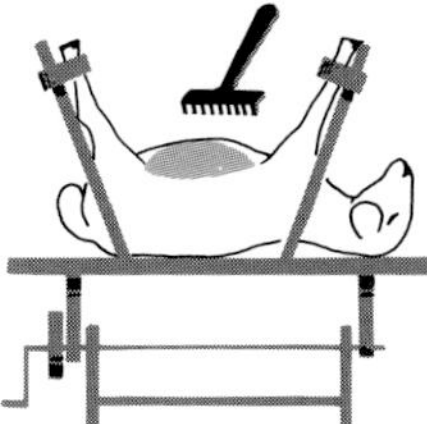

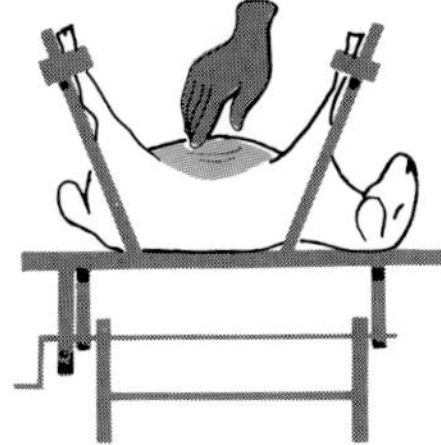

Inoculation of the seed-lymph drawn from laboratory-stock preserved in glycerin solution.

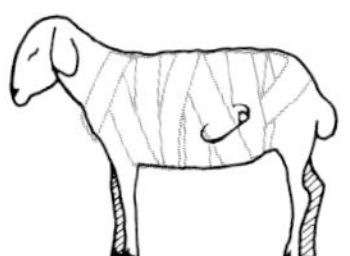

Sterile dressing around the animal's abdomen.

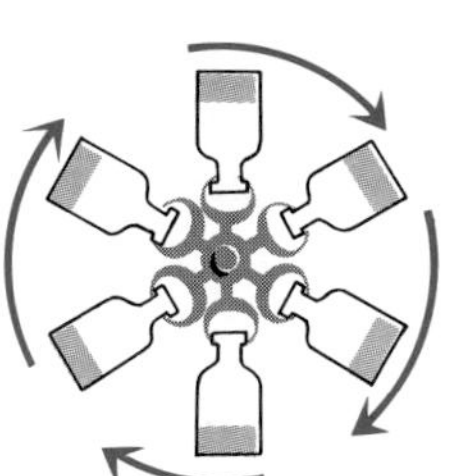

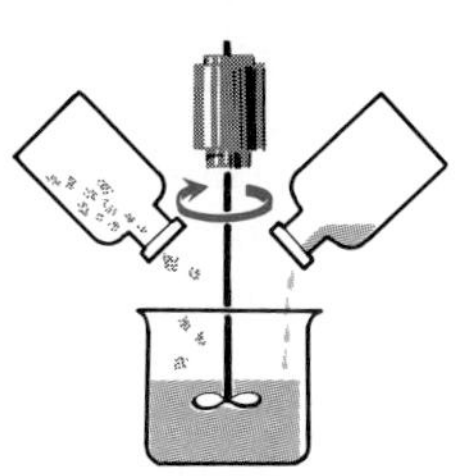

Above: *Homogenization* with buffer solution and *slow-speed centrifugation* to eliminate the tissue fragments and the main part of the bacteria from the harvest.

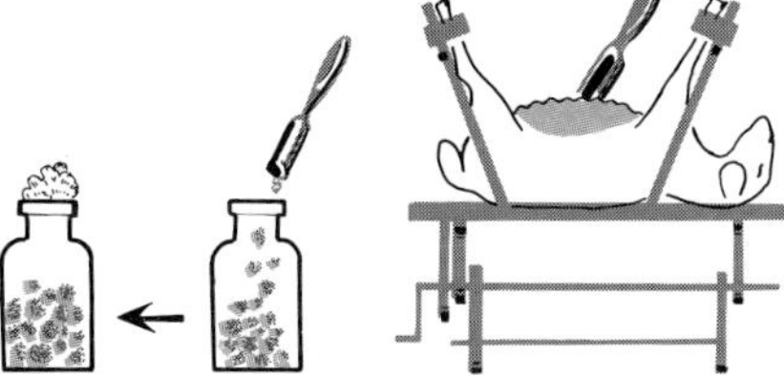

Harvest of the virus, four or five days after inoculation; tissue fragments are included in this harvest. Storage of the virus material at −20 to −70°.

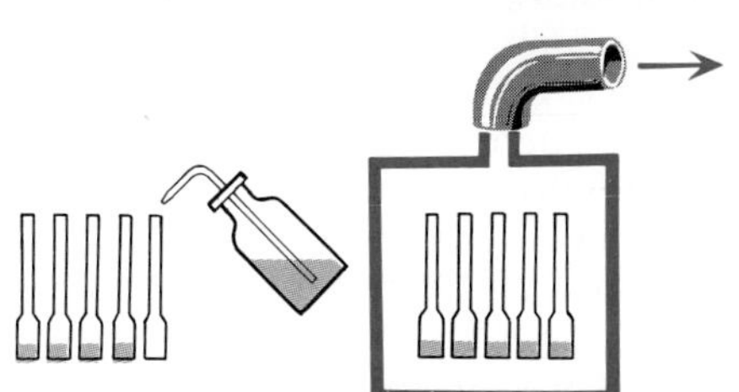

Freezing of the vaccine virus at −70° centigrade and *vacuum drying*, at a temperature progressively raised to +20° centigrade.

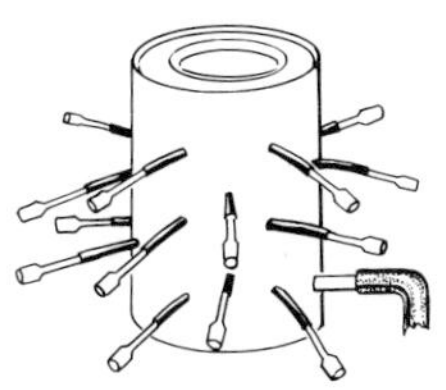

Vacuum pump

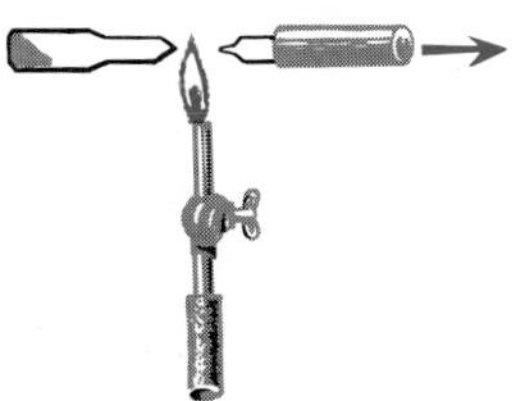

Sealing of ampoules under vacuum.

The result of all these operations is a stable powder which dissolves easily. It remains effective for years if stored below freezing point and for some weeks at tropical atmospheric temperatures.

VACCINES

Suspensions of dead or attenuated pathogens, or their toxic products, are classified as *vaccines.* Recognized as a vital factor in reducing the threat of communicable diseases, vaccines are capable of provoking antigen-antibody reactions with little or no discomfort to the recipient of the antigenic material. Whenever the vaccine consists of bacterial toxins rather than the bacteria themselves, the resultant vaccine is known as a *toxoid* (denatured toxin). The toxicity of these materials is removed without diminishing their immunizing potential. It is likely that most readers of this text have, at some time in their lives, received toxoid for protection from diphtheria and tetanus.

The extent to which the threats of smallpox, pertussis (whooping cough), diphtheria, and poliomyelitis have substantially lessened is indicative of the importance of vaccines to human well-being. In the middle 1920's, for instance, more than 55,000 cases of smallpox were reported in the United States. By 1971, largely as a result of mass immunization programs, not a single case of smallpox was reported in this country. While this dreaded disease has been largely eliminated in the United States and Europe, there are still areas of the world—India, for example—where smallpox persists as a threat to health and life.

The recent history of diphtheria is striking. During the 1930's more than 30,000 cases and 3,000 deaths were recorded in a single year. Since this period, widespread use of diphtheria toxoid has greatly reduced the incidence of this infection. Since 1971 about 200 cases of diphtheria were identified in the United States, and indications are that the disease will continue to decline.

Although it is true that periodic outbreaks of poliomyelitis have occurred since the development of a successful vaccine, most of the victims have proved to be those who had never received a full series of inoculations. Dr. James Peavy, Texas State Health Commissioner, reported in September 1966 that of the total of 43 cases of poliomyelitis reported in the United States in 1965, 14 occurred in his own state. Of the 43 stricken Americans (all infants and children) 35 had never received polio vaccine. Similarly in 1971 an outbreak of polio occurred in Texas causing some deaths among those children who were either not vaccinated or did not complete the series of vaccinations. Apparently, one of our nation's major concerns should be to make people aware of how they may protect their health by the utilization of vaccines. Furthermore, the medical facilities and services essential for such protection should be made available to all people. Experience has demonstrated that in those areas where intensive immunization programs are underwritten and conducted, the disease is virtually nonexistent. It is entirely possible that the conscientious and determined use of oral polio vaccine will, within the next generation, practically eradicate this disease throughout the world. The introduction of the Enders measles vaccine in 1963 is producing similar results.

Rubella epidemics occur in the United States about once every ten years. The disease is usually over in three days and there are no lasting effects—

Fig. 9-8. *Hearing loss is one of the main physical defects of rubella syndrome children, who may have multiple impairments at birth because their mothers had German measles during the first three months of pregnancy.* (*Merck, Sharpe & Dohme*)

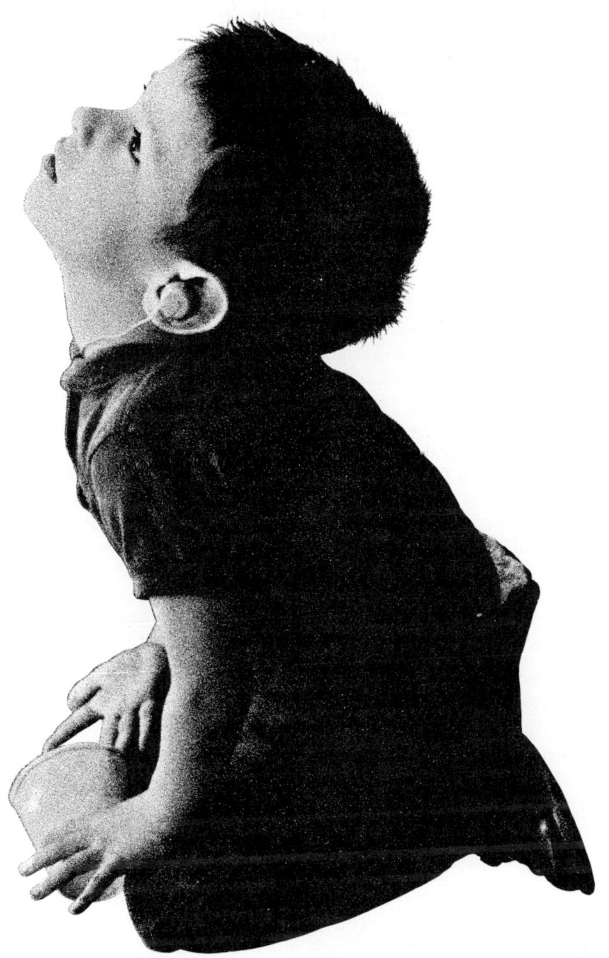

unless the patient was a woman early in her pregnancy. Then the effects of the disease on her unborn child can be devastating. As a result of the 1964–1965 rubella epidemic 50,000 children either died in the womb or were born with a loss of hearing, impaired vision, congenitally damaged hearts, or mentally retarded. Very often these children have several of these impairments and are multihandicapped. The need for protection was met in June 1969 when the first rubella vaccine was licensed. This vaccination program, like the others, is based on the well-established epidemiological principle of "herd immunity." The herd immunity approach calls for vaccinating enough people of the community to produce a large percentage of immune persons so that a disease would be unable to spread in epidemic fashion. Children are targets of the vaccination program since 90 per cent of cases occur among children in the lower grades. There has been some question as to the long-term effectiveness of the program. One study suggests that periodic serological surveys of children vaccinated should be implemented to determine whether or not these children remain safe from rubella as they approach their childbearing years. Continued research for a more effective long-lasting vaccine continues.

Artificial immunization is presently available for many more diseases than our discussion would indicate. Pertussis, tetanus, influenza, typhoid fever, and tuberculosis are examples of other diseases for which prophylaxis (a vaccine) is used in the United States. The American Academy of Pediatrics has suggested an immunization schedule which, in its judgment,

Table 9-1. ***Revised Schedule for Active Immunization And Tuberculin Testing of Normal Infants And Children in the United States***

2 mo.	DTP[1]	TOPV[2]
4 mo.	DTP	TOPV
6 mo.	DTP	TOPV
1 yr.	Measles[3]	Tuberculin Test[4]
1–12 yr.	Rubella[3]	Mumps[3]
1½ yr.	DTP	TOPV
4–6 yr.	DTP	TOPV
14–16 yr.	Td[5]	and thereafter every 10 years

[1] DTP—diphtheria and tetanus toxoids combined with pertussis vaccine.

[2] TOPV—trivalent oral polio virus vaccine. The above recommendation is suitable for breast-fed as well as bottle-fed infants.

[3] May be given at 1 year as Measles-Rubella or Measles-Mumps-Rubella combined vaccines (see Section (p. 127) Rubella and Section (p. 88) Mumps for discussion of age of administration.

[4] Frequency of repeated tuberculin tests depends on risk of exposure of the child and on the prevalence of tuberculosis in the population group.

[5] Td—combined tetanus and diphtheria toxoids (adult type) for those over six years of age in contrast to diphtheria and tetanus (DT) containing a larger amount of diphtheria antigen.

Tetanus toxoid at time of injury: For clean, minor wounds, no booster dose is needed by a fully immunized child unless more than 10 years have elapsed since the last dose.

For contaminated wounds, a booster dose should be given if more than 5 years have elapsed since the last dose.

Routine smallpox vaccination is no longer recommended.

Approved by the Committee on Infectious Diseases
October 17, 1971

Source: "Report of the Committee on Infectious Diseases, *Red Book,* 16th edition (Evanston, Ill: American Academy of Pediatrics, 1971), p. 5.

represents the soundest course of action for those seeking artificial immunizations.

Some Communicable Disease Problems

Influenza and Pneumonia

The United States Public Health Service and other official health agencies combine the data on influenza (flu) and pneumonia when reporting on the incidence and severity of either disease. Both of these conditions affect the respiratory system and are commonly referred to as "clinical companions." That is to say, an attack of the flu can and does lead to pneumonia, especially if the victim represents a high-risk group. Influenza predisposes the lungs to later bacterial infections, including pneumonia, and whenever a flu epidemic strikes there is a corresponding increase in pneumonia deaths.

Though these diseases are not the killers today that they were in past years, they are the only acute diseases remaining among the major causes of sickness and death in the United States. Both usually take their heaviest toll among infants and the elderly. As the percentage of citizens age 65 and over increases, we can expect influenza and pneumonia to continue as major health problems. This will, in fact, be the case, unless effective control measures are developed and applied in our society.

Influenza is an acute infection of the upper respiratory tract resulting from invasion by one of several filterable viruses. At least three virus types (Types

Fig. 9-9. *Electron micrograph of flu virus particles magnified 12,625 times. (Center for Disease Control)*

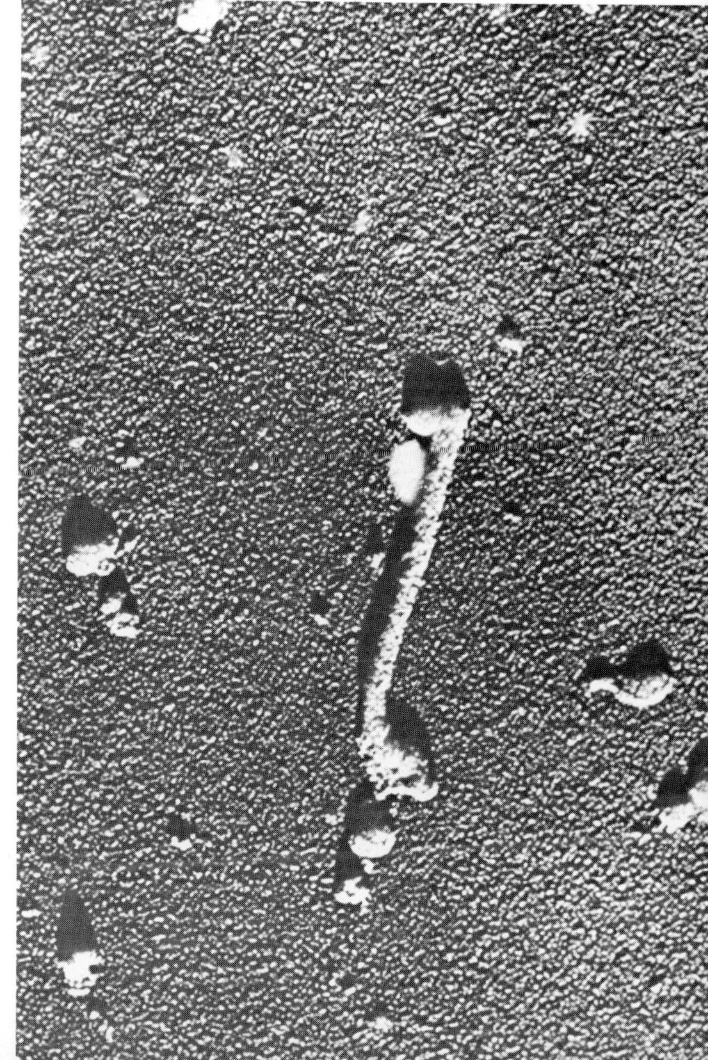

A, B, and C) have been identified and are classified in the myxovirus group. It appears that several distinct strains of virus make up each of the A and B types. Influenza C virus is less common than either of the other major types and generally leads to milder forms of the disease. One or more of the four strains of Type A virus cause outbreaks of influenza nearly every year in the nation. Type B influenza has been most elusive to health-science investigators, as it appears that the virus changes its form frequently. The unpredictable character of Type B viruses has baffled researchers in their efforts to develop a successful immunization.

An acute and highly infectious disorder of the upper respiratory tract, influenza typically manifests itself from 24 to 72 hours (incubation period) after the virus has entered the host. The early symptoms mimic those of the common cold, with accompanying chills, achiness (especially in the back and limbs), and prostration. Influenza is a self-limiting disease and typically runs its course in two to three days. In many cases, however, a nonproductive cough and general feeling of weakness persist long after the disappearance of other symptoms.

Invasion by an influenza virus is believed to stimulate the production of antibodies which are specific for that particular virus strain. The immunity thus conferred appears to last for varying lengths of time in different individuals. Those who are afflicted with more than one attack of influenza in a given season are very likely to be victims of more than one virus type. To date, effective vaccines are available for the prevailing strains of Type A and Type B viruses. The periodic emergence of new virus strains has resulted in the presently available inoculations' being only partially successful in controlling the disease. The ultimate in flu prophylaxis would be a single vaccine with the capability of immunizing individuals to all forms of the virus. Medical authorities do not at the present time recommend routine immunizations for the general population. Special risk groups, including the very young and the elderly, and those suffering from chronic cardiac, respiratory, metabolic, renal, and neurological disorders, are commonly advised to receive inoculations. There is some evidence that pregnant women show a greater tendency to develop pulmonary complications following influenza, and many medical authorities consider these individuals as a risk group.

The most recent severe epidemic of flu in the United States occurred in 1918–1919, during the pandemic (world wide epidemic) which caused an estimated 20,000,000 cases of influenza and pneumonia and resulted in 850,000 deaths. Since this tragedy, the number of deaths from these diseases has decreased steadily.

In 1957 the world was alerted to a major outbreak of influenza in China, where hundreds of thousands had been stricken. Known popularly as Asian Flu, the disease was caused by a Type A virus, immunologically distinct from previously known strains. The World Health Organization responded to the emergency by charting the movement of the epidemic from one country to another. Fortunately, the efforts of the World Health Organization enabled the United States and other nations to prepare for the epidemic onslaught. The United States Public Health Service was able to prepare a vaccine and inoculate millions of Americans. Estimates of the effectiveness of the 1957 vaccine indicate that approximately 50 per cent of those inoculated were protected from the disease.

For the young adult the major dangers from influenza do not involve serious illness. Bed rest is recommended for a quicker recovery, with many physicians sometimes prescribing additional therapy, depending on the needs of the individual.

Infectious Mononucleosis

Known popularly as "mono" and the "kissing disease," mononucleosis affects an estimated half a million young people each year. The majority of these cases are found in the 15- to 30-year-age group, with a slightly greater incidence among males. Mononucleosis is not a new disease. As early as 1889, Emil Pfeiffer described an epidemic of "glandular fever," a disease remarkably similar to that now known as mononucleosis. This term was first used to describe glandular fever in 1920.

In spite of the fact that medical personnel have known about this curious disease for more than three-quarters of a century, it remains largely a medical mystery even today. For example, the causative organism is generally believed to be a virus, though none has been identified. Its unknown etiology is further complicated by the fact that attempts to transmit the infection from one person to another via blood, stool samples, and nasopharyngeal secretions have not been very successful. The term "kissing disease" implies that mononucleosis is transmitted by way of respiratory discharges. Yet, medical research has not determined that this is the actual mode of transmission.

The mononucleosis syndrome is variable and the common symptoms include enlargement of lymph nodes (usually the cervical nodes are involved), sore throat, headache, and irregular fever (commonly ranging from 100 degrees to 103 degrees, or higher). Frequently these symptoms increase in intensity during the first week of the illness and will be severe enough to convince the patient that a medical consultation is advisable. Examination by a physician may reveal noticeable enlargement of the spleen. In some cases, a chaotic condition of lymphocytes is noted and is helpful to the physician in diagnosing mononucleosis. A new diagnostic test has been developed that utilizes blood serum from suspected mono victims and blood from horses. Reportedly, blood serum from an infected individual causes a clumping of red blood cells in horse blood. This diagnostic technique is still being studied and researchers are encouraged by its effectiveness and simplicity. Because of the dangers of liver or spleen involvement, mononucleosis should be treated by a physician. Typically, the discomforts of mononucleosis persist from two to eight weeks. In many cases, the individual does not feel acutely ill, but his physician should prescribe a daily regimen.

Hepatitis

Hepatitis (inflammation of the liver) is an acute infection and its syndrome commonly includes fever, loss of appetite, nausea, malaise, and abdominal discomfort, sometimes followed by jaundice. Jaundice, a yellowish tinting of the skin and sclera, results from the appearance of certain bile salts in the blood. The discoloration lasts for varying lengths of time. There are, however, many cases of hepatitis in which this symptom does not appear. Whether jaundice is or is not present, the convalescent period may extend for weeks or months.

The presence of antibodies found in gamma globulin of pooled blood suggests that the majority of adults have probably had this type of infection and not even been aware of its presence. Although its effectiveness is questioned by many authorities, immune serum globulin may be administered to those who have had contact with the disease. There is some evidence that these inoculations may provide passive immunity lasting from six to eight weeks.

Our concern in this section will be infectious hepatitis, as a distinction must be made between this disease and its close relative, serum hepatitis (homologous serum jaundice).

Infectious Hepatitis has a reputation as one of the most serious communicable diseases in the United States. Actually, it is not a new disease, but has only in recent years gained public attention. Known variously as "yellow jaundice," "camp jaundice," "infectious jaundice," and "catarrhal jaundice," this condition is known to have been common during the Franco-Prussian War. There were nearly 20,000 cases among Union forces in the Civil War. More recently, in both world wars, hepatitis posed a serious threat to the Allies, the case rate being as

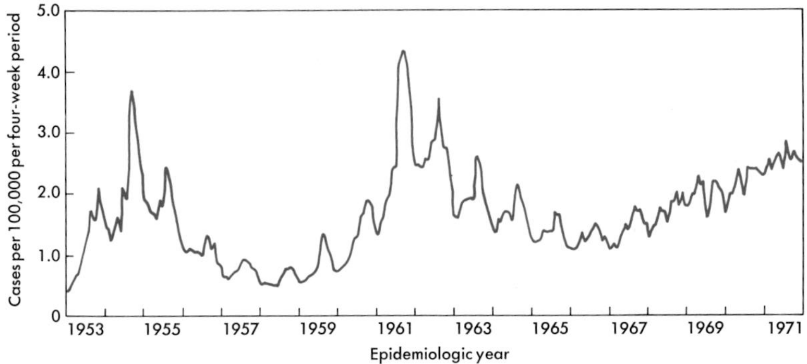

Fig. 9-10. Viral hepatitis cycle—a high incidence of hepatitis appears to recur periodically. (Center for Disease Control)

high as 35 per 1000 men in some theaters of war. Our inability to cope with outbreaks of the disease and the extended period of rest usually required for convalescence placed a heavy demand on our overseas hospitals in particular.

In temperate zones, infectious hepatitis becomes more prevalent in the late summer months and typically reaches it peak in late fall or early winter. It is essentially a disease of children and young adults and often causes prolonged incapacitation.

Complete information on this disease is lacking because of the inability of virologists and other researchers adequately to identify and cultivate the causative agent. To date, most experimental work has had to be done on human volunteers because of the difficulty of artificially transmitting the disease to laboratory animals. The exact manner by which infectious hepatitis is transmitted is poorly understood, though the medical community generally agrees that it might possibly be transmitted via respiratory discharges. Curiously enough, efforts to demonstrate Virus A in nasopharyngeal secretions have been largely unsuccessful. The most common source of infection is contaminated fecal material, and the usual mode of transmission is via the intestinal-oral route. Perhaps the reason why the disease appears to be most common in children is that many in this age group have not yet formed basic hygienic practices such as washing the hands after using the bathroom and washing before meals. A further reason for our lack of total control of hepatitis is that contaminated food, water, and milk have been known to be reservoirs of infection for epidemics.

Serum Hepatitis is caused by a virus (Virus B) that is different from infectious hepatitis (Virus A) and appears to be transmitted only by subcutaneous, intramuscular, and intravenous injection. The incidence of serum hepatitis was on the decline until recent years. The drug abuse problem with its widespread injected use of heroin and amphetamines has caused a resurgence in the incidence of this disease. The prevalence had been reduced largely through routine screenings of individuals who donate blood and as a result of intensified efforts to sterilize instruments used when various kinds of injections are administered. The relatively recent use of disposable hypodermic syringes and needles has undoubtedly reduced the number of those who might otherwise have been infected by contaminated equipment.

Venereal Diseases

Ironically, the incidence of venereal diseases has been rising throughout the world. The increased incidence started about 20 years after effective treatment in the form of penicillin was discovered in the mid-1940's. There was a significant spread of venereal disease in the early 1940's during World War II. With the discovery and introduction of penicillin as a form of treatment, both syphilis and gonorrhea receded in incidence. The expected demise of these diseases was not to occur, however. Starting in the late 1950's there has been a steady and alarming increase of venereal disease. There has to date been little understanding of the significance and consequences of this unnecessary scourge. Positive efforts, however, to eliminate this ignorance are currently being made, as many school systems are becoming involved in instructional programs to familiarize young Americans with the nature of the venereal diseases.

All of the venereal diseases are highly infectious and spread by direct contact with an infected individual. The nature of this contact nearly always involves intimate sexual relations. Chancroid lymphogranuloma venereum, granuloma inguinale, syphilis, and gonorrhea make up this group of dreaded diseases. Because the latter two venereal infections are most common and present the greatest challenge to public health authorities in the United States, the discussion here will be limited to them.

Syphilis. In 1957 the reported number of cases of syphilis reached a low of 6,251. By 1965 the reported cases of syphilis reached 23,250, and has hovered around the 20,000 mark since. Lest the reader be misled by these statistics, it must be emphasized that they represent only those cases of syphilis *reported* to public health officials. Many authorities estimate that the number of new cases of each year to be as high as 140,000. The reluctance of physicians to report the incidence of such cases and patients unaware that they have the disease are

Table 9-2. ***Primary and Secondary Syphilis and Gonorrhea Reported Cases and Rates per 100,000 Population****
United States, Fiscal Years 1957, 1963–1971

	Primary and Secondary Syphilis			***Gonorrhea***		
Year	*Number of Reported Cases*	*Rate per 100,000 Population*	*Percent Change from Previous Year*	*Number of Reported Cases*	*Rate per 100,000 Population*	*Percent Change from Previous Year*
1957	6,251	3.8	—	216,476	129.8	—
1963	22,045	11.9	+ 9.8	270,076	145.7	+ 3.7
1964	22,733	12.1	+ 3.1	290,603	154.5	+ 7.6
1965	23,250	12.3	+ 2.3	310,155	163.8	+ 6.7
1966	22,473	11.6	− 3.3	334,949	173.6	+ 8.0
1967	21,090	10.8	− 6.1	375,606	193.0	+12.1
1968	20,182	10.3	− 4.3	431,380	219.2	+14.8
1969	18,679	9.3	− 7.4	494,227	245.9	+14.6
1970	20,186	10.0	+ 8.1	573,200	285.2	+16.0
1971	23,336	11.5	+15.6	624,371	307.5	+ 8.9

Data: U.S. Public Health Service.

*Source: *Today's VD Control Problem 1972* (New York: American Social Health Association, 1972).

 factors in the discrepancy between reported and actual incidence.

Syphilis is caused by treponema pallida, a corkscrew-shaped organism (spirochete) that requires both moisture and body temperature to grow and reproduce. These critical requirements are satisfied by the warm, moist surfaces of the mucus membrane of the oral cavity and the genitourinary system. Syphilis is also known to enter the body when infectious material is introduced into cuts or other breaks in the skin. Conditions of temperature and moisture are so vital to the survival of the spirochete that direct contact is almost always the manner by which the infection is transferred. It is quite unlikely that the organism could live for more than a few seconds on inanimate objects such as toilet seats. It is generally agreed that almost all cases of syphilis are transmitted as a result of direct contact during sexual intercourse or other intimate sexual activities.

Shortly after contact with the treponema, the newly infected individual harbors the organisms in his lymphatic system. Before the primary symptoms appear, the infection reaches the bloodstream. Usually the symptoms of primary syphilis are evident in about three weeks, but may not appear for three months following contact.

A certain element of risk is involved whenever one attempts to describe a classical disease syndrome. Deviations from the pattern described herein are common and certainly should not be reason for a person to postpone medical attention at the first suspicion of venereal disease. As a rule, venereal

Fig. 9-11. Treponema pallidum, the causative organism of syphilis, as seen against a dark background referred to as the Dark Field. (Reproduced with permission of Technical Information Services, State and Community Services Division, Center for Disease Control, Health Services and Mental Health Administration, Department of Health, Education and Welfare.)

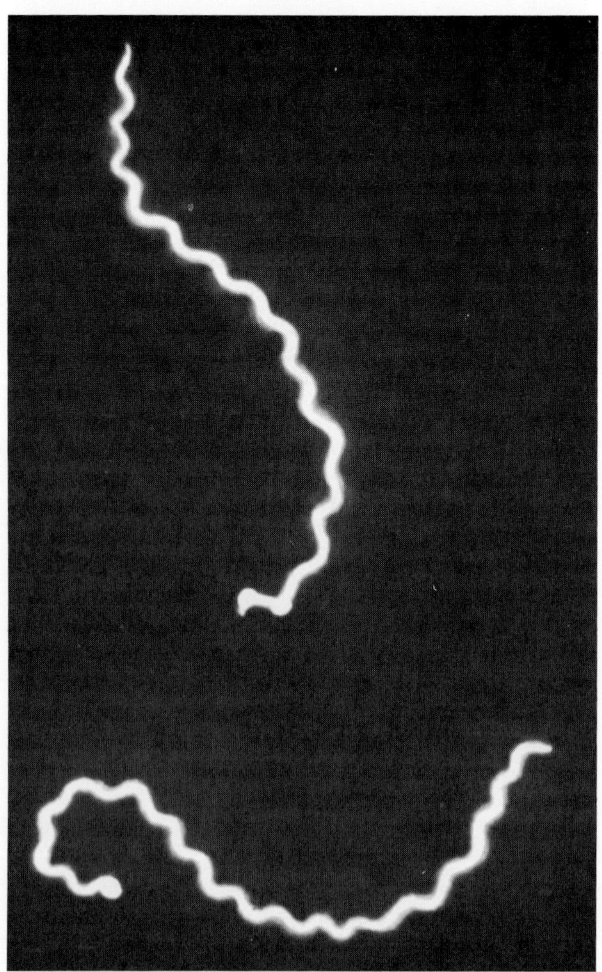

diseases are most easily cured in the early stages and become progressively less responsive to therapy as the infection persists.

The development of the syphilis infection may be conveniently divided into four major stages:

Primary Syphilis. The initial symptom is oftentimes a chancre. This lesion is usually a hard, painless papule, although some may be soft and irritating. The chancre is a highly communicable source of the disease and is usually located in the ano-genital region, but many appear on the lips, tongue, finger, or wherever the spirochete first entered the body.

Curiously, the presence of a chancre is not always detected by the infected person for the following reasons:

1. The chancre may be located internally, as in the urethra or vagina. Cervical chancres are fairly common and are frequently overlooked in even superficial medical examination.
2. Occasionally lymphoid tissue becomes inflamed and characteristic swelling of lymph nodes occurs and may be present in the absence of a chancre.
3. The development of a chancre may be suppressed as a result of antibiotic therapy for another disease.

In all of these instances the disease would continue to develop, though its presence might not be noted for weeks or months.

Many syphilitics pass through the primary phase of their infection without being aware of their condition. Even when the chancre is noticed, it quickly heals even without treatment. Spontaneous disappearance of the chancre misleads many into believing that they must be rid of the infection. This assumption is most unfortunate, because the infection is permitted to continue its devastation at a time when it is most amenable to antibiotic therapy.

During the primary stage, the organisms may not be present in the blood in sufficient force to show a positive reaction in a serological examination (blood test). It is, therefore, possible to harbor an early syphilis infection and still react negatively to blood tests. If the physician and patient suspect that this is the case, frequent blood tests are recommended until a firm diagnosis has been made. Needless to say, the patient should refrain from intimate sexual contact until his physician is convinced that syphilis is not present.

Secondary Syphilis. Secondary symptoms may appear as soon as three weeks or as late as six months after the appearance of primary symptoms. The nature of these more advanced symptoms varies greatly from one patient to another, but those appearing most commonly are a non-itchy rash covering the entire body or confined to the hands and feet, headache, mild fever, sore throat, and alopecia (hair falling out in patches). Infectious lesions may appear on the ano-genital surfaces, and mucous patches may be evident on the membranes of the mouth. The disease is highly contagious in this stage of its development, and it is possible to spread the infection to others by kissing or other intimate contact. It should be noted that the symptoms associated with this period may be confused with those of other diseases. For this reason syphilis is sometimes referred to as

Fig. 9-12. Infectious syphilis outbreak, Fort Worth, Texas 1971. (Today's VD Control Problem 1972. *Published by American Social Health Association*)

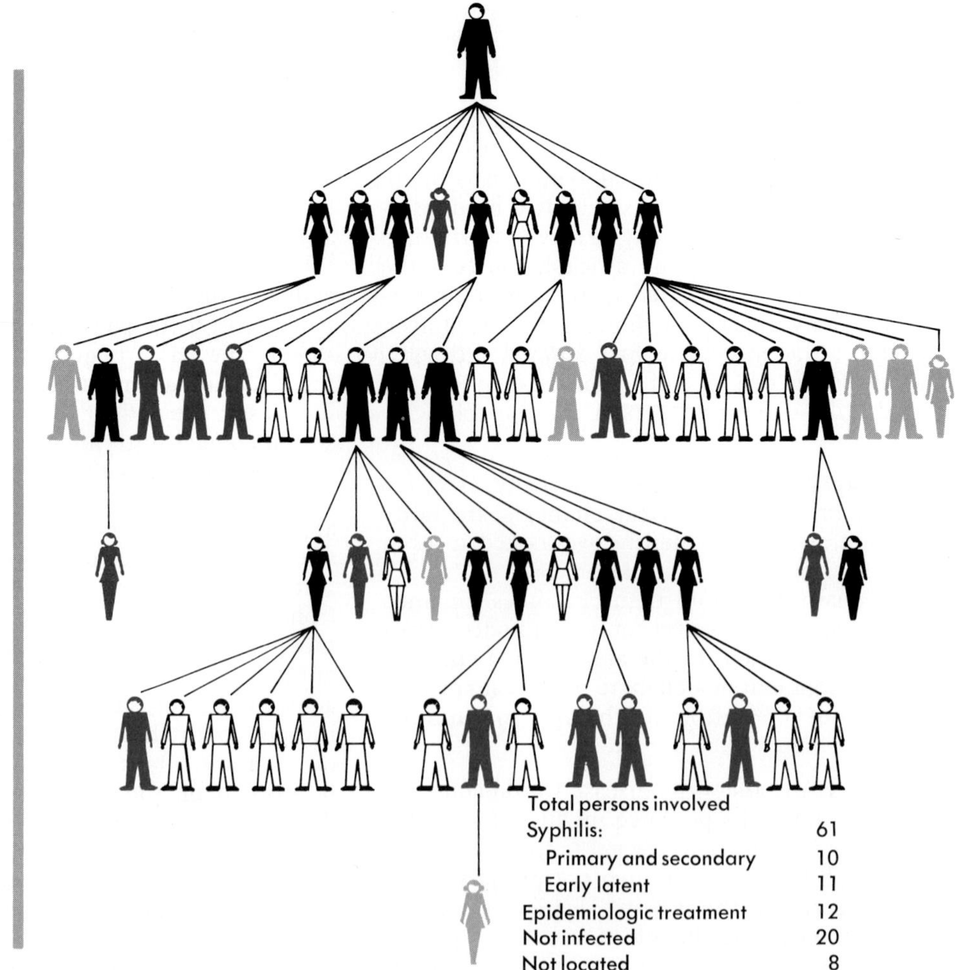

Fig. 9-13. *Syphilis "the great imitator"—The rash of secondary syphilis shown here must be distinguished from measles, dermatitis, and other conditions causing similar skin eruptions.* (*U.S. Public Health Service*)

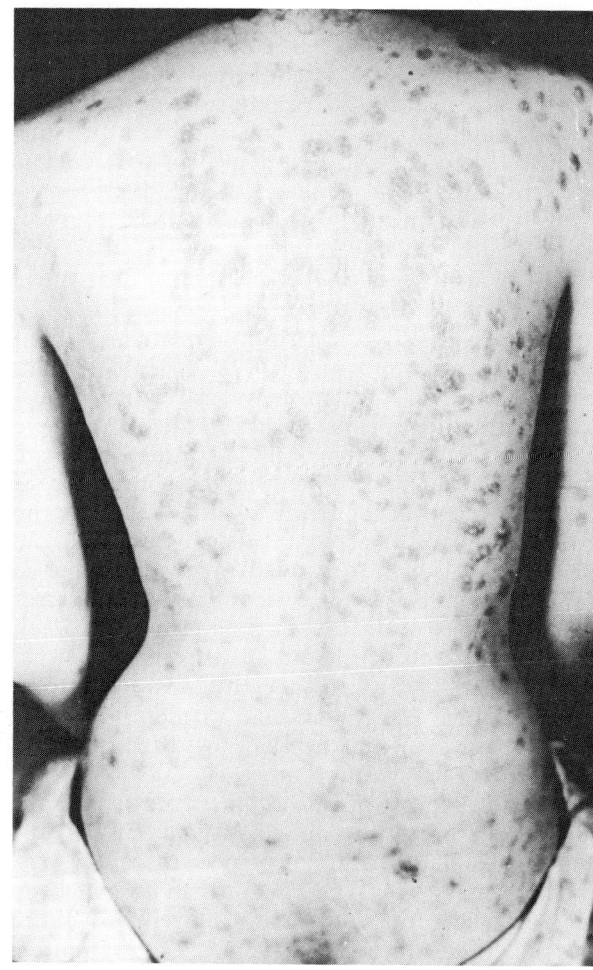

the "great imitator." Sometimes the rash, sore throat, and other discomforts are so mild as to go unnoticed. Whatever the case, these symptoms will eventually disappear without treatment, and the infection is then permitted to continue on its insidious course of destruction.

Serological examinations are highly reliable in diagnosing syphilis that has progressed to this point, and antibiotic therapy is very effective in curing secondary syphilis.

Latent Syphilis. Because the treponemae pallidae settle down in clusters in various parts of the body, no symptoms are evident. The syphilitic may feel perfectly normal during a period that extends from five to twenty years or longer. As is true in the secondary stage of syphilis, blood tests are reliable in detecting the disease during the latent period. Whether the latent disease is or is not communicable has not been definitely determined. Most authorities agree, however, that after the first year of the infection its communicability via sexual intercourse is reduced considerably.

The term "latent" is often considered to have the same connotation as dormant. When referring to latent syphilis, it is incorrect to view the infection as one of dormancy. The absence of overt signs of illness during this period is certainly not indicative of the insidious internal damage to organs, the central nervous system, bones, and other structures.

Late Syphilis. When syphilis is permitted to go untreated, the victim eventually may develop the tragic, chronic, and disabling conditions associated with long-term syphilis infection. The symptomatic manifestation of late syphilis depends on the extent of damage incurred by body structure during the latent period. The United States Public Health Service has reported that of untreated syphilitics, approximately 7 per cent will suffer cardiac disorders, 4 per cent will be crippled or paralyzed, 2 per cent will experience severe mental disturbances (paresis), and nearly 1 per cent will be blinded. These unfortunate afflictions, as well as the thousands of deaths resulting from syphilis, have made this the most devastating of the venereal diseases.

Although syphilis cannot be inherited, if a woman with syphilis becomes pregnant it is possible for her unborn child to develop congenital syphilis. The placental barrier is effective in filtering many toxic substances, but treponema pallida is able to penetrate this natural defense. Whenever the conception of the child occurs at approximately the same time the mother becomes infected with syphilis, it is likely that the child will be harmed unless treatment is administered. Apparently the spirochete passes through the placenta at about the eighteenth week of gestation. Adequate treatment of the mother before this time will protect the child from infection. If the mother's infection is four or more years old, it is quite possible for the baby to escape infection without therapy of any kind.

Occasionally, a woman becomes infected rather late in her pregnancy and the symptoms go unnoticed. Under these circumstances the child may exhibit symptoms of syphilis at birth or at some later date. Ordinarily the symptoms of congenital syphilis resemble those of secondary syphilis. Many children are stillborn or born with severely handicapping conditions such as blindness, skeletal deformities, and neurosyphilis.

The most effective way of reducing the frequency of congenital syphilis is to require serological examinations of pregnant women. In fact, the majority of states require such measures. This is apparently not the final solution to the problem, for even today thousands of pregnant women do not receive adequate prenatal care. Perhaps in years to come, legislation, education, and better distribution of medical personnel and facilities will result in the eradication of this tragic form of syphilis.

Penicillin remains the preferred medication for treating all stages of syphilis. In those few cases in which patients are allergic to penicillin, other equally effective antibiotics may be prescribed by the physician. The objective of antibiotic therapy is to maintain a high level of penicillin in one's bloodstream to destroy all of the syphilis microorganisms and eliminate the infection. The goal is more easily attained when treatment is begun early, preferably during the primary stage of the disease. When the infection is untreated and allowed to progress, increasing doses of antibiotics are required over longer periods in order to eliminate the disease.

Even individuals suffering from advanced cases of syphilis may benefit from antibiotic treatment. Central nervous system disorders, syphilitic heart, and other organic damage resulting from late infection cannot, however, be repaired by even the best antibiotic therapy.

Another disheartening observation frequently

made today is that from 3 per cent to 7 per cent of syphilitics adequately treated with antibiotics suffer relapses, without being reinfected. At the moment, the cause or causes of these relapses are unknown and justifiably of great concern to physicians. This phenomenon suggests that the spirochete may sometimes develop a resistance to penicillin, although medical authorities do not believe that this is the case. At any rate, in view of the frequency of relapses, successfully treated syphilitics should be encouraged to have periodic blood examinations for at least two years following their cure. Unlike most other communicable diseases, syphilis can strike the same individual more than once. Apparently, the immune mechanisms that characterize measles, chickenpox, and mumps do not operate with syphilis.

Following the isolation and identification of treponema pallida by Schaudinn and Hoffman in 1905, Wassermann and his colleagues developed (in 1906) the first satisfactory serologic test for detecting syphilis infections. Wasserman's original procedure was rather complex and it has since been simplified and improved upon. Today the Wasserman Test is still of great value in the diagnosis of syphilis. Of course, additional diagnostic laboratory tests have been in use in recent years.

Gonorrhea. In both sexes, gonorrhea is essentially a disease of the genitourinary system. Since 1957 there has been an accelerating incidence of the disease from a reported incidence of 216,476 to an excess of half a million. Estimates are that actual incidence is far in excess of a million cases. The group with the highest venereal disease rate is the 15–24-year-age group. Some health authorities have described venereal disease as being "out of control"

Fig. 9-14. Communicable diseases —number of Reported Cases in the United States, 1970. (U.S. Public Health Service)

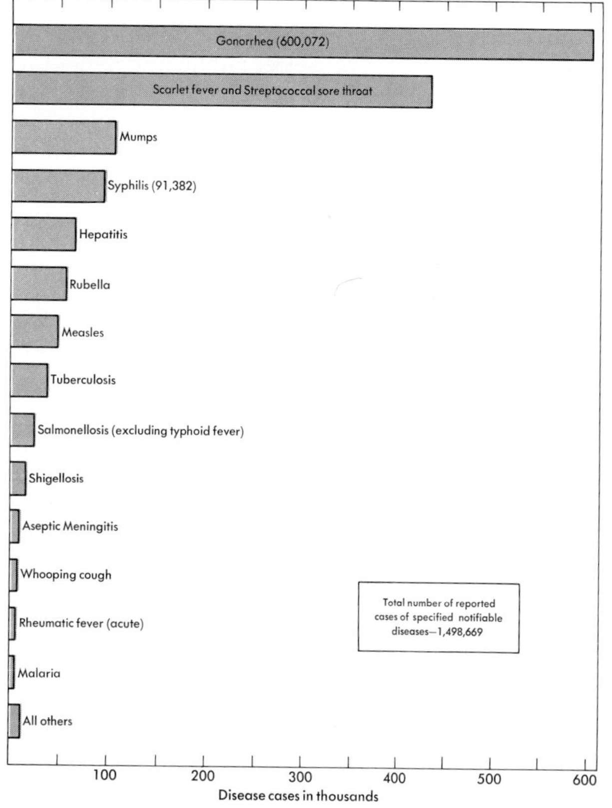

 . . . others have described it as being "epidemic". Suffice it to say that only the common cold exceeds it in terms of incidence. Better public understanding and community health programs to counteract the devastation of gonorrhea are now in order.

The microorganism responsible for gonorrhea is the gonococcus, a bacterium discovered by Neisser in 1879. Intimate sexual contact (nearly always sexual intercourse) is the manner by which the causative agent is transmitted. The disease remains communicable until it is cured.

Unlike syphilis, gonorrhea is usually an infection of the sex organs and their adjacent structures. In women, the infection ordinarily starts in the vagina, and if untreated, progresses to the uterus and fallopian tubes, where it may cause inflammation and adhesions, blocking the passage of ova from the ovary. Obviously, in such cases sterility may be the consequence. Gonorrheal infections in males begin in the urethra, causing widespread inflammation and irritation. If allowed to progress, the infection may eventually involve the testes and convoluted tubules, resulting in sterility. In those relatively uncommon cases where untreated gonorrhea invades the circulatory system, the gonococci may invade the body's connective tissue. The result of this is inflammation of joints, which may lead to gonorrheal arthritis, or inflammation of cardiac tissue. The latter condition may lead to severe heart disorders. Generally speaking, however, the total impact of untreated gonorrhea is much less damaging to the individual than is untreated syphilis.

The incubation period of the disease is short, with initial signs and symptoms usually developing within three to four (at times 9 days or longer) days following contact. Men often experience burning sensations, especially when voiding urine, as soon as three days following contact and a pus-like discharge from the penis may be observed. This discomfort is apt to intensify upon urination as the inflamed urethra (urethritis) is irritated by urine. Females, however, often do not experience such early discomfort. The inflamed vagina is somewhat less sensitive than the penis and obviously is apart from the female urinary system. Therefore the burning irritation so common in males in early gonorrhea is typically absent in females. Furthermore, the internal reproductive system of the female makes the discharge of pus less obvious than in males. In one sense, these sexual differences are unfortunate because they so frequently lead to delayed diagnosis and treatment of the infection.

Women usually experience their first discomfort from gonorrhea several months after contact, when the fallopian tubes become inflamed. The usual symptoms at this time are pain in the lower abdominal region.

There are many causes of urethritis in males and vaginitis in females. By no means does the presence of a viscous discharge necessarily indicate a gonorrheal infection. Any abnormal discharge should be referred to a physician so that accurate diagnosis can be made. Sometimes discharge in males accompanies a bladder infection that should be treated immediately. Vaginitis, with an accompanying discharge, is indicative of an abnormal condition not necessarily gonorrhea. Improper hygienic practices are a common cause of these infections.

A positive diagnosis of gonorrhea results when gonococci are detected in samples of secretions from the reproductive system. Very often the organisms are not observed in a routine microscopic examination of the samples. In such cases the culture should be incubated for three or four days and reexamined. Even this procedure may not yield positive results, and it is sometimes necessary to take several cultures. At the present time promising research is being conducted to produce a blood test for the detection of gonorrhea which would make the testing easier and faster.

One very important difference between gonorrhea and syphilis is the extent to which their respective causative agents respond to penicillin therapy. In discussing syphilis, it was mentioned that penicillin therapy in syphilitic control appears to be as effective today as it was when penicillin was first used to treat syphilis in 1943. Gonorrheal infections, on the other hand, are "fast becoming refractive to penicillin. It is not known whether this is due to the nature of the organism, which closely resembles the meningococcus and which organism is also becoming resistant, or whether the use of long-acting antibiotics in the treatment of venereal disease has produced a type of organism which now requires, in some instances, high blood levels to destroy it."[3] Medical authorities have become alarmed over the increasing amounts of penicillin required to cure some gonorrheal infections. Perhaps one day, if present trends continue, gonorrhea will not respond to any program of penicillin therapy. The implications of such a development pose serious threats to our venereal disease control programs.

Whenever a case of gonorrhea is diagnosed, the physician should also perform routine serological examinations for syphilis. Experience has shown that these two venereal diseases often infect an individual simultaneously. Were the gonorrheal diagnosis positive and no serological studies initiated to determine the presence of a syphilis infection, the routine antibiotic therapy for gonorrhea might obscure the symptoms of syphilis. In past years, this occurrence was fairly common and a concurrent syphilis infection was allowed to progress in the unsuspecting patient. Physicians are quite aware of this possibility now and routinely conduct blood tests for all individuals infected with gonorrhea.

Years ago, gonorrhea of the newborn was not uncommon. Infected mothers were responsible for infection of their infants because the infectious material was introduced into the child as it passed through the birth canal during delivery. In most cases, these infant infections involved the eyes, and a condition known as gonorrheal ophthalmia often led to blindness. Today, with our increased understanding of gonorrheal infections, solutions of silver nitrate or penicillin are routinely administered to the eyes of infants to prevent infection. This control measure has greatly reduced the incidence of gonorrheal ophthalmia and blindness in infants.

[3]Ibid., p. 24.

208 Developments in Venereal Disease Control

The advent of penicillin (1943) as an effective cure for syphilis was greeted with unprecedented enthusiasm by physicians and public health personnel, and each year from 1943 to 1958 the incidence of syphilis decreased. Suddenly, in 1959, the downward trend of syphilis and gonorrhea reversed itself and the United States experienced an upsurge of both venereal diseases. The increased frequency of these diseases has continued at an alarming rate, particularly in the teenage and young adult groups.

Many authorities have speculated as to the reasons for the unanticipated increase, and their explanations include:

> . . . the record of all-time low rates plus the ease and effectiveness of treatment had lulled physicians into a false sense of security regarding the relative importance of the disease; in turn, physicians had become desensitized to the need for considering syphilis when making a differential diagnosis; the disease itself had become more difficult to recognize; serious deficiencies had developed in such diagnostic aids as serologic tests and darkfield examinations; the medical schools and hospitals had reduced their clinical training in syphilis below an irreducible minimum; the organism had become more virulent, especially in relation to the increased use of penicillin.[4]

In addition, some feel that the advent of "the pill" replacing the condom as a birth control measure has also removed the condom as a protective device as far as protection from venereal diseases is concerned. Increased male homosexual activity appears to have made its contribution to the problem, with more relaxed attitudes toward heterosexual activity making an even greater one. Studies show that only approximately 3 per cent of the VD cases are related to prostitute contacts.

In response to the resurgence of venereal disease, public health leaders have suggested several measures to control and finally eliminate the venereal disease problem. They follow:

1. Increased local, state, and federal funds to expand present control efforts.
2. Enactment by state legislative bodies of laws requiring the reporting of all cases of venereal disease by all laboratories.
3. Required serological tests on all routine hospital admissions.
4. Support of venereal disease education programs in school and colleges.
5. Initiation and expansion of courses in venereal disease management in medical schools.
6. Intensification of research efforts to develop effective gonorrhea and syphilis vaccines.
7. Expansion of behavioral science research that will contribute to the control of venereal diseases.
8. Encouragement to physicians to report all cases of venereal disease.

Those working in public health VD programs find that individuals with VD are often inhibited from

[4]New York State Department of Health, "The Resurgence of Venereal Disease," *Health News,* Vol. 40, No. 6 (June 1963), p. 10.

seeking treatment or reporting who their sexual contacts were out of concern that moralistic judgments may be made with regard to how they contracted the disease. This is also a factor with physicans who do not report cases of VD in order to "protect" their patient.

Physicians and public health personnel recognize that venereal disease must be treated as a disease with moralistic judgments left to others if they are to handle this problem effectively. A number of state legislatures recognizing this aspect of the problem have passed legislation making it possible for minors to seek VD treatment without requiring that the physician inform the parent. In essence, it is essential that treatment personnel and facilities be easily and comfortably approached if the VD problem is to be reversed. These measures are realistic and attainable and the key to their success is largely an aroused and concerned public. It is entirely within the realm of possibility to eliminate venereal disease as a blight on our society.

The Unfinished Task

Though tremendous progress has been realized in understanding and combating the communicable diseases, those caused by viruses still represent a major challenge to medical research. By comparison with bacterial infections, viral diseases such as influenza and the common cold are not as well understood.

The number of viruses known to affect man and animals has been estimated at roughly 500 to 600. Approximately 150 of these, including the influenza viruses and those that cause the common cold, affect the respiratory tract and pose serious problems to Americans and people in other areas of the world. Present virus research efforts are rapidly contributing to our fund of knowledge and offer new hope against many of our virus enemies.

In 1956 it was discovered that a protein substance called interferon was developed in the body in response to the presence of certain viruses. When the level of interferon in the body is raised, it appears to increase bodily resistance to viral infection. Animal experimentation thus far conducted seems to confirm this phenomenon. Since the effects of interferon are not believed to be specific (research results indicate that it may be effective against many viral diseases), some scientists believe that interferon may serve as a basis for the development of a universal vaccine effective against many viral infections. The search for better disease control continues.

Review Questions

1. Describe the progress man has made in the control of communicable disease.
2. How can you distinguish between control of a disease and its eradication? What kind of effort would be necessary to eradicate a disease?
3. Define: (1) morbidity, (2) mortality, (3) incidence, (4) prevalence, (5) vectors, (6) immunity, (7) antigen, (8) antibody.

4. Distinguish between an active and a passive immunity.
5. What have been some of the difficulties in the development of preventive measures for influenza?
6. What is known about the etiology of mononucleosis? Why is "kissing disease" possibly a misnomer for this condition?
7. How do infectious and serum hepatitis differ? What have been some of the inhibiting factors in dealing effectively with the problem of infectious hepatitis?
8. Why is syphilis a difficult disease to detect and effectively treat? Why is it often referred to as the "great imitator?"
9. What can be the effects of advanced cases of syphilis?
10. Why is the detection of gonorrhea particularly difficult in the female? What can be the detrimental effects of this disease?
11. What are the implications of the increased resistance of gonorrheal infection to penicillin therapy?
12. What are some of the suggestions that have been made by public health leaders to bring our expanding venereal disease problem under control?

Chapter 10
Constitutional and Degenerative Diseases

It is a common misconception that the study of chronic and degenerative diseases is of interest to the older members of our populace because only they are affected by them. Though these diseases are more prevalent among our older population, their incidence is higher among our children and youth than is generally recognized. Many times, the incidence of chronic or degenerative conditions later in life can be prevented by a change in living patterns at an earlier age.

The chronic and degenerative diseases are of increasing public health concern since they have become the major cause of death in the country. In the 1900's tuberculosis, pneumonia, diarrhea, and enteritis were the leading causes of death. At the present time, heart disease, cancer, stroke, and accidents top the list. As we have gained greater control over the communicable diseases, people have survived to those ages when heart disease, cancer, and stroke are more prevalent.

Research effort and increased medical services are being focused on these leading causes of death. The acceptance of premature death from disease is being tolerated less and less. The term "died of natural causes" is rapidly becoming obsolete. Those "natural" causes are now being identified as disease entities, with treatment procedures being developed to correct them and, more important, preventive measures used to eliminate or forestall them.

Cardiovascular Diseases

Cardiovascular diseases, which are responsible for more than half of all deaths that occur in the United States, deserve our primary attention. There is an increased incidence of cardiovascular disease in those countries that have raised their standards of living and have gone from malnutrition to overnutrition and from rural to urban living with its inherent stresses, sedentary life, and pollution. Cardiovascular disease is increasingly being recognized as an "affliction of civilization."

ARTERIOSCLEROSIS AND ATHEROSCLEROSIS

Arteriosclerosis is commonly referred to as hardening of the arteries. Changes take place, as a result of this condition, in the middle layer of the artery wall, which causes a loss of elasticity and contractility. Atherosclerosis, which is the most common form of arteriosclerosis, is a condition in which fatty substances are deposited on the inner lining of the artery. These individual deposits are referred to as atheromas. As more and more of the atheromas are formed, they tend to increase in size and gradually narrow the channel through which the blood flows. The roughening of the lining of the artery through this process facilitates the forming of blood clots. The accumulation of fatty tissues in the lining of the arteries may ultimately result in the blocking of these blood vessels. This is particularly important when it happens to the coronary arteries of the heart or the cerebral arteries of the brain. A technique used for measuring the degree of blockage has been developed. It is called phonoangiography, and works well with arteries near the body surface. In essence a highly sensitive microphone detects the turbulent

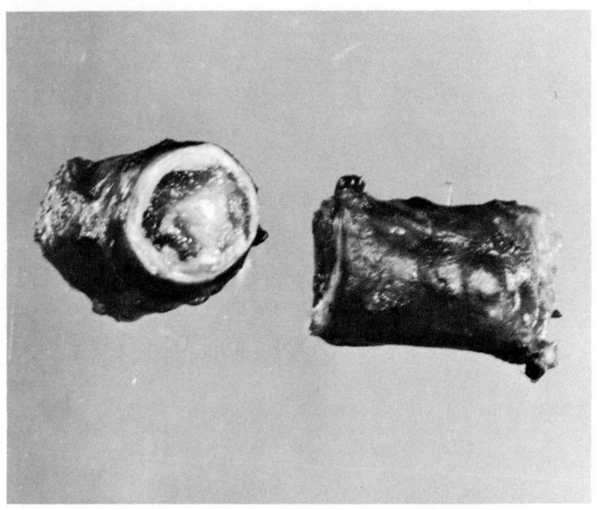

Fig. 10-1. Atherosclerosis, known to be one cause of heart attack, has been associated with elevated levels of cholesterol in the bloodstream. Here is a human artery plugged by an atherosclerotic lesion, an important component of which is white fatty cholesterol. (National Institutes of Health)

sounds made by blood flowing through vessels partially clogged by atheromas. Normally blood flows almost without sound.

There are a number of factors associated with atherosclerosis. Heredity sometimes plays a role in one's susceptibility to this condition. Studies have shown that there are familial tendencies to develop high cholesterol levels and therefore an increased possibility for the incidence of atherosclerosis.

Age is another factor. A major portion of persons with atherosclerosis are in their middle and later years. In most countries throughout the world the incidence of arteriosclerotic disease has increased significantly in the 45 to 54-year-age group.

The incidence of this artery disease is lower in women than in men. This is particularly reflected in cardiac mortality rates where women enjoy a 10- to 20-year period of grace before arteriosclerosis and heart attacks become a significant cause of death. Female sex hormones (estrogen) protect the woman from arteriosclerosis until menopause after which she becomes as vulnerable as men.

A much-publicized factor leading to atherosclerosis is the level of cholesterol found in the blood. This is a fatty substance which when found abundantly increases the chances of this disease. There are many unknowns concerning this substance which the body manufactures and which is found in most animal fats we eat. It was felt at one time that simply eliminating or reducing high cholesterol foods from the diet would solve the problem. However, the Framingham, Massachusetts, heart disease study (discussed later in this chapter) has indicated that there is no discernible association between diet and blood cholesterol levels. The long controversy over whether an effort should be made to modify the levels of saturated fats in the American diet continues.

Other factors associated with higher rates of atherosclerosis are inappropriate diets leading to obesity, lack of exercise, hypertension, and smoking. A team of surgeons from the University Medical Center in Cleveland, Ohio, reported that they knew smoking was known to accelerate arteriosclerosis but never before had they seen such dramatic evidence of the harmful effects of cigarette smoking even where blood cholesterol levels had been reduced with drugs. They were describing a study of 102 patients who underwent blood vessel surgery. Nine remained heavy smokers and all suffered blockage damage to their rebuilt arteries a year or more after their operations. No such problems occurred among the other patients who did not smoke or who smoked pipes or cigars in moderation.

Coronary Thrombosis (Myocardial Infarction)

The coronary thrombosis, or heart attack, may be caused by a blood clot in a coronary artery. Such a blood clot would be known as a thrombosis. A closure of the artery may also be effected by an accumulation of atheromas. Closure of an artery by either one of these causes will deprive that part of the heart of blood. The muscle tissue of the heart is thus deprived of oxygen and nutrient material

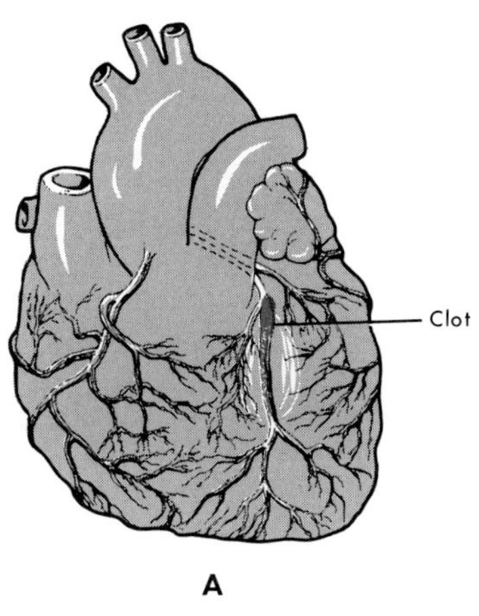

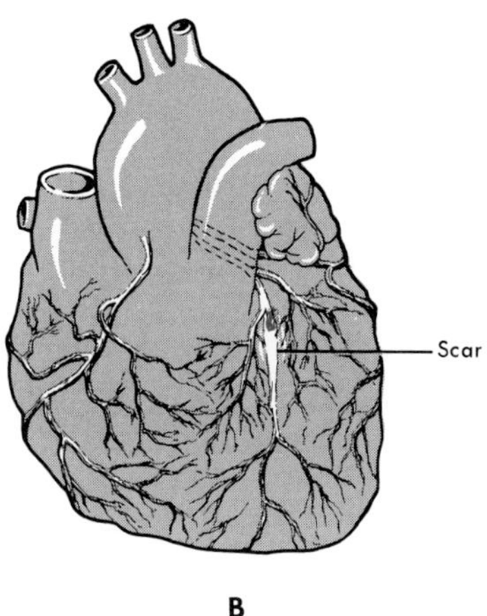

Fig. 10-2. **A.** *White cells are clearing away the dead tissue. Scar tissue is beginning to form at the edges of the damaged area (just below the clot). The patient must remain quiet because during the first several weeks there is danger that this weak spot will rupture.* **B.** *Tough scar tissue has formed. The patient begins to resume activities. He must keep his weight down, avoid severe mental and physical strain, and stop smoking. Moderate physical activity is encouraged. If all goes well, the patient may be in excellent health and free of symptoms in a relatively short time.*

necessary for maintaining its life. Fortunately, most closures of coronary arteries occur in the smaller vessels. The result is that most heart attacks are not fatal.

Symptoms of a heart attack will often include painful sensations of pressure in the chest. These sensations sometimes spread to the arms, throat, or back and may persist for long periods of time. Sudden and intense shortness of breath will often accompany the condition, along with sweating and possibly loss of consciousness. Nausea may sometimes be a symptom that can be mistaken for acute indigestion. Only a physician should make the diagnosis.

Complete rest is usually prescribed following a coronary, whose duration may last from several weeks to months, to permit the healing process to take place. The injured portion of the heart forms a weak area in that muscular organ. A scar must form and toughen during this period of rest. A new supply of blood is also sent into the area around the injury through the development of new blood vessels that branch out into the affected part. This growth of new blood vessels into the injured area is known as *collateral circulation.* Loss of excessive weight and a modification of the diet is usually part of the therapy for a coronary patient. Such a patient is usually advised to stop his smoking habits. Anticoagulants (heparin) are sometimes used to prevent the formation of additional blood clots.

Fig. 10-3. The rhythmic beating of the heart is recorded on the electrocardiogram (ECG). The high points in the tracing represent ventricular contractions. These are preceded by indications of the actions of the auricles. Deviations from the normal ECG tell the physician that something is wrong. (Courtesy Sam R. Mason, M.D.)

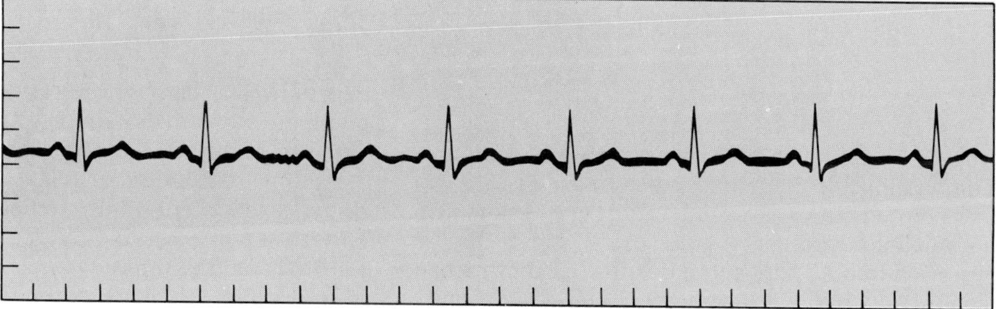

Fig. 10-4. Causes of a stroke.
A. *Hemorrhage, or bleeding. If an artery wall breaks down as a result of injury or inherent weakness or disease, blood seeps into the surrounding tissue instead of flowing in its normal channels. Although the most dangerous, this kind of stroke is less frequent.*
B. *Thrombosis, or clot formation. Because of a diseased condition in an artery or vein, a clot of blood may form at some point, and grow in size until it finally plugs the vessel completely.*
C. *Embolism, or traveling clot. A blood clot formed somewhere else in the arterial system (most commonly in a diseased heart), may break loose, be pumped into a brain vessel and block it.*

Thrombosis and embolism are frequent and the most common causes of strokes. Fortunately they are also the conditions doctors now have good prospects of controlling.
D. *Compression. A tumor or swollen tissue may press upon a blood vessel to the point where it stops the flow of blood. Since brain tumors, however, are relatively rare, this condition is the least common source of a stroke.*

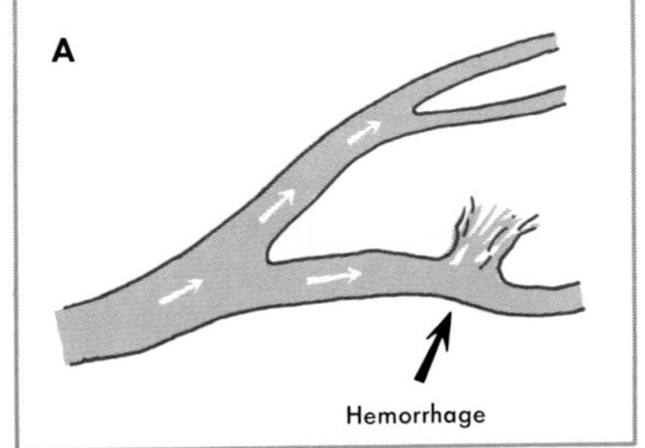

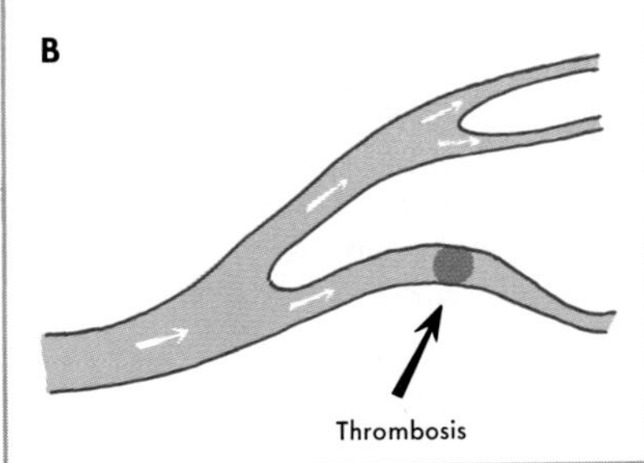

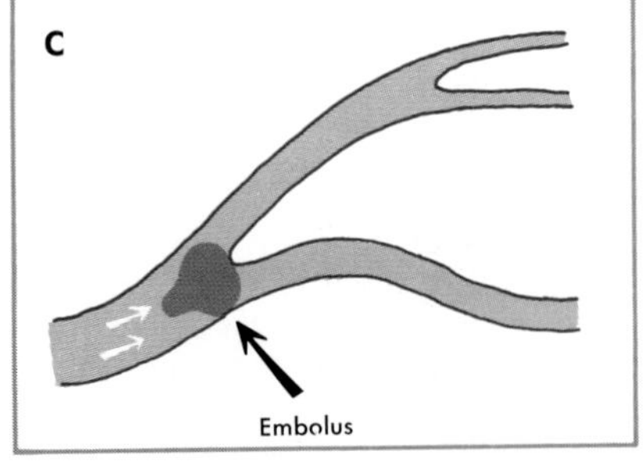

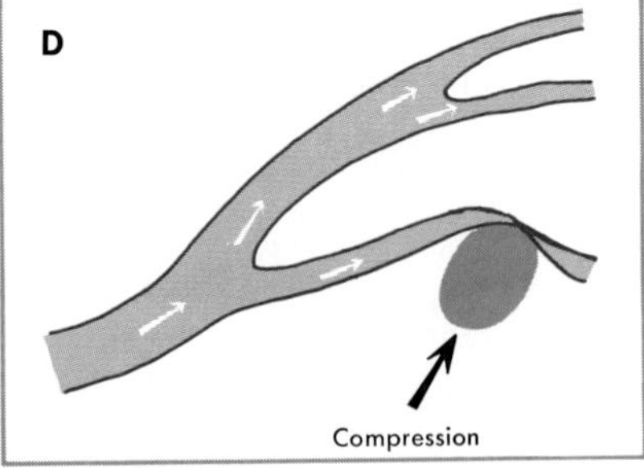

Angina Pectoris

Angina pectoris is a term for cardiac insufficiency. The relationship of angina and coronary disease was first pointed out by Edward Jenner, better known for his smallpox vaccine. Angina is really not a disease but a symptom. It is an indication of diminished blood supply to the heart muscle. The person usually experiences a feeling of tightness or pressure in the chest and sometimes pain or a tingling sensation that extends to either shoulder or upper arm. These symptoms usually occur following exercise or emotional excitement; they reflect the inability of enough blood (carrying oxygen and nutrient material) to reach the muscle tissues of the heart in order to feed it properly. During the intervals between the angina attacks, the patient is not aware of any discomfort and claims to feel fine. X ray and listening with a stethoscope reveal no abnormality. Even an electrocardiogram will be normal in one-third of the patients with angina. However, the electrocardiogram will sometimes show nontypical irregularities or abnormalities suggestive of coronary insufficiency. In these cases the patient might be given a controlled exercise tolerance test which will in all probability bring on an angina attack. The angina patient is, in essence, forewarned that he has an atherosclerotic condition of the arteries of his body. Management of this condition is generally through loss of weight, exercise, and controlled diet. Because present evidence suggests that there is a cause-and-effect relationship between smoking and atherosclerosis,[1] this patient is usually advised to stop his smoking habit. Nitroglycerine or other forms of nitrate are often prescribed before exercise to dilate the coronary arteries and prevent an angina attack.

Stroke (Cerebrovascular Disease)

A stroke occurs when the blood supply to a part of the brain is significantly reduced or completely cut off. As a result, nerve tissue in the brain is not able to function. Those parts of the body which this brain tissue controls will also cease functioning. A stroke, therefore, can result in a variety of effects including loss of speech, memory, or paralysis of various parts of the body. There are several causes of stroke. A stroke may be caused by a hemorrhage resulting from an injured or diseased artery wall. The blood seeping into the surrounding brain tissue will inhibit its functioning. A thrombosis or a clot can also cause a stroke by blocking off a vein or an artery. An embolism, or traveling clot, may become lodged in a smaller blood vessel and have a similar effect. Thromboses and embolisms represent a more common cause of stroke. Compression of a blood vessel can be another cause of stroke. A tumor or a swollen tissue can press upon a blood vessel to the extent that it stops the flow of blood through it. Fortunately, this is a rare occurrence.

There are sometimes warning episodes that will lead a diagnostician to suspect a developing stroke condition. Numbness, dizziness, and confusion are many times indicative of small strokes that precede more significant episodes. Approximately one-third of all strokes can be traced to blood vessels of the neck that have become clogged due to the formation of atheromas. Surgical removal of this material will correct the condition.

The American Heart Association states, " . . . for the first time, suggestive evidence linking cigarette smoking and strokes was shown. The stroke death rate was 40 per cent higher in men aged 55–64 who smoked cigarettes, as compared with nonsmokers. In this same disease category, incidentally, the risk proved unexpectedly greatest for women. Female

[1]Jack P. Strong, M.D., "More Artery Hardening Found at Post-Mortem in Coronaries of Cigarette Smokers" in American Heart Association *Heart Research Newsletter*, Vol. XI, No. 4 (Fall 1966).

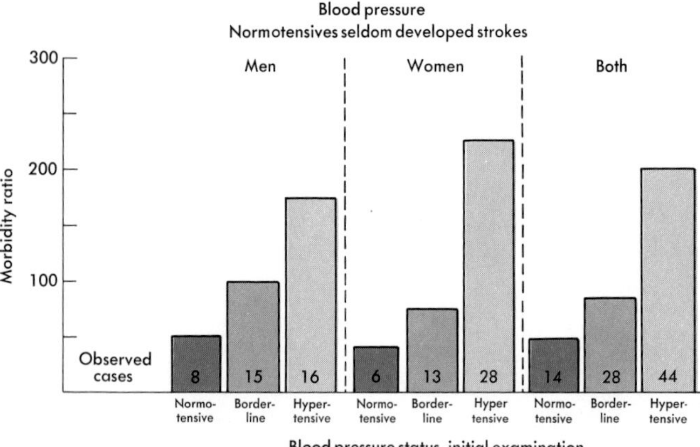

Fig. 10-5. "Epidemiology of Stroke." (Public Health Service Publication, National Heart Institute, Bethesda, Md.)

smokers in all age groups had up to twice the stroke death rate of nonsmoking women."[2]

An individual's susceptibility to stroke increases noticeably when the person suffers from hypertension. Their risk is four times greater than those individuals with normal blood pressure. This is also supported by a study done in Washington whereby 88 per cent of the hypertensive deaths below the age of 60 were blacks. Hypertension appears at a younger age, is more severe, and results in a higher mortality rate, more commonly from stroke rather than coronary artery disease, in the black population.

The presence of diabetes also increases the risk of stroke among men. It follows, then, that a combination of diabetes and hypertension is an extremely dangerous one and makes individuals six times more prone to having a stroke than normal persons.

It becomes obvious that stroke or cerebrovascular disease is merely a small part of the larger problem of cardiovascular disease. A new preventive approach to this disease seems imperative, for once the brain is damaged, recovery or return to normal is difficult, if achieved at all. If the stroke-prone individual is identified early and preventive measures are pursued, it is probable that many strokes could be forestalled or thwarted completely. The measures for the prevention of stroke seem to be the same as those indicated for the prevention of coronary heart disease.

[2]"AHA Highlights Heart Risks of Smoking," *The American Heart,* Vol. XVII, No. 2 (Spring 1967).

Hypertension (High Blood Pressure)

Blood pressure is the force exerted by blood against the walls of the vessels. This force or pressure is measured by a sphygmomonometer and consists of two readings. The higher reading is the systolic pressure recorded during the heart's pumping stroke. The lower reading is the diastolic pressure recorded when the heart is relaxed and refilling between beats. Blood pressure readings vary with individuals and range from 120/80 to 140/90. These would be considered normal. However, figures are not absolute and the physician considers all factors before labeling a reading normal or high. For example a reading of 160/90 may be serious in an individual 20 years old, but normal for a 50- or 60-year-old. Blood pressure increases with age, and in adults a good index of normal systolic blood pressure is 100 plus your age in years.

The causes of primary hypertension (or essential hypertension) are generally unknown. It is more common and less serious than secondary hypertension but if left untreated can become a more serious problem. In secondary hypertension the causes are known and usually involve a renal (kidney), vascular (blood vessel), or endocrine malfunction. One of the contributing factors to primary hypertension appears to be heredity. For example, it has been documented in numerous scientific studies that the incidence of hypertension among the black population is far higher than among whites. A family history of hypertension is a common finding.

Though these findings suggest it is an inherited characteristic, there are familial patterns of living that could be making entire families susceptible, not solely owing to the genetic makeup. Another contributing factor is the emotional makeup of the individual. The tense, nervous person who consistently overreacts to stressful situations is highly susceptible to hypertension.

An accusing finger has been pointed to the trace metal cadmium. In autopsies of individuals who suffered from hypertension the level of cadmium in the kidneys was much higher than those individuals with normal blood pressure. An experiment with rats that were fed trace quantities in their water since birth showed that they accumulated higher levels of cadmium in their kidneys and developed hypertension very similar to humans. Of great significance was the fact that the condition could be reversed by giving rats certain chemicals that combined with the cadmium to form a compound more easily excreted by the kidneys. How applicable these studies are to human hypertension is yet to be established.

There is an intimate relationship between arteriosclerosis and heart attacks with hypertension. Uncontrolled hypertension hastens the development of atheromas which in turn increases the risk of heart attacks and stroke from blocked vessels. Uncontrolled hypertension also forces the heart to pump harder, and in extreme cases the strain may cause heart failure. Though we can neither prevent nor cure hypertension, enough is known about the many facets of the disease that reasonable control over the condition is possible.

Hypertension can sometimes be treated successfully by diet control. Very often the overweight person who diets successfully and returns to a normal weight will also return to a normal blood pressure. The restriction of salt in the diet lowers blood pressure for the obese as well as the thin person in about one-third of the cases with hypertension. When hypertension does not respond to changes in living patterns, the physician today has at his disposal a myriad of drugs or combinations of drugs designed to lessen tension, dilate blood vessels, encourage the kidneys to excrete salt, or block nerves that prevent the reflex that constricts the vessels. As a result of improved diagnostic and treatment techniques the death rate from hypertension has decreased by nearly 50 per cent during the past ten years.

Wide-ranging epidemiological studies on the incidence and mortality due to coronary heart disease are helping to identify the high risk coronary person. Factors such as diet, stress, exercise, smoking, family history, blood cholesterol, hypertension, electrocardiogram abnormalities, among others, are being carefully studied. One such investigation in The Framingham Study which began in 1948 and continued for twenty years. Five thousand persons participated in the study which centered in the Framingham Union Hospital in a Boston, Massachusetts, suburb. The study uncovered vulnerable persons on their way to coronary attacks through the use of a coronary risk profile. Information for the profile was gathered from laboratory findings, physical exercise information, personal habit reports, and electrocardiogram readings. The subjects were followed as they

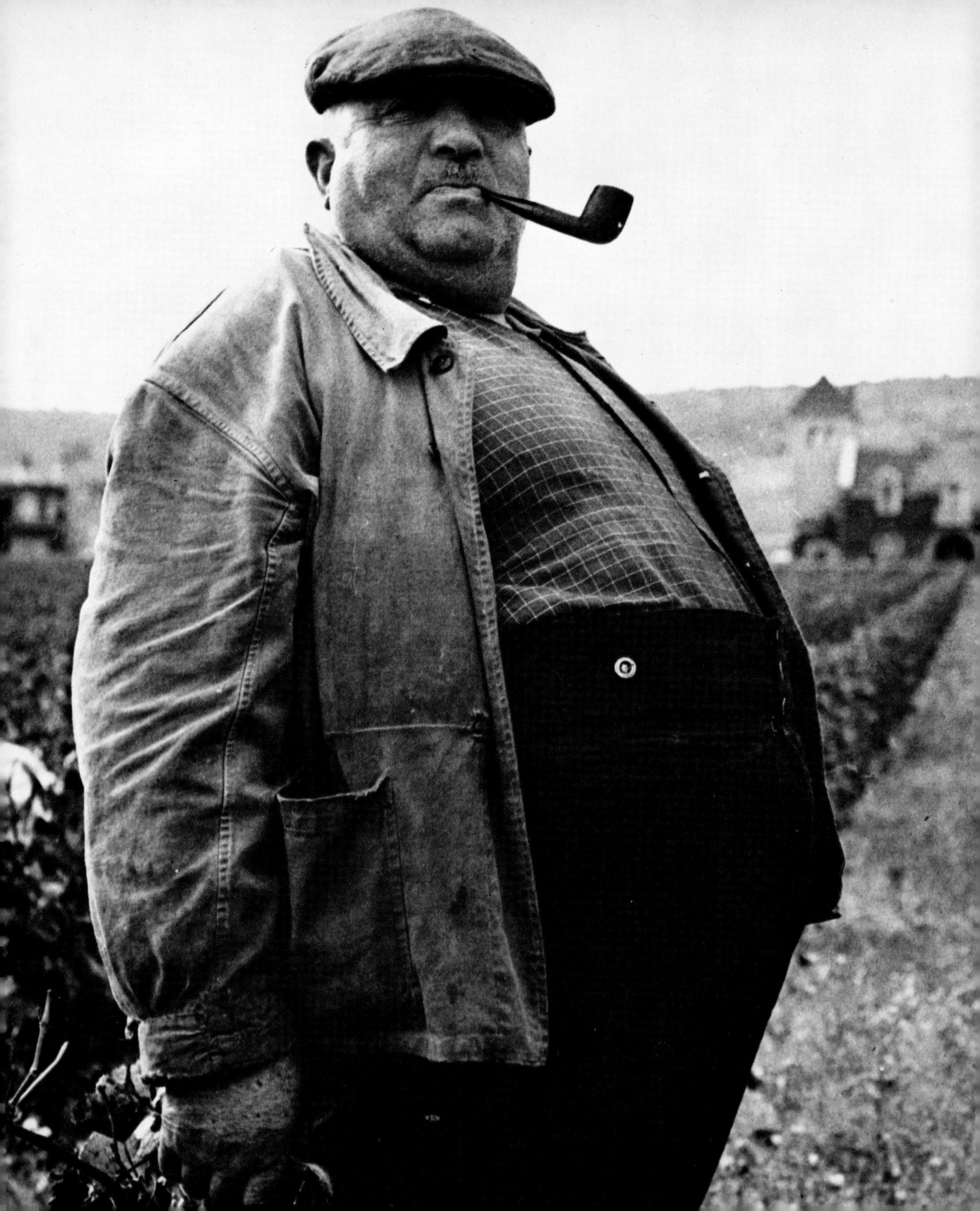

Fig. 10-6. Overweight predisposes a person to hypertension. (Paul Almasy)

aged and acquired disease conditions and were compared with themselves at an earlier age. The advantage of such a long-term study is that most participants are now in their sixties and their profiles for other chronic diseases is of considerable scientific value.

The intensive effort in the area of cardiovascular disease exemplified by the research activities cited is beginning to have its effects. The mortality rate from this cause has leveled off and even shown some signs of declining; nevertheless, it remains the number one killer of our adult population.

Rheumatic Fever and Rheumatic Heart Disease

Rheumatic fever is a disease that sometimes follows a streptococcal infection. It is estimated, however, that 90 to 97 per cent of streptococcal infections do not develop into rheumatic fever. Rheumatic fever, in turn, may or may not result in rheumatic heart disease. Rheumatic heart disease, however, does develop often enough to account for much of the cardiovascular disease among the young people of this country. It is estimated that approximately 500,000 children between the ages of 5 and 19 have this condition. The etiology of this disease is not completely understood. It is recognized that a streptococcal infection precedes a rheumatic fever attack. Prevention of the disease is therefore aimed at preventing recurrent streptococcal infections through the administration of antibiotics, because the body, instead of developing a resistance to the streptococcus, seems to become more vulnerable to each recurring attack. The damage to the heart in this condition is done by the scarring of the valves between the auricles and the ventricles. The bicuspid or mitral valve on the left side of the heart is the one that is usually most seriously affected. The disease may also cause damage to the endocardium, which is the inner lining of the heart. Surgical procedures have been developed that permit the cutting of the scar tissue which inhibits the proper functioning of the valves. Now, with the heart-lung machine, surgeons are given a dry field to work in and can replace entire valves with artificial ones.

Because there is no specific cure for rheumatic fever, drugs such as penicillin and cortisone are used to relieve symptoms and inflammation. The amount of bed rest that would be required varies with individual patients. It may be a matter of weeks or sometimes months. How much activity a person with rheumatic heart disease may be permitted will depend on the amount of damage done to his heart. Many rheumatic fever children recover and will live normal lives, provided that they receive proper medical care. Because rheumatic fever can be prevented through the utilization of penicillin or sulfa drugs, it is at the present time the only major form of cardiovascular disease that we have the specific knowledge to prevent.

Congenital Heart Defects

Congenital heart defects represent malformations that occur in the structure of the heart or the large

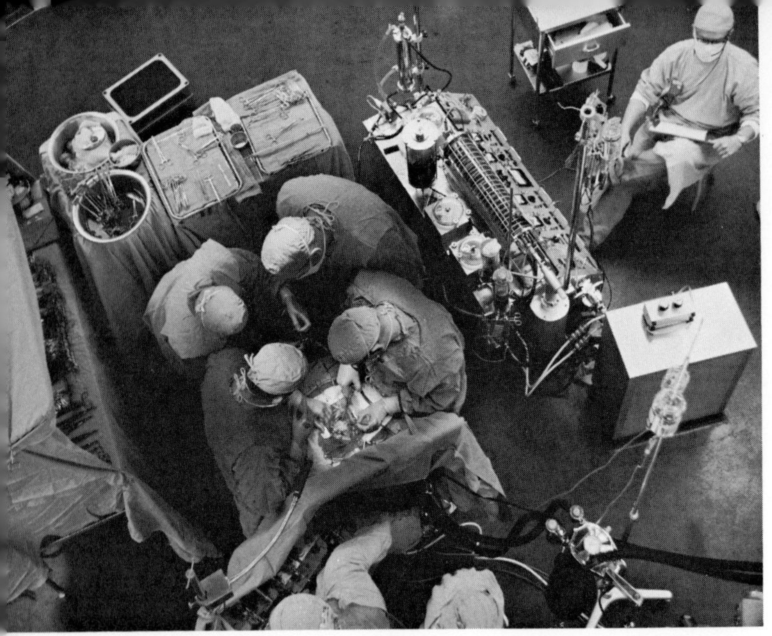

Fig. 10-7. Dramatic progress has been made in the development of techniques for repairing hearts which are imperfect at birth and for correcting harmful defects which sometimes result from illnesses such as rheumatic fever. Surgeon-scientist teams at the Public Health Service's National Heart Institute, like the one seen here, have played a leading role in developing and perfecting these lifesaving open-heart surgery methods. To the right of center is seen part of the heart-lung machine, the operating room tool which has made these complicated heart repairs possible by taking over the heart's blood pumping and oxygenating functions during surgery. (National Institutes of Health)

blood vessels associated with it. Although these defects may be present at birth, they are many times not detected until childhood or even adulthood. The causes of congenital heart defects are generally unknown. There appears to be a hereditary factor associated with some. Others are believed to be caused by viral diseases such as German measles during the first trimester of pregnancy. In a study conducted by Dr. Aloss J. Beuren, of the University of Gottingen, Germany, it was found that vitamin D in excessive amounts during pregnancy could severely damage the functioning of the fetus heart by narrowing the aorta and thereby obstructing blood flow.

A blue baby is one that has a malformation of the heart or of the major blood vessels near the heart. These conditions prevent his blood from getting enough oxygen, resulting in the skin and lips taking on a bluish tinge (cyanosis). These malformations are varied. In some cases a congenital heart defect may involve openings between walls of blood vessels or of chambers within the heart itself. It may involve a narrowing or constriction of a blood vessel or a valve inhibiting blood flow. Sometimes several of the above-mentioned malformations combine to form a more serious problem.

The development of the heart-lung machine has made it possible to operate more effectively on the heart. The machine permits the blood to bypass the heart, giving the surgeon a dry field to operate in. Stopping the heart by cooling it with ice is another new technique that permits the surgeon to operate on the organ when it is not in motion. Of the 30,000 to 40,000 children born each year with heart defects, it is now estimated that 75 to 80 per cent of them can be helped by surgery.

Varicose Veins

Varicose veins are a result of the breakdown of the valves in those veins found just below the skin. These valves may break down because of an inherent weakness due to heredity. The valves may also be destroyed because of phlebitis, which is an inflammation of the vein. The result is bulging, distorted veins that appear mainly in the legs. This condition is common in both sexes, but somewhat more so among women, the difference being sometimes attributed to the women's tight garters or undergarments that permit the flow of blood into the leg, but inhibit its flow back to the body. The increased blood pressure that this creates in the veins helps to break down the valves in the blood vessels. Varicosed veins also seem to be more prevalent in people whose occupations require that they stand for long periods of time. Overweight and pregnancy are additional contributing factors in varicosed veins. After the termination of a pregnancy the varicosed veins become much less marked. The use of elastic stockings prescribed by a physician seems to help this condition in that this garment is supportive of the outside walls of the veins. Weight reduction also is helpful in that it relieves some of the pressure on the veins of the legs. Surgery is used as a corrective measure either to remove the affected vein or to ligate it, which is the tying off of the vein. Because of the greater possibility of recurrence with the latter method, the removal or stripping of the vein seems to be the more effective procedure.

Cancer

Cancer is best described as a group of diseases that have a characteristic of abnormal cell growth. Cancer is not so much a disease of the body as it is a disease of the cells. The cells of any living organism are under the control of a regulating mechanism that permits its birth, life, ability to reproduce, and death. The rate at which this happens is carefully controlled. When something goes wrong with this controlling mechanism, and cell division becomes much more rapid, tumors then develop. When these tumors are malignant, their atypical cancer cells can erupt into the blood and lymphatic systems and be carried to various parts of the body. This spreading of cancerous cells is known as *metastasis* (me-TAS′-ta-sis). What happens to the controlling mechanism that permits this wild growth of cells is for the research scientist to discover. The cancer cells are not only produced more rapidly but are different in their nature. Their structural differences are such that they can in many instances be recognized under the microscope.

Although the specific causes of cancer are unknown, a number of related contributing factors and possible causes have been identified. Overexposure to radiation has been found to be a predisposing factor to the development of cancer. A higher incidence of leukemia has been found among those infants who were X-rayed in prenatal life. Radiologists who in the past did not properly protect themselves while X-raying patients have also had a higher cancer rate. Excessive exposure of the skin to the sun is also a factor in the increased incidence of skin cancer. The levels of safe radiation exposure are still being determined and in some instances debated by authorities in the field. A more judicious use of medical and dental X rays has resulted. For high-incidence groups in which tuberculosis is being sought, a simple tuberculin test is recommended as a first procedure. If the results of this test are positive, then a chest X ray is recommended.

One of the best-documented studies of the relationship of exposure to radiation and cancer incidence is being conducted in Japan. The Japanese being carefully studied are those who were in Hiroshima and Nagasaki and exposed to the intense radiation of the atomic bombs set off over those cities that ended World War II in 1945. Those receiving the heaviest doses of radiation are eight times more likely to contract leukemia (cancer of the blood), with cancer generally occurring ten times more frequently. Even those Japanese exposed to a lesser degree of radiation have a higher incidence of cancer of the thyroid, uterus, and bone. In the early 1980′s the young survivors of the atomic explosives will reach an age when the cancer incidence is expected to increase sharply. To what extent their previous exposure to excessive radiation will effect the cancer incidence in that group is a foreboding that remains to be seen.

A good deal of research is now going on to explore the relationship of viruses and cancer. A number of animal cancers have been identified as having been produced by viruses. There is suspicion that these microorganisms also play a role in the development of some human cancers. To date, however, no specific virus has been identified as being cancer-producing in man. The recent association of a herpes-type virus with Burkitt's lymphoma (cancer of the lymph glands occurring primarily in African children), and the Baylor University researchers noting a herpes-type II virus present in 83 per cent of cervical cancer patients provide new tools for investigations along this line.

The relationship of hormones to cancer has become suspect. There have been spontaneous recoveries from terminal cases of cancer which were attributed to changes in the hormonal environment. The use of hormone treatment in cancer of the breast, uterus, or prostate is already well established. At the other end of the spectrum there is some belief that vaginal cancer in young women up to age 22 may be a direct result of the administration of estrogenic hormones to their mothers during pregnancy. Though cancer as a disease cannot be inherited, with the exception of retinoblastoma,[3] it appears that a predisposition to some types of cancer may be. A physician's study of recent family history may give some clues as to preventive measures that one might take. Certainly, where a parent or grandparent has been claimed by lung cancer, one should view cigarette smoking with a jaundiced eye.

Various chemicals have been identified as being carcinogenic (cancer-producing) in nature. Coal tar colors that were used as color additives at one time have been identified as among these types of chemicals. Chimney sweeps in England, for instance, have a higher incidence of skin cancer, which is related to their contact with soot. A high incidence of cancer of the bladder among dye workers has been traced to aniline dyes. Studies have also shown arsenic to be a cancer-producing agent, particularly cancer of the skin. Chronic irritations of various types have also become suspect as possible cancer-producing factors. Even omissions in the diet have been demonstrated to be related to the incidence of cancer of the liver in communities of South Africa and Java, where vitamin B is lacking in the diet. The incidence of leukemia is 20 times as frequent in patients suffering from Down's syndrome (mongolism) as in the normal population. An abnormality of chromosome 21 appears in patients with a certain type of leukemia, though it is not the same as found in Down's syndrome (mongolism). The relationship between this type of cancer and this genetic abnormality remains unsolved.

While the research scientists are looking for the specific causes of cancer, the epidemiologist can perform the function of identifying those factors that are responsible for triggering certain cancers. The identification of these factors and where they occur in our environment can play a very significant role in the prevention of this disease.

[3] "Retinoblastoma" is usually found in children under the age of four and is considered to be a congenital tumor. The aim of treatment is to save not only the life of the patient but the vision of at least one eye.

As reported by the National Advisory Cancer Council,

It is believed that the core of the cancer problem is in the cell: on the one hand, for the conversion of a normal cell to a malignant one; and on the other, for the reversal of the malignant change, or destruction of malignant cells without harm to normal ones. Further, many investigators believe that the malignant transformation has its origins in the genetic-protein synthesizing system of the cell; that is, in DNA (deoxyribonucleic acid), the master chemical which contains genetic information coded into its structure, and RNA (ribonucleic acid) which receives instructions from DNA and oversees the synthesis of proteins, including enzymes that catalyze, or govern the speed of specific biochemical reactions.

Damage to the genetic apparatus may be the key factor in the transformation of a normal cell to a cancer cell. Support of this concept comes from information that some of the chemical carcinogens are known to react with nucleic acids, that radiation can alter DNA, and that viruses are themselves composed of DNA or RNA. Furthermore, certain tumor-inducing viruses have recently been found to cause an increase in the enzymes of the cell concerned with the synthesis not only of the DNA of the virus progeny but also of the DNA of the cell itself.[4]

Sites of Cancer

Cancer of the Skin is easily detected, diagnosed, and treated. This is a site of cancer that a physician can view easily. He can check telltale signs of the disease such as moles and skin blemishes that change in size or color, or a sore that does not heal. Construction workers, sportsmen, and farmers seem to be more prone to the development of cancer of the face, neck, and hands because of their greater exposure to the sun. Fair-skinned people are also more susceptible.

In spite of the fact that this type of cancer can be easily detected, diagnosed, and treated, approximately 5,000 unnecessary deaths per year can be attributed to it.

Lung Cancer is now a leading cause of cancer death among men. The recovery rate from this disease is very low, with approximately 4 per cent of the males and 8 per cent of the females recovering. The incidence of lung cancer among women has doubled in the last 22 years. The lung cancer death rate among American men is three times greater than it was in 1947 and partially accounts for the general increase in the male cancer death rate from 280 per 100,000 population in 1947 to 304 deaths per 100,000 population in 1970.

Diagnosis of this condition is difficult and often too late. Persistent hoarseness, coughing, and spitting up of blood may be symptomatic of the condition.

Cancer of the Stomach. There has been a 40 per cent decrease in the last twenty years in cancer of the stomach, for reasons that have not been determined. Persistent indigestion and bloody discharge with bowel movements are the prime symptoms related to this condition.

Cancer of the Colon and Rectum. Together, cancers of the colon and rectum make up the second

[4] *Progress Against Cancer 1966,* A Report by the National Advisory Cancer Council (Washington, D.C.: U.S. Dept. of Health, Education and Welfare, National Cancer Institute).

Fig. 10-8. Clinical data prove that regions with the most sunshine have the highest incidence of skin cancer. (U.S. Dept. of Commerce, Weather Bureau)

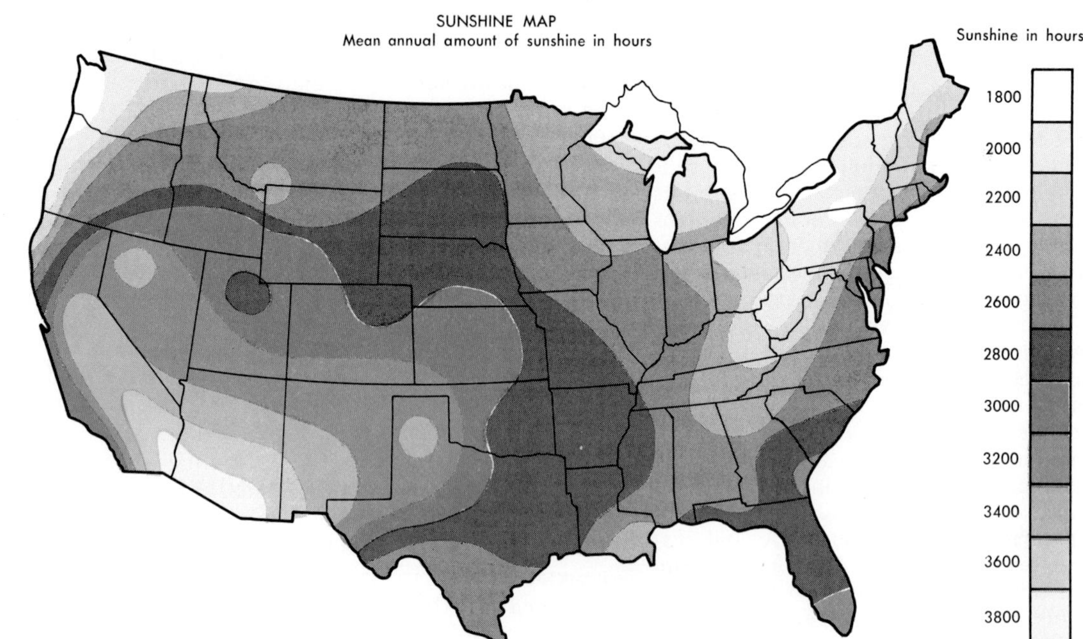

leading cause of cancer death in the United States. Approximately 93 per cent of cancer of the colon or rectum occurs in people over 45 years of age. Three out of every four of these afflicted people can be saved for it is a highly curable disease when detected early. Digital and proctoscopic examinations should be routinely included in annual physical checkups as a means of early detection.

Breast Cancer lends itself to early detection through breast self-examination, mamography (a special breast X ray), and thermography (a heat sensitive photograph of the breast). Hopefully a newly devised test involving cell examination of fluid extracted from a breast will reveal early irregularities of cell growth similar to the Pap smear for cervical cancer. Approximately 95 per cent of all breast cancers have been detected by women themselves. For this reason it is important that all women be properly

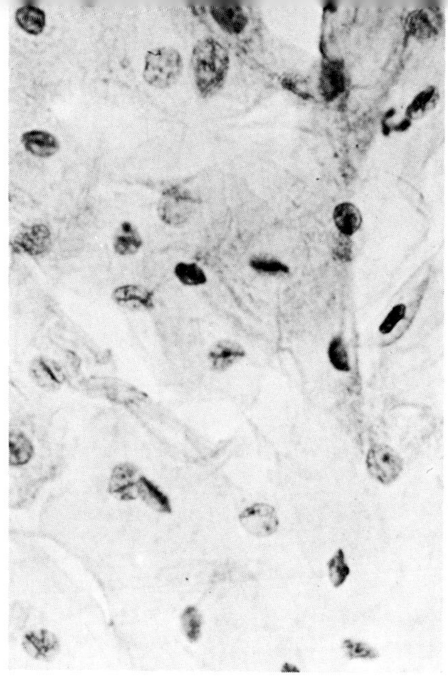

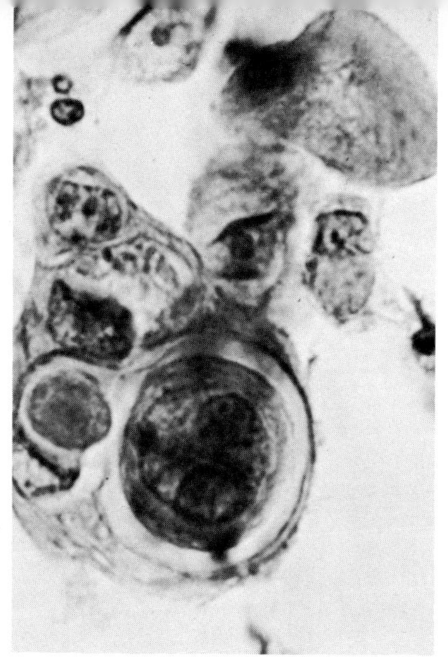

Fig. 10-9. Pictured above are the cells taken in "Pap" smears of the cervix of uterus. The cells on the left are normal, the cells on the right cancerous. (National Institutes of Health)

instructed with regard to this procedure. Lumps or thickenings in the breast are sometimes symptomatic of this disease. It must be remembered, however, that most lumps appearing in the breast are not cancerous in nature. Nevertheless, all irregularities should motivate the individual to confirm this with a medical opinion. Bleeding from the nipple and swollen lymph nodes under the arm pit are also possible signs of this disease. Treatment for breast cancer usually involves surgical removal (mastectomy) of the involved breast and surrounding tissues and lymph nodes. Sometimes radiotherapy and hormonal therapy are also utilized. Male hormones and adrenal cortical hormones inhibit advanced breast cancer. Female hormones (estrogens) are given to postmenopausal patients only. It is the leading cause of death among women.

Cancer of the Uterus. Uterine cancer is a malignancy that can occur in the cervix (neck of the uterus) or the body proper (corpus) of the uterus. Most uterine cancers occur in the cervix, and there seems to be no age limit. After age 45, however, cancers of the corpus of the uterus tend to be most prevalent. Deaths due to cancer of the uterus have been significantly reduced since the introduction of the Pap (Papanicolaou) test. The test consists of removing and examining cells from the vagina and from the cervix of the uterus. The microscopic examination of the cells will indicate whether cancer or precancerous cells are present. The cure rate for this type of cancer is exceedingly high, provided it is detected early enough. Entire communities have organized for action to bring the women in for their yearly Pap smear. Some hospitals have initiated the policy of doing a Pap smear on every female admitted regardless of the reason for admission. The importance of early detection and prompt treatment has been substantiated by the fact that the cure rate has risen from 38 per cent to 50 per cent in the last 25 years. The overall cancer rate among women has decreased from 294 per 100,000 population in 1947 to 256 per 100,000 population in 1971. The general decrease of cancer among women was attributed to a drop in uterine cancer as well as stomach and rectal cancers.

Cancer of the Prostate. The function of the prostate gland is to secrete a thick alkaline fluid which aids the sperm cells to get through the acid environment of the urethra. Incidence of cancer of the prostate is highest in men over 55 years of age. Black men are 65 per cent more likely to suffer from cancer of the prostate than whites. Frequent, thorough rectal examinations in men over 40 are helpful in detecting the disease early. Blood in the urine or in the ejaculate are significant signs. These symptoms, however, may be indicative of a number of other conditions including the bacterial infection of the prostate, bladder, or other related structures. Treatment for prostatic cancer, where the cancer is limited to a small nodule or hard area in the gland itself, is usually surgical removal. However, when the cancer extends beyond the prostate gland itself, alteration of the hormonal balance is carried out, either through surgical removal of the testes (orchiectomy) and possibly the administration of female hormones (estrogens).

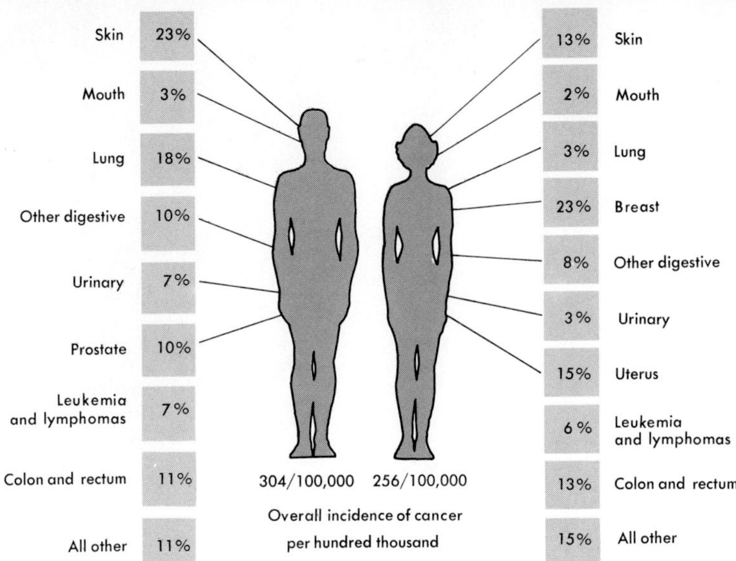

Fig. 10-10. Cancer incidence by site and sex. (American Cancer Society)

Cancer of the Blood, or Leukemia. Leukemia is the leading cause of nearly half of the deaths due to cancer in children between the ages of 3 and 15. This is a cancer of the blood-manufacturing organs, the bone marrow, spleen, and lymph glands. Its presence is detected by large numbers of white blood cells or the presence of immature blood cells. The acute form of leukemia occurs in younger people, and the survival period of this form of the disease is now five years or more. This has been made possible with the use of a barrage of drugs. Some of these drugs are called inducers and bring about a remission of the disease, with a second group of drugs used to help maintain the remission. The chronic type of leukemia occurs usually after 25 years of age. The patient with this disease may survive for ten years or more. Through the use of drug therapy, physicians have managed to obtain some control over leukemia. Steroid hormones and cytotoxic drugs are among those used in chemotherapeutic procedures. Blood transfusions are also utilized as a means of controlling anemia. Optimism has been expressed that effective drug therapy will soon be possible for the control of this condition.

Cancer of the Lymph Glands is a cancer that arises in the lymphatic system and is characterized by enlarged lymph glands. Hodgkin's disease is one of several malignant disorders of the lymphatic system that affects adults between the ages of 20 and 40. It is a relatively uncommon type of cancer.

If lymph glands should remain enlarged for three weeks or more, a physician should be seen so that a biopsy (the microscopic examination of body tissue to determine the presence of cancer cells) may be performed. The progress of the disease is slow and the person affected may live a normal life for many years, provided he is under treatment with drugs and/or X rays.

The American Cancer Society has developed a list of seven danger signals for cancer. These signs will in most cases be indicative of *other* malfunctions rather than the presence of cancer. However, they should be brought to the physician's attention for his investigation and diagnosis. The warning signals are:

1. Unusual bleeding or discharge.
2. A lump or thickening in the breast or elsewhere.
3. A sore that does not heal.
4. Persistent change in bowel or bladder habits.
5. Persistent hoarseness or cough.
6. Persistent indigestion or difficulty in swallowing.
7. Change in a wart or a mole.

Treatment for Cancer

With each cancer patient, the physician has the problem of deciding what treatment is best for that individual. In making this decision, he must take into account the type of cancer, the location, the patient's age, and general health. Consideration of these factors will lead him to recommend one of three basic forms of treatment or a combination of them.

Surgery is one of those basic forms of treatment. If the surgeon decides to perform the type of operation that is meant to cure the patient, then he will completely remove all of the cancerous tissue or organ, including surrounding tissues to which the cancer may have spread. Some scientists are wary of the term *cure* in dealing with cancers. They prefer instead the concept of control of cancer, where the cancer cells are held in check rather than allowed to grow to the point of destruction. Cancer surgery may also be designed to remove certain hormonal sources such as the ovaries, adrenal glands, or the pituitary gland. This is done in those cases where a diseased organ depends on these hormones. Such an operation might be performed in an effort to check breast cancer in a woman by the removal of the ovaries. Cancer surgery is sometimes done in an effort to relieve pain. Such an operation would sever nerves to the cancerous area as a way of making a patient more comfortable. Surgery is also used as a diagnostic procedure as part of a biopsy. This involves the removal of a bit of suspicious tissue from the body. It is then prepared by certain laboratory procedures and examined under a microscope. The microscopic examination will reveal whether or not the cells are cancerous or in a precancerous state. Preventive surgery is also done to remove certain types of polyps, moles, gallstones, or any chronically infected or ulcerated area that the physician judges to be precancerous in nature. The removal of tissues in the body that are in a precancerous state is receiving a good deal more attention as a preventive measure with this disease. Improvements developed in surgery have helped to make this form of treatment more effective. This has involved not only improvements in surgical techniques, but in the general care of the patient during and after operations.

Radiation is a second type of treatment for cancer. Two general types of radiation are used, namely, X rays and radio isotopes. From studies that have been done, man has learned that amounts of radiation that have relatively little effect on normal tissues can cause considerable damage to cancer tissue. For this reason it has been utilized as a form of treatment for this disease. The radiation may be beamed into the body from an outside source or placed directly on or in the body. Radio isotopes are used in the form of either solids or liquids. In either form they are placed as close as possible to the cancer. In recent years X-ray machines have been improved and made more efficient. Their rays are more penetrating than they have been in the past and there is less scattering of radiation throughout the body. The result is that a smaller zone of normal tissue is thus irradiated.

It is well known that radiation can cause cancer as well as cure it. For this reason the complex techniques involved in radiology must be performed with skill and caution. It has also been observed that different cancers react differently to various kinds of radiation. As is true of other diseases and treatments, patients react rather individually to them. Though there is a good deal to be learned about radiation treatment, it remains as one of the most effective procedures we have in combating cancer.

Chemotherapy is the most recently developed treatment for cancer. A great deal of research is going on in this area in attempts to find drugs that will effectively stop malignant growths. Drugs developed thus far have in some instances slowed cancerous growths or stopped them for periods of time. A wide range of drugs have been utilized in attempts to stop or retard tumor growths. They include such items as hormones, cell poisons (cytotoxic drugs), and metabolic antagonists. Even antibodies can now be counted among the new anticancer drugs.

Hormones have been rather effectively used in affecting cancer growth in those tissues that are influenced by body hormones. Sites such as the breast, prostate gland, and uterus are such areas. The attempt is made to change the hormonal environment in which the cancer has grown, with the hope that this change will affect its growth. Thus, male hormones or androgens are sometimes effective in treating breast cancer in women, and estrogens prove helpful in cases of metastasized prostatic cancer in men. Cortisone and ACTH are other hormones that have been used in treating cancer of the blood-forming organs. Their values here have sometimes been limited and have resulted in only symptomatic improvement in some patients.

Cell poisons or cytotoxic drugs are designed to interfere with the reproductive process of cancer cells. They have managed to produce at least temporary relief in patients with Hodgkin's disease and those with cancers of the blood-forming tissues, such as leukemia. Because these drugs damage normal cells as well as cancerous ones, they have limited use.

Metabolic antagonists interfere with the vital life processes of cancer cells by acting as "counterfeit building blocks." These antagonists resemble materials that are needed by the cancer cell in order for it to develop and reproduce. The utilization by the cancer cell of this counterfeit material results in its being slowed down in terms of its growth.

Each year, thousands of drugs are screened and tested to determine their value as anticancer medications. For example, The National Cancer Institute scientists have reported successful drug treatment of a rare but highly malignant type of cancer (choriocarcinoma). The malignancy arises from the placenta during or after pregnancy. Methotrexate and the antibiotic actinomycin D resulted in a complete remission of the disease in 74 per cent of the study group used.

Drugs are sometimes helpful used singly, in combination with other drugs, or in addition to surgery and radiation. More and more there seems to be an attempt to combine the beneficial effects of various approaches to treatment.

Cancer Research

Cancer research is divided into three basic areas. First is basic research, which deals with the study of the fundamental structure, function, and chemical makeup of cells. It is hoped that greater knowledge in this area will lead to further understanding of changes that take place in the cancer cell, the causes of these changes, and possibly preventive measures that might be taken here. Secondly, we have clinical research which includes the study of various means of treating the disease. Constantly new methodology is being sought with regard to surgery, the use of radiation, drugs, and hormones. New and improved detection techniques are constantly being worked for so that other Pap tests may be developed for other types of cancers that will help to give us earlier detection and higher cure rates. This is exemplified by the work of a Russian scientist, Professor G. Abelev, who detected the presence of a particular embryonic protein in the blood of animals with primary liver tumors. Using his method in the Soviet Union and some South African countries where primary liver cancer is widespread, it is possible to diagnose the various types of liver tumor and differentiate between them.

Preventive research is a third area in which work is being done. Here investigation is going on with regard to immunology, and researchers hope to discover natural defenses in the body that may already exist and can be stimulated to produce resistance to cancer. A new and still experimental treatment called immunotherapy is gaining some attention in the medical community. In essence it awakens the body's natural defenses against cancer as well as other diseases. In some cases this is being done by deliberately exposing patients to attenuated tuberculosis bacilli (BCG vaccine). The BCG vaccine seems to have the ability to turn on the individual's immune system which in some cases attacks the cancer cells. There have been cases of spontaneous cures or remissions in cancer, which brings up the question of the role of immunology in these cases. It is also apparent that some people are more resistant to cancers than others. Why this is so is of concern to the immunologist.

The recent viral associations with human cancer presents the hope that vaccines in the future may be utilized as a preventive to the disease. The epidemiological approach is another facet of preventive research. The epidemiologist investigates those environmental factors that may be responsible for cancer. Epidemiological studies hope to explain why skin and lip cancers are twenty times more common among white people in the southern half of the United States than among white people in the northern part of the United States; why there is more uterine cancer among women in China and India than in other parts of the world; why breast cancer is eight times more common among women in Israel than among the women of Japan; why single women and married women who do not breast-feed their babies have a higher incidence of breast cancer; why liver cancer is responsible for half of all cancer deaths among the Bantu in Africa, and yet accounts for less that 4 per cent of cancer deaths in Europe; why stomach cancer accounts for 50 per cent of cancers among men in Japan, while the rate is about 10 per cent in the United States, and even less in other parts of the world. These represent some of the questions facing the epidemiologist working with cancer. The answers may lie with differences in the atmosphere, nutrition, personal habits, or a hundred and one other possible internal or external environmental factors. This type of research is significant because it will many times lead to preventive measures that can be taken even before specific knowledge with regard to the disease is substantiated. We learned, for instance, to prevent smallpox before we isolated the smallpox virus. This has occurred with a number of other diseases. The epidemiologist offers us similar hope with regard to cancer.

The Outlook for Cancer

In the early 1900's, few cancer patients had any hope of cure. By the 1930's, some progress had been made, but still fewer than one in five could be saved. At the present time, of every six persons that develop cancer two are being saved and one could have been saved if proper treatment had been received in time. In other words, about one-half of those who currently develop the disease should be saved by early diagnosis and treatment. This represents, then, one of the immediate objectives in reducing the mortality rate from this condition. The Strang Cancer Clinic in New York examined patients without apparent symptoms for twelve years and found that they have a cure rate of 85 per cent for cancer of the colon and rectum. The national average is 30 per cent. The University of Minnesota Detection Center reports that those cancers diagnosed in routine checkups have a cure rate twice that of patients who see doctors after symptoms have appeared. The implications here for routine checkups and early detection are obvious. A new approach that is being used to facilitate early diagnosis involves ways of identifying persons or groups with high-risk susceptibility to particular types of cancers. For example, this could mean routine chest X rays for every male

Fig. 10-11. Cancer strikes one in four. (American Cancer Society)

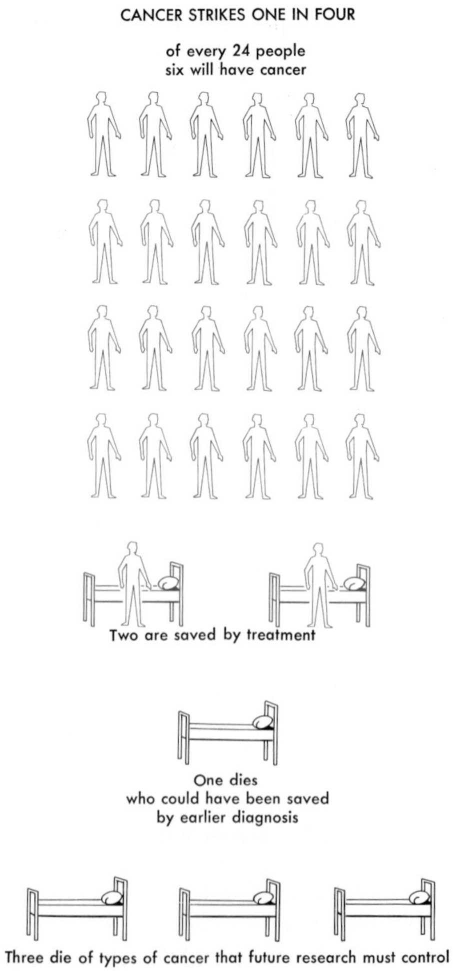

cigarette smoker over forty, and yearly physical examinations for women after menopause. There are implications in this approach for increased detection facilities, the training of personnel to man them, and a more objective attitude on the part of the general public. With regard to cancer, the unfortunate attitude still persists that what one does not know will not hurt him. The fact remains that of every twenty-four persons, six will develop cancer. In order to save three of these six, instead of the current two, we must make the most effective use of treatments, facilities, and medical personnel now available.

Neurological Disorders

Epilepsy

Epilepsy refers to repeated episodes of sudden overactivity of the nervous system. The episodes are associated with convulsions (or seizures) and lapses in consciousness. The EEG (electroencephalograph) is able to record the abnormal brain wave patterns developed in this disorder. Most causes of these convulsive disorders are idiopathic (cause unknown). In some known cases, it has been found that tumors or blood clots from traumas, infection of the meninges, or strokes are responsible. Faulty development of brain tissue during fetal life, birth injuries, deficient amounts of sugar and oxygen, high fever in young children, or defects in cerebral circulation are also possible causes. Though there may be a hereditary factor associated with some of the less understood forms of this disorder, it apparently is not associated with known causes of epilepsy, such as injury and disease. Seizures occurring in epilepsy vary greatly. The *grand mal* type of seizure is often initiated by an aura, and the person sees flashing or colored lights and senses an unpleasant odor. The eyes and head turn to one side, and this is sometimes a warning of an oncoming attack. This is followed by convulsive movements. During the seizure, it might be helpful to remove furniture or any other objects against which the person might hurt himself during his thrashing moments. After the seizure, the person may have a headache or feel tired and sleepy.

In the *petit mal* type of seizure, the person may do nothing more than develop a blank stare for a short period of time. Sometimes the stare is as brief as the blinking of the eyes. This type of epilepsy is usually idiopathic and more prevalent in young girls. The inattentive child or one who falls easily and drops things may in some instances prove to be suffering from petit mal convulsive episodes. Petit mal seizures can occur as often as two hundred times a day.

The *psychomotor* type of seizure usually results in purposeful motions that are not relevant to the situation, such as chewing or smacking of lips. Psychomotor episodes seem to be more prevalent among males. The incidence of the seizures is less frequent than in petit mal, but they may last from between three to five minutes. Sometimes disrobing becomes part of the actions taken during the seizure, with the result that the person is mistaken for a sexual deviate. In all three of the types of seizures described, total amnesia is part of the attack. In focal or Jacksonian seizures, involuntary actions may start in one part of the body, such as a foot or hand, and migrate upward to other parts. These attacks will often occur without loss of consciousness.

In the treatment of epileptics, drug therapy has been a very effective control. There are a number of anticonvulsant drugs used in varying combinations, dependent upon the symptoms and the reactions of the patient. It is felt that these types of drugs will ultimately be the answer to the complete control of this disorder. The difficulty, however, is that only one out of five epileptics at the present time is under a physician's care. Surgery is sometimes effective when the epilepsy is due to a brain tumor. Removal of the tumor returns the person to normalcy. Surgery is also used to remove brain tissue that serves as a focal point for epileptic reactions. This can be done only in those people suffering from psychomotor seizures and whose focal points are in an accessible part of the brain. In the vast majority of instances, this results in a complete cure of the condition. Maintaining emotional balance is important to the epileptic in that stress will often precipitate seizures. Some epileptics are sensitive to alcohol and therefore must restrict their use of it. Others have seizures triggered by flashing lights. Automobile driving for these people, then, can become dangerous. The biggest problem to the person suffering from a convulsive disorder is often the "normal" person, who does not understand his condition. He has to face the prejudicial actions and ignorance on the part of the society he lives in. Convulsive disorders are often not well understood, being erroneously confused with mental illness or feeblemindedness. This is one disorder in which some people feel that the sufferer is more handicapped by the regressive attitude of society than by his disability. While this attitude appears to be changing, many epileptics still face the possibility of chronic unemployment and poverty.

Cerebral Palsy

Cerebral palsy is a brain-centered disorder affecting the muscles. Because of damage to the motor area of the brain, cerebral palsied individuals are not able to control the voluntary muscles of the body. There are approximately 550,000 cerebral palsied persons in the United States. All the causes of cerebral palsy are not known; however, some causative factors have been identified. Rubella (German measles) contracted by the mother in the first trimester of pregnancy is one of them. Other causes include trauma, prematurity, Rh factors, anoxia (a lack of oxygen), and congenital malformations. The relationship of inheritance as a causative factor in cerebral palsy is receiving increasing attention.

There are several types of cerebral palsy, the most common being the *spastic* type. Spastics have a great deal of muscle tenseness and excessive contractions, making coordinated movements difficult. The *athetoid* type is characterized by slow, involuntary, and unorganized movements. The spastic and athetoid types represent 80 per cent of the cerebral palsy population. A mixed form of cerebral palsy occasionally occurs, severely incapacitating the individual. *Ataxia* is a third type of cerebral palsy in which a disturbed sense of balance is present. This usually will result in many falls. The fourth type is characterized by tremor, in which one or more limbs of the body may be affected. The shaking makes use of the hands and feet most difficult. A fifth type is characterized by rigidity of one or more limbs of the body. The rigid muscles resist movement and therefore make people so afflicted slow moving.

Many cerebral palsied individuals will have normal or above-normal intelligence. This is oftentimes masked by their inability to express themselves easily because of their muscular conditions. Preventive measures with regard to cerebral palsy center around good prenatal care, the reduction of premature deliveries, and the prevention or reduction of neonatal anoxia. The control of Rh incompatibility and the prevention of accidents can also serve as preventive measures.

Multiple Sclerosis

Multiple sclerosis is a disease that affects the nervous system. It attacks the myelin sheath of the nerve and in doing so leaves scar tissue; hence the term sclerosis. The myelin sheath has the function of insulating the nerve fiber and preventing the overflow and loss of the nerve impulse. Since the disease can affect many parts of the nervous system, it is called *multiple.*

The onset of this condition is usually between the ages of 20 and 40 years. Symptoms that will appear when the myelin is destroyed in parts of the body will include partial or complete paralysis, numbness, double vision, slurring of speech, staggering, and general weakness. In the more advanced stages of the disease, problems in speech, swallowing, and loss of bladder or bowel control occur. The disease is not necessarily consistent in its progress. There will be periods of deterioration followed by temporary remissions. The prognosis for the disease varies, with most patients being ultimately disabled. In some people, the disturbance is relatively mild, permitting them to live long and productive lives. In the majority of cases, however, the life-span is shortened.

Muscular Dystrophy

Muscular dystrophy is a disease in which there is a degeneration of the striated or voluntary muscles of the body. In this condition the nerves are not affected. The number of persons afflicted with this disease is not known, but it is estimated that approximately 200,000 have the condition. More than one-half of these are children between the ages of 4 and 15. The cause or causes of muscular dystrophy are unknown, although there is general agreement that a hereditary basis exists in all types of the disease. Some research indicates a possibility that those so afflicted have the inability to utilize vitamin E. This and other theories with regard to causation are being investigated. The prognosis for the disease varies a great deal, dependent upon the type of dystrophy.

Types of muscular dystrophy are broken down into four basic categories. One is *childhood dystrophy* (pseudohypertrophic), found almost exclusively in the male. Its onset is at anywhere from 2 to 10

Fig. 10-12 Which of the two children is retarded? Answer: They both are. From their confident smiles one can ascertain that others have regarded them with the respect and humaneness due all human beings. Self concepts are made not born. (*N.Y.S. Dept. of Mental Hygiene; Photo by Julian A. Belin*)

years of age. Muscles that become involved are the gluteals, abdominal and back muscles, as well as the muscles of respiration. The prognosis here is poor, with the great majority of individuals afflicted dying before the age of 20. A second type is the *facio-scapulo-humeral* type of dystrophy. The age of onset may vary anywhere from 10 to 18 years of age. Muscles of the hands and forearms are affected, as well as those of the neck, and some facial muscles. Prognosis for this condition is poor. It progresses slowly, with the ultimate involvement of the muscles of mastication. *Myotonic dystrophy* has its onset at anywhere from 15 to 80 years of age. It is initiated by weakness in the hands and forearms and may involve the muscles of the face and neck. Myotonic dystrophy progresses slowly, and its final involvement of the respiratory muscles causes death. A fourth type is *ophthalmoplegic dystrophy*, in which a hereditary history of the disease is found in approximately one-half of the cases. The age of onset is anywhere from 1 to 40 years of age. The muscles primarily involved here are the ocular, facial, and neck muscles. Prognosis for this type of dystrophy is good. Though it may be a disabling disease, it ordinarily is not fatal. While research holds the ultimate key to the prevention and treatment of this disease, we as a society have the responsibility to do everything possible for the present generation of patients now afflicted. There unfortunately seems to be at the present time the same kind of apathy about rehabilitation of the muscular dystrophy patient as there was approximately twenty years ago about those suffering from cerebral palsy. Rehabilitation programs for patients with dystrophy try to make the individual as self-sufficient as possible, physically, vocationally, and psychosocially. Successful rehabilitation programs keep dystrophy patients vocationally occupied longer and better adjusted for many years beyond the time that they could possibly be without this kind of help.

Parkinson's Disease

The cause of Parkinson's disease still remains elusive. It is generally agreed, however, that damage to the cells of a little-known part of the brain results in a disease that affects more than one million elderly Americans. This nerve disorder is sometimes referred to as shaking palsy, since an involuntary tremor, muscle rigidity, slurred speech, and a hasty forward leaning gait are among its symptoms. A drug called L-dopa (short for Levo-dihydroxyphenylal anine) has proved effective in the treatment of Parkinsonism. The possibility that the drug may also have some usefulness in treating certain forms of cerebral palsy is being explored.

Mental Retardation

The term *mental retardation* describes an effect rather than a given condition. "The mentally retarded person is one who, from childhood, experiences unusual difficulty learning and is relatively ineffective in applying whatever he has learned to the problems of ordinary living; he needs special

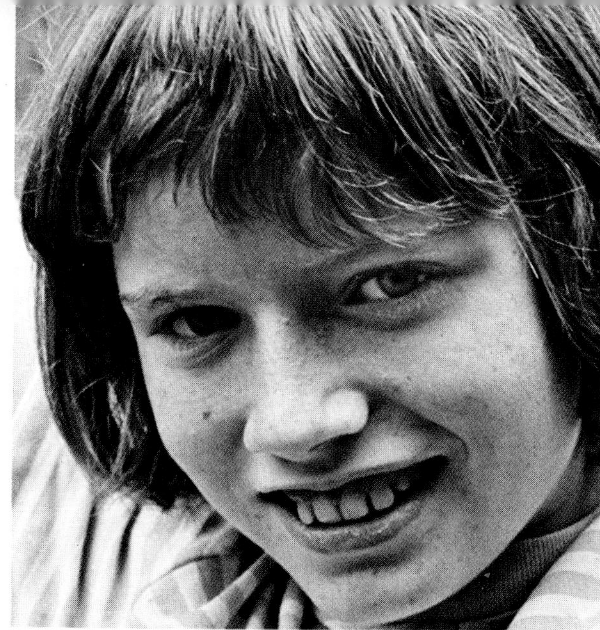

training and guidance to make the most of his capacities, whatever they may be."[5]

Some Causes of Retardation

Mental retardation has many different causes which may manifest themselves *before* birth, *during* birth, or in early *childhood.*

Brain development may be impaired by chemical substances before the child is even born. This was demonstrated with phenylketonuria (PKU). It has also been docomented that the intake of too much Vitamin D by pregnant women is responsible for mental retardation. Another cause would be the development of abnormal chromosomes as in Down's syndrome. The viral attack of rubella (German measles) may leave the fetus with multiple handicaps one of which may be mental retardation. The Rh incompatability of the parents may cause retardation. In the process of fetal growth the malformation of the brain structure itself may begin, with the resulting condition of hydrocephalus (an accumulation of fluid within the cranium causing a great enlargement of the head.) In these instances, the mental retardation is congenital (existing) at birth and is considered a birth defect.

Mental retardation may occur *at* birth. During difficult deliveries there may be an injury or a reduction of oxygen supply to the infant's brain. Modern obstetrics have made significant contributions toward minimizing these as factors, particularly when prenatal care has been sought by the mother.

A "normal" child may become retarded as a result of such diseases as measles (rubeola), meningitis, encephalitis, whooping cough, scarlet fever, or other diseases causing high fever. Accidents such as a blow on the head or lead poisoning as a result of ingesting pieces of lead-based paints or window putty may cause retardation.

"There is a growing recognition, documented by studies, that the role of nutrition during pregnancy and immediately thereafter has great significance on the intellectual development of the infant as well as the infant's physical growth."[6]

Attitudes Toward the Retarded

Societal attitudes toward the retarded have been undergoing considerable change. The era of hiding the retarded child in the home and having feelings of shame and guilt are rapidly disappearing. A more enlightened populace is recognizing that the many unknown causes of retardation make this a condition that could occur in any family. Where feelings of shame exist, it is often because the parent erroneously feels responsible for the child's state. Thus it is that the parents' feelings of guilt are expressed in feelings of shame for the child. In recent years, greater understanding of these conditions has resulted in more objective and positive responses to

[5] *Facts on Mental Retardation,* National Association for Retarded Children, Inc.

[6] Sally K. Livingston, "What Influences Malnutrition," *Journal of Nutrition Education,* Vol. 3, No. 1 (Summer, 1971).

the problem. New and concerted efforts are being made to develop each retarded child to the maximum of his potential.

Comprehensive Programs for the Retarded

In order to diagnose mental retardation early, many communities have diagnostic and treatment clinics. These clinics often offer appropriate therapy for the retarded where needed. Home visit programs are often provided so that parents may be counseled with regard to their child's condition and potentialities.

Special education classes in schools provide a curriculum for the "educable" children. The IQ's of these children range from 50 to 75, with most growing up to be self-sufficient adults because of the education now provided them. This group makes up the bulk of the retarded. Special classes are provided for those children whose IQ's range from about 30 to 50. These children are referred to as "trainable." Their curriculum prepares them to care for themselves and to do less complex work tasks.

A third group of retardates consists of those that are severely or profoundly retarded. Their condition is complicated by a higher incidence of physical handicaps. The multiple-handicapped child is difficult to care for at home. For this reason these individuals are often institutionalized where they may be better cared for.

Except for the severely retarded or multiple-handicapped, most retarded children are raised at home. They do better in a home environment where enlightened parents and community accept them. When one looks past the handicap to see the children beneath it, one realizes that the needs of these children are the same as those of any other. Love and acceptance are basic to their emotional development.

There are over 2 million retarded persons of work age in this country, and this figure is expected to grow. In the interests of the individuals involved as well as the national economy, it is important for retardates to be vocationally trained. Their contribution will be an increasingly significant one. It can only come about, however, with parental and community investment of time and effort in the training of the retarded leading to personal and vocational growth and worth.

Research

At the present time, research is our greatest hope for the prevention of the bulk of the cases of retardation. The research being conducted is as varied as the causes of this handicap. Some modest gains have already been made in the preventive area. We now have a vaccine for measles (rubeola), a childhood disease that can cause not only mental retardation but hearing loss as well as a number of other afflictions. Universal use of the measles vaccine should eliminate this disease as a cause. Likewise, the development and mass distribution of the German measles (rubella) vaccine should eliminate this viral infection and its deleterious effects.

Advances that have been made in modern obstetrical care are responsible for a similar contribution.

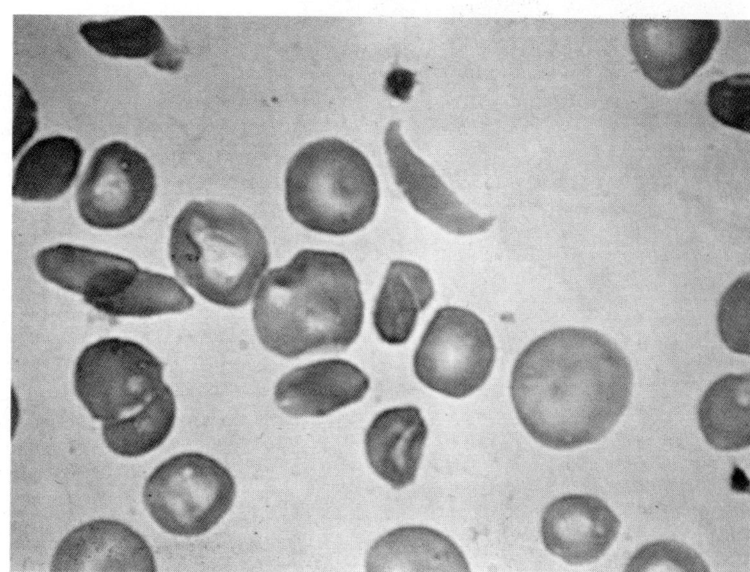

Fig. 10-13 In sickle-cell anemia the abnormal structure of the hemoglobin causes the red blood cells to pucker or assume a sickle shape. (Carl Pochedly, M.D., Director of Pediatric Hematology Dept., Nassau County Medical Center, East Meadow, N.Y.)

Birth injury is not nearly as common as it used to be. Good prenatal care has also reduced the incidence of premature birth, which carried with it a higher incidence of retardation. There is now the awareness that malnutrition during pregnancy and infancy has a relationship to mental retardation. Where parents have an incompatible Rh blood factor, many a child's life and mental capacity have been saved by an amniocentesis, which alerts the physician to the problem before real damage occurs. The results that research can produce have been exemplified by work done with phenylketonuria (PKU) and galactosemia.

Research efforts will no doubt continue to make contributions to the prevention of retardation. These efforts deserve the enthusiastic support of the community they will serve. In the meantime, we have the obligation and need to utilize effectively that information we already possess in the area of prevention and rehabilitation of the retarded.

Genetic Diseases

More than 1,600 human diseases caused by defects in the content or the expression of the genetic information in DNA have been identified. Some of these diseases are very rare; others, such as cystic fibrosis and sickle-cell anemia, are relatively common and are responsible for much illness and death. It has been estimated that more than 25 percent of the hospitalizations of children are for illnesses with a major genetic component.[7]

[7] *Scientific American*, Vol. 225, No. 5 (November, 1971), p. 34.

Through new developments in biochemistry and cell biology man will be better able to control disease entities that have ravaged families for centuries. The initial discovery that cells from patients can grow and be studied in tissue cultures was a most important one, for as these cells grow, they continue to show the abnormal function of a gene, if one exists. The most significant application of this knowledge is seen in prenatal genetic diagnosis. It has been demonstrated that the technique known as *amniocentesis* (see Chapter 6) can diagnose some genetic diseases prior to birth through examination of the chemical composition of the amniotic fluid itself or the cells that are found in the fluid.

The most obvious genetic diseases are those involving chromosomal abnormalities; however, the vast majority of these diseases results from more subtle defects in the genes. Such a defective gene may *not* set in motion the production of certain enzymes that are essential for the body's biochemical reactions.

Sickle-Cell Anemia

Sickle-cell anemia is an inherited disease affecting our black population almost exclusively, though it has been seen rarely in white families of Mediterannean origin (Italian, Greek). The abnormal structure of the hemoglobin causes red blood cells to pucker or assume a sickle shape. These twisted cells cannot pass through the capillary walls and often pile up eventually to block the flow of blood to body tissues. These red blood cells are also very fragile and are rapidly destroyed. "Their life span may be only

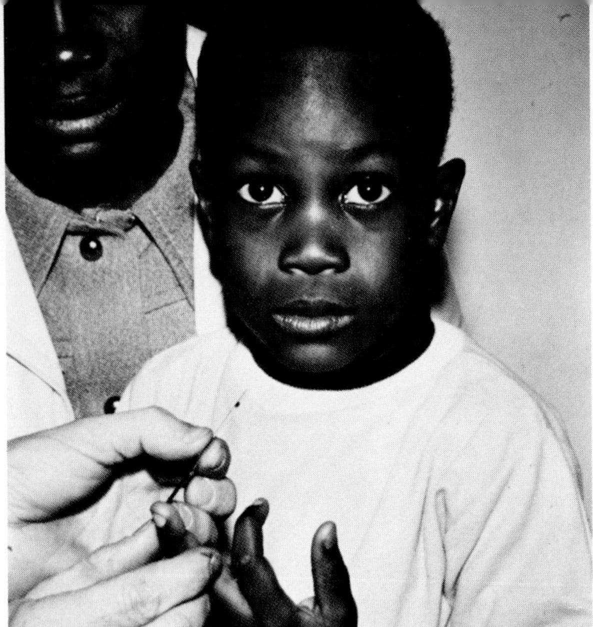

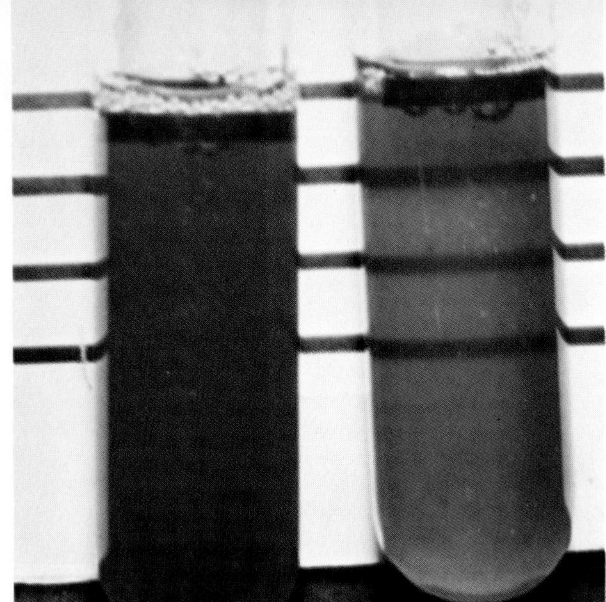

30–40 days instead of the normal 120 days. Although a person with Sickle Cell Anemia can produce new cells at a rapid rate, he becomes anemic because the rate of destruction of cells is greater than that of production."[8] When the flow of blood to body tissues is hampered by the blockage of these sickled cells, the person is said to be suffering a sickle-cell crisis. These periodic attacks of acute pain, anemia with weakness, nausea, and jaundice are the plight of the person suffering this disease.

The sudden deaths of four black recruits stationed in El Paso, Texas, were attributed to severe sickling of the blood cells as determined by autopsies. It was felt that the combination of stress and high altitude were contributing factors in bringing on the crises. Many doctors feel all blacks should be screened for this inherited blood trait before undergoing basic training, surgery, or participation in strenuous athletics. Individuals with the disease and those merely carrying the genetic trait are advised against flying in unpressurized airplanes or engaging in any activity that might cause a moderate lack of oxygen, since a lowered amount of oxygen may lead to a sickling crisis.

It has been confirmed by studies conducted in Africa and the Mediterannean basin that sickle-cell hemoglobin makes the person more resistant to malaria. Throughout history those with sickle-cell hemoglobin thus had the advantage of surviving in malaria-infested areas and had the opportunity to pass on this characteristic to their offspring. It is estimated that 2 out of every 25 black Americans are carriers of the sickle-cell trait. Only 1 out of every 400 actually has the disease. When both the mother and father are carriers of the sickle-cell trait, out of every 4 children they have, chances are that 1 will have sickle-cell anemia; 2 will be carriers of the trait; and 1 will not have either the disease or the trait.

The Sickledex Test is used in mass screening for sickle-cell anemia. A positive reaction may mean the individual has either sickle-cell anemia or carries the trait. If a positive Sickledex is recorded, the person would then undergo additional tests which would determine whether the person had the disease.

Physicians now warn known carriers of the disease who are contemplating marriage what the disease risks are for any children born to them. This is one of the genetic diseases that *cannot* as yet be detected through amniocentesis. However, since the development of a simple blood test, the implications for *prevention* by genetic counseling are greatly increased. It has been noted in certain communities where massive screening has been conducted that there is a great need for mental health counseling in addition to the genetic counseling. The feelings of helplessness and hopelessness that result with the diagnosis of sickle-cell anemia are feelings that people must be helped to cope with. With improved treatment methods, hospitalization, and antibiotics to curb infections, the life-span of these patients has been increased considerably, though it remains as a low 20 years of age. The disease is most severe in

[8] Carl Pochedly, M.D., "Sickle Cell Anemia: Recognition and Management," *The American Journal of Nursing*, Vol. 71, No. 10 (October, 1971).

Fig. 10-14. This child is being tested for sickle cell anemia. In the Sickledex solution, blood with sickle hemoglobin becomes cloudy and opaque (left test tube) indicating the child has either the trait or the disease. In this case further testing confirmed sickle-cell disease. The child shown died shortly after this picture was taken. (Dr. Carl Pochedly, Director of Pediatric Hematology Dept., Nassau County Medical Center, East Meadow, N.Y.)

the young; once adolescence is reached, the sickling crises are not as severe and do not occur as frequently. Continued identification through education, routine testing, and follow-up programs remain essential.

Cystic Fibrosis

This is a disease that was not recognized until thirty years ago. At the present time, because of better knowledge and better diagnostic techniques, it is ranked as one of the leading causes of death among children. Cystic fibrosis is an inherited disease of children which affects the externally secreting glands of the body, including sweat and mucus glands. Instead of the mucus glands secreting the normally free-flowing fluid, they give off a mucus that is thick and sticky. Its effect is to clog and block the various ducts of the body. The thick mucus interferes with such bodily functions as breathing and digestion. In 80 per cent of the cases of cystic fibrosis the ducts of the pancreas become clogged with these secretions, inhibiting the flow of enzymes necessary for digestion. While the child's appetite may be enormous, his inability to digest some foods will result in early signs of malnutrition. In more severe cases of this disease, patients are born with their intestinal tract completely obstructed by an accumulation of thick puttylike material in the digestive tract.

Chronic lung disease is a common complication of cystic fibrosis. The thickened mucus tends to block the passages of the lung, clogging air sacs and making breathing increasingly difficult. This sticky material also lodges in the branches of the windpipe and acts as an obstruction. Bacterial infections occur repeatedly, leading to progressive, irreversible lung damage and sometimes lung collapse. The complication of acute lung infections many times results in the patient's succumbing to pneumonia.

It has been noted that the cystic fibrosis patient has an excessive loss of salt. This may result in heat exhaustion during the summer months if extra salt is not taken.

Studies strongly suggest that cystic fibrosis is transmitted through a recessive gene. This means that both parents have to be carriers of the gene in order for one of their offspring to inherit the disease. When both parents are carriers of the recessive gene, there is a one-in-four chance that any child born to them will have cystic fibrosis. Tests have been devised for the early detection of the disease. The most common test is aimed at detecting the abnormally high salt content of the patient's perspiration. Early detection is necessary so that the condition may be treated before irreparable harm can be done to the child's organs. The test can be conducted while the baby is still in the newborn nursery, with the contents of the perspiration analyzed within minutes. These tests are usually performed after the first two days of life; test results are not reliable before that. Unfortunately cystic fibrosis cannot as yet be detected in the fetus by an amniocentesis. However, the presence of certain granules in the amniotic fluid of women who had previously given birth to children with cystic fibrosis has encouraged scientists to believe that prenatal detection is not far off.

It is estimated that there are as many as 10 million carriers of the disease in the United States, and that one child in every 1,000 is born with the condition. The primary concern in the treatment of these patients is to combat lung infections through the use of antibiotics and physical therapy, because about 90 per cent of the deaths from cystic fibrosis are due to chronic lung disorders. Mist tents are frequently used as a means of liquefying mucus and helping to clear the respiratory tract while the patient sleeps. Further treatment procedures include giving the patients commercially prepared pancreatic extracts to take the place of those enzymes not present in their digestive tract. Extra salt is also given to counteract the excessive salt loss in the perspiration. Though the death rate from this disease is still quite high, the outlook is becoming increasingly favorable. An increasing percentage of afflicted children are now surviving through adolescence to young adulthood. Continued research and the development of newer treatments are the hopes for the future.

Phenylketonuria (PKU)

Phenylketonuria is a congenital metabolic disease. It is caused by the inability of the body to metabolize properly one of the essential amino acids, namely phenylalanine. The amino acid phenylalanine is normally converted to tyrosine by the enzyme phenylalanine hydroxilase. It is the absence of this particular enzyme that causes the difficulty. Without it, phenylalanine is abnormally broken down into phenylketone bodies that cause damage to the brain in the young child, resulting in mental retardation. The incidence of the disease was first estimated to be anywhere from one in 20,000–40,000 births. However, recent extensive screening programs have shown that the incidence is approximately one in every 10,000 births.

Phenylketonuria is transmitted through a recessive gene. It is estimated that 1 in every 70 persons is a carrier. When two carriers of the disorder marry, they will transmit to their offspring the recessive gene in accordance with the Mendelian laws of genetics. The expectation is that 1 child will be a phenylketonuric; 2 will be carriers; and 1 will be a noncarrier of the gene.

A test that has been developed for the detection of phenylketonuria is the Guthrie blood test. This procedure detects the presence of phenylketone bodies found in phenylketonurics. With this testing technique, a drop of blood is taken from the child's heel shortly after birth, with the blood proving to be diagnostic at this early time. Under the sponsorship of the Children's Bureau of the Department of Health, Education and Welfare, a nationwide screening program was instituted in 1963 for the early detection of phenylketonuria.

Treatment of the disease thus far is through dietary management. Because phenylalanine is an essential amino acid, it cannot be excluded from the diet completely without ill effects. However, in the dietary management of phenylketonuria there is a drastic restriction of phenylalanine intake. With controlled amounts of the amino acid, the child will usually grow and develop without the expected re-

Fig. 10-15. Testing for phenylketonuria: A drop of blood from this child will be examined for the presence of phenylketone bodies. (N.Y.S. Health Photo by M. Dixson)

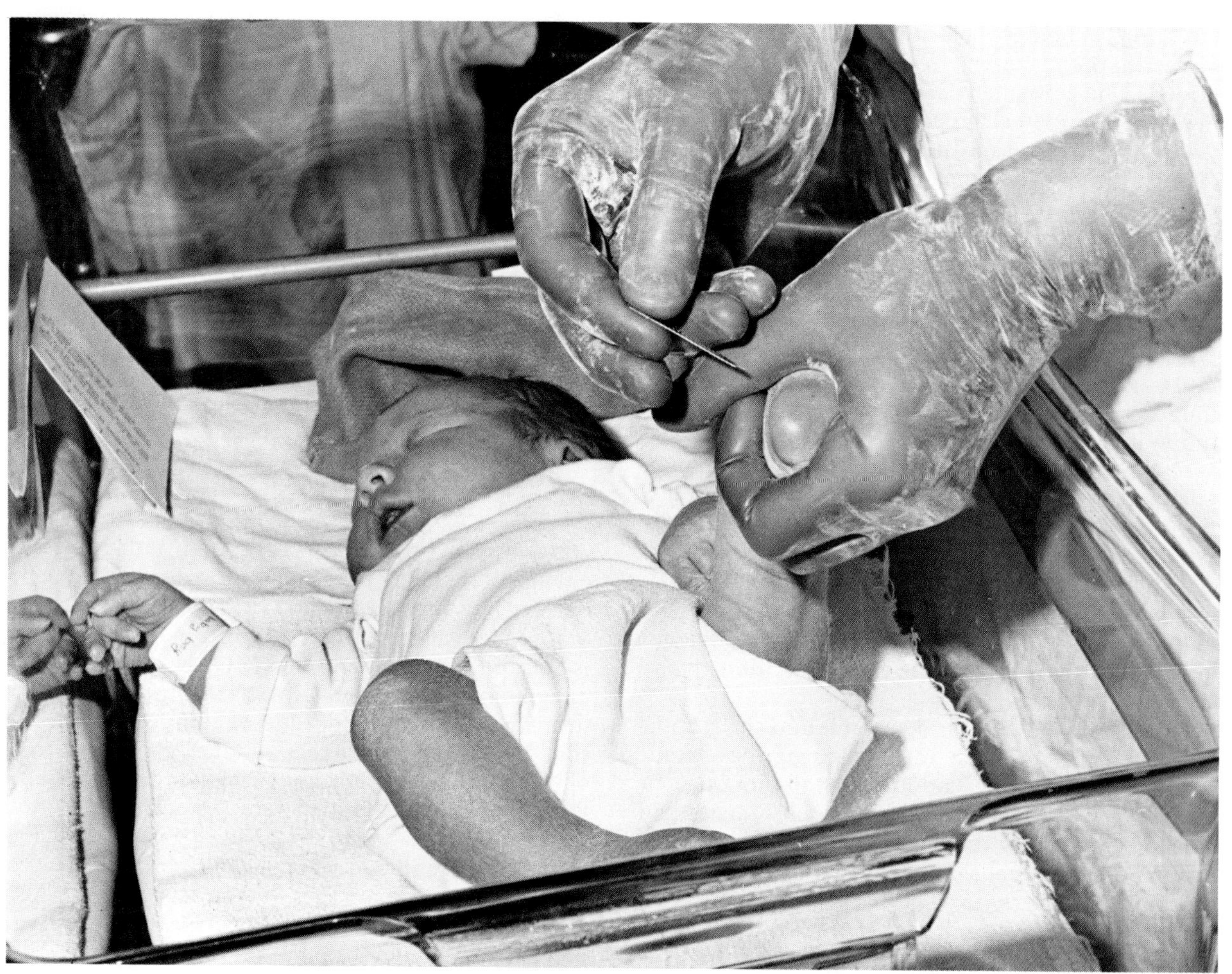

tardation. Whether dietary control is the complete answer to the management of PKU is yet to be determined. The low phenylalanine diet is a pasty formulalike commercial preparation. As the child grows older, keeping him on this profoundly unattractive dietary regimen becomes most difficult. How long a child must be kept on this restricted diet will probably vary with individuals. Definite conclusions can be drawn only after physicians have had more experience in dealing with this disorder. The regulation of the diet must, of course, be done under a physician's care. Phenylalanine levels of the blood must be checked periodically to make sure that the diet is meeting the needs of the particular individual.

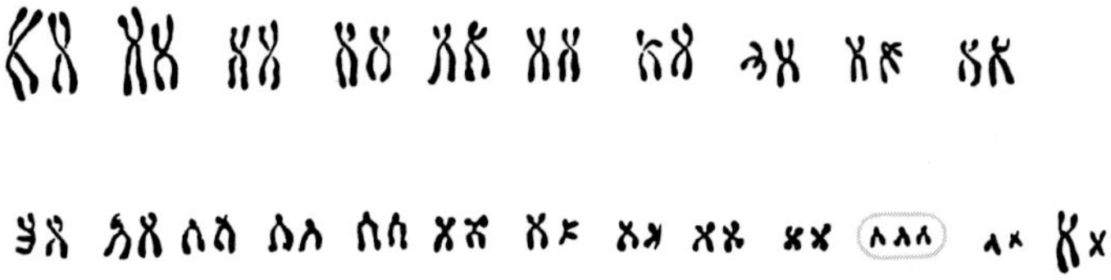

In addition to those characteristics related to mental retardation, phenylketonurics are often found to have schizoidlike personalities (withdrawn, with feelings of persecution and periods of incoherency). A patchy type eczema and/or convulsions may accompany the condition. Electroencephalograms are abnormal in 80 per cent of the cases tested. Phenylketonurics are usually blue-eyed and more blond than their parents.

Because this disorder is detectable and the retardation often preventable, a number of states have made it mandatory (by legislation) that all newborn be screened for this condition. Some physicians had voiced reservations about legislating a medical procedure that was considered by many to be in its experimental stages.

It has also been found that there is such a thing as maternal phenylketonuria. In some cases, the mother is a phenylketonuric and has a high level of phenylalanine in her blood. When such a woman is pregnant, the high serum phenylalanine level will cause damage to the brain of the unborn child. This child will then, of course, be born mentally retarded. It has been suggested that perhaps all mothers of retarded children be tested for phenylketonuria as a means of preventing the birth of additional retarded children. These mothers are in many instances individuals who are not severely retarded but may have a mental capacity that is normal or just below normal. Where a mother is a phenylketonuric, physicians find that they can sometimes protect the unborn child by placing the mother on a low phenylalanine diet during her pregnancy.

Tay-Sachs Disease

Another genetic disorder associated with a specific enzyme deficiency is Tay-Sachs disease. Severe retardation, blindness, and early death, usually before 3 or 4 years of age, are the results of a massive accumulation of lipids in the brain. This occurs because an enzyme needed to break down fats properly was not developed in the child. One of the peculiarities of this disease is the fact that about 85 per cent of the children it affects are from Jewish families of Eastern European origin. An elaborate system of detection has been undertaken to detect and prevent new cases of this disease. Blood tests of both partners are performed prior to marriages among Jews. When both husband and wife are found to be carriers all their pregnancies are monitored by amniocentesis. The

Fig. 10-16. *The diagram shows the abnormal additional chromosome found in Down's syndrome (mongolism).*

Fig. 10-17. *A comparison of the normal hand and foot prints with those of the mongoloid child. (March of Dimes)*

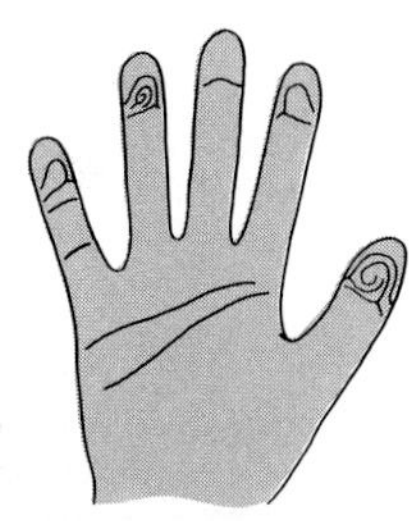

The left hand print of a normal child shows whorls on the thumb, a radial loop on the index finger, and ulnar loops on the ring and little fingers. There are two flexures in the little finger and two palmar creases.

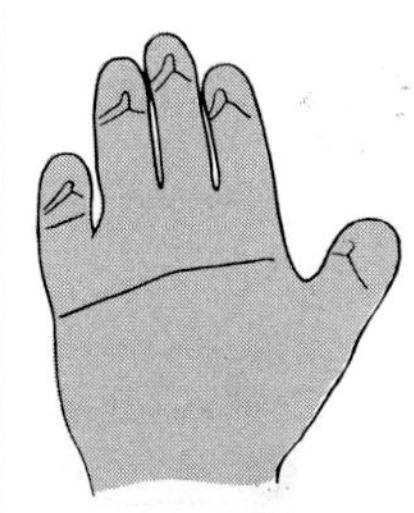

Hands of children with Down's syndrome show many more ulnar loops and most have a single ("simian") palmar crease. The hands of Down's syndrome patients are often short and stubby with little fingers curving inward.

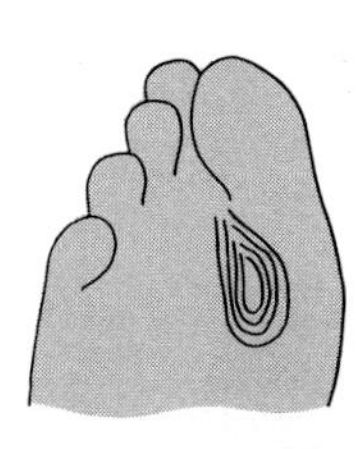

The left foot of a normal child shows characteristic whorls or loops in the "ball" of the foot, called the hallucal area.

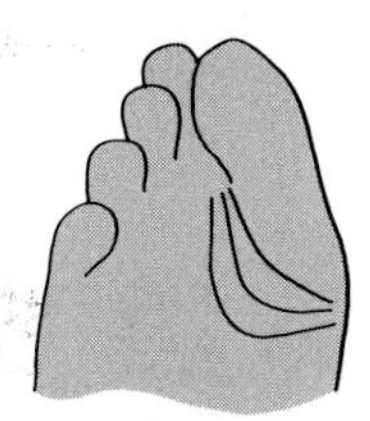

Foot of Down's syndrome child shows tibial arches instead of whorls or loops in the same area.

scientist who discovered the defective form of the enzyme followed twenty pregnancies in women known to be carriers. Seven of the twenty fetuses were affected with the disease, and in all seven cases the women chose to end the pregnancies through abortion.

Galactosemia

Galactosemia is an inherited disease caused by the absence of an enzyme required to convert galactose (a sugar substance found in milk) to glucose (a simple sugar the body can utilize). As a result, too much galactose accumulates in the body tissues, particularly the brain. Eventually the level becomes toxic and causes cataracts, liver damage, and brain damage resulting in mental retardation. With biochemical analyses of the amniotic fluid, the mother's diet can be modified prior to the birth of the baby. The diet of the newborn is also controlled and the disease arrested.

Down's Syndrome (Mongolism)

Mongolism is a common form of retardation that is genetically caused by abnormal chromosome formation. Where there should be only two of the 21st chromosome, there are three. Standard trisomy is the name used to describe this most common form of Down's syndrome that affects 1 out of every 600 births.

This type of Down's disease is rarely familial; that is, there seems to be no family pattern of mongoloid children. It does, however, appear more commonly in children born of older women. For example, in women 20 to 30 years of age, the risk of occurrence is 1:1500; in women 35 to 40, the risk is 1:600; and in women 45 or older, the risk of occurrence is 1:60. In mongolism the back and front of the head are flattened, making the forehead seem large. Oriental eyes are an added characteristic. The hands are often stubby, and the hand prints show definite characteristics different from normal prints. The child's degree of retardation may range from moderate to severe, and curiously enough genetically confirmed mongoloids are notoriously susceptible to leukemia.

Sex-Linked Genetic Diseases

Some disease traits are determined by genes carried on the X chromosome and are called sex-linked, or X-linked. In such disease entities the defective genetic characteristic is transmitted from the heterozygous female (one who does not *have* the disease but carries the defective gene) to half her sons (Fig. 10-18). If the male is affected with the disease none of his sons will get the disease; however, all of his daughters will be heterozygous carriers (Fig. 10-19). Going a step further, if an affected male marries a heterozygous female, then their female child will display the disease as well as the male child. Remember, however, that the male child inherits the trait from the mother, since there is no male-to-male transmission of an X-linked trait (Fig. 10-20).

A typical example of an X-linked recessive trait is the disease hemophilia. In this disease there is a

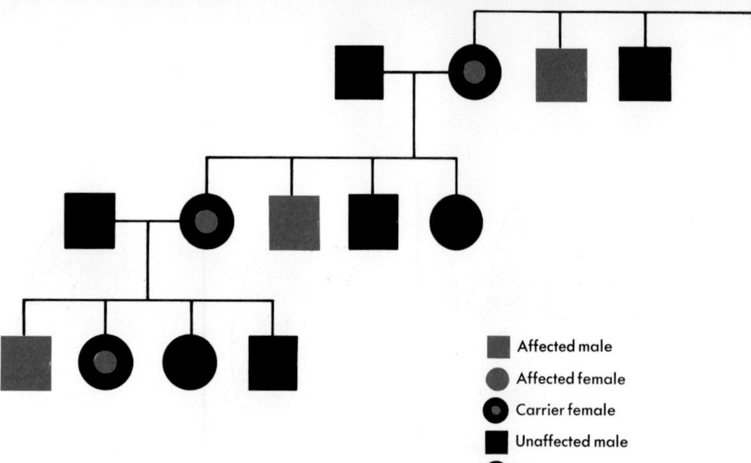

Fig. 10-18. In X-linked disease entities the defective genetic characteristic is transmitted from the heterozygous female (one who does not have the disease but carries the defective gene) to half her sons. (Genes in Families and in Populations, *The National Foundation, p. 6.*)

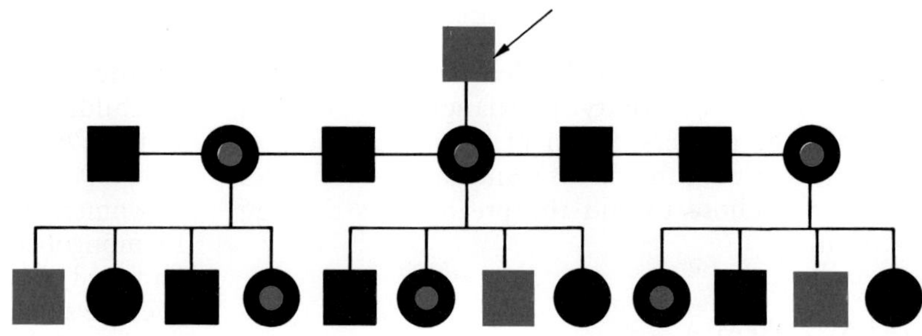

Fig. 10-19. If the male is affected with the disease none of his sons will get the disease; however, all of his daughters will be heterozygous carriers. (Genes in Families and in Populations, *The National Foundation,* p. 6.)

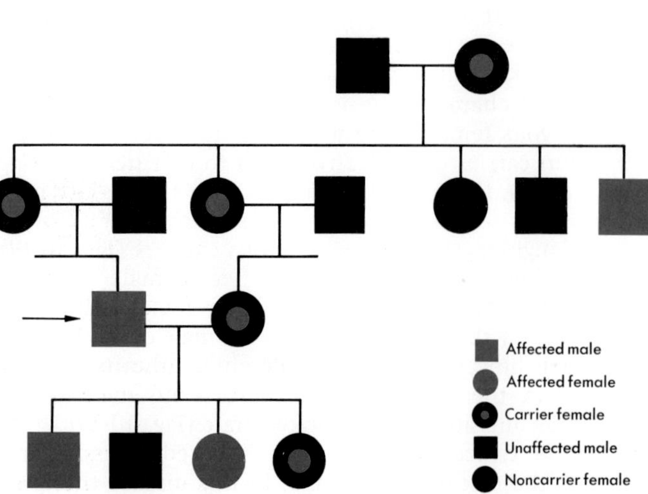

Fig. 10-20. Going a step further, if an affected male marries a heterozygous female, then their female child will display the disease as well as the male child. Remember, however, that the male child inherits the trait from the mother, since there is no male-to-male transmission of an X-linked trait. (Genes in Families and in Populations, *The National Foundation, p. 6.)*

deficiency of a protein factor required for blood clotting. This results in prolonged bleeding as a result of injury, however mild it is. Color blindness, a certain form of muscular dystrophy, and more than 50 other diseases are known to be inherited this way.

There are now implications for prevention of these diseases through amniocentesis. If it is determined that the fetus in utero is female, then the possibility of the disease is ruled out even though half of those females will be carriers. If it is determined that the fetus is male, he may either be affected by the disease or be normal.

A Chromosome Registry

The New York State Health Department's Birth Defects Institute has compiled via computer a Chromosome Registry that contains information on persons in New York State who have rare inherited diseases. A physician concerned about a patient with a particular genetic disease can consult the Registry and find out quickly if there are similar cases elsewhere in the state and compare notes with the physicians in charge of such cases. This should permit physicians to provide better care to their patients and also prove a valuable aid in research. Ultimately it is hoped to have a nationwide Registry.

Other Constitutional Diseases

Diabetes

Although significant progress has been made in the control of diabetes, it is still the eighth leading cause of death and the third leading cause of blindness. It is estimated that approximately 4 million Americans have diabetes. Half of these cases are undetected. There are two types of diabetes: diabetes mellitus and diabetes insipidus. Diabetes insipidus is believed caused by a dysfunction of the pituitary gland resulting in abnormal thirst and hunger. It tends to occur in people over 40 who are overweight. The etiology of this disease is not well understood. Diabetes mellitus is caused by the insufficient production of insulin by the islets of Langerhans in the pancreas. This type of diabetes has its onset in childhood or adolescence and is sometimes referred to as the juvenile form of diabetes. The result of this insufficiency of insulin is the inability of the body to properly utilize carbohydrates as a source of fuel. The lack of insulin has a number of effects, such as raising the blood sugar level, inhibiting the conversion of sugar to glycogen, and accelerating the conversion of glycogen to sugar. The tissues of the body also find it more difficult to utilize sugar. As a result of all this, sugar is found in excessive amounts in the bloodstream and thereby excreted in the urine. This sometimes will result in an excessive loss of water and salt as well. Because sugar is not being utilized as a source of energy, the body will increasingly utilize proteins and fats for this purpose. The incomplete by-products of protein and fat combustion may also prove harmful. One of the harmful effects is to accelerate the hardening of arteries. An objective of early detection of diabetes, therefore, becomes the prevention of premature arteriosclerosis.

Symptoms in cases of diabetes may go unrecognized. Where they do appear, they generally consist of constant hunger, thirst, and frequent urination. A tired feeling, loss of weight, itching, changes in vision, and slow healing of cuts may also be symptomatic of this disease. Tests for the detection of diabetes usually consist of urinalysis and blood analysis. Glucose tolerance tests are sometimes administered as an additional method of checking for this disorder. The person is given a concentrated amount of glucose to drink. Periodic testing of the urine and blood is then done to determine how well the body handled this concentration of sugar intake. Heredity ranks as a primary contributing factor for this condition. The predisposition for the development of diabetes is apparently passed on through a recessive gene. Studies have also shown that where diabetes has appeared after 40 years of age, overweight appears to be associated with the condition. The sex of the individual may be another factor, in that women have one-third more chance of developing diabetes than men. It has also been noted that four-fifths of the diabetics are over 40 years of age. Diabetes that develops in later life is usually milder, whereas its incidence in children is usually more severe.

Many cases of diabetes can be controlled through diet alone. Where medications are necessary, it has been found that some cases respond to oral drugs such as diabanese or orinase. These are sulfonylureas. Their major function is to stimulate production of insulin in the still active parts of the pancreas. In the most severe cases insulin by injection is required. In these cases, the individual must develop a balance between the carbohydrates taken in the diet, the amount of insulin injected, and the amount of exercise participated in. The diabetic must live a rather well-regulated life so as to keep these three factors in proper balance. Athletes who are diabetics will often have available a source of carbohydrate to replace the amount of this nutrient expended during exercise. The failure to keep a balance between carbohydrates and insulin in the body can result in two dangerous diabetic reactions. The first of these is *diabetic coma,* or *acidosis.* In this condition, there is a lack of insulin present in the body, with the result that sugar and starches cannot be burned. This in turn, results in an excessive breakdown of fats, with the production of ketone bodies in amounts greater than the body can use. Diabetic coma may be slow in onset. It is characterized by nausea, pain in the abdomen, thirst, deep breathing, and a pungent breath odor.

The second diabetic reaction is *insulin shock,* or *hypoglycemia,* which results from taking too large a dose of insulin, eating too little food, or exercising too much. Any of the preceding three factors will result in the presence of too much insulin in the body for the amount of carbohydrate. This can be remedied by the individual's taking a source of carbohydrate such as sugar or orange juice. The onset of insulin shock may be rather sudden, the symptoms being hunger, weakness, paleness, and drowsiness. The diabetic who can feel the reaction setting in can usually correct it by taking some carbohydrates. Diabetics who pass out from either reaction should receive medical help as soon as possible.

Many diabetics carry identification cards indicating the need for medical help should they suffer from either diabetic coma or insulin shock. Too often, diabetics who are in difficulty are mistaken for people who are intoxicated and are in many instances ignored. A diabetic suffering from either reaction could be in very serious difficulty.

Before the development of insulin, a diabetic in need of surgery was in real danger. Now, in a controlled case of diabetes, surgery need not be much more of a risk than for the normal nondiabetic. Controlled diabetes need not interfere with childbirth, either. However, it has been found that where a woman is a prediabetic, the disease may manifest itself during pregnancy. The greatest hazard in childbirth is to the fetus, particularly in the last three months of pregnancy. Some physicians choose to make an early delivery in such cases via Caesarean section. It may also be mentioned here that the presence of sugar in urine after the delivery of a child may not be symptomatic of diabetes but merely due to the presence of lactose from breast milk.

Allergies

An allergen is a chemical substance leading to an abnormal response called an allergic reaction. This reaction will often cause the release of histamine. Histamine, when released from the cells, may cause dilation and congestion of the blood vessels, forcing fluids from these blood vessels into the surrounding tissues of the body. This may result in a swelling of tissues (edema) or the development of hives on the skin. It may also cause a spasmodic contraction of some involuntary muscles of the body. If these muscles are in the bronchial tubes, asthma may be the result.

The causes of allergies are many and varied. There are airborne substances such as pollen, molds, insect fragments (hairs, stings, and scales of insects), dander or dandruff of dogs, cats, horses, or even mice. Ingested substances such as foods are possible causes, with milk, strawberries, and shellfish examples of more common allergens. Drugs of various types will also, at times, cause allergic reactions. The increasing sensitivity of many people to penicillin is characteristic of this. Injected materials such as a wasp or bee sting, insulin, and vaccines of various types may contain substances that become allergens for some people. The extent of this can be exemplified by the fact that more people die from allergic reactions to insect bites than from poison snake bites in this country. During a 10-year period ending in 1959, venomous snakes killed 138 persons, while hymenopterous insects—bees, wasps, hornets, yellow jackets, and fire ants—killed 229. Death was attributed to bees in 124 persons, to wasps in 69, to yellow jackets in 22, to hornets in 10, and to ants in 4. The interval of time between the sting and death, recorded in 208 of the 229 fatalities, was less than an hour in 80 per cent of the victims. The suddenness of death has focused attention on emergency measures and desensitization procedures.[9] Current stud-

[9] "Bites and Stings," *Therapeutic Notes.* Vol. 73 (Detroit, Mich.: Parke, Davis & Company, May–June 1966), p. 59.

 ies continue to substantiate this initial finding. There are also contact substances that will cause allergic reactions, such as poison ivy, orange rind, and certain fabrics. Just about any substance has a potential for the development of an allergic reaction in a given individual.

Asthma is one of the more common allergic reactions that we see. Three million people in this country suffer from this condition. It results in general shortness of breath, coughing, wheezing, and even choking. Asthmatic attacks can be caused by a spasm of the bronchial muscles, the swelling of the bronchial mucous membrane, or the clinging of plugs of phlegm to the bronchial tubes. During an asthmatic attack, the individual, in essence, is attempting to breathe through a constricted opening. A complication of this condition can be emphysema, in which air is trapped in the lungs and cannot be properly exhaled. The child suffering from asthma will in most instances not outgrow the condition. Something should be done to attempt to correct the asthmatic reaction before the individual suffers physical, social, and economic difficulties which in turn may precipitate emotional problems.

The history and examination of the person are prerequisites to allergic management. Skin tests are often done to determine the varied substances to which a person may have a positive allergic reaction. Knowledge of the history of the patient's reactions of an allergic nature are most important at this stage. Controlling the allergy may mean doing such things as getting rid of the dog, cat, or certain types of clothing. It may also mean the installation of a filtering apparatus to filter out molds, pollens, or dust in the home that might be causes of the reaction. If certain kinds of foods are implicated, then substituting for these foods in the diet becomes necessary. This is sometimes difficult in infants who are allergic to milk.

Treatment for allergies may take various forms and should be administered by an allergist, the medical doctor best trained to treat these conditions. A process of desensitization is sometimes used where people are allergic to airborne substances. This process is accomplished by the use of a small amount of allergen; the doses are gradually increased over a period of time to help the individual develop an immunity. These types of vaccines are developed by allergists for their patients' specific allergies. Cortisone and ACTH are hormonal substances that are sometimes used to help people over an acute phase of their allergy. A change in climate or location is also helpful in allergy management if a given mold or ragweed is the cause. It is also recognized that an emotional factor is often associated with allergic reactions. People who are overanxious and emotionally insecure suffer a higher incidence of this disorder.

There is a great need for allergy research. The relationship of emotional factors, climatic conditions, and hormone changes to allergies is not completely understood. The role of bacteria and viruses and their connection with these kinds of reactions need more study. As a population that is being exposed to a wider and wider variety of food, drugs, fabrics, and other substances, we can probably look

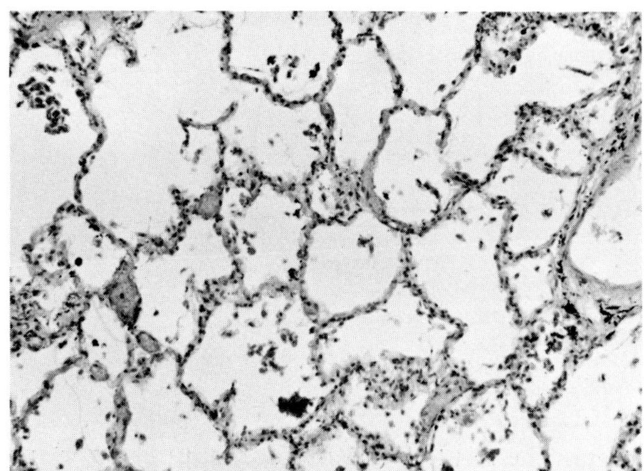

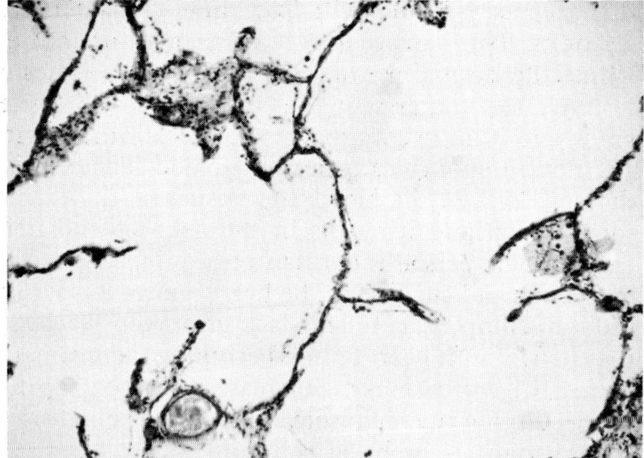

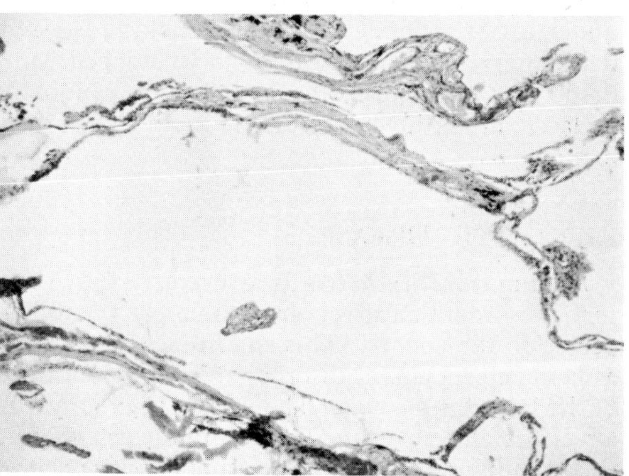

Fig. 10-21. The pictures show the progressive damage (by rupture) of the alveoli or air sacs of the lung as it occurs in emphysema. (Oscar Auerbach)

forward as a group to increased incidence of sensitivities as a result of this increased exposure.

EMPHYSEMA

Emphysema is a chronic lung disease more common than cancer and tuberculosis combined. Emphysema is the fastest-rising cause of death in the United States. In 1949 the death rate from this disease was 2.1/100,000 population; in 1960 it rose to 6.0/100,000 population; and in 1967 it reached 12.9 deaths/100,000 population. Alarming estimates indicate that over 10 per cent of our middle-aged and elderly Americans are afflicted with this disorder. The disease is more common among men than women.

There has recently been a link between an enzyme (Alpha$_1$-antitrypsin A_1AT) deficiency with a particular kind of emphysema. This inherited deficiency seems to affect a greater percentage of female patients than is generally seen in the normal emphysema population. It is too early to make any conclusive statements concerning the genetic studies. However, the hope that genetically identifying susceptible portions of the population and preventing or eliminating cigarette smoking in this high-risk group may serve as a major step in stemming the tide of this disease.

In this disease the lungs are inflated with air that the victim cannot expel; hence the term "emphysema," which is a Greek word meaning inflating or puffing up. Chronic irritation of the bronchi often causes obstructions that trap air in the lungs behind them. The result is that less of the lung is working. The air sacs of the lungs may also be damaged by this trapped air and will lose their characteristic elasticity. This damage may be permanent in nature. While the normal person breathes fourteen times a minute, the emphysematous person may breathe anywhere from twenty to thirty times a minute and still not get enough oxygen in the blood. The carbon dioxide level in the blood and tissues of these persons is high and it results in sluggishness and irritability. The person is constantly gasping for breath, wheezing, and coughing. The heart pumps harder in order to compensate for the lack of oxygen reaching the tissues, with heart failure becoming the ultimate hazard. Cigarette smoking increases the risk of dying from pulmonary emphysema and is a much greater hazard than atmospheric pollution.

Methods of treatment for this disease are currently under investigation. Cessation of smoking is essential if progress of the disease is to be stopped. Lung tissue that has already been destroyed cannot be replaced or repaired by current methods of treatment.

Rheumatic Diseases

Rheumatoid Arthritis is a severe type of rheumatic disorder that affects approximately 4½ million people in the country. This condition is recognized as being a generalized disorder and not one limited to the joints of the body. The disease, therefore, can affect the entire person. The cause of this affliction is still unknown. It is most commonly developed by young adults between the ages of 20 and 40, although cases of the disease may appear later in life. A form of the disease known as juvenile rheumatoid arthritis may even be found among the newborn. This type of arthritis can be most crippling, because it can do damage to the ligaments and coverings of joints and muscles as well as to some of the organs of the body. The joints of the hands, wrists, elbows, knees, ankles, and feet are often involved. These joints are weakened and distorted by the affliction. The onset of rheumatoid arthritis is in many cases rather insidious in nature. The earliest symptoms very often are nothing more than fatigue, accompanied by a loss of appetite and weight and sometimes a numbness of the hands. It is oftentimes weeks and even months after the vague symptoms appear that the aching of the joints begins. These symptoms are most commonly experienced in the morning upon rising. The involvement of joints is usually symmetric in that if a finger on the right hand is affected, the same finger on the left hand will also be affected. A curious thing about rheumatoid arthritis is that although it may persist in the patient for weeks or months, it may at times suddenly go into spontaneous remission, with its symptoms and effects disappearing. This sudden remission of the disease that occasionally takes place is responsible for so called "cures" that some quacks like to take advantage of. Spontaneous relapses of the disease may also occur. Treatment for the arthritic is aimed to prevent contraction and deformity of joints as well as to relieve discomfort.

Osteoarthritis is usually attributed to wear and

tear, although it many times follows injuries and other diseases of the joints. This condition tends to occur in the weight-bearing joints of the body and occurs more frequently in those patients who are overweight or obese. Such patients are usually placed on a regimen that will result in weight reduction so as to take some of the strain off these joints and slow down the degeneration of the articular cartilage. A good deal of research with regard to osteoarthritis is aimed at uncovering the unknown factors related to the speeding up of the degenerative process in cartilage metabolism. Nutritional, genetic, and endocrine factors are being scrutinized to discover the role they play in determining the resistance of cartilage to wear and tear.

Gout is a rheumatic disease in which typically only one joint is affected, usually in the lower extremities. The condition is accompanied by severe pain and swelling, redness, and warmth about the joint affected. The sensitivity of the affected tissue is such that the mere vibration caused by someone walking in the room may cause unbearable pain. With treatment the pain can be terminated almost immediately, and in many instances the recurrence of an acute attack prevented. Without treatment, however, the acute phase of the illness may go on for days or weeks. The gout is caused by an excessive production of uric acid. For some reason, too little of it is eliminated through the kidneys. The tendency toward the development of an excessive amount of uric acid seems to run in families and is presumed to be an inherited factor. Many attacks of acute gout occur for no apparent reason. A number of patients have noted that acute attacks of gout seem to follow stressful situations in their lives, including traumatic incidents, dietary excesses, infections, or even surgery. It is interesting to note that an ancient drug called colchicine, discovered by the Greek physician Alexander of Tralles, in 550 A.D., is found to have dramatic effects in relieving the inflammation and pain in gout. Though this drug has been used for centuries, its action is still not well understood. Because excessive amounts of uric acid precipitate gout conditions, physicians will restrict those foods that are rich in purines from which uric acid is derived. Examples of these foods are sweetbreads, anchovies, liver, and kidney. People trying to lose weight by adhering to diets high in proteins and fats (or ketogenic diets) tend to raise the levels of uric acid in their systems, sometimes bringing on a gout crisis. It has in the past been generally believed that alcoholic beverages were guilty of precipitating such attacks, but research in this area has shown no relationship between the two. The prognosis for gout is quite favorable. The patient who seeks early medical help should be able to avoid the crippling effects of the disease and to enjoy considerable relief from medication during the acute phases.

Some types of arthritis have been found to be caused by specific types of bacteria. In these cases the disease is treated with an antibiotic and is cured. This brings up the possibility that there may be other infectious agents responsible for other forms of arthritis. Should this be the case, the identification of the specific agent or agents involved can lead ultimately to more effective treatment of the disease.

Fig. 10-22. The hand of a person with gout, showing the effects of the disorder before and after treatment. (The National Institute of Arthritis and Metabolic Diseases)

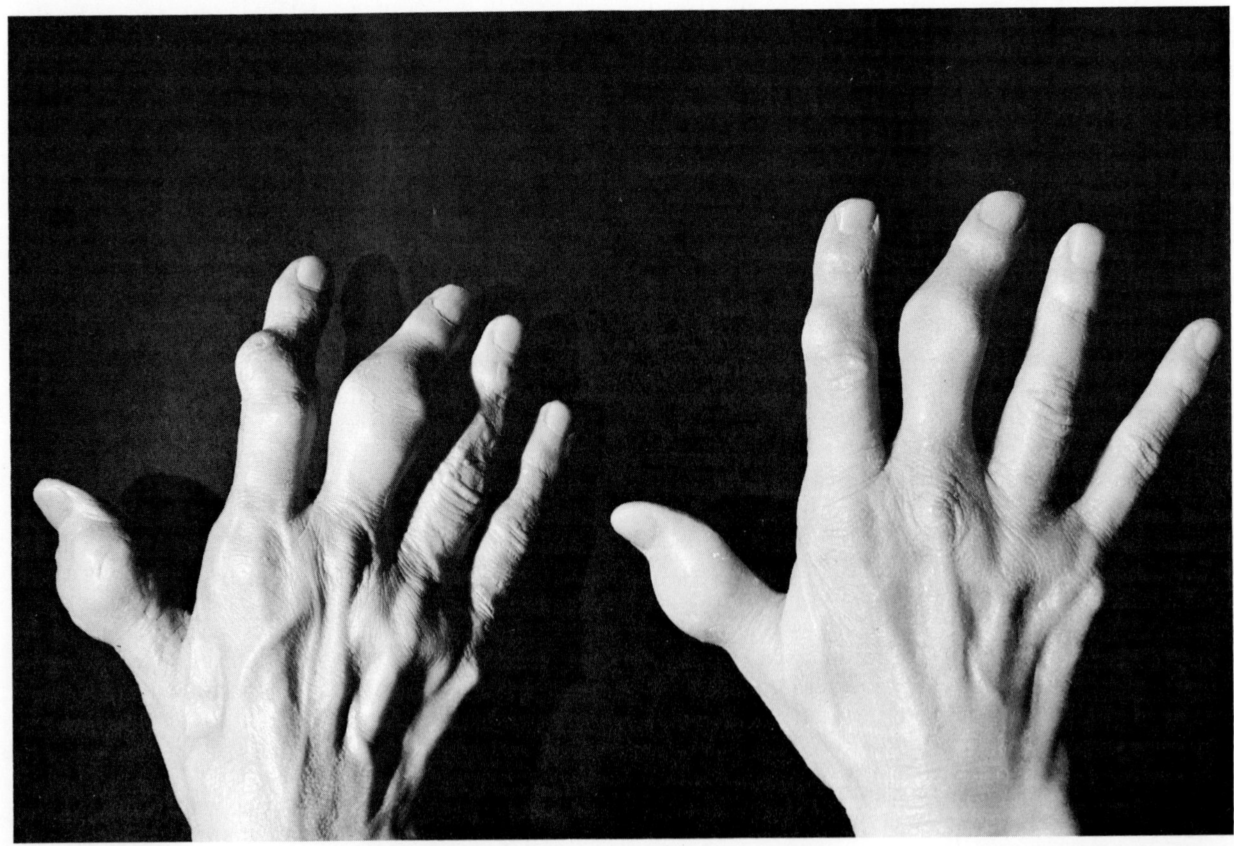

Biochemical research is developing clues to other possible causes of arthritis. Researchers feel that they are not too far away from important breakthroughs in this area that could lead to more specific preventive and treatment measures.

Review Questions

1. Describe arteriosclerosis. What are the factors related to the development of this condition?
2. What is a coronary thrombosis; angina pectoris? How are these conditions related to arteriosclerosis?
3. What are some of the varying causes of strokes? Describe some of the warning signals that may precede this condition.
4. How have advances in surgical procedures improved the prognosis for individuals with rheumatic heart conditions?
5. Describe the various types of congenital heart conditions. How has modern surgery improved the survival chances of children so afflicted?
6. What factors can contribute to the development of human cancer? With which forms of cancer has there been significant medical progress?
7. Explain the contribution that can be made by the epidemiologist in the discovery of environmental factors related to cancer causation.
8. How has the public attitude toward cancer been changing? What is the outlook for cancer control in the future?
9. Distinguish between diabetic coma and insulin shock. Identify the two types of diabetes. What differences in these two disorders are now recognized?
10. What are some of the many causes of convulsive seizures? How are these reactions largely controlled?
11. What preventive measures can be taken to reduce the incidence of cerebral palsy? How do these types of conditions differ?
12. What is an allergy? What are the varied approaches used to alleviate or correct allergic reactions?
13. Describe the lung changes that take place in emphysema. What causative factors have been related to this condition?
14. Describe cystic fibrosis. Why is early detection necessary? What kinds of treatment procedures have been developed for this condition?
15. What are the purposes of rehabilitation programs for people with muscular dystrophy?
16. How do rheumatic diseases differ? What is known about the causes of these conditions?
17. Mental retardation is an effect rather than a given condition. Explain.
18. How can genetic counseling control the incidence of sickle-cell anemia?

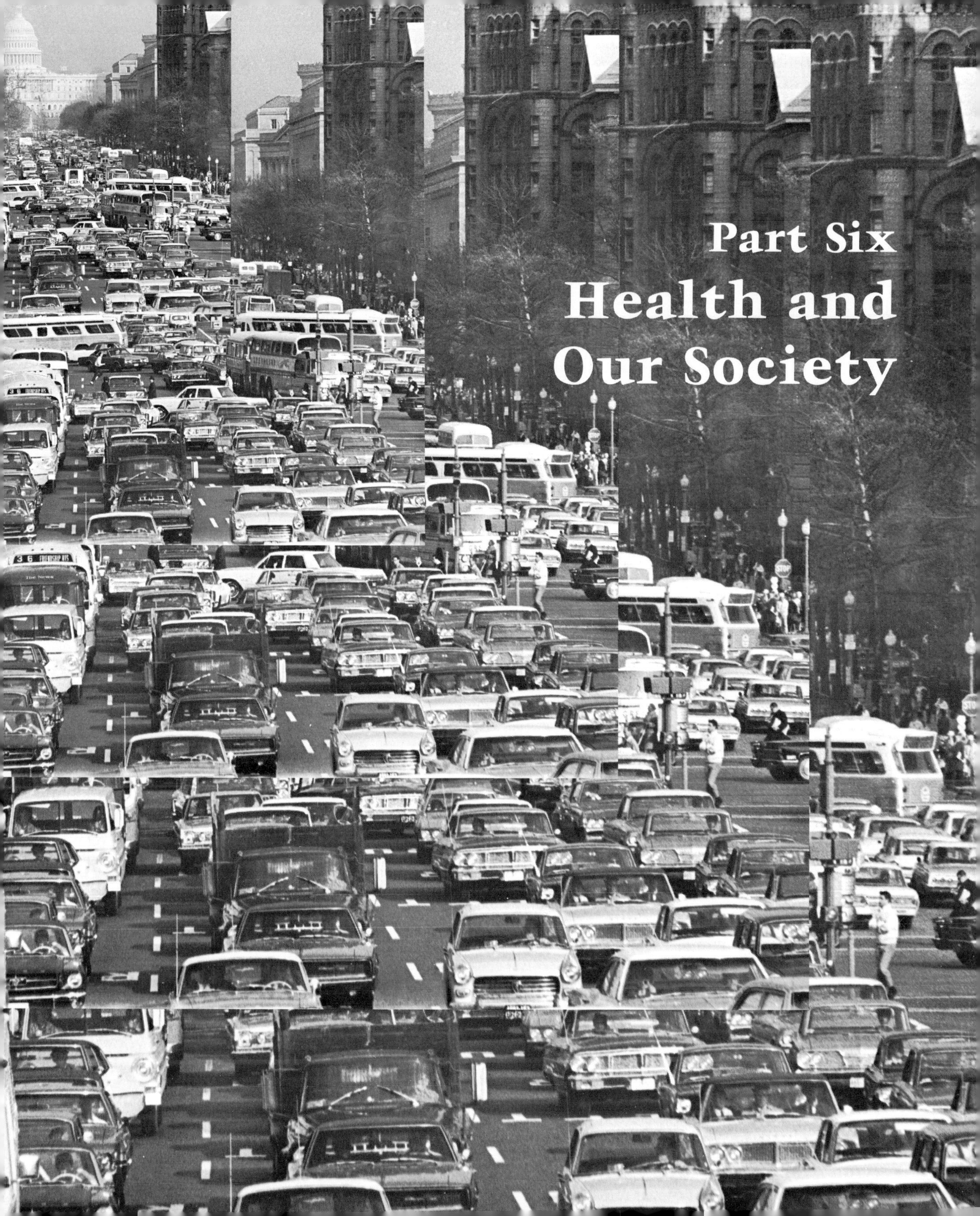

Part Six
Health and Our Society

Chapter 11
Consumer—Beware!

In a competitive, industrialized society it is expected that each industry will attempt to sell its products more successfully than its competitors. The major and predominate focus is the financial health of the particular commercial company. The question that must be asked is, Does this basis for modus operandi in the health area serve the best interests of all segments of society? There are several issues that stand forth. There are those who sell fraudulent health products and services as well as those who *oversell* legitimate health products and services. What are the responsibilities of government in the protection of the consumer? What are the ways in which the consumer can protect himself? In the purchase of health care services some new directives and issues emerge for the consumer. As stated by Dr. Vernon E. Wilson,

> Perhaps of even greater long-range significance for preventive medicine and health maintenance is the new emphasis on consumer health education. It is apparent to anyone who views the health scene in broad perspective that the greatest single untapped potential for reducing the unnecessary use of health resources and adding manpower at very low cost is the patient himself and his family. Activating this powerful resource is one of the critical challenges before us. . . . In each individual case—which is where it counts—the individual himself is the ultimate decisionmaker. Preventive medicine has a secondary but vitally important role. For it is the business of preventive medicine to help activate him toward the choice that is in his best interest.[1]

[1] Vernon E. Wilson, "New Initiatives in Prevention," *Preventive Medicine*, Vol. 1, No. 3 (August 1972), 289–290.

Quackery: The Backwash of an Uninformed Public

The judgment of the American as a consumer of health products and services is notoriously poor. The National Health Test given by CBS television in 1966 confirmed this with test results indicating that basic health knowledge was generally inadequate in this country. A study conducted by the Food and Drug Administration in 1972 confirmed that Americans have some strange ideas about maintaining their health. They expect vitamins to give them added energy and even prevent cancer and arthritis. Many carry on self-medication based on ignorance. The lack of health education either as courses of study in our schools or as part of public education programs has resulted in a woefully uninformed American. This fact, coupled with the misrepresentation of health products and services, has created the most lucrative con game in this country. It has now reached such proportions that it is causing concern and alarm among physicians and other health professionals. An amount of $250 million a year is spent on quack devices for arthritis alone and this is just a fraction of the "market."

Research has not provided medical science with treatment that will result in the complete rehabilitation of all cases of arthritis. Medical treatment in its present stage can, however, relieve pain associated with the condition and prevent a great deal of crippling, particularly where arthritis cases are treated early.

Because arthritis is a painful condition and a com-

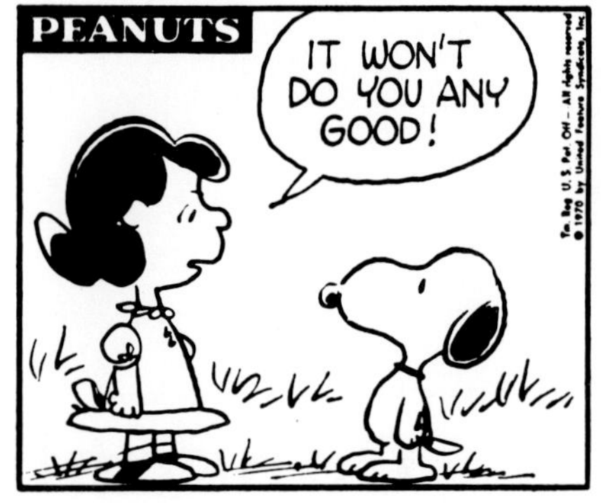

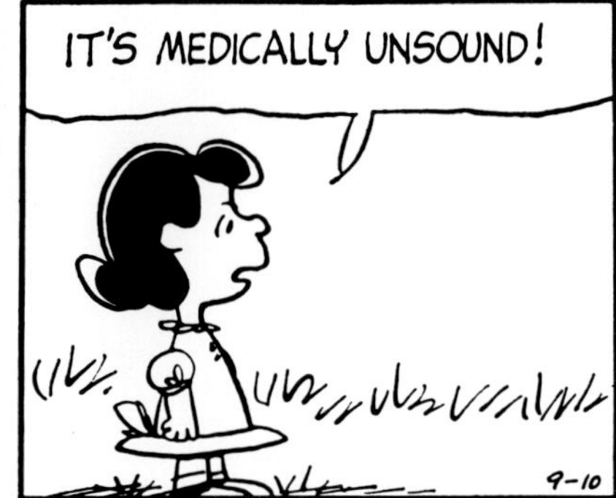

Fig. 11-1. "It's medically unsound!" Peanuts cartoon by Charles M. Schulz. (© 1970 United Feature Syndicate, Inc.)

plete cure is not available, many arthritics reach out for the "miracle" cures offered by the quack. It has been found that 14 out of 100 arthritics have been sold vibrating devices that are either useless or harmful, as well as glorified aspirin at exorbitant prices. Arthritis is a condition that often follows an erratic course, with occasional remissions and recurrences. When a remission occurs following the use of a fake product, the arthritic is misled into thinking that he has found an effective treatment.

Fraudulent practices in the area of cancer "cures" are also many and varied. The delays they cause in reaching legitimate treatment often makes the differences between life and death. When the person with a terminal case of cancer seeks out the quack, the only visible result is the exchange of money that takes place.

Probably the oldest form of cancer "treatment" is the use of a salve or similar concoction that is supposed to draw the cancer right out of the body. For the cancers that are deep inside the body pills or injections are offered by the quack in a mimicking of modern medical procedure. Some of the nostrums sold have been found to contain substances that actually accelerate cancer growth. Others have been found to contain laxatives. A widely used quack treatment is the giving of injections of plain water to cancer victims. The fees for the injections are usually several hundred dollars. Other frauds sell "shots" that are supposed to be vaccines. In recent years a number of "cancer curing" diets have also evolved. To add to the shenanigans, a variety of mechanical devices that give off varied colored lights and make impressive noises have been sold as cure-alls. The fleecing of ailing older people who have limited savings is undoubtedly the cruelest of hoaxes.

How difficult it is to determine what is fraudulent was exemplified by the Krebiozen case. Dr. Andrew Ivy, a well-known physiologist, was scientific adviser for the Krebiozen Research Foundation, producers of the drug Krebiozen. Claims were made that the drug could cure cancer, resulting in its wide use and sale. Government investigation of the drug showed that Krebiozen contained creatine, a common body substance that had no effect on cancer. Early in 1967 a "cancer vaccine" was being used on 1000 terminal cancer patients in Cleveland, Ohio. The Food and Drug Administration halted the testing in spite of testimony from several dozen patients indicating they benefited from the medication. As in the Krebiozen case, the vaccine was never subjected to controlled studies and therefore the company was violating federal regulations governing the testing of new medicinal substances in man. Though the users may well have been terminal cases with "nothing to lose," the government's argument was that unless stringent regulations were enforced, nothing would prevent the wholesale indiscriminate testing and human experimentation that would take place by every well-meaning saviour of mankind. It would appear that human life, even in its terminal stages, deserves a greater dignity than what usually proves to be the clumsy, unscientific efforts of the overzealous.

A wide range of devices with flashing lights and

YOU'RE JUST FOOLING YOURSELF!

EVERYONE CRITICIZES MY COPPER BRACELET
SCHULZ

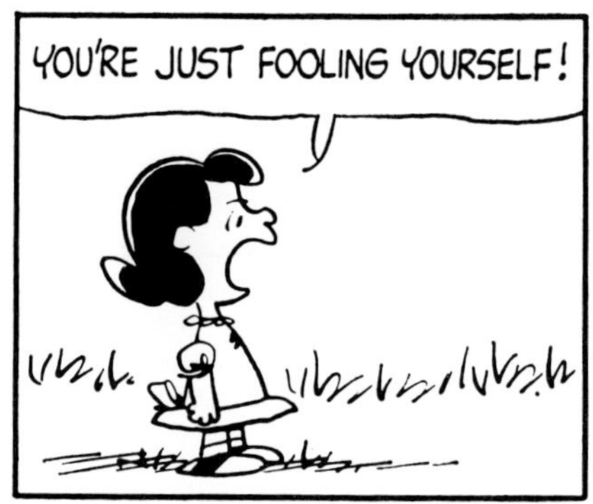

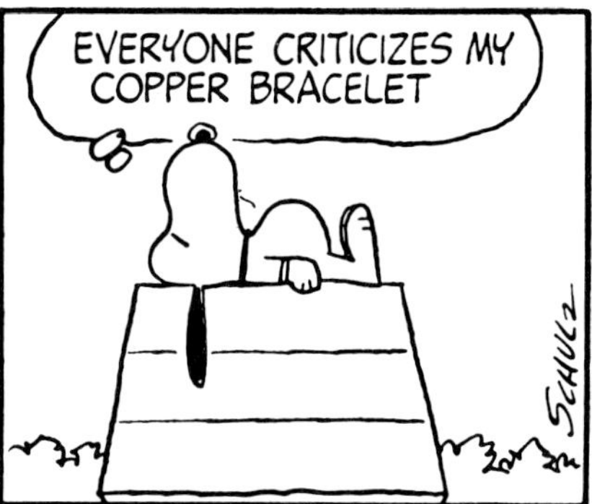

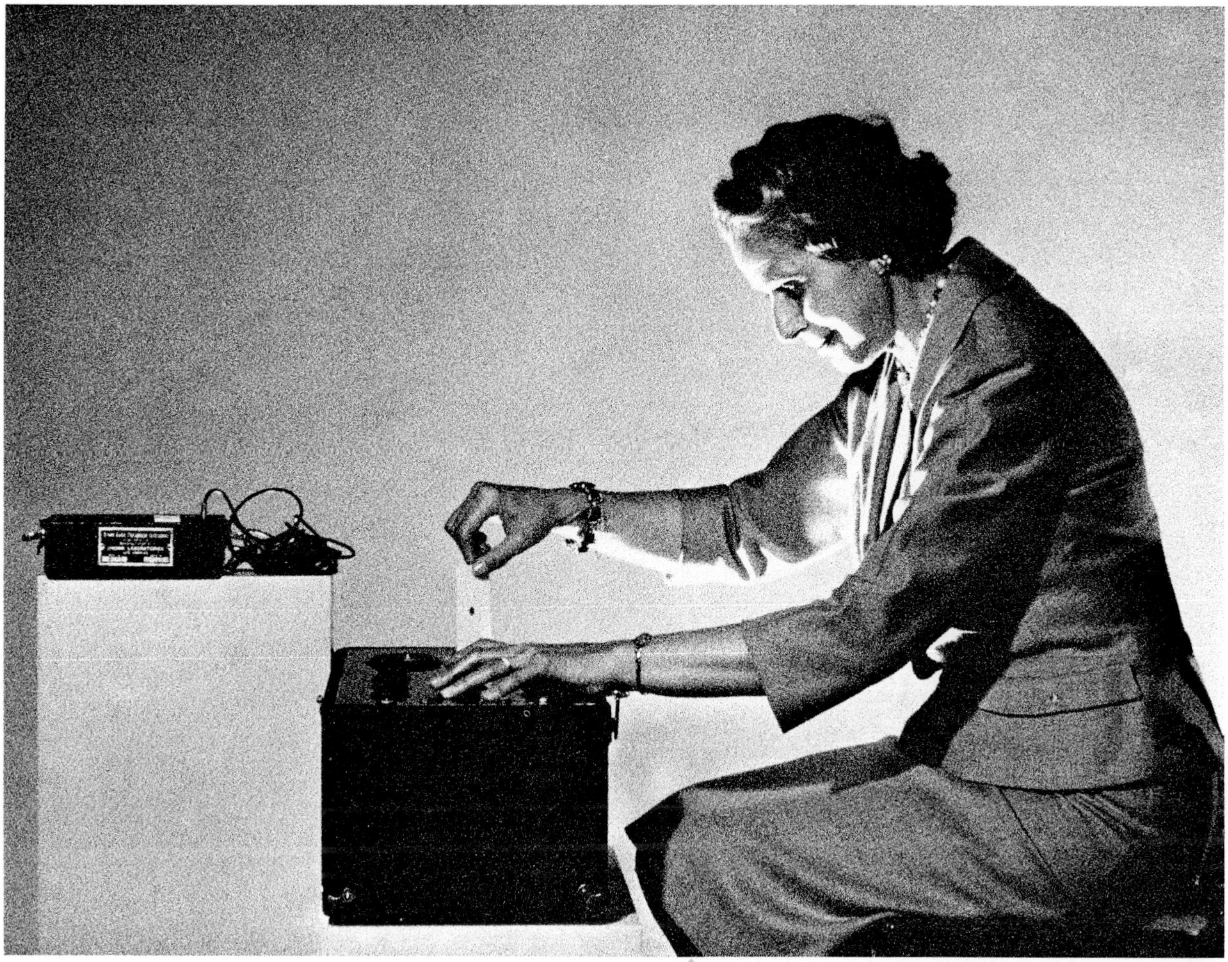

Fig. 11-2. For almost 30 years this fraudulent device was used by Ruth Drown, a chiropractor from Los Angeles, for the diagnosis and treatment of disease. Patients sent in a drop of blood on a piece of blotting paper and the machine tested it for any disease. Once diagnosed, the disease was treated by radiation sent out by the same machine. Combined efforts of the FDA and officials of the State of California finally put this fraud out of business. (FDA)

ozone-generating mechanisms have been sold with the promise of curing just about everything.

"Doorbell doctors" are busy selling vitamin and mineral supplements. They incorporate in their sales talk professional-sounding jargon and are usually quite free in giving medical advice. They are too often successful in selling needless dietary supplements. It is estimated that approximately 50,000 such salesmen prey upon the American public with misleading information and needless products.

The sales of so-called health foods have been increasing. Examples of these are yogurt, which has the same nutritional value as milk, or blackstrap molasses, which consists of the impurities gathered from the refining process of sugar. The iodine that is found in kelp tablets is supplied in adequate amounts in natural sea foods and iodized salt. Producers of so-called health foods try to imply that the American food supply is nutritionally deficient. This is obviously not true. Other fraudulent products include air purifiers that are supposed to treat diseases such as tuberculosis, pneumonia, and influenza. "Tired blood" tonics are supposedly sold for iron deficiency anemia, whose symptoms resemble a large number of other conditions, including pernicious anemia. This is a disorder that could prove to be fatal if not properly diagnosed and treated. A number of cosmetic preparations have been sold with the promise that they will restore youthful attractiveness.

In addition to the monetary loss exacted by these practices, the health of many people is being endangered. Fraudulent devices and services often keep a patient from the legitimate, early diagnosis and treatment that would have saved his life. "Your money and your life" is an appropriate summation of the situation.

Testimonials represent a basic means of selling nostrums and quack services. They are often written by deluded people who were told they had a dread disease and were subsequently "cured" by a quack device or treatment. Such diseases are easy to cure when the person does not really have them in the first place. The person's account of a situation cannot be described as being scientifically accurate; he is merely reporting his impressions. The routine reminds one of a clever person performing some sleight-of-hand tricks. What the person "sees" is quite different from what actually happened. One study also indicated that 75 per cent of the testimonials are from people who are now deceased.

Legitimate health services do not rely on testimonials to justify the worth of their services, but on well-established research procedures and their resultant scientifically accurate findings. Ulcer cures, wrinkle removers, royal jelly (for the restoration of sexual potency), seawater, kidney remedies, high blood pressure treatments, various hormones, and hazardous diabetes treatments are all part of a lucrative, dangerous business called quackery. It is at best unfortunate, if not disgraceful, that this problem exists to the extent that it does in our society. We have perhaps exhibited too great a tolerance for practices that are wasteful and a threat to the health of the American people. It is time to educate the population as a first line of defense against quackery.

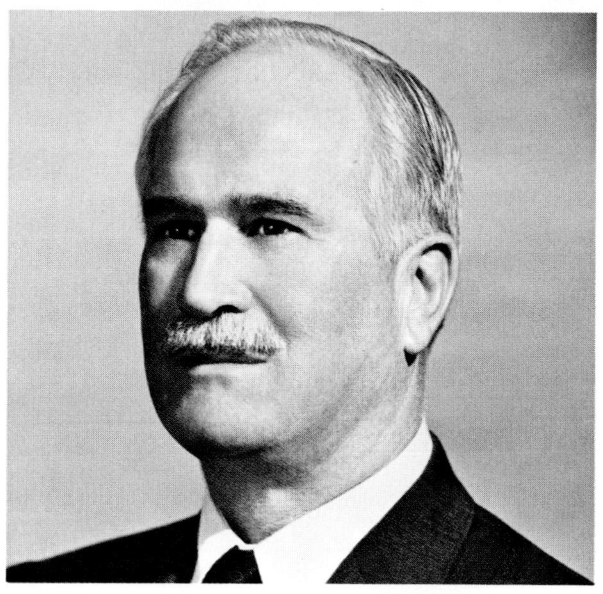

Fig. 11-3. Hollis S. Ingraham, M.D., Commissioner of Health, N.Y.S. Dept. of Health. (N.Y.S. Health Photo by M. Dixson)

Quackery's Areas of Gray

At a symposium on quackery, Dr. Hollis S. Ingraham, the New York State Commissioner of Health, stated the following:

> I have set as my goal to attempt a definition that captures the unwholesome essence of health quackery—the gray fringes as well as the deep-dyed fraud. I hope to demonstrate that while all quacks practice quackery, not all quackery is perpetrated by quacks. While the vicious peddler of a cancer cure may fit at the darkest edge of the spectrum, innumerable shades of lesser quackery also tend to erode the public's health.
>
> Note how often the suggestion of scientific respectability is woven into patent medicine promotion, "Actual clinical tests prove . . ." "A new medical report tells us . . ." "In tests by doctors . . ." "Medical authorities say . . ." The thinking mind rebels at these insinuations of authority. What doctors? Which medical authorities? Whose survey? How many of these scientific trappings could withstand a penetrating analysis?
>
> Is it less quackish to publish a book like *Calories Don't Count* than it is to write it? Can a publisher take much pride in having one of his titles atop a best seller list when that book is *Arthritis and Common Sense*, a discredited thesis written by an unqualified layman?
>
> Are the electronic media totally free of quack attitudes? I suggest that there is a touch of quackery in the radio or television executive's tolerance of much medical nonsense that is piped into the American home.
>
> Quackery is a misrepresented health insurance—especially policies peddled to the aged that are so riddled with loopholes that they offer almost no protection at all.
>
> Is there something akin to quackery in the views of some tobacco industry spokesmen regarding smoking and health? How else are we to interpret their rejection of the overwhelming evidence that cigarette smoking can cause lung cancer and greatly increase deaths from coronary heart disease?
>
> Do I detect a quackish tone in the negative attitudes of some automobile manufacturers towards building safety features into their product?[2]

Perhaps it is time to review *all* fraudulent consumer health practices. It does not take one long to find out that advertisements in television, radio, newspapers, and the magazines make a real attempt to lead the consumer into the practice of self-diagnosis and self-medication. The mass media have been quite successful in selling the public on the habitual use of unnecessary drugs that take the form of alkalines, laxatives, pain relievers, vitamins, tonics, and so forth. When millions of dollars a year are spent in this country on proprietary drugs, one begins to wonder what is *really* wrong. Is it that we must be ever alert to the wiles of the advertisers who are leading people into the excessive and indiscriminate use of drugs? Or is it time that we ask why this kind of situation exists? What of the drug industry? Does it not have a responsibility not only to label its product properly but to advertise it honestly as well?

Let us take a look at some of the malpractices. A mouthwash advertisement implies that the product will help prevent the common cold. Enter petri dish with half the dish treated with the mouthwash. The

[2] Hollis S. Ingraham, "Quackery," New York State Congress on Health Quackery (April 1965), pp. 3–8. Sponsored by the Medical Society of the State of New York.

number of bacteria that grow on the mouthwash side of the dish are practically nil, while many bacteria grow on the other side. The fact is that the common cold is *not* caused by *bacteria* but by viruses.

One gargle manufacturer advertised his product as being effective for the treatment of sore throats and bleeding gums. The ineffective treatment of a sore throat caused by a streptococcal infection could delay legitimate treatment and become a possible "contribution" to the development of nephritis or rheumatic heart disease.

Aspirin is sold under various brand names as well as guises. In some cases it is buffered; in others caffeine and phenacetin are added. False claims with regard to its speed of absorption by the body or its pain-relieving effectiveness are then made, with even more inappropriate elevations in its price. Adding other substances has a doubtful effect on the performance of the drug. Aspirin is aspirin!

Many eyewashes are advertised as relievers of that "tired eye feeling" (no relation to tired blood). They also imply that the eye should be cleansed periodically for further relief. The eyes do not need to be cleansed any more than the digestive tract does (the neurotic fixation on cleanliness does not die easily). Human tears, the fluid layer that covers the eye, not only soothe it best, but also have mild antiseptic qualities as well. Again, should the person experiencing eye discomfort be reaching for an eyewash or finding out what is wrong?

The amount of sound information that reaches the American public is a mere trickle compared with the deluge of misinformation. Radio and television are often sources of misleading and false health information. Books on health topics found on best seller lists contain reams of invalid information. The person who relies on his physician for health information finds that he sees him all too infrequently or only *after* he becomes ill. Many of our schools add to the problem by omitting from their curricula health instruction that is concerned with the many vital health issues of our society. The school, the agency that should serve as a major source of health information, often fails to do so. The health consumer is thus ripe for plucking.

The Ethical (Prescription) Drug Industry

There are probably few, if any, industries whose usefulness to society exceeds that of the ethical drug industry. Its leaders have emphatically and often stated its concern for the public welfare. In recent years, however, a number of questions have been raised concerning the drug industry that warrant examination.

The drug industry has been the most profitable in the United States. Its profits after taxes are about twice the national average for all industries. While it has never been a crime to make money in this country, complaints about drug prices and other practices of the drug companies prompted the late Senator Kefauver and his Senate subcommittee to look into the matter in 1960. One of the factors related to drug price was the manner in which prescription drugs were sold. When a drug is purchased under a brand name, its price is many times higher than if the same drug were bought by its generic name. (The "generic name" refers to the chemical ingredient in the drug. The brand name refers to the name given to a drug by a particular company. Thus several brand name drugs of different companies can all contain the same generic drug.)

Buying a drug by its generic name, however, is not simple. Getting the family physician to prescribe drugs by generic name is not easy. The drug industry carries on a massive advertising campaign aimed at the physician to get him to write brand names on prescriptions rather than generic names. A drug is put out in so many forms, combinations, and brand names that the busy physician finds it difficult to keep up with them all. The result is that he finds it easier to follow the leads given by the drug industry via its medical advertisements and detail men (drug salesmen), and to prescribe the more expensive brand name drug. It is estimated that out of every ten dollars spent on a drug, three dollars goes for pharmaceutical advertisements aimed at physicians.

One recipient of the usual drug company mail who testified before the subcommittee was Dr. James E. Bowes, an obstetrician from Salt Lake City, who had become so annoyed by the sheer volume of circulars and samples pouring into his office daily that he had got hold of a postal scale and weighed every piece of material he received over a two month period. "The results soon began to look fantastic," he reported. "It would take two railroad cars, one hundred and ten large mail trucks, and eight hundred postmen to deliver the daily load of drug circulars and samples to doctors if mailed to a single city."[3]

[3]Richard Harris, *The Real Voice* (New York: Macmillan, 1964).

The American drug industry has claimed that the high cost of drugs is due in great part to research that they conduct. Investigation has shown that most new drugs are developed in other countries or by independent or governmental efforts. Many drug industries find research too costly. Though they do some, they would rather concentrate on marketing a new product or developing variations of it.

As the hearings continued, Kefauver brought on several former drug-company employees, including a number of doctors. One of these, Dr. A. Dale Console, who had been Squibb's medical director for five years, remarked that the companies were always talking of the great number of research failures they had for every success, and said, "This is true, since it is the very essence of research. The problem arises out of the fact that they market so many of their failures." Kefauver asked him if, in his opinion, much of the industry's research led to the marketing of drugs that were useless or worse. "I think more than half is in that category," Dr. Console answered. "And I should point out that with many of these products it is clear while they are on the drawing board that they promise no utility. They promise sales."[4]

After reviewing drug industry research, a *Science Digest* writer commented:

In drug industry parlance, the word (research) is a catch-all including these activities: learning to copy another firm's successful drug; developing new dosage forms of established drugs; devising packaging changes; making slight, but patentable, alterations in the molecule of a drug someone else has patented (called "me-too re-

[4]Ibid., p. 79.

Fig. 11-4. *Right are shown two nine-week-old baboon fetuses. The one on the left shows normal development while the one on the right demonstrates thalidomide-induced deformity of the limbs, ear, and spine. (Dr. Andrew G. Hendrickx and Dr. Leonard R. Axelrod—Photo by Gerard T. Rote, Jr.)*

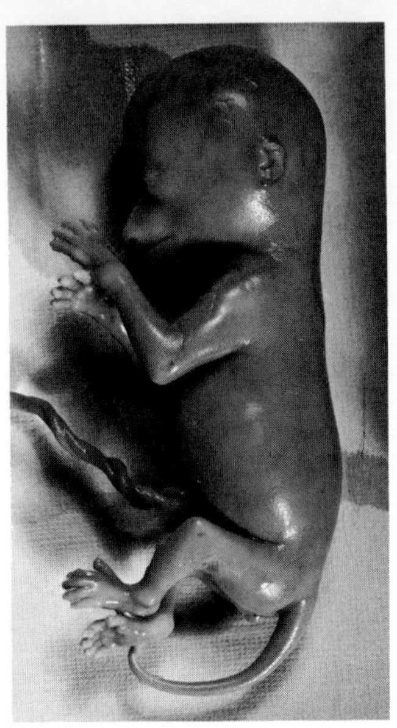

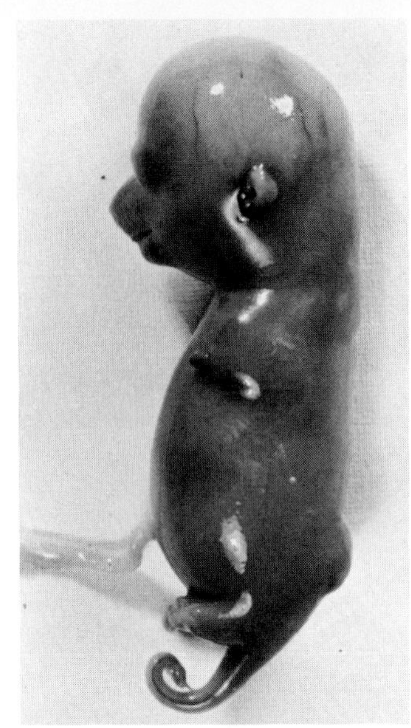

search"); developing large-scale production processes; patent searches—and looking for completely new drugs.[5]

The safety and efficacy of drugs being marketed also came under serious questioning. Side effects of drugs were not being properly reported to physicians by the drug industry, and testing procedures of the drug compounds for new drugs were also found faulty.

One of the first reserpine derivatives was marketed early in 1956 with the claim of "no known contraindications." This was so preposterous a statement about a powerful chemotherapeutical agent that the manufacturer was forced to withdraw the claim, but not before he made a killing (fortunately only in dollars). But equally misleading claims persist. For example, Dr. Frank J. Ayd, Jr., a widely respected psychiatrist, testified before a House Committee headed by Congressman John Blatnik about Pacatal, a tranquilizer with which serious side effects had been reported in Norway and Germany. The side effects included a few instances of agranulocytosis, a rare blood disease which is fatal in about 40% of the cases. An article in the British Medical Journal also warned against its widespread use. Dr. Ayd tested Pacatal on his patients and reported to the firm that hired him, Warner-Chilcott, that, while effective, it presented some dangers. In promoting the drug the company "edited" his findings so as to present them in a more favorable light. When the psychiatrist protested, he was dropped out of future ads, but not before his name had been used in thousands of mailings.[6]

[5]Bruce H. Frisch, "Kefauver's Last Interview," *Science Digest* (November 1963), pp. 10–18.

[6]Alek A. Rozental, *The Crisis in American Medicine* (New York: Harper & Row, 1961), p. 102.

After thorough Senate committee hearings on the drug industry, the Kefauver-Harris Drug Amendments Act of 1962 was proposed. These amendments seemed to have no chance of adoption by Congress until the news of the thalidomide tragedy broke. Thalidomide was used in Europe to prevent nausea in early pregnancy. The drug, it was found, caused deformed births. Babies were being born without parts of limbs and, in some cases, no limbs at all. Dr. Frances Kelsey of the FDA prevented a major medical tragedy in this country by refusing approval for the sale of this drug in the United States and asking for more testing information on it for further assurance as to its safety. In the interim, the tragic qualities of thalidomide became known. The need for stronger drug legislation became a public mandate, and consumers had every reason to hail the passage of the Drug Amendments of 1962 as a major advance in the cause of safe, effective, and honestly promoted drugs.

Senator Kefauver's committee initially started the drug industry investigation in an effort to determine why drug prices were so high. While the legislation stimulated by Senator Kefauver and his group resulted in major reforms with regard to insuring drug safety, the part of the bill dealing with drug prices was omitted. Senator Kefauver intended to investigate further the proprietary (over the counter) as well as the prescription drug prices. The committee hearings indicated that a few large drug companies seemed to have undue influence on drug costs. Drug prices in Europe, it found, were well below those in the United States; this included those drugs sold in

Europe made by American drug companies. Senator Kefauver's untimely death in the early sixties interrupted his work. In this day of increasing medical care costs, the question of drug prices remains very much at issue.

The High Price of Drugs on the Legal Market

"For years the American people have been forced to pay the highest prices for drugs—prices which fall most heavily on those who are least able to afford them—the sick, the poor, and the aged."[7] In hearings held by Senator Nelson, he found that the Eli Lilly Company sold 100 tablets of Darvon to druggists in the United States for $7.02. The same product was sold in Ireland for $1.66 and to pharmacists in England for $1.92. The Ciba Pharmaceutical Company charged druggists $39.50 for 1000 tablets of Serpasil, a drug used to lower blood pressure. The same drug ordered by the U.S. Defense Department under the generic name of Reserpine, cost 60¢ per thousand. Pfizer charged $20.48 for 100 tablets of Terramycin (an antibiotic) in this country, $4.63 in Brazil, and $3.68 in New Zealand.

One of the most outrageous examples of price gouging is the tranquilizer meprobamate, a widely prescribed drug sold under the trade names of Miltown and Equanil. The holder of the patent on this drug is Carter-Wallace, Inc., a pharmaceutical manufacturer based in New York City. Although this firm sells meprobamate under the trade name, Miltown, it does not and never has produced its own meprobamate either in bulk or in final dosage form. Carter-Wallace buys the bulk material from foreign manufacturers for resale to U.S. manufacturers and for use in the meprobamate tablets it sells under its own name. Carter-Wallace was buying this drug in bulk at 87 cents a pound and selling it to domestic manufacturers at $23.80 a pound, a markup of about 2,600 percent.[8]

Of added interest is the case described in *Consumer Reports* of Osco Drug Inc., a retail chain of 178 pharmacies in 17 states. Osco Drug Inc. took the unprecedented action of posting the prices of prescription drugs in their drugstore windows. "The Illinois Board of Pharmacy began proceedings to suspend the licenses of Osco pharmacists on charges of 'gross immorality.' Rival pharmacists telephoned Osco's director of professional services and called him a 'prostitute' and a 'traitor.' Pharmacy associations spoke out publicly against the Osco program and, in several states, threatened to demand revocation of Osco pharmacy licenses."[9]

The American Pharmaceutical Association has taken the position that the posting of prices of prescription drugs is inconsistent with its code. It denies that its motivation is economic gain and insists that the public health and welfare are its sole concern.

Part of the Osco Drug Company's motivation to post its prices came from a Department of Health,

[7] *Parade* Magazine, January 21, 1973.

[8] *Congressional Record,* Proceedings and Debates of the 93rd Congress, Omnibus Drug Bill S. 966, February 21, 1973.

[9] "Drug Pricing and the Rx Police State," *Consumer Reports* (March 1972), 137.

 Education, and Welfare report from its Task Force on Prescription Drugs, which stated in part, "If a patient is to maintain the right to select a pharmacy, he also has a right to know the prices it charges and to compare these with other prices."[10]

Other Issues Concerning the Drug Industry

The ethical drug industry has at times been accused of nonethical behavior. Back in 1966 Dr. James L. Goddard, the then newly appointed commissioner of the FDA, spoke bluntly of the drug industry's practice of submitting slipshod data on new drugs to the FDA. He said:

> I have been shocked at the materials that come in. . . . In addition to the problem of quality, there is the problem of dishonesty in the Investigational New Drug stage. . . . I will admit there are gray areas in the IND situation.
>
> But the conscious withholding of unfavorable animal or clinical data is not a gray-area matter.
>
> The deliberate choice of clinical investigators known to be more concerned about industry friendships than in developing good data is not a gray-area matter.
>
> The planting in journals of articles that begin to commercialize what is still an Investigational New Drug is not a gray-area matter.
>
> These actions run counter to the law and the ethics governing the drug industry.[11]

[10]Ibid.

[11]Speech before Pharmaceutical Manufacturers Association, 1966.

The drug industry's response to the charge was that Dr. Goddard was overemphasizing "isolated instances without acknowledging the integrity and responsibility which our industry has consistently demonstrated."[12]

A few years later a scandal in drug testing which involved prison inmates of several southern states precipitated some legislative actions by Senator Gaylord Nelson of Wisconsin. It seems an enterprising physician, who had no formal education or training in pharmacology, was hired by several drug companies to carry on testing of new drugs. In fact it was estimated that this doctor had made between 25 to 50 per cent of the initial new drug testing in the United States, with little or no medical supervision of the studies. The National Communicable Disease Center released its extensive investigation of this physician and made known the records attributing an epidemic of viral hepatitis to blood plasma programs that were operated by him in the prisons of Alabama, Arkansas, and Oklahoma. Outraged by this scandal, Senator Nelson proposed legislation to impose more rigorous tests on experimental drugs and to make mandatory that these tests be carried out by the federal government, and *not* by the drug companies. While drug companies would have to pay the costs of federal testing, they would have no jurisdiction over the selection of scientists who were testing their product. Senator Nelson further stated that

[12]"Rx for Drug Industry," *New York Times*, April 10, 1966.

It is equally clear that there is imperative and urgent need for a better system for the testing of drugs prior to their approval for marketing. Steps must be taken to reduce the possibility of bias to a minimum. Testing of drugs should be done by specialists who have no direct relationship with the manufacturer, who cannot benefit financially from the results, who are not motivated even subconsciously by the desire to get anything but the truth. We must remove the responsibility for testing drugs from the applicant who has a financial interest in the drug. This responsibility must be placed with an evaluating group which has no interest at all in whether or not the drug gets into the market other than the interest of the public.[13]

More recently Ralph Nader's Health Research Group developed a report that had some disturbing allegations. It "criticized FDA's practice of allowing drug-company officials free access into FDA offices, and using "consultants" with possible conflicts of interest to perform duties identical to those of line officers."[14] The report continues:

It is well known to medical officers that drug company officials are constantly in the corridors of FDA, walking into the scientific staff offices expecting immediate attention. The reason for industry's presence in FDA halls is similar to that of detail men in doctor's offices: to persuade doctors to make drug decisions on the basis of factors other than the scientific evidence before the doctor. Drug men's freedom of access to FDA personnel not only contributes to a division backlog, but is a potential danger to the scientific judgment of the medical officers responsible for the safety of the American drug supply.[15]

[13]*Congressional Record,* Proceedings and Debates of the 92nd Congress, Vol. 117, No. 166, November 4, 1971.

[14]*U.S. Medicine,* April 15, 1972, 1601 18th Street N.W., Washington D.C. 20009.

The great number of drugs marketed by the drug industry continues to add confusion and problems to the scene. At the present time there are some 21,000 drug products on the market. This multiplicity of drugs exists because of the many brand name drugs that are marketed containing the same generic drug. Dr. Walter Modell one of this country's great pharmacologists has stated,

Simply because a drug is new, it is not necessarily better than those already available, safer or even just as good. Often, it is even less effective and sometimes more hazardous than the parent drug. But they also do harm by their very existence in the drug market. I take the stand that as a general principle everything that adds to the difficulty in dealing with and understanding drugs also makes drugs more dangerous. Thus, the excessive number of needless drugs constitutes a present danger. We can make the useful drugs both less dangerous and more efficient by weeding out the useless, the ineffective and the duplicates, and by so doing, make it possible for the physician to learn in depth about the potent drugs he will prescribe for his patients. We must add only those new drugs that really add something more than their mere presence.[16]

An added problem is identified by HEW's Task Force on Prescription Drugs.

[15]Ibid.

[16]*Drug Industry Antitrust Act:* Hearings, Subcommittee on Antitrust and Monopoly; Committee on the Judiciary, 87th Congress, 1st Session; Part I, AMA and Medical Authorities, p. 320.

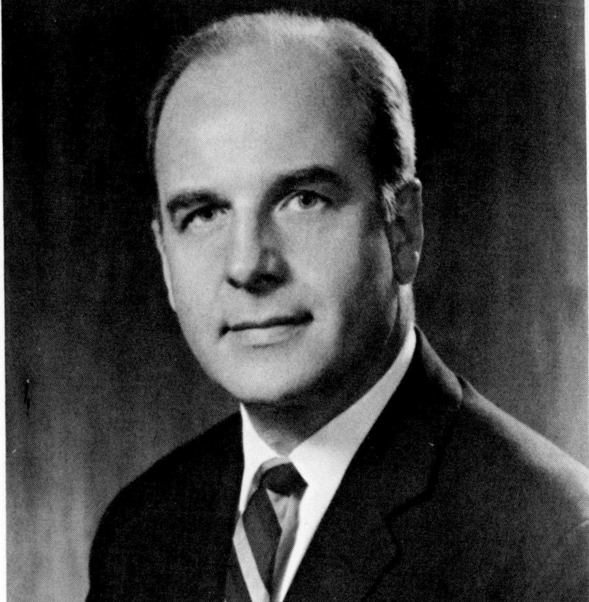

Fig. 11-5. Senator Gaylord Nelson of Wisconsin.

Upon entering private practice, the average physician, knowingly or unknowingly, becomes the key figure in drug marketing strategy.

He must choose from a very large number of competitive and often duplicative products.

He must deal with a very large amount of advice, biased or unbiased, from detail men, advertisements, and other forms of promotion.

Substantial efforts are made on his behalf by the drug industry and others to prevent any interference with his right to prescribe as he sees fit.

Finally, it is assumed that he has the training, experience, and time to weigh the claims and available evidence, and thus to make the proper selections.

Everything, of course, hinges on the validity of this final assumption.

We find that few practicing physicians seem inclined to voice any questions of their competency in this field. We have noted, however, that the ability of an individual physician to make sound judgments under these quite confusing conditions is now a matter of serious concern to leading clinicians, scientists, and medical educators.[17]

In order to correct the problems related to drug production, safety, testing, advertising, sales, research, and labeling, Senator Nelson proposed legislation (Omnibus Drug Bill S. 966) that would provide the following.

I—Sets up a National Drug Testing and Evaluation Center which will be reponsible for the testing of all drugs, both prescription and over-the-counter, that are now or will be marketed in the United States. The FDA must give approval prior to testing drugs on human beings and the results and conclusions of all tests will be made public. In order for a new drug to be approved, it must be demonstrated that the new drug is safer and more effective than a drug already on the market. As it has been the manufacturer's reponsibility in the past to bear the expense of a drug's testing, he will continue to bear the expense. However, there will be channels open for appeal if the manufacturer is dissatisfied with the testing procedure.

II—Provides for the publication of a compendium which will list all drugs available in the United States by both generic and brand names. Such a compendium would include, for each drug, the drug's purpose, side effects, dosages available, cost, as well as other relevant information. As such a compendium could eliminate the need for inserts with full prescribing information now required, the cost of the compendium would be borne by the drug industry. Supplements will be issued from time to time to keep the compendium as up-to-date as possible, and it is also provided that all drug labeling and advertising must conform with the information found in the compendium.

III—Establishes a committee which will compile a formulary of drugs necessary for good medical practice, for purposes of direct procurement by the Federal Government and reimbursement for all Government financed programs, indicating the best drug available for each therapeutic category, in order to assist the physician in his prescribing of medication.

IV—Gives the Secretary of Health, Education and Welfare the authority to require batch-by-batch certification of all drugs—when needed—which will include provisions prescribing standards and identity of strength, quality and purity, tests and methods to determine compliance with such standards, and other measures necessary for the public good.

[17] *Congressional Record,* Proceedings and Debates of the 92nd Congress, Vol. 117, No. 166. November 4, 1971.

V—Prohibits the distribution of sample drugs without the written request of the physician. Furthermore, the sale of sample drugs, either directly or indirectly, is prohibited.

VI—Is a general section providing that (1) potentially dangerous drugs will be labeled with the appropriate warning; (2) labeling of drugs will be required so that all active ingredients will be clearly labeled; (3) no drug salesman shall make any oral presentation regarding any drug until he has placed before the physician or pharmacist an FDA approved document about the drug; and (4) the Secretary of HEW shall approve all advertising in advance that appears in either the electronic media, or in any publication or advertising circular, for any drug. The Secretary will approve only advertising which does not mislead or misrepresent the product, either in text or layout.

VII—Is designed to protect the American public against excessively high and discriminatory prices for drugs through mandatory licensing of drug patents at a reasonable royalty.

Needed reform is always difficult to achieve. There are those who have vested interests, while the uninformed and the complacent are always ready to make their peculiar contributions. There is considerable doubt whether the Kefauver-Harris Drug Amendments would have become law without the "help" of the tragic thalidomide incident in Europe.

In 1937, when the sulfanilamide drugs were first introduced, a chemist at the suggestion of a salesman tried to put the drug out in liquid form. He used diethylene glycol as a solvent, which proved to be deadly and killed 108 people. A few simple tests would have proven the toxicity of the compound. The law at that time did not require even these kinds of simple testing procedures. An outraged public moved its representatives to put into effect the Federal Food, Drug and Cosmetic Act of 1938. It is disquieting to realize that a supposedly sophisticated society such as ours still relies on tragedy and disaster as a stimulant for progress. How long can we afford to do so?

Protection of the Consumer

Years ago when the marketplace was simple and uncomplicated, when bartering of services and produce was in order, the slogan "Let the buyer beware!" was the only protection one had. It was the individual's responsibility to make a good bargain. Today, the individual has less and less control over matters concerning his purchase of health products and services. As stated by Dr. James L. Goddard, all the consumer has is a great deal of faith.

"If the doctor is not qualified, they wouldn't let him practice."

"If the medicine is no good, they wouldn't let it on the market."

"If the lab is not accurate, they wouldn't give it a license."

"If the insurance doesn't cover it, they wouldn't allow the policy."

"If the records are wrong, they wouldn't put them into the machine."

"They" constitute the vast and highly sophisticated teamwork upon which the individual now instinctively relies because he has no alternative. This is especially so in the field of public health. The quality and integrity of his life, along with the lives of his unborn children and his aging parents, are intimately entwined with "them." "They"—and I suggest we include all our health professionals in this category—"They" are making decisions, setting standards, adjusting the environment, controlling production, forming judgments, and otherwise surrounding the individual citizen so that "consumer choice" is worthy of more careful examination.[18]

Let us look more closely at "They," namely the governmental and private organizations that endeavor to protect the consumer.

The Food and Drug Administration (FDA)

The major function of the Food and Drug Administration is the enforcement of the Federal Food, Drug and Cosmetic Act, which is designed to protect both the consumer and law-abiding manufacturers and dealers. This federal agency does *not* have responsibilities for the supervision of advertising of foods, nonprescription drugs, and cosmetics. They *do* have responsibilities for supervising advertising for prescription drugs. The FDA is a scientific law-enforcement agency. Its scientists test the toxicity of ingredients used in foods, drugs, and cosmetics and evaluate the potency and effectiveness of various drugs and vitamins. The FDA also has facilities and personnel to do extensive research. For these functions the FDA is staffed with bacteriologists, pharmacologists, biochemists, physicians, veterinarians, lawyers, and entomologists, among others. It has a total staff of approximately 6,300 working out of 20 major cities in the country. The FDA has a legal staff for the preparation of its court cases. All inspectors are responsible for the gathering of evidence for the prosecution of violations in the courts. Criminal prosecutions are made against individuals or firms responsible for violations. These involve the unsanitary food factory operation, shipment of filthy or decomposed food, shipment of substandard food and drugs, and the false or misleading claims for drugs and dietary supplements.

In 1970 there was again a major administrative reorganization of the Department of Health, Education and Welfare. The Public Health Service was reorganized into three functioning units which consisted of the National Institutes of Health, Health Service and Mental Health Administration, and the Food and Drug Administration. The FDA, as one of the three operating agencies of that service, itself began reorganization and evolved with six major Bureaus and two additional functioning units.

1. *Bureau of Foods* is responsible for the purity, safety, and wholesomeness of foods, food additives, colors and cosmetics. It conducts research designed to improve the detection, prevention, and control of contamination which might cause illness or injury conveyed by foods, colors, and cosmetics. It samples and tests for pesticide residues in food and enforces those tolerance levels that have been established by the Environmental Protection Agency.

[18] James L. Goddard, M.D., "Public Health and the Consumer." Delivered at the 63rd Annual Health Conference, May 24, 1967.

2. *Bureau of Radiological Health* is concerned with the protection against unnecessary human exposure to radiation from electronic products and in the healing arts.

3. *Bureau of Drugs* has the responsibility for overseeing the safety and efficacy of the nation's drug supply both prescription and over-the-counter (OTC) products. This bureau monitors the clinical tests of new drugs before they are put on the market and follows up the drug after its release for any unexpected side effects. Inspectors investigate drug plants to be sure ingredients are pure and facilities are complying with sanitation regulations, as well as the other facets of good manufacturing procedures which prevent errors in the drug production, labeling, and distribution. All batches of insulin and antibiotics for human use are tested for purity and potency. The FDA has authority over the advertising of prescription drugs only. These drug advertisements that are aimed at physicians must be truthful and fully informative. Advertising of OTC drugs on television and radio or in magazines and newspapers falls under the jurisdiction of the Federal Trade Commission.

4. *Bureau of Veterinary Medicine* requires that veterinary drugs, devices, and medicated foods be safe and effective to ensure the health and safety of the animal and to ensure the wholesomeness of the food derived from treated animals. Particular attention is given to residues of drugs found in the tissues of slaughtered animals.

5. *Bureau of Biologics* is responsible for assuring the safety, purity, and potency of biologic products which include vaccines, antitoxins, blood and blood products for human use.

6. *Bureau of Product Safety.* As of this printing, the Bureau of Product Safety will be separated from the FDA as a result of the signing of the Consumer Product Safety Act on October 28, 1972. The new agency will have jurisdiction over former FDA programs of the Hazardous Substances Act and the Child Protection and Toy Safety Act, the Flammable Fabrics Act, as well as the National Electronic Surveillance System (NEISS).

7. *Executive Director for Regional Operations* executes direct authority over all the nineteen FDA regional offices. It serves as the liaison for activities between FDA, state, and local agencies.

8. *National Center for Toxilogical Research* is not a bureau but a multiagency facility that will provide a national resource for projecting through animal studies the effects on man of an increasing array of chemicals in his environment. The FDA will administer the new facility but the Environmental Protection Agency and a number of other government agencies will utilize the center for assessing potential health hazards from chemicals in foods, drugs, and from environment sources. The following exemplify some FDA actions which benefit the consumer:

In 1972 the Food and Drug Administration announced a massive and unprecedented review program to ensure that the many thousands over-the-counter drugs (OTC, those sold without a prescription) were safe, effective, and had fully informative labeling for self-treatment of minor, symptomatic conditions. The FDA was concerned that many formulations did not have the claimed effect, or adequate instructions for effective use by the consumer. They were also concerned about those drugs that were promoted in deceptive and indefensible ways. The FDA set up expert panels to evaluate ingredients, dosages, and conditions for use of each of at least 26 basic classes of OTC products. These included such preparations as antacids, cough remedies, stimulants, laxatives, and analgesics. Since it was estimated that there were anywhere from 100,000 to 500,000 separate items, it was necessary to do the investigation by product categories. From this evaluation came monographs for each basic class of OTC drugs. Each product had to meet the standards of the monograph or be reformulated to meet the standards in order to gain approval. Sometimes this means reapplying through the FDA new drug application system.

This new investigative program was unprecedented in scope and intensity. It was designed to build a permanent system of offering all American consumers the best possible assurance that every OTC drug not only was safe and adequately labeled but that it did what the manufacturer claimed it would do for the relief of minor illnesses and discomfort.

Later in that year,

> The Food and Drug Administration published new findings from the National Academy of Sciences which took issue with the extent of the claims made for 14 brands of over-the-counter analgesics, including Bufferin, Nebs, and Tylenol. . . . While attesting to the pain-relieving capability of aspirin, the panel said the claims that Bufferin acts "twice as fast as aspirin" and "helps prevent the stomach upset often caused by aspirin" lacked supportive evidence. . . . The study also indicated that Darvon—the nation's most frequently prescribed drug—was of questionable effectiveness. . . . The efficacy of Darvon had been seriously challenged two years prior by medical researchers at the University of Chicago, who reviewed the 20 best studies comparing Darvon to other analgesics. They concluded that Darvon "is no more effective than aspirin or codeine and may even be inferior to these analgesics," and attributed the drug's wide popularity in large part to "promotional efforts which have included large expenditures for advertising in medical journals, detailing to physicians (visits to doctors by drug company employees), and distributing free samples."[19]

In a similar action the Food and Drug Administration has announced its conclusions concerning the effectiveness of certain mouthwash and gargle preparations. It concluded that there is a lack of substantial evidence that those preparations are effective for any of their labeled claims which relate to antimicrobial, antiseptic, germicidal, and analgesic uses. Examples of the type claims made for these products follow:

> "Effectively destroys bacteria that cause bad breath in the mouth—and stays active against bacteria for hours" . . . "combat cold symptoms and minor throat irritations" . . . "to help against the spread of infection" . . . "temporary

[19]"Aspirin: A Bitter Pill for the Ad Men," *New York Times*, April 23, 1972.

relief of minor sore throat and mouth irritations" . . . "long acting antibacterial action."[20]

THE FEDERAL TRADE COMMISSION (FTC)

The Federal Trade Commission has the responsibility of enforcing the Federal Trade Commission Act of 1938 and the Wheeler-Lea Amendment of 1938. It was the Wheeler-Lea Amendment that empowered the Federal Trade Commission to control false or misleading advertisements of foods, drugs, cosmetics, and devices via the mass media. It attempts to review advertisements that are beamed out over 4,000 radio and television stations as well as those that appear in published material.

This agency has been notoriously understaffed and lacks a realistic operating budget for the massive assignment that it has. Advertisements are not reviewed by the Federal Trade Commission *before* they are used. The understaffed commission must not only *find* the misleading or false advertisement; it has the additional task of proving it false. Before any *substance* can be used in a food or a drug, its safety must be proven by the company to the FDA *before* it is marketed. With *advertisements,* the situation is quite the *opposite.* When the FTC wants to question a pseudoscientific claim in an advertisement, it must develop a sound medical-legal case against it. Studies need to be conducted to disprove claims that the manufacturers have backed up by "tests" and often self-styled "research studies." When the FTC has finally prepared its case, it issues a complaint to the advertiser. The advertiser has thirty days to respond to the complaint while the selling of the product via fraudulent advertising goes on. The advertiser often appeals the complaint, which means that a hearing must now be scheduled on a busy FTC calendar. If the decision at the hearing goes against the advertiser, he can appeal the decision to the FTC—another delaying tactic. If the FTC denies the appeal and issues an order to cease and desist, the advertiser can now appeal to the courts. The court decision can be appealed all the way up to the Supreme Court. If the advertiser finally loses, he is fined up to $5,000, which represents a drop in the bucket for a firm carrying on a nationwide operation. Though the misleading advertisement is now stopped, the advertiser by this time has developed a new approach, which, if misleading, could start the cycle all over again. As reported in Ralph Lee Smith's book *The Health Hucksters,* "The FTC finally stopped Carters Little Pills from claiming directly or indirectly that the pills aided the liver. The case took sixteen years."[21] Meanwhile, practically a generation of Americans were purged of more than their money, for in essence Carters Little Pills are a laxative.

More recently the Federal Trade Commission came under close investigation by three young men

[20]Reprinted from Federal Register of August 4, 1970; 35 F.R. 12411. Department of Health, Education and Welfare, Food and Drug Administration (21 CFR Part 3) Labeling of Mouthwash, Mouth Freshener and Gargle Preparations.

[21]Ralph Lee Smith, *The Health Hucksters* (New York: Hillman-McFadden, 1961), p. 187.

who were dubbed "Nader's Raiders" by the newspapers. Their critique on the commission demonstrated to the increasingly dissatisfied consumer and taxpayer that something was amiss in this stagnant government bureau. "Cases of unadulterated thievery have stretched on and on before being resolved, while the offender reaped profits never to be returned and devised new schemes not covered by the cease and desist orders."[22]

The critique carefully outlined where the FTC was negligent in carrying out their assigned duties either by design or incompetence. In 1969 a presidential commission recommended to the President of the United States that, indeed, drastic reforms were needed in the FTC. In 1970 with a new chairman, the commission underwent some administrative reforms and structural overhauling. In some newer cases the commission called on the *manufacturers* to substantiate claims of safety, performance, and therapeutic value instead of assuming the burden of proof. The commission's tough new policy was demonstrated again in the spring of 1972 when Anacin, Bayer Aspirin, Bufferin and Excedrin were accused of misleading the public with false advertisements. Not only were the advertisements to "cease and desist" but the commission "called for two years of corrective advertising to remove the heavy veil of deception from the public eye."[23]

[22]Edward F. Cox, Robt. C. Fellmeth, and John E. Schulz, "The Nader Report" on the Federal Trade Commission (New York: Richard W. Baron, 1969), p. ix, Preface by Ralph Nader.

[23]"Aspirin: A Bitter Pill for the Ad Men," *New York Times*, April 23, 1972.

Another example of the FTC's more vigorous policy has been its battle against the J. B. Williams Company, makers of Geritol. This governmental agency concluded that the advertisements for Geritol were deceptive because most people suffering vague, tired feelings were not helped by the product. The Geritol makers violated a series of "cease-and-desist" orders while the case seemed hopelessly stalled in the courts. After almost 14 years of battling, a Federal judge in 1973 fined the Williams Company $812,000 for deceiving the public into thinking that their product was a panacea for that "tired blood" feeling. These are excellent examples of how constructive, intelligent criticism can bring about changes within our institutions.

The Federal Communications Commission (FCC)

The Federal Communications Commission is charged with the responsibility to see that the airways are used in the public interest. Although this kind of mandate implies almost limitless powers to prevent commercial abuses, it is rarely used. It has not only permitted misleading advertisements but also recognized quacks who reach the public through these media.

The realization that the television commercial as the country's biggest drug pusher is beginning to take hold. In 1972, the FTC urged the FCC to develop regulations mandating "counter-advertising" and "to provide free time for broadcasting replies to commercials that raise issues of current public importance."[24] Heretofore, this had been done only with cigarette advertising until 1971 when cigarette commercials on radio and television ended. Now, however, enlightened consumer groups are demanding honest advertising for all products as well as issues. For example:

> a Washington-based consumerism group called the Stern Community Law Firm filed a complaint with the FCC after the three networks rejected a counter-commercial dealing with the 1971 recall of some 2 million Chevrolets with defective engine mounts. The Stern-produced spot lists recalled models and warns: "If you have one of these Chevrolets, it could cost you your life. Get it to a Chevrolet serviceman . . . slowly."[25]

Another countercommercial displays samples of six top-selling analgesic products while the commentator says, "The American Medical Association has found remedies like these to be either irrational, not recommended or unsound."[26]

Hopefully, the countercommercials will force the advertiser to rid his ads of the misleading and deceptive information. However, some advertisers are threatening to withdraw their advertising from television rather than have their product attacked by countercommercials, as did the tobacco industry.

[24] *National Clearinghouse for Smoking and Health,* February 1, 1972.

[25] *Newsweek,* June 5, 1972, p. 65.

[26] Ibid.

THE POST OFFICE DEPARTMENT

The Post Office Department's Division of Fraud and Mailability can act against parties attempting to use the United States mail for the purposes of fraud. The Fraud Statute empowering the Post Office to take action in these cases was enacted by Congress in 1872. The Post Office can issue a fraud order to a company that is sending through the mail materials with the intent to defraud. The aged legislation on the basis of which the Post Office operates inhibits it from taking consistently effective action because of its many loopholes. The Post Office may be successful in stopping the sale of a fraudulent product through the mails and yet be unable to prevent a mail circular from going through announcing where the product is available.

THE BETTER BUSINESS BUREAUS

As stated by Mr. Hugh Jackson, President of the Better Business Bureau of metropolitan New York:

> The Bureaus continue to have as their first and primary purpose the promotion of action to assure that advertising and sales representation shall be truthful, informative and responsible, and that these goals shall be reached, to the maximum extent possible, through the processes of voluntary business self-regulation. But they have also taken on the responsibility of seeking to assist both business and consumers through the handling of thousands of individual complaints where members of the consuming public feel that they have been unfairly treated in eco-

nomic transactions of all types. And in many more thousands of instances, they have become information centers to which the public, as well as business itself, may turn for free and impartial factual information on the reliability of companies or business offers based on the files developed by the Bureau through knowledge and experience with the companies inquired about. The Better Business Bureaus have, to an increasing degree, sought to advance the objective of responsible and ethical practice by widespread education of the public.

. . . We are ready, willing and able to work in close cooperation with governmental authorities in those instances where voluntary self-regulation does not succeed or where we uncover actual fraud or flagrant misrepresentation. Our friends and colleagues from the field of government can attest to the closeness of this relationship and the fact that many of the matters with which they must deal are brought to them, with facts and evidence, by the Better Business Bureau.[27]

Professional Organizations

The American Medical Association, the American Dental Association, as well as others set standards of education and performance for their members. They also concern themselves with fraudulent practices with regard to services and products in their areas. The American Medical Association's Department of Investigation checks on practices in medical quackery. Its Council on Foods makes studies of manufactured foods. The Council on Physical Medicine reports on nonmedical devices and apparatus that are sold to the public, physicians, and hospitals. The Council on Dental Therapeutics sets standards and approves dental products. These professional organizations work closely with the federal agencies in their efforts to control fraudulent practices.

Evaluating Health Information

Making judgments with regard to advertisements and claims for health products and services is not easy. Some questions a person might ask in the evaluation of health products and services are:

1. Do they lead one to self-diagnosis and self-medication?
2. Are services being sold on the basis of personal testimonials?
3. If research findings are quoted, who did the research? Were they done by qualified and unbiased people?
4. If authorities are quoted, who are they?
5. If literature is presented, is it acceptable to medical, dental, and public health professionals?
6. Does the sales appeal play on fears, or superstitious beliefs?
7. Is the sponsor of the product or services a recognized, bona fide organization?
8. Is the product offered as a cure-all or as a sure cure for cancer, arthritis, or heart disease?

Where doubts exist with regard to health products and services, they should be checked out with the family doctor, the local health department, the Better

[27] "Quackery," New York State Congress on Health Quackery (April 1965), pp. 48–49. Sponsored by The Medical Society of the State of New York.

Business Bureau, or the school or college health educator. Well-recognized organizations occasionally put out publications evaluating certain kinds of health information that is of value to the consumer. The Arizona Dietetic Association, Inc., has made available a publication to help individuals choose reliable books on nutrition. The opening statement of this publication indicates that,

> Nutrition books are being published in growing numbers, and they run the full gamut of reliability. Some are excellent, many are misleading and faddish in approach, and others are false and unreliable. There is no official censorship of substandard books. Readers are exposed to the poor along with the good. The result is that food quackery has flourished and its teachings have become a serious potential danger to health.[28]

Some books that were RECOMMENDED for the general public were listed as follows:

Deutsch, R. M., *The Family Guide to Better Food and Better Health,* Des Moines, Iowa, Meredith Corp., 1971, $7.95.

(Reviewed J.N.E., Fall 1971: Recommended for reading by the interested layman. Dr. Philip White of the A.M.A. wrote "This book fills a void that has existed all too long. Until now there has been no totally acceptable, comprehensive book on nutrition for the layman. I think now we have one. The book will do much to help those who seek a positive approach to good health. It likewise should dissuade others from going the way of the food faddist.")

(Reviewed J.A.D.A., November 1971: This book is surely an answer to those professional persons who have long asked: "What nutrition book can I refer to my patients and/or friends?" It will also help those professionals who have difficulty in speaking in "lay" nutrition terminology. Teachers, social workers, nurses and other non-nutrition professionals alike should find this a valuable reference.)

Fleck, Henrietta, *Introduction to Nutrition,* New Jersey, The Macmillan Co., Second Edition, 1971, $8.95.

Commended for being up-to-date. It is clearly written, attractive and well organized. A good nutrition reference.

White, Philip L., *Let's Talk About Food,* Chicago, American Medical Association, Second Edition, 1970, paperback $1.00.

By giving answers to frequently asked questions, authoritative nutrition information is presented on a wide range of subjects of interest to the public.

Those books NOT RECOMMENDED according to this publication were:

Fredericks, C., and Bailey, H., *Food Facts and Fallacies; The Intelligent Person's Guide to Nutrition and Health,* New York, The Julian Press, 1965, $5.95.

(Evaluated C.N.A. Library Committee: This book presents the authors' own interpretation of the findings of research as applied to human disease. Many of the concepts are unsound. Their acceptance and application

[28]*Nutrition Books for Lay Readers: Recommended, Recommended for Special Purposes. Not Recommended,* The Arizona Dietetic Association, Inc., Education Section, Compiled 1972.

by the public could result in delay in seeking proper medical advice and treatment.)

Hunter, B. T., *The Natural Foods Cookbook,* New York, Simon and Schuster, 1961, $4.95.

(Evaluated C.N.A. Library Committee: Emphasis is placed in all recipes on "natural foods"—whole grains rather than refined flours, honey rather than refined sugar. There is no reason to question that the recipes are reliable and the foods tasty. However, the implication that good nutrition depends on the exclusive use of "natural foods" is not tenable.)

Hunter, B. T., *Consumer Beware, Your Food And What Has Been Done to It,* New York, Simon and Schuster, 1971, $8.95.

(Reviewed J.N.E., Fall 1971: This book cannot be recommended for the consumer for whom it is intended, nor is it an accurate reference book for the professional educator. The book is a one-sided attack on just about all aspects of the food industry. Although there are many threads of truth in the book, to attempt to answer all the charges and half-truths, point out the errors both in editorial content and typography, and bring the book up-to-date would mean writing another book.)

Stillman, Dr. Erwin Maxwell, and Sinclair, Sam., *Doctors Quick Weight Loss Diet,* New York, New York 10017, Dell Publishing Co., 1970, paperback $1.25.

Davis, A., *Let's Eat Right to Keep Fit,* New York, Harcourt Brace and Jovanovich, 1970, $5.50.

The author's account of how good nutrition can be obtained, why the Davis diet is prescribed, and what the consequences are of failure to meet the dietary standards constitutes a confusing mixture of fantasy, fact, inconsistency and outright error.

Davis, A., *Let's Get Well,* New York, Harcourt, Brace and World, Inc., 1965, $4.50.

(Evaluated Chicago Nutrition Association Library Committee: This book is a confusing combination of fact and fiction. There is a surfeit of documentation on some of the basic findings of nutrition, but the interpretations of such findings are over-simplified and the conclusions drawn, as to treatment of disease, are often at variance with accepted medical practice.)

Other Books of the Same General Character by the Same Author: *Let's Have Healthy Children, Let's Cook It Right, Vitality Through Planned Nutrition.*

At a luncheon in the spring of 1972, Adelle Davis was confronted by nutritionists, educators, consumer advocates, and food manufacturers. Her statements concerning premature births and a lack of Vitamin E were challenged by a high-ranking official of the Food and Drug Administration. When asked why she advocated doses of Vitamin A and D that were known to be toxic in some people, she replied, "I accept your criticism, and promise to be more careful hereafter."[29]

Consumers Union, a nonprofit organization, is another organization with the consumer's interest at heart. It is responsible for a monthly publication

[29] "Adelle Davis vs. the Scientists," *The Washington Post,* May 4, 1972.

called *Consumer Reports* in which all kinds of consumer commodities are evaluated. These products, ranging from vacuum cleaners to contact lenses, are rated after careful laboratory and use tests, thus enabling the consumer to get the best product for his money. Medical doctors serve as consultants to Consumers Union and make judgments on matters of health and medicine. Their comments are based on the study and findings of many research scientists and research institutions. The Consumers Union publication, *The Medicine Show,* is concerned with health-related products and services. The following statements represent the nature of their evaluations.

On Medicines for Colds

The latest fads in the hotly competitive cold remedy field concern not ingredients so much as dosage forms—the sustained-release preparations, of which *Contac* is one of the most heavily advertised, and the aerosol medications such as *Congestaid* and *Pertussin.* The latter release a spray compounded of menthol (a mild anesthetic), glycols (antibacterial agents long ago shown to be without therapeutic value when sprayed in the air), and flavoring oils. Even if the ingredients were effective medications, common sense would make one wonder how anyone could get a large enough dose from the room air with these products. There are, in fact, no published reports of controlled trials indicating that either preparation can give the relief from congestion that is claimed.[30]

[30]*The Medicine Show* (Mount Vernon, N.Y.: Consumers Union, 1971), p. 20.

On Gargles for Sore Throats

The chief claims in TV commercials for *Isodine Gargle* have been that it "stops sore throat pain fast" and "reduces inflammation."

Most sore throats are the result of infection with either bacteria or viruses. With respect to the latter, an antiseptic gargle is an obvious waste, since viruses as they are found in the throat tissues cannot be destroyed or inhibited by any known antiseptic. Many bacteria, on the other hand, *are* susceptible to destruction or inhibition by antiseptics. But the germs that the gargles reach are not important in terms of disease.[31]

On Cosmetics

. . . In this remarkable world, you are invited to lubricate the skin with a product whose prime action removes fats and oils (*Dove* detergent bar). You can be tranquilized by a simple antiperspirant ("Ice Blue" *Secret*). And you can cure dishpan hands by washing dishes (*Ivory Liquid*).

All these exaggerations are embellishments attributed for promotional purposes to products of basically limited usefulness. Common sense says the products cannot possibly do all that is claimed for them. Why, then, does not the Federal Trade Commission step in?

For one thing, most cosmetics claims are not susceptible of proof, either true or false; what researcher would care to find proof, for example, of the claim that a cosmetic can make your body "a scented column of silken smoothness and your presence a sheer delight"?[32]

[31]Ibid., p. 27.
[32]*The Medicine Show* (Mount Vernon, N.Y.: Consumers Union, 1963), p. 187.

Many articles and editorials in *Today's Health* magazine evaluate health products and services. Innumerable publications of this type are also available from the Food and Drug Administration, the United States Public Health Service, official health agencies, and various voluntary health agencies (American Heart Association, American Cancer Society, National Mental Health Association, and others).

The Practitioners of Health Care

Preparation for the profession of medicine requires four years of college work and an additional four years of medical school. This is followed by a one- or two-year internship. All physicians must be licensed by the State Board of Medical Examiners before they can practice within that particular state. Reciprocity between some states exists; however, where it does not, the physician who may already be practicing in one state must take the state board examinations of the new state to which he intends to move in order to practice there. National board examinations are the basis for state licensing in three-fourths of the states. The physician thus trained is usually referred to as a general practitioner or family doctor. This physician may refer a patient with a complex problem to a medical specialist who has specific preparation in depth in a particular area of medicine.

The medical specialist requires advanced specialized training plus practice in the specialty for two or more years. The physician must in addition pass an examination by an American Examining Board.

To check the credentials of a physician, one need only refer to the American Medical Association Directory found in any local library. The AMA Directory will indicate if the physician involved has a membership in the local medical society and the AMA, and if he is certified by the appropriate specialty board (be it for the area of pediatrics, internal medicine, obstetrics, or any of the others). The Directory will also indicate fellowship in the American College of Surgeons or the American College of Physicians. In choosing a family physician, another criterion to be considered is whether the doctor is continuing postgraduate work in his area of specialization to help him keep up with current developments in his field. How thorough the physician may be is another criterion for evaluation. The doctor who leaves no stone unturned is less likely to make an avoidable error of omission.

Types of Medical Specialists[33]

Allergist. One who treats and diagnoses body reactions which show hyper-sensitivity to drugs, pollens, foods, animals, or other things (a subspecialty of internal medicine).

[33]Definitions of medical specialists have been adapted or quoted from *Stedman's Medical Dictionary*, 20th ed. (Baltimore: The Williams & Wilkins Company, 1961); *Today's Health* (January 1963), pp. 12–13; W. W. Bauer, ed., *Today's Health Guide* (Chicago: American Medical Association, 1965); *Health Careers Guidebook* (Washington, D.C.: U.S. Govt. Printing Office, 1965).

Anesthetist or Anesthesiologist. One who administers an anesthetic to effect a loss of consciousness (general anesthesia) or a loss of sensation in a specific location (local anesthesia).

Cardiologist. One having special knowledge and experience in the diagnosis and treatment of heart disease (a subspeciality of internal medicine).

Dermatologist. A practitioner who specializes in the diagnosis and treatment of cutaneous lesions and the related systemic diseases; a "skin specialist."

Endocrinologist. One who deals with the internal secretions of the ductless glands and their physiologic and pathologic relations.

Epidemiologist. One who specializes in the study of the determinants and distributions of disease prevalence.

Family Physician. One who specializes in a new area called Family Practice. This area of specialization deals with preventive medicine for the entire family.

Gastroenterologist. A specialist in the diseases of the digestive system.

Gerontologist or Geriatrician. One who specializes in the science of the physiologic and pathologic changes incident to old age.

Gynecologist. The physician who specializes in the branch of medicine which has to do with the diseases peculiar to women, primarily those of the genital tract, as well as female endocrinology and reproductive physiology.

Internist. A physician trained in internal medicine, which is the medical specialty concerned with illnesses of a nonsurgical nature, mainly in adults.

Neurologist. A specialist in the nonsurgical treatment of diseases of the nervous system.

Neurosurgeon. A specialist in the diagnosis and surgical treatment of the nervous system.

Obstetrician. One who is skilled in the medical care of a woman during pregnancy and in childbirth and the interval immediately following.

Ophthalmologist or Oculist. A specialist in diseases and refractive errors of the eye.

Orthopedist or Orthopedic Surgeon. One who specializes in the branch of surgery that has to do with the treatment of chronic diseases of the joints and spine and the correction of deformities.

Otolaryngologist. A specialist in the diseases of the ear and larynx.

Otologist. A specialist in the diseases of the ear.

Otorhinolaryngologist. A specialist in the diseases of the ear, nose, and larynx.

Pathologist. A specialist in the identification of disease through the analysis of body tissues, fluids, and other body specimens.

Pediatrician. A medical practitioner who specializes in the prevention, diagnosis, and treatment of diseases in children.

Plastic Surgeon. The physician who specializes in the branch of operative surgery that corrects or repairs deformed or mutilated parts of the body.

Proctologist. A specialist in the science that deals with diagnosis and treatment of the colon, rectum, and anus.

Psychiatrist. A specialist who deals in the interpretation and treatment of mental and personality disorders.

Radiologist. A physician who is skilled in the diagnostic and therapeutic use of X-rays and other forms of radiant energy.

Rhinologist. A specialist who deals with the disorders of the nose.

Surgeon. A specialist who treats diseases through operative measures.

Urologist. The physician who specializes in the study, diagnosis, and treatment of diseases of the genito-urinary tract.

Dental Specialists

Dentists are individuals trained to care for the health of the mouth, teeth, and supporting tissues. The degrees of DDS (Doctor of Dental Surgery) or DMD (Doctor of Dental Medicine) are awarded after completion of a course of study at approved dental schools. The dentist today is becoming more and more allied with the field of medicine. His early training parallels that of the medical student, with great emphasis on the basic sciences. This background is necessary because of his key role in the detection of oral cancer and in the dental treatment of patients with diabetes, hemophilia, or allergies. Because he is licensed to prescribe drugs, he needs to have a background parallel to that of the medical student.

State board examinations must be passed in order for a dentist to practice. Graduate schools offer specialization in particular areas of dental medicine. Following are a few of the dental specialists with a brief description of each:

Endodontist. One who specializes in the diagnosis and treatment of diseases of the pulp (or nerve) of a tooth. This specialty embraces methods of pulp conservation as well as tooth retention once infection at the root has developed.

Orthodontist. The dental specialist who is concerned with the correction and prevention of irregularities of the teeth and malocclusion of the jaw.

Pedodontist. One who specializes in the treatment of dental ills of children.

Periodontist. A dentist who specializes in the treatment of the supporting tissues of the teeth.

Prosthodontist is concerned with the construction of special appliances (dentures, bridges, crowns) to compensate mechanically for oral deficiencies such as tooth loss and cleft palate.

Osteopathy

Osteopathic Physician (Doctor of Osteopathy, D.O.). A practitioner licensed to practice medicine and surgery who includes in his treatment some elements of manipulative therapy, which must not be confused with the adjustments and manipulations practiced by the nonmedical chiropractor. Today the osteopathic physician is recognized as having training comparable to the medical general practitioner. He is licensed to practice osteopathic medicine and surgery in all states. In some states the osteopathic and medical associations have merged. The American Osteopathic Association has resisted such a move on the national level for fear that it would merely be absorbed by the larger American

Medical Association and lose its distinctive recognition of the function of the musculoskeletal system in health and disease.

Initially, osteopathic practice was based on the theory that malfunction was related to disalignment of the body. It has since developed philosophy, training, and practices that are more closely related to the medical profession. Osteopathic medicine encompasses all phases of medicine, for example, anesthesiology, dermatology, internal medicine, neurology, and so forth. There are 6 osteopathic colleges in the United States. In addition to the provision of four years of training, the student serves a year of internship in one of 263 osteopathic hospitals, and has the option of specializing in any of the specialties with postgraduate training.

Nonmedical Specialists

Optician. A craftsman who is skilled in the grinding of lenses according to the prescription of the oculist or optometrist, and properly sets these lenses in the frames.

Optometrist. A graduate from a school of optometry and licensed in all fifty states to measure visual acuity and to prescribe glasses and other nonmedical measures.

Orthoptist. A technician trained to correct defects of the ocular muscles through eye exercises and visual training as prescribed by the oculist.

Podiatrist. One who engages in the specialty that includes the diagnosis and treatment (either medical, surgical, mechanical, or physical) of the diseases, injuries, and defects of the human foot. A number of podiatrists are affiliated with hospitals and are generally recognized as being a paramedical profession. The National Association of Chiropodists in 1958 decided to change its name to the American Podiatry Association. While Podiatry (Podiatrist) and Chiropody (Chiropodist) are synonymous terms, Podiatry is now the preferred one.

Psychologist. An individual without a medical background who concerns himself with applying scientific methods to the study of human behavior. He may be a *School Psychologist* and perform such duties as testing, classifying, and counseling of students. If he is a *Clinical Psychologist,* he has earned a Ph.D. and has completed a supervised internship at a psychiatric clinic. If the clinical psychologist meets the standards set by the American Psychological Association, he is then qualified to diagnose and treat behavior disorders, usually through testing and other psychological diagnostic devices, without the use of medication.

Chiropractic

One of the most controversial groups in the health care field in the United States is that of chiropractic. Most medical doctors view them as akin to quacks; chiropractors view themselves as being the professional equals of medical doctors; others view their status as somewhere in between the first two assessments. Basic to the issue is the theoretical basis of chiropractic practice.

As stated in *Your Health and Chiropractic:*

These four principles make up the bedrock of chiropractic practice.

1. Anatomical disrelation can create functional disturbances in the body.
2. Disturbances of the nervous system are primary factors in the development of many disease conditions.
3. Spinal subluxations (minor displacements of spinal bones) are a specific cause of nerve irritation or interference.
4. The viscero-spinal principle: nerve irritation at the spine may lead to a disturbance in the function of one or more internal organs of the body.[34]

In sharp contrast to the above, Ralph Lee Smith in his publication, *At Your Own Risk: The Case Against Chiropractic,* questions leading physicians concerning chiropractic theory and practice:

"In your experience have you ever found the 'foramina or apertures between the vertebrae, through which the nerve branches issue from the spinal cord' narrowed and causing pressure upon a nerve or nerves? If so, under what circumstances?"

Dr. R. R. Bensley, Director of the Department of Anatomy of the University of Chicago responded, "In a period of twenty-nine years, during which time I have been Director of this Department, we have never found in our dissecting rooms a single instance in which the foramen or aperture between the vertebrae through which the nerve branches issue from the spinal cord have been so narrowed as to cause pressure upon nerves."

"In your judgment is it possible to reduce a subluxation or misalignment of the vertebrae and thus relieve pressure upon nerve branches by manipulation of the hand' "?

Dr. Dean Lewis, Surgeon-in-Chief of Johns Hopkins Hospital, said, "In my judgment it is not possible to reduce subluxation or misalignments of the vertebrae and thus relieve pressure of the nerve branches by manipulation of the hand."[35]

The American Public Health Association put forth in their journal the following statement concerning chiropractic and naturopathy:[36]

Chiropractic and Naturopathy

Chiropractors are licensed to practice throughout the United States (except in Louisiana and Mississippi). Naturopaths are also licensed in at least six states and the District of Columbia. These practitioners provide primary health care to a segment of our population, treating a wide range of diseases and conditions, including infectious diseases, heart conditions, and cancer, along with the musculoskeletal conditions for which they are commonly known and which are believed to be the major part of their practice.

The Department of Health, Education, and Welfare, at the instruction of Congress, recently conducted an intensive study of these two professions. On the basis of its findings, which are fully documented in the report, the department concluded that:

> Chiropractic theory and practice are not based upon the body of basic knowledge related to health,

[34]Thorp McClusky, *Your Health and Chiropractic,* (New York: Pyramid Books, 1962), p. 17.

[35]Ralph Lee Smith, *At Your Own Risk: The Case Against Chiropractic* (New York: Trident Press, 1969), pp. 144–145.

[36]Naturopathy is a healing art that relies on nature's forces. Water, air, sunlight, electricity, exercise, rest, and diet are prescribed in combinations suitable for each patient to cure disease.

> disease, and health care that has been widely accepted by the scientific community. Moreover, irrespective of its theory, the scope and quality of chiropractic education do not prepare the practitioner to make an adequate diagnosis and provide appropriate treatment. Therefore, it is recommended that chiropractic and naturopathic services not be covered in the Medicare program.

It appears that the practice of chiropractic and naturopathy constitutes a hazard to the health and safety of our citizens. The American Public Health Association therefore urges:

1. That Congress amend Title XIX of the Social Security Act to specify that federal funds not be used to match state Medicaid expenditures for chiropractic or naturopathic services.
2. That Congress not amend Title XVIII of the Social Security Act to permit coverage of chiropractic or naturopathic services in the Medicare program.
3. That state legislatures and health agencies not include chiropractors and naturopaths under state health programs.
4. That states reevaluate their existing licensure program for chiropractors and naturopaths to determine whether such licenses should be further restricted or abolished, and that existing restrictions be more rigorously policed.
5. That professional and consumer groups undertake appropriate consumer education on the hazards of unscientific health care including chiropractors and naturopaths.[37]

[37] *American Journal of Public Health,* January 1970, American Public Health Assoc., Inc., Resolutions adopted by the Governing Council of the APHA, 1969, p. 179.

Harry Schwartz, science writer for *The New York Times,* asks the question:

> "Why, then, has chiropractic been able to grow, to gain state recognition and licensure in 48 of the 50 states, to mobilize substantial Congressional support for Medicare recognition of chiropractic, and—most recently—to win 'insurance equality' in New York?"
>
> In part the answer is that chiropractors are tenacious, skillful and patient lobbyists. But in part, too, there is no doubt that a significant number of Americans believe chiropractors have helped them, are willing to give testimonials to chiropractic, and to support chiropractors' political pressure on state and national legislators.
>
> Many people who come to their offices, doctors know, have primarily psychological rather than organic ailments. They can often be helped by anybody willing to listen to their troubles, be sympathetic, and do something—such as the laying on of hands that has an old tradition—which convinces the sufferer he is being helped.
>
> Another factor is the self-limiting nature of many diseases, the fact that many ailments end and suffering disappears after a time regardless of whether a person has received any kind of help.
>
> Finally, of course, there is the possibility that with respect to some back disorders—such poorly understood entities as low back pain, for example—chiropractic manipulation may be useful. Some neurosurgeons and orthopedists warn, however, that chiropractic manipulations may sometimes worsen a back problem.[38]

The American Public Health Association suggests

[38] "Chiropractic: Is the Name of the Game 'Flimflam'?" *New York Times,* July 18, 1971.

that states should reevaluate existing licensure programs for chiropractors to determine if such licenses should be further restricted or abolished and that existing restrictions be more vigorously policed. An example of the restrictions that exist in licensure laws for chiropractors can be found in New York State law. An exerpt from this law follows:

§ 6558. Rights of licensed practitioners

1. Each duly licensed practitioner who shall have complied with the provisions of this article, shall have the right within this state to practice chiropractic as defined in this article.[39]

2. The practice of chiropractic, as herein defined, is hereby declared not to be the practice of medicine, or osteopathy, or physiotherapy within the meaning of the laws of the state of New York defining the same, but nothing in this article contained shall be construed to restrain or restrict any licensed physician or osteopath, or physiotherapist in the practice of his profession.

3. A license to practice chiropractic shall *not* [italics mine] permit the holder thereof:

a. to practice obstetrics, psychiatry or any medical, surgical or paramedical specialty or sub-specialty;

b. to perform surgery of any kind or to reduce fractures or dislocations;

c. to treat for any of the following conditions: any infectious diseases such as pneumonia, any communicable diseases listed in the sanitary code of the state of New York, any of the cardio-vascular-renal or cardio-pulmonary diseases, any surgical condition of the abdomen such as acute appendicitis, or diabetes, or any benign or malignant neoplasms.

d. to prescribe, administer, dispense or use in his practice biologicals, drugs, medicines, sera, vaccines or hormones;

e. to use any diagnostic or therapeutic methods involving chemical or biological means or the use of electrical devices, except those devices approved by the board as being essential to the practice of chiropractic; or

f. to use radio-therapy, fluoroscopy, or any form of ionizing radiation except X-ray which may be used only as provided in this subdivision; (i) X-ray shall only be used for the purposes of chiropractic analysis; (ii) such use of X-ray shall be confined to persons over the age of 18; and (iii) the area of such X-ray exposure shall not extend below the level of the top of the first lumbar vertebra. The requirements and limitations with respect to the use of X-ray by chiropractors shall be enforced by the state commissioner of health and he is authorized to promulgate rules and regulations to carry out the purposes of this subdivision. Chiropractors shall retain for a period of three years all X-ray films taken in the course of their practice, together with the records pertaining thereto, and shall make such films and records available to the state commissioner of health or his representative on demand. Added L.1963, c. 780, § 1, eff. July 1, 1963.

Index to Notes

Laboratory analyses and examinations

1. Diseases, treatment of

Chiropractors are not authorized to diagnose or treat patients for disease.

[39]Definition of chiropractic according to Article 132, Section 6550, New York State Education Law: "'The practice of chiropractic' means a method of detecting and correcting, by manual or mechanical means essential to the practice of chiropractic, structural imbalance, distortion, or subluxation in the human body for the purpose of removing nerve interference and the effects thereof, where such interference is the result of or related to distortion, misalignment or subluxations of or in the vertebral column."

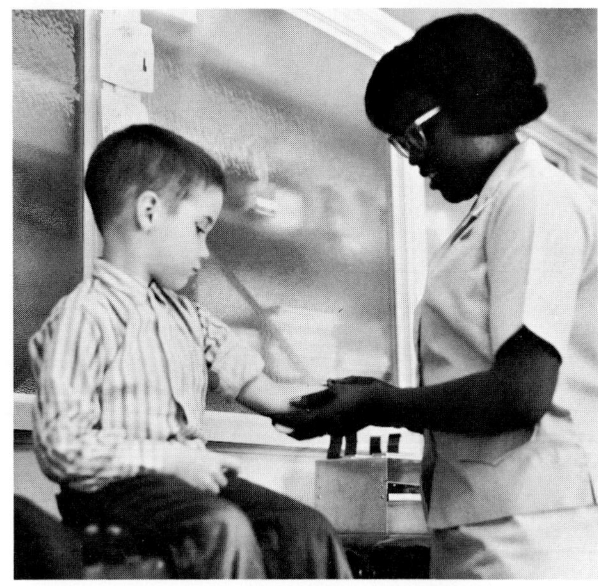

Fig. 11-6. An allied health professional, a member of the health care team. (N.Y.S. Dept. of Health)

It could be a fruitful exercise to review the state licensure laws for varied health professional groups to determine the legal limits of their professional practice.

While chiropractors accuse physicians of inflexibility in not recognizing chiropractic, physicians are equally dismayed at chiropractors who refuse to recognize the value of eminently successful medical procedures such as immunization programs. Epidemics of smallpox, diphtheria, and polio have been reduced to almost zero incidence, not through the spinal manipulations to reduce subluxations, but through programs of immunization. As stated by Dr. Andrew V. Friedrichs of the Department of Pathology and Bacteriology at Tulane University: "the chiropractors advocate . . . that all immunization and inoculation for polio, tetanus, typhoid, smallpox, diphtheria, to name a few, and many other diseases which are combatted by immunization and inoculation, be discarded, to be replaced by manipulation of the spinal column, to normalize the flow of nerve impulses."[40]

The Department of Health Education and Welfare developed a Report on chiropractic. Some of their conclusions include:

1. There is a body of basic scientific knowledge related to health, disease, and health care. Chiropractic practitioners ignore or take exception to much of this knowledge despite the fact that they have not undertaken adequate scientific research.
2. There is no valid evidence that subluxation, if it exists, is a significant factor in disease processes. Therefore, the broad application to health care of a diagnostic procedure such as spinal analysis and a treatment procedure such as spinal adjustment is not justified.
3. The inadequacies of chiropractic education, coupled with a theory that de-emphasizes proven causative factors in disease processes, proven methods of treatment, and differential diagnosis, make it unlikely that a chiropractor can make an adequate diagnosis and know the appropriate treatment, and subsequently provide the indicated treatment or refer the patient. Lack of these capabilities in independent practitioners is undesirable because: appropriate treatment could be delayed or prevented entirely; appropriate treatment might be interrupted or stopped completely; the treatment offered could be contraindicated; all treatments have some risk involved with their administration, and inappropriate treatment exposes the patient to this risk unnecessarily.
4. Manipulation (including chiropractic manipulation) may be a valuable technique for relief of pain due to loss of mobility in joints. Research in this area is inadequate; therefore, it is suggested that research based upon the scientific method be undertaken with respect to manipulation.[41]

The Changing Nature of Health Care

Anyone who has ever watched television is familiar with the character "Doc" from the western "Gunsmoke." "Doc" was a trusted friend in the community. His mere chin-rubbing presence assured every-

[40] Ralph Lee Smith, *At Your Own Risk*, p. 151.

[41] HEW Report of Chiropractic, pp. 196–197.

one that needed help was at hand. In addition to his ability to probe for bullets in human beings (a Dodge city avocation!), he also delivered babies and treated a variety of folk for a variety of ailments aided only by the pitiful few aids he carried in his little black bag—a kind of nineteenth-century "trick or treat" medical approach. It was an era when a great many people died of "natural causes," with equal numbers recovering from their ailments for the same reasons. With the advent of the twentieth century, medical research produced voluminous amounts of new medical information. Since no one man could master such great amounts of knowledge, this resulted in physicians' specializing in specific areas of medical care as well as the development of varied allied health professional groups who became part of the health care team. The twentieth century also brought forth sophisticated (and expensive) diagnostic and therapeutic equipment that the individual doctor could not afford to buy. In the last few decades, there has therefore been a definite trend toward increased medical group practice. With the increased sophistication in respect not only to knowledge but to diagnostic techniques, there has been emphasis on laboratory and technical procedures in the prevention, diagnosis, and treatment of disease. Not only did group practice make it easier to obtain expensive equipment but it also facilitated hiring of allied health staff. The sharing of this equipment and staff is not only an economical move but makes available to each physician a greater capacity for quality medical care. In group practice, there seems to be a greater emphasis on preventive medicine. There is greater opportunity for comprehensive physical examinations to catch disorders in their early stages before they are dangerous, or through health education to prevent them in the first place. Such practice also provides more free time for the doctors involved. Vacation time, as well as time for further study, can be scheduled much more easily because there are others to cover for the missing physician. In addition, it provides the doctor with the professional stimulant of working closely with other branches of medicine and leads to some healthy exchanges of information as well as philosophy. A possible disadvantage in this kind of arrangement is that some medical men find it difficult to work as part of a team. In addition, from the physician's point of view solo practice is usually a more lucrative one and can often produce greater monetary benefits than group practice. There are also dangers with regard to the doctor-patient relationship. Where a number of physicians are involved in the care of the patient, a more impersonal doctor-patient relationship may develop.

There are many variations of group practice. These might include groups of a few doctors or many doctors, with varied combinations of general practitioners and specialists. The majority of the groups operate on a fee-for-service basis (the patient attends the clinic for a particular medical service and upon receiving it pays the fee). The Mayo Clinic in Rochester, Minnesota, and the Lahey Clinic in Boston exemplify this kind of arrangement. Other group practice is financed by the prepayment insurance plan that involves comprehensive coverage. The

New York City Health Insurance Plan (HIP) exemplifies this kind of group practice. The original purpose of HIP was to care for the municipal workers in New York City; however, others may now join the plan. It has some thirty-two medical centers. People who join this plan have a choice of physicians within each of these groups. A number of them work for HIP on a part-time basis with a private practice on the side. This organization boasts a department of health education stressing education as one of its aspects of preventive medicine.

Recent scientific advances as well as socioeconomic developments indicate that there will be a further growth of medical group practice. This form of medical practice is increasingly acceptable to both physicians and the general public.

Financing Costs of Health Care

There have been dramatic increases in the cost of health care in this country. In 1950 the average health care expenditure for an individual was $79 a year; by 1970 this amount rose to $324. At the present time approximately $70 billion a year is spent on health care, more than five times spent two decades ago. While 50 per cent of the rise in costs reflects an increased population and greater utilization of health services, the other 50 per cent in increased costs reflects higher prices.

Through the years it has been noted that *direct* payments for medical costs have been reduced as a result of broader health insurance coverage. In 1950, 9.7 per cent of medical costs were covered by insurance benefits; by 1960 this rose to 24.2 per cent. The objective is to have this kind of coverage extend to 90 per cent of health care costs.

Voluntary Health Insurance

There are five basic types of health insurance policies that are generally offered by insurance companies. These are:

Hospital Expense Insurance. Coverage provides to some degree for room and board in addition to drugs, anesthetics, and the use of the operating room. General nursing care is also covered. Coverage may be for maximum periods of 60, 90 or 100 days. Hospital expense insurance is the most popular one, with more people being covered by this kind of protection than any other type.

Surgical Expense Insurance. This type of coverage pays part or all of the surgeon's fee for a given operation. The policy will usually list various kinds of operations and the amount it will allow for each. There are variances in the amounts allowed for operations and these, of course, are covered by varying insurance premiums. This type of insurance is often combined with hospital expense insurance.

General Medical Expense Insurance. This type of coverage will pay part or all of the physician's bills other than for surgery. It will cover a doctor's call at the hospital or the home or for patient's visits to the physician's office. Often this kind of policy will include diagnostic, X ray, and laboratory fees. The policy will indicate the amount that is payable as well as the maximum number of calls that it will cover.

Major Medical Expense Insurance. This type of coverage is to provide payment for exceedingly heavy medical and hospital bills. It is intended to prevent the wiping out of a persons' savings and the possibility of being thrown into debt. This type of policy picks up where hospitalization and surgical plans leave off. Costs in excess of these plans are covered by major medical policies taking care of physicians' fees, hospital bills, nursing care, drugs, and any other expenses arising out of treatment in or out of the hospital. These policies may pay up to 10,000 dollars or more in medical expenses. In order to keep the premiums of major medical insurance within reasonable limits, they may contain a deductible provision similar to deductible auto insurance whereby the policyholder will pay a certain amount before the policy takes over. In some instances, the deductible feature of the policy may be combined with a coinsurance clause. The policyholder in this case may pay 25 per cent of costs past the initial deductible amount, with the insurance company paying the remainder or 75 per cent of major medical costs. Major medical insurance is the most recent type of health insurance as well as the fastest-growing one.

Loss of Income Insurance. This type of insurance helps to replace income that is lost during a period of illness or disability, and is usually written for the family breadwinner. It permits the family to pay its rent, buy its groceries, and cover its basic costs of living. Its benefits usually begin a week or two after the illness or disability occurs. Some policies, however, call for 30-, 60-, or 90-day waiting periods before payments start. Insurance of this type that provides 50 per cent of regular salary is considered good. Many families plan to pay the costs of minor illness out of their regular income and rely on health insurance for coverage for longer disability periods.

Federal Health Insurance Programs

Medicare (Title 18), enacted in 1966, is a health insurance program for older people. The *basic* part of this plan is financed through social security payments during a person's working years. At the age of 65, the person is eligible to receive medicare benefits that include hospital and nursing home care, home visits by nurses, and limited out-patient services in hospitals. The purpose of the program is to provide paid-up health insurance for older people for the time in their lives when they need it most.

The *voluntary* portion of Medicare is financed by a modest monthly premium payment by the individual. This part of the program helps to defray costs of doctor bills, X rays, and other diagnostic tests, surgical supplies, and various therapeutic appliances, iron lungs, or artificial limbs, physical therapy, and drugs.

When an aged person with Medicare cannot pay his portion of medical costs under this plan, he may be helped by the Kerr-Mills Medical Assistance program (Medicaid). This program is operated by the states and subsidized by the federal government. Criteria to determine if a person is in need of financial assistance vary from state to state. If a state decides that a patient is indigent, it would under this plan pay for the patient's portion of Medicare costs.

Title 19 of the Social Security Act established a federal-state program for health care of the needy and medically indigent. Persons eligible for medical aid under this program would include the aged, the blind, the disabled, and medically indigent children under 21. It also provided that states participating in the Kerr-Mills program must provide, as a minimum, five kinds of services:

1. Inpatient hospital services.
2. Outpatient hospital services.
3. Doctor's services.
4. Nursing home services.
5. X ray and other laboratory services.

Title 19 serves as a supplement to Medicare by providing the states with additional assistance to pay for the premium of the voluntary portion of Medicare for those aged who are in need. It may also pay for the patient's share of the Medicare bill.

Inequities in Health Care

Those of us who are dedicated to the cause of public health are today faced with a cruel paradox. On the one hand, our colleagues in health-care research have fashioned for us new tools for combating disease and premature death; they have made enormous progress in devising new techniques, inventing new lifesaving procedures, discovering new drugs to aid in the prevention, diagnosis and treatment of disease, and in giving us an opportunity for a meaningful, positive health experience even in chronic illness. On the other hand, we are often frustrated by our inability to make available and accessible to all our people the full measure of comprehensive health-care services that scientific medicine has made possible. This paradox represents today's greatest challenge for all who work in the field of health care. It is a challenge to our ingenuity and resourcefulness to organize and administer new patterns for providing the total complex of high-quality health care and to find the financing needed to make these services available to all our people.[42]

Within our population we have groups who do not have access to adequate medical care. They include the unemployed, the disabled, and their families. There are also the "medically indigent," a group who are otherwise self-supporting but who cannot afford the added costs of medical care. It is ironic to note that those groups most in need of health services are also least capable of purchasing them. There have also been disparities in the quality of medical care among the poor and those in rural areas as compared to the higher-income groups of the urban areas. This has in part been due to inequities in the distribution of physicians, other health personnel, and facilities.

The national average physician-to-population ratio is 150 to 100,000. This is the number once cited by a Surgeon General as that necessary to protect the health of the people. But in many areas of our Nation, mostly in inner-

[42]"Closing the Gaps in the Availability and Accessibility of Health Services." *The 1965 Health Conference of the New York Academy of Medicine*, Vol. 41, No. 12 (December 1965), p. 1201.

ADULT MEDICAL
CLINIC
EVERY WEDNESDAY
3-5 P.M.
7-9 P.M.
CHILDREN'S CLINIC
EVERY TUESDAY & THURSDAY
2-4 P.M.
AT THE
HEALTH CENTER

Fig. 11-7. We have within our population, groups who do not have access to adequate medical care. (N.Y.S. Dept. of Health)

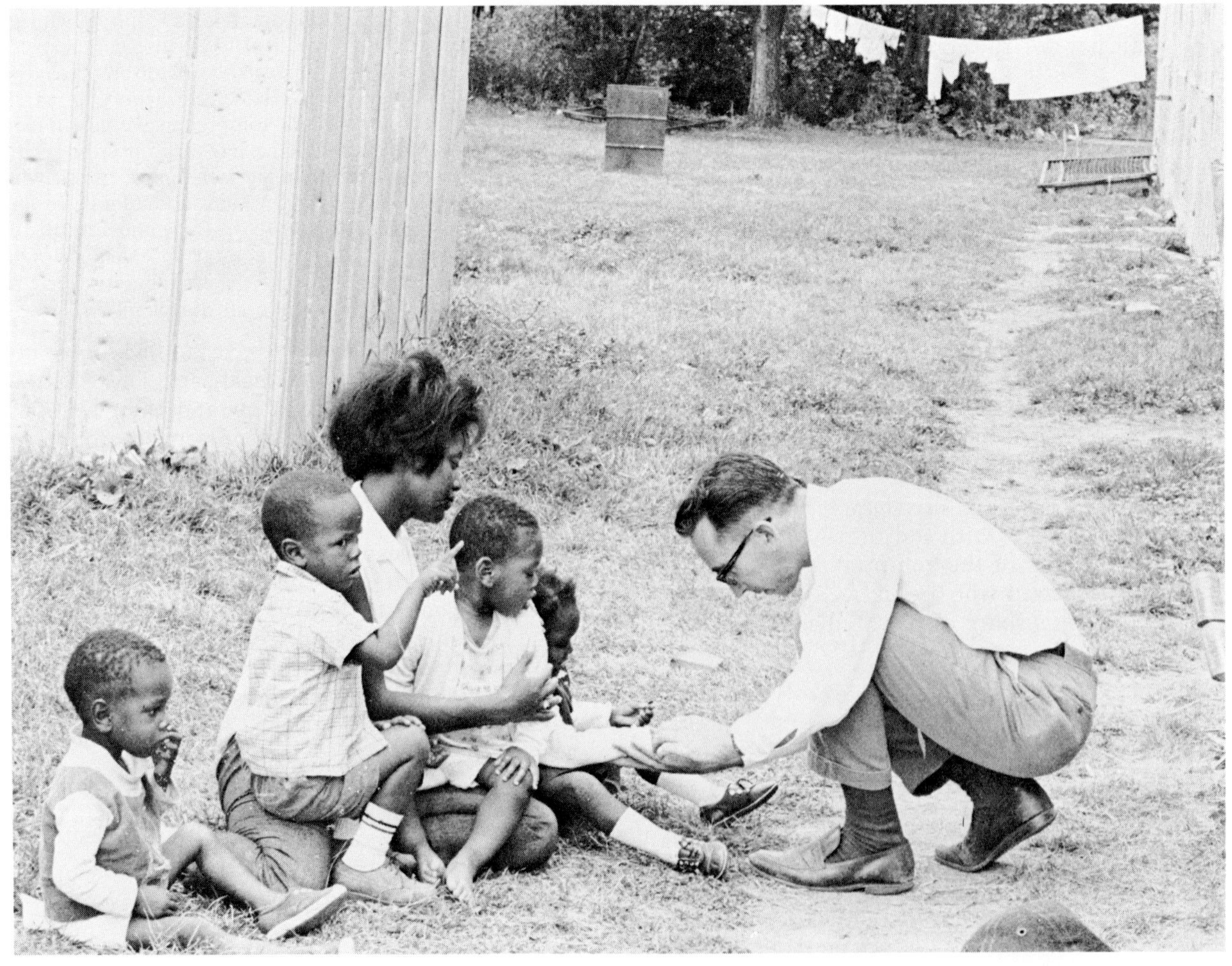

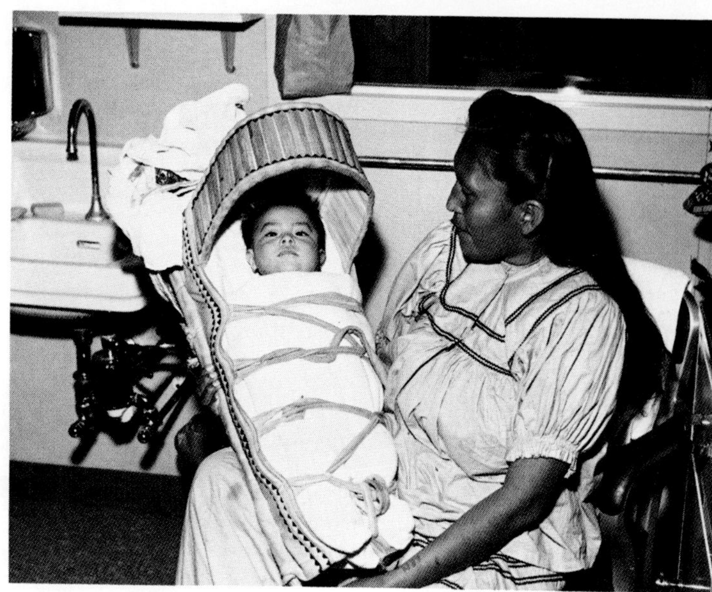

Fig. 11-8. Apache mother visits the health clinic with her baby. (Indian Health Service, Dept. of Health, Education and Welfare)

city and rural areas, there are far fewer than 150 physicians per 100,000 people. In the Kenwood area of Chicago, for example, there are five physicians per 100,000 people. And in the South Bronx in New York City, in East Los Angeles, and in central St. Louis, the ratios are less than 50 to 100,000. In the rural areas similar situations prevail. In all of Kansas there are only 108 physicians per 100,000 population. In one five-county area, this decreases to less than 45 to 100,000. In Mississippi the figures are 88 to 100,000, with certain areas decreasing to less than 20 to 100,000. The facts are then quite clear—health care is simply not available to many Americans.[43]

Though the major medical centers will continue to be located in high population urban areas, a system of primary treatment available to all population groups needs to be developed. In addition, a system for referring those in need of the more sophisticated services of the medical centers must be made available.

A major factor inhibiting the availability of medical care has been its skyrocketing costs. In the decade 1960–1970 the costs of hospital care rose 170 per cent and physicans' fees 60 per cent, as compared to an average rise of 30 per cent in consumer prices during that same period. Some have concluded that the rising costs of medical care have even made the middle- and upper-middle-income Americans medically indigent.

[43]William R. Roy, M.D., *The Proposed Health Maintenance Organization Act of 1972.* Sourcebook Series Volume 2, Science and Health Communications Group, 1730 Rhode Island Ave., N.W. Washington, D.C. 20036.

The problem has been further aggravated by shortages of physicians and other health personnel. As both voluntary and government health insurance plans proliferated, greater demands for health care have placed added strains on an understaffed health care system.

Why has the health care system witnessed an increase in the cost of care? Why does the health care system remain inflationary and inefficient? The answer must be *incentives.* There is not an individual, or group, or corporation, or governmental agency in our society that is responsible for controlling health care costs. Instead, the more services a provider's patient uses, the more it is paid.[44]

In essence the health care delivery system is rewarded for *treating* illness, but not for *preventing* illness and maintaining a healthy population.

In addition, the manner in which some health insurance is written causes the inappropriate use of already strained medical care facilities. For example, an individual in need of an X ray series finds that the cost of this procedure will be covered by his health insurance only if he is hospitalized for it. If the X rays are done on an outpatient basis, then he has to assume the costs. He naturally seeks to be hospitalized for the X rays, resulting in not only the inappropriate use of the hospital but the unnecessary costs of a hospital stay. There is need therefore to redesign the organization of medical care delivery *and* the way it is financed.

[44]Ibid., p. 10.

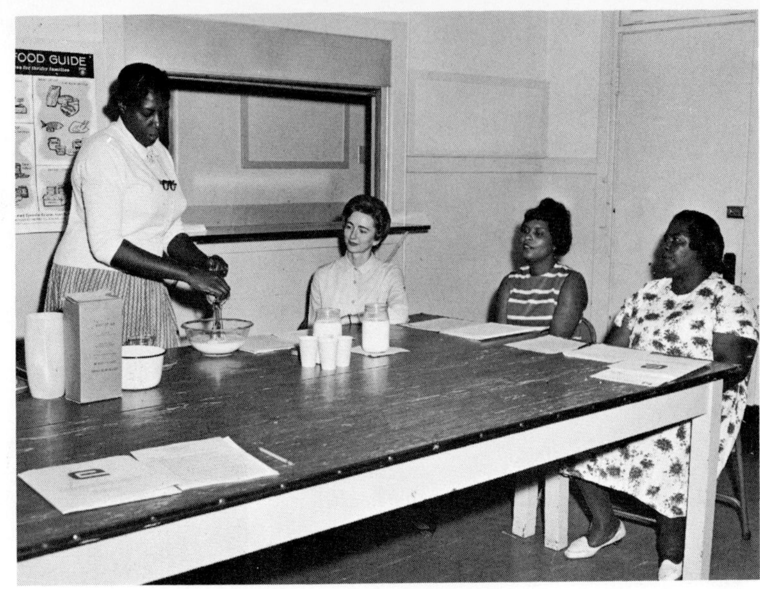

Fig. 11-9. Health educators and dieticians are becoming increasingly a part of the preventive medical team. (N.Y.S. Dept. of Health)

A Look to the Future

We are entering an era that will be marked with a level of health consciousness and action that is unprecedented. It will be accentuated with an increasing intolerance for preventable disease and infirmity and an increased desire for higher levels of health. There will be greater and more widespread demand for high-quality medical care. Some rather startling changes are already taking place, not only in the practice of medicine, but in the manner in which it is organized and financed.

The practice of medicine as an individual enterprise is being transformed into one involving highly organized teams of health personnel operating in groups and/or in hospitals with the latest of modern equipment. Open heart surgery, for example, is not undertaken by an individual doctor, but by a team of physicians, nurses, and technicians in a hospital where a heart-lung machine is available as well as other facilities and equipment needed for this advanced operative procedure. Those who advocate that medical group practice be related to medical or hospital centers appear to be responding to the dictates of advancing technology and knowledge. The highly expensive and complex preventive diagnostic and therapeutic equipment and personnel can no longer be duplicated in each doctor's office, but must be centrally located in the community.

Specialism in medicine is also resulting in the development of a large number of allied health professions. They include medical librarians, statisticians, health educators, social workers, and dieticians, among others. This broad development of allied health professional personnel is partially due to a reduction in the number of physicians in proportion to our growing population. It is expected that the population will continue to outgrow the number of doctors who will be graduated from our medical schools. Increasing emphasis on comprehensive care and preventive medicine is another reason for the expected proliferant development of the allied health professions. The physician already represents less than 10 per cent of the health personnel in a developing "health industry."

The concept of comprehensive care is one that has been gaining momentum. It refers not only to diagnosis, treatment of disease, and rehabilitation, BUT *to the promotion of health and the prevention of disease as well.* This approach is in sharp contrast to that in which a person would seek out a doctor only *after* illness has occurred and oftentimes when the illness has reached a terminal stage. The increase in the number of allied health personnel gives the physician more time for patient care, thus compensating somewhat for the doctor shortage. It also escalates the potential in the area of preventive medicine. It makes possible testing by the technician, for example, counseling by a social worker, educating by the health educator. These are functions that the overworked physician has less and less time for. Preventive medicine is on the threshold of universal acceptance. Although there will probably always be a need for therapeutic medicine, perhaps the following poem will indicate the need for greater medical and health emphasis on the *preventive* aspects.

The Parable of the Dangerous Cliff

Twas a dangerous cliff, as they freely confessed,
Though to walk near its crest was so pleasant;
But over its terrible edge there had slipped
A duke, and full many a peasant.
The people said something would have to be done,
But their projects did not at all tally.
Some said, "Put a fence 'round the edge of the cliff;"
Some, "An ambulance down in the valley."

The lament of the crowd was profound and was loud,
As their hearts overflowed with their pity;
But the cry for the ambulance carried the day
As it spread through the neighboring city.
A collection was made, to accumulate aid,
And the dwellers in highway and alley
Gave dollars or cents—not to furnish a fence—
But an ambulance down in the valley.

"For the cliff is all right if you're careful," they said;
"And if folks ever slip and are dropping,
It isn't the slipping that hurts them so much
As the shock down below—when they're stopping."
So for years (we have heard), as these mishaps occurred
Quick forth would the rescuers sally,
To pick up the victims who fell from the cliff
With the ambulance down in the valley.

Said one, to his plea, "It's a marvel to me
That you'd give so much greater attention
To repairing results than to curing the cause;
You had much better aim at prevention.
For the mischief, of course, should be stopped at its source,
Come, neighbors and friends, let us rally.
It is far better sense to rely on a fence
Than an ambulance down in the valley."

"He is wrong in his head," the majority said;
"He would end all our earnest endeavor.
He's a man who would shirk this responsible work,
But we will support it forever.
Aren't we picking up all, just as fast as they fall,
And giving them care liberally?
A superfluous fence is of no consequence,
If the ambulance works in the valley."

The story looks queer as we've written it here,
But things oft occur that are stranger.
More humane, we assert, than to succor the hurt,
Is the plan of removing the danger.
The best possible course is to safeguard the source;
Attend to things rationally.
Yes, build up the fence and let us dispense
With the ambulance down in the valley.[45]

[45] The author of the poem is unknown. Quoted from *Farm Safety Review* (May–June 1966), published by the National Safety Council.

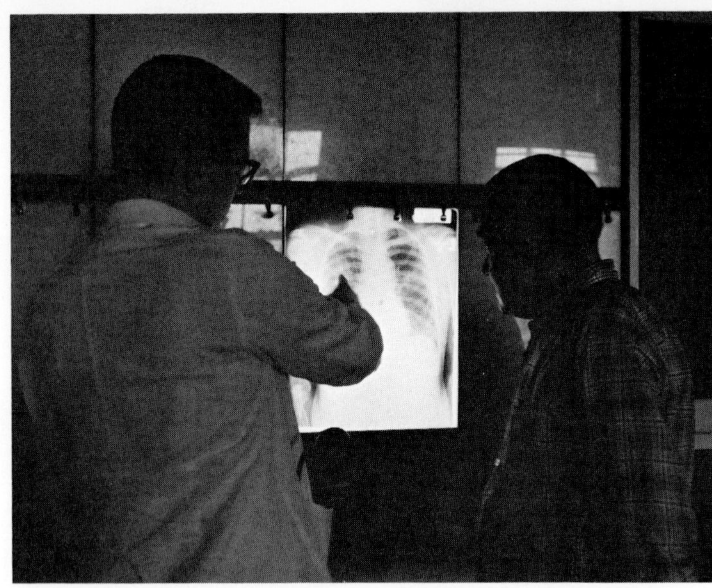

Fig. 11-10. Here is "The ambulance down in the valley . . ." (*N.Y.S. Dept. of Health*)

Fig. 11-11. but where is the "fence 'round the edge of the cliff?" (*N.Y.S. Dept. of Health*)

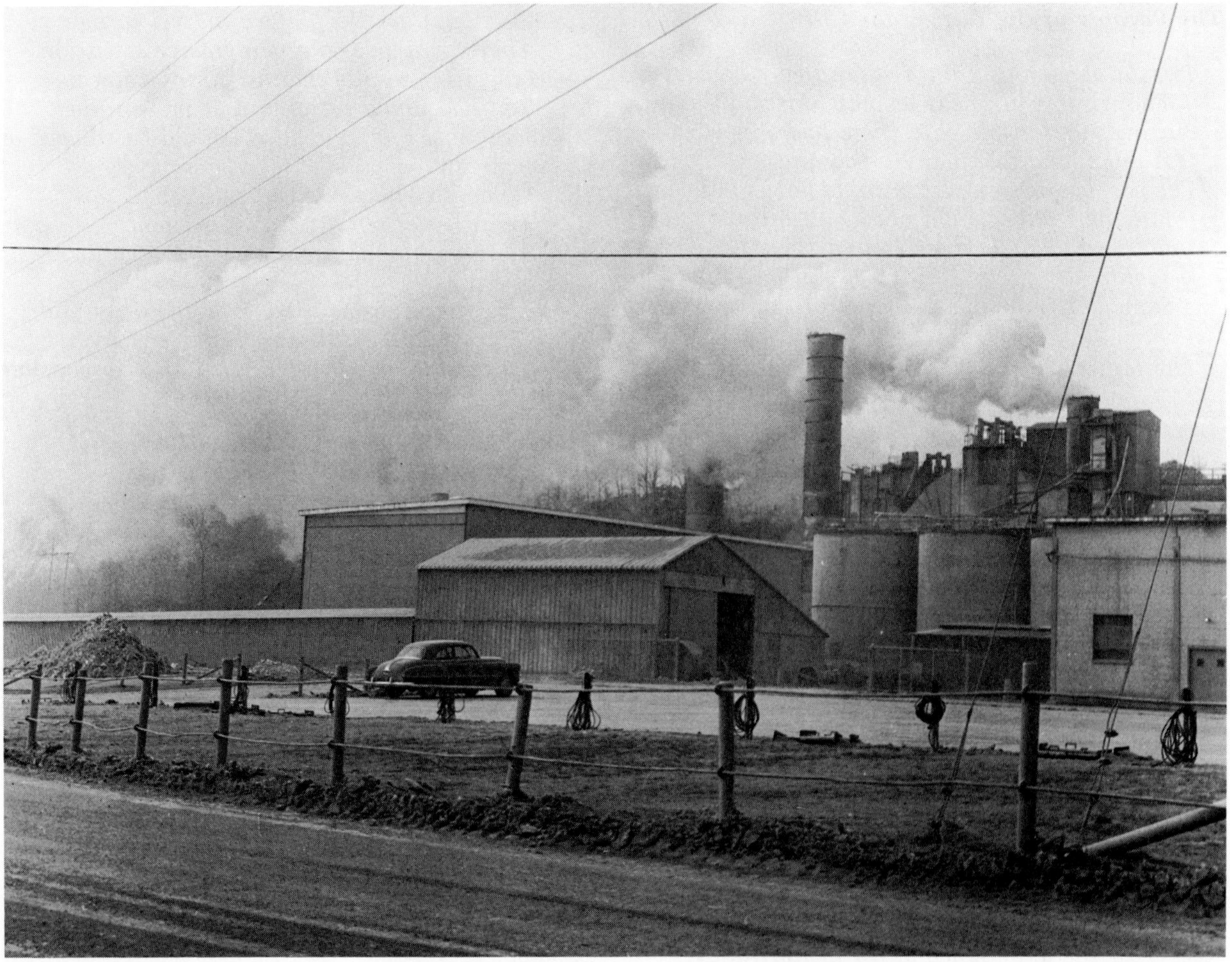

A community-based group of medical and allied health specialists with complementary skills and a concentration of preventive diagnostic and therapeutic facilities has a great potential for high-quality medical care. It is this kind of thinking that has led the federal government to give impetus to the development of a new medical care delivery system with the above ingredients.

The new medical care delivery system of the United States will consist of a series of Health Maintenance Organizations.

> An HMO, in addition to accepting payment for health care, assumes responsibility for actually providing health care services to its members. This is the major difference between an HMO and traditional indemnity health insurance such as Blue Cross/Blue Shield and Aetna. Indemnity insurance pays for health care if it can be found; an HMO provides the services itself. Since it controls the delivery mechanism itself, an HMO, unlike indemnity insurance, is in a position to guarantee the availability, accessibility, and continuity of care.[46]

The Health Maintenance Organizations will be in the form of prepaid health insurance financed by a varied combination of individual, employer, and government contributions. They will also feature group medical practice. Changes in medical care delivery have been stimulated by governmental activity in the form of legislation as well as finances.

With the developing philosophy that medical care is not a privilege but a right of the citizen, increased governmental activity in this area seems inevitable. As stated by Mencher, "We have permitted ourselves the luxury of debating for a longer period than any other western industrial nation the issue of government responsibility in this connection."[47] The developing thesis of our society appears to be one stating that we will educate according to ability and medicate according to need. The ultimate medical care goal, in whatever form it may take, will be to provide high-quality comprehensive health services for all.

Review Questions

1. How does one explain the extensive quackery problem prevalent in the United States?
2. Why does the Food and Drug Administration firmly enforce the federal regulations governing the testing of new drugs or vaccine, even when they are being used on terminal cases?
3. What can be identified as some of quackery's areas of gray? Why may this problem be of greater concern than outright quackery?
4. What is the role of the Food and Drug Administration in the protection of the consumer?
5. What are the responsibilities of the Federal Trade Commission? How is this federal agency handicapped in its efforts to carry out its assignment effectively?
6. What were the significant issues raised by the late Senator Kefauver's Senate subcommittee investigation of the drug industry?

[46] *The Proposed Health Maintenance . . .*, op. cit., p. 13.

[47] Op. cit., p. 1357.

7. What criteria should be used in the evaluation of health information and products? Identify those organizations that help the consumer in their evaluation.
8. Describe the professional preparation of the medical doctor. What kind of examination must he pass to practice in a state to become a specialist?
9. Why is the osteopathic physician generally recognized as comparable to the medical doctor who is a general practitioner?
10. Identify the various areas of specialization in dentistry. Describe the functions of each.
11. Define: (1) optician, (2) optometrist, (3) orthoptist, (4) podiatrist, (5) psychologist.
12. What have been some of the questions raised with respect to the quality of training of chiropractors?
13. What are the significant changes taking place in the organization of medical care?
14. What are the basic types of coverage found in health insurance policies?
15. Describe the factors that have resulted in the inequities of health care in this country.
16. How have the advances in the medical sciences actually resulted in greater medical care needs?
17. Describe the basic and voluntary portions of Medicare (Title 18).
18. What are the trends in medical care administration and practice? How do you envision the practice of medicine in the United States in the future?

Chapter 12
Drugs in Our Society

Take thou this vial, being then in bed,
And this distilled liquor drink thou off;
When presently through all thy veins shall run
A cold and drowsy humour; for no pulse
Shall keep his native progress, but surcease;
No warmth, no breath, shall testify thou livest;
The roses in thy lips and cheeks shall fade
To paly ashes, thy eyes' windows fall
Like death when he shouts up the day of life;
Each part, depriv'd of supple government,
Shall; stiff and stark and cold, appear like death;
And in this borrowed likeness of shrunk death
Thou shalt continue two-and-forty hours,
And then awake as from a pleasant sleep . . .[1]

Man has used drugs in one form or another for thousands of years. There is evidence that drugs were used even before 2100 B.C. Man, in his early use of drugs, thought that demons caused pain and that drugs capable of casting out these demons had magical qualities. Even today there are exaggerated notions as to the effectiveness of some drugs, as exemplified by the term "miracle" drugs used in referring to antibiotics. Although pain-relieving and sleep-producing drugs were known to man since 400 B.C., they were not used for surgery until the nineteenth century. The utilization of drugs for this purpose could have prevented much suffering.

[1] William Shakespeare, *Romeo and Juliet*, Act IV, Scene I, from *The Complete Works of Shakespeare*, ed. by George Kittredge (Boston: Ginn, 1936), p. 1035.

Through trial and error our forefathers discovered a number of useful drugs. Opiates, digitalis (a blood vessel dilator), ephedrine (a stimulant), and reserpine (a tranquilizer) are examples of drugs that came to us from primitive medicine. Many of the early drugs that were used had no real effect on the ailments they were supposed to relieve. People using them felt better simply because they thought they were being helped. This is still true today, of course, in too many instances where the use of self-prescribed drugs often indicates a kind of self-doting.

Modern Drugs and Their Contributions

Man has always had the fond dream of finding a drug that would counteract every disorder that plagued him. Man would rather be told that there is a vaccine or drug that will prevent or cure a disease than be asked to follow a specific regimen of diet or exercise that would accomplish the same thing. Significant advances have been made in the discovery of a number of chemical substances that have proved to be quite helpful in the prevention and control of many diseases. Antibiotics like penicillin destroy disease-causing bacteria. Other drugs control inflammatory reactions found in arthritis or convulsions related to epilepsy. Pain-relieving drugs range from fairly simple substances like aspirin to the powerful opiates. Mood drugs such as stimulants can help individuals out of depressive states, while the tranquilizers can have a quieting effect. Diuretics help the body to get rid of excess fluids, and antihistamines are used to control allergic reactions. The effect of all this has been a major contribution to life expectancy, which has increased from 47 years in 1900 to approximately 70 years in 1966. It is estimated that more than 5 million Americans are alive today as a result of the changes in the mortality rate in the last three decades. More than 90 per cent of the prescriptions that are now written are for drugs that did not exist 25 years ago. Approximately 800 to 900 drugs are extensively used by the general public in the United States at this time.

The nature of drugs varies considerably. A number of them come from plants. Penicillin, reserpine, and quinine would serve as examples. Others are obtained from animals, as in the development of vaccines. Most drugs, however, are chemical compounds that are developed in the laboratory.

The human body is, in essence, a chemical factory that produces drugs of its own in the form of hormones and enzymes. These substances have the function of controlling various body processes such as growth, digestion, and activity. The introduction of "foreign" drugs into this chemical factory often results in unexpected reactions called *side effects* that can many times prove harmful. Side effects can be as mild as a slight rash and as severe as convulsive death. How a drug will affect a particular person can never be completely predictable, because each person's body chemistry varies. A physician's supervision in the use of more powerful drugs is naturally a wise idea. These more powerful drugs are usually classified as prescription drugs.

Prescription Drugs

Prescription drugs, also referred to as *ethical* drugs, are those that can be bought only with a prescription from a medical doctor, a doctor of dentistry, or an osteopath. The Dunham-Humphrey Amendment of the Federal Food, Drug and Cosmetic Act forbids the filling of a prescription not authorized by these professionals. Dosages of prescription drugs are based on the person's age, height, weight, and his condition of health, among other things. In essence, the drug in this case is a rather personal thing. The giving of a prescription drug to someone else because he appears to have the same or a similar ailment in effect constitutes the practice of medicine without a license. It is at best foolhardy to attempt to diagnose an ailment when even the well-trained physician is hard put at times to accomplish this task.

The Kefauver-Harris Amendments of 1962 to the basic Federal Food, Drug and Cosmetic Act also require that a true and non-misleading brief summary of information as to side effects be included in prescription drug advertisements, thus forging another link in the chain of protection for the patient. However, the chain is broken by the patient himself if he attempts to obtain an illegal refill of his prescription. By law, a pharmacist may refill a prescription only on specific instructions, written or oral, from a physician. The physician chooses the drug after evaluating the possible side effects in relation to the hazard of the disease being treated. Use of the drug beyond the period of time originally intended, or use for another purpose, or for another patient, would short circuit the protection built into the law.[2]

[2]"FDA Memo for Consumers, CM-7" (Washington, D.C.: U.S. Dept. HEW, Food and Drug Administration).

Nonprescription Drugs (or Proprietary Drugs)

Nonprescription drugs are those that are sold "over the counter" or without a prescription. The law requires that these types of drugs have directions on the label with regard to their use. These directions should be followed carefully because any drug, if misused, can have deleterious effects. Typical warnings that may appear on the label would refer to:

1. Its safe use.
2. When *not* to use it.
3. When it should be discontinued.
4. When to see a doctor.

They usually read as follows:

> Don't apply to broken skin.
> Do not exceed recommended dosage.
>
> ---
>
> Do not drive or operate machinery while taking this medication.
>
> ---
>
> Discontinue use if rapid pulse, dizziness, or blurring of vision occurs.
>
> ---
>
> WARNING
> If pain persists for more than 10 days or redness is present, or in conditions affecting children under 12 years of age, consult a physician immediately.

Nonprescription drugs should be used for minor and short-term ailments. Any continuing illness or symptoms should be referred to a physician. It is wise never to become a steady user of *any* drug unless it is recommended by a doctor.

Drug Abuse

There are many ways to leave this world. All people in one manner or another "escape" temporarily through such things as daydreaming, sleep, or alcohol. Others escape permanently through death or irreversible psychotic conditions. Some use drugs as a temporary escape only to find their ensuing addiction to be rather permanent. It is perhaps analogous to the astronaut who leaves his spaceship for a brief venture into space and finds that he cannot return. He is rather ironically "trapped" in the vast regions of outer space. The drug user likewise is "trapped" in his fantasy world, never quite returning to a substantive reality. The escape becomes the entrapment.[3]

Drug abuse refers to the inappropriate use of drugs taken without medical advice, obtained illegally, or used in amounts that constitute a danger to the individual as well as the community.

The scope of drug abuse is an ever-widening one as the number of new drugs keeps increasing. An inherent danger in the improper use of these drugs is the development of drug dependence best described in terms of drug addiction or habituation. The World Health Organization has defined these terms as follows:

Drug Addiction is a state of periodic or chronic intoxica-

[3]John S. Sinacore, New York State Health Education Syllabus.

tion produced by the repeated consumption of a drug (natural or synthetic). Its characteristics include:

1. an overpowering desire or need (compulsion) to continue taking the drug and to obtain it by any means;
2. a tendency to increase the dose;
3. a psychic (psychological) and generally a physical dependence on the effects of the drug;
4. an effect detrimental to the individual and to society.

Drug Habituation (habit) is a condition resulting from the repeated administration of a drug. Its characteristics include:

1. a desire (but not a compulsion) to continue taking the drug for the sense of improved well being that it engenders;
2. little or no tendency to increase the dose;
3. some degree of psychic dependence on the effect of the drug, but absence of physical dependence and hence of an abstinence syndrome;
4. a detrimental effect, if any, primarily to the individual.[4]

Dr. Lindesmith, an authority in the social psychology of drug addiction, views addiction somewhat differently than does the World Health Organization as expressed in its definition. He feels that the key factor in addiction is related to the psychological craving for opiates when the individual realizes how potent these drugs can be in relieving the distress caused by withdrawal illness. He illustrates the point by asking one to

> imagine that a large amount of morphine has been unknowingly introduced into the water supply of a small community. In a few months the residents would become physically dependent on the morphine and would experience pain or discomfort whenever they failed to drink enough of the opiate water. In all likelihood, however, few if any of the residents would attribute their distress to a lack of water or morphine, nor would they recognize their pains as withdrawal distress, but would probably attribute them to rheumatism or arthritis or any number of ailments that normally beset human beings. Once a person moved away from the community the discomfort would eventually disappear. On the other hand, if a person learns that there is morphine in the water, attributes withdrawal distress to it and drinks the water to relieve the distress, then he is addicted—he has become "hooked."[5]

It is significant to note that a number of drugs that were hailed as safe when first discovered and introduced were later found to be addictive, strongly habituating, or harmful in other ways. Drugs demand a respect for their therapeutic values when properly used and for the dangers they present to health and life itself when abused. An aura of respect for drug agents does not pervade our society at the present time, as evidenced by increased drug dependence, drug intoxication, and death.

[4]"Report of the Task Force on Addictions," Section on Mental Health, New York State Planning Committee on Mental Disorders. June 1965.

[5]"Riddle of Addiction," Broadcast #6065—June 2, 1963, University of California, Radio-Television Administration.

Who Are the Drug Abusers and Why?

It is too often a presumption on the part of the older segments of our population that drug abuse is associated with the young. At the same time younger groups in the population see obvious widespread instances of drug abuse among their elders. In order to draw attention to our drug-oriented society Dr. Alton Dohner identified drug abusers as follows:

They are not all young. Neither are they all hippies, nor all hippies drug abusers. Drug abusers are physicians who recklessly prescribe amphetamines and tranquilizers rather than helping individuals learn to cope adequately with normal anxiety, frustration, depression and fatigue. Drug abusers are pharmaceutical companies who advertise their products to deal with "the everyday problems of anxiety and tension."

Drug abusers are truck drivers who take amphetamines for long runs; they are workers who use amphetamines to stay awake for night shifts or a second job. Drug abusers are students who use amphetamines to stay awake for studying.

Drug abusers are housewives who use amphetamines to give them the energy to complete everyday chores or allegedly to cut appetite and enable them to lose weight. Drug abusers are housewives and workers who live on tranquilizers and sleeping pills. Drug abusers are parents who give tranquilizers and diet pills to their children without a physician's prescription.

Drug abusers are businessmen who must have a martini with lunch; they are fathers who need a drink immediately upon returning home from the day's routine. Drug abusers are "the hidden alcoholic"—the housewives who drink several times each day.

Drug abusers are persons who smoke one or more packs of cigarettes per day. They are persons who drink 10 to 16 cups of coffee or endlessly consume cola drinks each day. Drug abusers are persons who take 20 to 40 aspirin tablets daily strictly for a mood effect.

Drug abusers are children and adolescents who sniff glue, gasoline, thinners and solvents. They are young people who try spices, their parents' medicines, nitrous oxide or unknown tablets in search of a high.

Drug abusers are high school and college students who continue to smoke pot or take LSD, mescaline and STP for alleged consciousness-expansion. Drug abusers are social dropouts who shoot heroin or amphetamines. They are businessmen, doctors, lawyers, etc., who daily take morphine or Demerol to avoid pain. This pain may be real or imagined, social, vocational, physical or psychological.[6]

After reflecting on the above statement it becomes difficult to describe inert chemicals as problems. Drugs are not the problem—people are! "After all, Adam and Eve have never been described as having had an 'apple problem'!"[7]

It is interesting to note that many of the motivations for drug abuse are common to young and old alike. Neither does it make much difference (from a health point of view) whether a drug is a legal or illegal one. Drugs are all potentially harmful ranging from marihuana to heroin among the illegal drugs,

[6]V. Alton Dohner, "Drugs Are Not the Problem," *Compact*, Vol. 4, No. 3 (June 1970), p. 21. Published by the Education Commission of the States.

[7]Gustave B. Timmel, "Description of a Drug Studies Course Taught in a College Camp Setting," *Journal of Drug Education*, Vol. 2, No. 1 (March 1972).

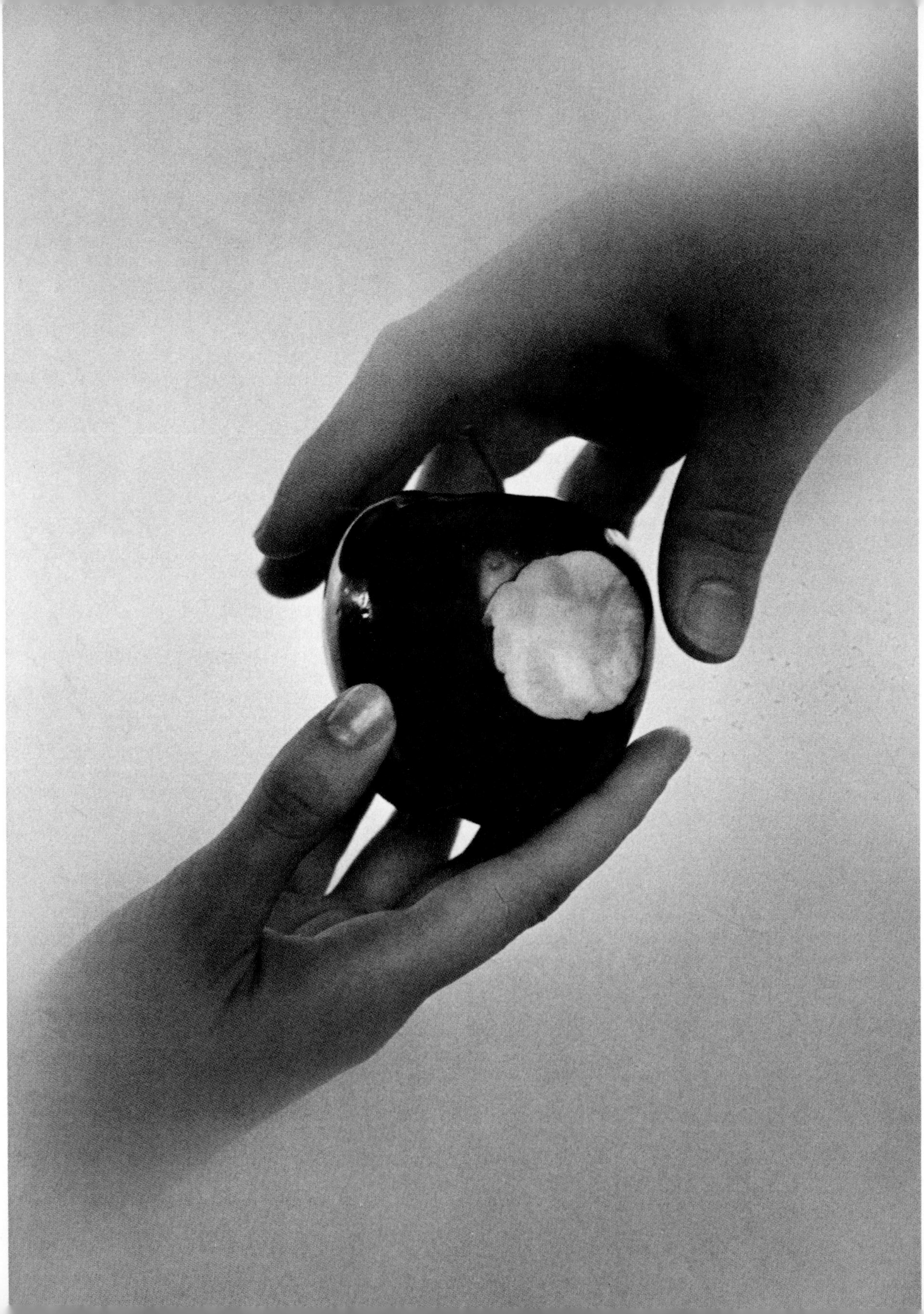

Fig. 12-1. It becomes difficult to describe inert chemicals as problems. Drugs are not the problem—people are! "After all, Adam and Eve have never been described as having had an apple problem!" (Robert M. Lightfoot III)

and from aspirin to barbiturates among the legal ones. The issue of drug abuse has often been emotionalized by an attempt to identify some drugs as being those of the young (i.e., marihuana) and others associated with the adult, (i.e., alcohol). Yet surveys have shown the drug most commonly used and abused by young people is alcohol, whereas marihuana has been increasingly tried by adults. It is important to note that the issue at hand is not really drugs. In recent years the phenomenon of alienation has played a significant role in the drug scene. Groups of young people questioned and rejected the established institutions of our society such as the church, schools, government, industry, and marriage, among others. The hypocracies of our society were laid bare for public discussion. Hair styles and manner of dress differed greatly from those of the establishment. These groups also sought out drugs for use that were different from those of the establishment. Drugs such as marihuana and LSD thus became a part of new subcultures.

With some groups the use of drugs became a part of a search for spiritualism. They felt that organized religion failed to meet their spiritual needs and sought to find God and self-identity through the medium of drugs. Some were seeking the love ethic of early Christianity which they felt organized religion only parroted and our society too infrequently reflected. They rejected material wealth as a primary objective of life and tried to substitute love of man. They also turned to the drugs used by primitive religions to aid their search and their cause. The results of these ventures were often overromanticized and overly publicized with the results that the users were enticing others to find themselves and God through the medium of drugs. It is at best ironic that they appeared to mimic one of the giant industrial corporations of the "materialistic" establishment whose motto is, "A Better Life Through Chemistry!" Perhaps love, like good wine, does not need the help of the alchemist.

The easy availability of drugs has no doubt served as a provocateur of drug abuse. Both illegal and legal drugs have been readily available for those who have sought them out. It must also be pointed out that the number of drugs made available by the pharmaceutical industry in recent decades runs in the thousands. Drugs have also been sold through television commercials as solutions to all of life's problems. They put you to sleep, wake you up, speed you up, slow you down, help you to compose yourself, take care of headaches, overeating, family problems, and so forth. In fact one advertisement indicated that they had invented a new disease. They then described some vague generalized symptoms and indicated they would not have invented a disease if they did not also have the cure—namely their product. The result of all this huckstering has been the development of a drug-oriented society seeking a pill for every ill. The situation was further complicated by physicians who were seduced by pharmaceutical detail men to overprescribe and badgered by patients for unneeded prescriptions.

We have in essence turned loose in our society thousands of potent chemicals without any real attempt to inform lay people or professionals what constitutes rational use of those substances. They were in fact foisted on the public as cure-alls. Add to this the mystique that surrounds some of the illegal drugs such as LSD and marihuana and the huge profits associated with heroin-trafficking and the stage has been set for massive drug abuse.

Perhaps most curious of all are the adult drugstore junkies whose purses, pockets, and medicine cabinets are lined with a wide variety of drugs but who are so terribly concerned about the drug abuse problem amongst their youth. On the other hand we have young people who think they are doing their own thing by taking drugs without realizing how establishment-oriented they really are!! An age of technology and mass media has also been an age of noncommunication. In an era of fast-changing values, we have been a society seeking direction and leadership. As stated by Dr. Donald B. Louria:

> The whole fabric of our society is in an upheaval. We appear to have lost our goals and are suffering from mass bewilderment. This sickness can best be cured with inspiring leadership. We need leaders who will define and articulate our major problems, establish goals, offer constructive solutions, and then forcefully lead our nation, especially the young, toward those objectives. At present, this country has too few such leaders, and at every level of our political structure we are dominated by self-aggrandizers and publicity seekers, by mediocrity, ineptitude, corruption, and laziness. We assassinate or ignore our best potential leaders, allow political office to be a playground for the rich, reward incompetence or political servitude by promotion to a judgeship, encourage our prosecutors to use their offices for political gain, and select our leaders on the basis of charisma, demagoguery, and shibboleth.[8]

Stimulant Drugs

The *amphetamines* are usually referred to as "pep" pills. Their intake serves to stimulate the central nervous system. Because they act as body stimulants and depress appetite, they are sometimes used by overweight people. They are also used in inhalers because they help to reduce the swelling of mucous membranes when one is suffering from a common cold. The stimulant drugs help develop a sense of well-being in people suffering from feelings of depression. Overdoses of amphetamines can result in the loss of judgment. People under their influence many times feel capable of performing impossible and oftentimes dangerous feats. College students often use "pep" pills to stay awake in order to cram for an upcoming examination. The feelings of well-being developed by the drug often give the student the impression that he has done well in the exam. This is, unfortunately, too often not substantiated by the grade received. How efficient study can be under these circumstances of masked fatigue is questionable. The numbers of students who have fallen asleep during exams or missed the exam because they overslept indicate other problems that are related here. Continued abuse of the drug can also result in hallucinations

[8]Donald B. Louria, M.D., *Overcoming Drugs* (New York: McGraw-Hill, 1971), p. 205.

and a psychotic state. It has been found that truck drivers who habitually use these drugs to stay awake on long trips will occasionally have hallucinations. They imagine that they are being attacked by animals or experience other frightening episodes and become involved in severe and tragic highway accidents. Some people who have little understanding of the potentialities of drugs will often use barbiturates to sleep and amphetamines to wake up. The alternate use of these drugs often leads to an overdosing with both, which can result in serious mental illness or barbiturate poisoning. Though the amphetamines are not addicting drugs, they create a psychic dependence (habit forming).

Thousands of women using amphetamines as a means of reducing weight often find the drug may create more problems than it solves. Because the drug reduces appetite and gives the person a feeling of well-being as an extra added reward, it can appear to be a pleasant way to lose weight. However, once the person stops taking amphetamines she usually goes back to the same old overeating and underexercising habits with a resultant weight gain. The real problem starts when that feeling of well-being becomes *the* reason for taking the drug, and the weight problem used as the excuse for needing the "medication." The question that inevitably comes to mind is if the person does not have the willpower to restrict food intake and increase physical activity, how can he have the willpower not to misuse the sirenlike temptations of potent amphetamines?

The Harris-Dodd Act (an amendment to the Federal Food and Drug Act) in an attempt to control this abusive practice forbids the excessive refilling of dangerous drug prescriptions. The amphetamines and barbiturates are classified as dangerous drugs. This legislation also requires that records be kept of the manufacture, sale, and distribution of these drugs.

The Hallucinogenic Drugs

The term *hallucinogenic* refers to a group of drugs that can affect the mind, causing visions and hallucinations. They are sometimes referred to as consciousness-expanding drugs. Some can have comparatively mild effects, but others can precipitate a psychotic state. They range from marihuana to LSD.

Marihuana

Few issues have stirred as much controversy as marihuana has. It became obvious even to the casual observer that more was involved in the issue than the pharmacological effects of the drug.

> The symbolic aspects of marihuana . . . may be at the heart of the marihuana problem. . . . It was youth-related at a time in American history when the adult society was alarmed by the implications of the youth "movement": defiance of established order, the adoption of new life styles, the emergence of "street people," campus unrest, drug use, communal living, protest politics, and even political radicalism. In an age characterized by the so-called generation gap, marihuana symbolizes the cultural divide.
>
> For youth, marihuana became a convenient symbol of disaffection with traditional society, an allure which sup-

plemented its recreational attraction. Smoking marihuana may have appealed to large numbers of youth who opposed certain policies or trends, but who maintained faith in the American system as a whole. In a time when symbolic speech is often preferred to the literal form, marihuana was a convenient instrument of mini-protest.[9]

Federal law added to the controversy and confusion when it inappropriately categorized marihuana some 35 years ago as a narcotic. This equated it in the minds of many with drugs as dangerous as heroin. Many adults responded with great concern for the young using such a drug. There were other adults for whom marihuana spelled rebellion, and a serious personal and societal threat. Many of these people would probably react with disappointment if marihuana were conclusively proved to be an innocuous, harmless drug. For them, the issue lies not in the drug, but its other representations.

The range of strength of marihuana is considerable. It is comparable to the alcoholic beverages ranging from beer to hard liquor. The active ingredient in marihuana is tetrahydrocannabinol (THC). The amount of it present determines the potency of the marihuana. The variety of marihuana (bhang—India) generally found in this country is of low potency. Ganja (India) is a higher grade of marihuana obtained from the flowering tips and leaves of the plant and is of somewhat higher potency. When the pure resin is removed from the leaves of the female *cannabis sativa* plant (a weed of the hemp family), a more potent source of THC is derived. This gummy-like substance is what *hashish* (Charas—India) is made up of and is 5 to 10 times more potent than the strongest marihuana generally found in this country.

Most of the marihuana entering the country comes from Mexico, although the plant can be grown in the United States. Marijuana is usually smoked in the form of cigarettes, causing degrees of intoxication. It creates feelings of pleasant drowsiness, visual distortions, and heightened suggestibility. The person may believe he is experiencing increased sexual desire. The latter is considered related to the drug's lowering of inhibitions rather than to any aphrodisiac effect. In other instances, the drug may cause nervousness and anxiety.

It has been noted that marihuana will adversely affect reaction time, visual and time perception, and intelligence test scores. It also causes a reddening of the conjunctivae. Since this is a means of identifying the marihuana smoker, dark glasses have often been used to hide this reaction. There have been instances where a person developed "pink eye," an infection of the conjunctivae, and found himself in more difficulty than anticipated. Current research also indicates that marihuana apparently does not affect hearing acuity, memory, verbal or musical abilities. To date, there appear to be no long-term physical effects from marihuana smoking except for respiratory tract irritation. Those who have studied the effects of tobacco in terms of broad-scale incidence of emphysema and lung cancer predict that chronic

[9] *Marihuana: A Signal of Misunderstanding,* The Official Report of the National Commission on Marihuana and Drug Abuse (New York: New American Library, 1972), p. 10.

smoking that involves inhalation will inevitably cause damage to sensitive lung tissue. They feel that this may be particularly true as related to the enforced inhalations of the marihuana smoker. Research is obviously needed to substantiate these predictions.

The psychosocial implications of marihuana use have more substantive concern related to them than the physical implications of the drug. While marihuana is not *physically* addicting, it can for some be psychologically addicting. *It is not so much the drug that has this property as it is the personality that seeks and needs a chemical escape.* At the present time there are some 9 million people who have used alcohol and ensuing alcoholism as an escape from their problems. The fear is that broad-scale unrestricted use of marihuana will exact a societal price in the form of 9 million potheads.

The stepping-stone theory has been one idea that has persisted in the minds of some people who believe that marihuana leads to the use of harder drugs. Pharmacologically there is nothing in marihuana that would lead to heroin use. It may be that those who seek chemical solutions to personal problems are unsatisfied with marihuana and thus seek out harder drugs. One positive correlation that does exist is that those buying marihuana place themselves in contact with the illegal drug market who have harder drugs as part of their wares.

Laws related to marihuana have in recent years become more lenient, helping to break it away from its undeserved categorization with drugs as potent as heroin. In 1972 the National Commission on Marihuana and Drug Abuse recommended that legal penalties be exacted only for those selling the drug and eliminating penalties for the user. There are some groups who take the stand that the only alternative is the legalization of marihuana. The latter does not appear to be an action that will be taken until more extensive short- and long-term research on marihuana and its more potent cousin, hashish, have been conducted. The liberalization of marihuana laws to make them more compatible with the pharmacological effects of the drug will probably be a continued trend.

Mescaline, Psilocybin, LSD: The More Potent Hallucinogens

The sources of the more potent hallucinogens vary, although their effects are similar. Mescaline is derived from the buttons or tops of the peyote cactus found in the southwestern part of the United States and in Mexico. Psilocybin, a somewhat more potent drug, comes from the Mexican mushroom (Psilocybe Mexicana). Some of the people of Mexico and Central America have used mushrooms during religious ceremonies, just as southwestern Indians have the peyote buttons. The purpose of the drug in these ceremonies is to bring the person into closer contact with these peoples' concept of God.

LSD (lysergic acid diethylamide tartrate) is a derivative of ergot, a rye fungus, and can also be produced synthetically. Though tasteless, odorless, and colorless when dissolved in water, it is one of the most powerful chemical agents known to man. One ounce of LSD can serve as an average dose for 300,000 people. The drug was discovered by Dr. Albert Hofmann, a Swiss chemist, in 1938. It was not until 1943 that Dr. Hofmann accidentally ingested some of the drug and experienced, as a result, fantastic visions which included a kaleidoscopic array of vivid colors, with objects appearing wavy and deformed. Occasionally he felt as though he were outside his own body. Other descriptions of the drug's effects include the following:

> The marked heightening of the sensation of color is usually one of the first manifestations, so that ordinary reds and blues, for example, become astoundingly vivid and flowing. New colors, difficult to put into appropriate words, are seen. They swirl around the individual with great vividness. Fixed objects fuse and diffuse; there is often a perpetual flowing of geometric designs and one sensation merges into another and one sense into another so that the individual may say he can taste color; touch sound. The body image is distorted and ordinary sounds increase profoundly in intensity. There is a sense of intense isolation and depersonalization so that "me" as an individual disappears and the user feels he is fused with all humanity and with his environment. Time stands still and many give themselves up to what they describe as an experience of inexpressible ecstasy.[10]

Some regard the experience as an erotic one, while others attach religious meanings to it, claiming a better understanding of God, the universe, life, and death. Under the influence of the drug there appears in some instances to be the ability to look into one's unconscious. In experimental work that is being done, psychiatrists are attempting to use this phenomenon as a way of helping mental patients and alcoholics to develop greater insight into their emotional problems. To date the use of LSD in treating emotional problems has not proved promising.

Although some LSD reactions are pleasurable and perhaps even helpful with the guidance of the trained professional, others are not. Some people have experienced the most terrifying of hallucinations, mental disorganization, and overwhelming feelings of panic. Many such persons have been hospitalized with acute psychosis. Strong tranquilizers are used on such patients in attempts to suppress the effect of the LSD. Others who are made to feel omnipotent by the drug have attempted to fly out of windows several stories off the ground, or have walked out in front of speeding cars.

The unstable personality seems to be most negatively affected by the drug in uncontrolled situations. It also appears to be this kind of personality who is most attracted to the illicit use of LSD or other hallucinogens. The result may be a prolonged psychotic condition in the user. The effects of the drug may also recur weeks later without the taking of additional amounts of the substance. One user suddenly became a flying horse a month after an LSD episode. Fortunately, the users of the drug have generally been the immature, who do not have serious responsibility for others. One shudders at the thought of having one's surgeon or airline pilot suddenly become preoccupied with kaleidoscopic swirls

[10]Donald Louria, M.D., *Nightmare Drugs* (New York: Pocket Books, 1966), pp. 45–46.

of vivid colors, touch sound, taste color, and feel literally beside himself. If we were to become a society of "acid heads" (LSD users), who would be left to watch the store?

The illicit use of LSD has alarmed health authorities and legislators alike. The result has been that Congress has passed legislation providing strong penalties for the manufacture, sale, or possession of the drug. A number of states, including New York, California, and Nevada, have enacted similar laws. An unfortunate effect of the sensationalism that has surrounded LSD is the suppression of research. Researchers often do not want to "get involved" when this kind of interest is associated with a drug. The federal government is currently serving as the LSD source for a small group of highly qualified researchers.

Experimentation with monkeys has shown that LSD can have permanent damaging effects on the animals' minds. A study by Drs. Jose Egozcue and Samuel Irwin revealed a high incidence of chromosomal damage in LSD users. One of the chromosomal abnormalities seen in the LSD user was a type associated with chronic leukemia. The only subject in the control group in the study to show chromosomal damage was a person who underwent fairly extensive X ray treatment several years before being tested. Drs. Egozcue and Irwin plan to study women LSD users to determine if there is a higher spontaneous abortion rate in the group and if they transmit the chromosomal defects to their offspring. Though LSD is not an addicting drug, its potential for harm is apparently great.

The Addicting Drugs

BARBITURATES

Barbiturate drugs are sedative, prescription drugs that are used medically to help people to relax and sleep. (The names of these drugs usually end in "al," as in phenobarbital, luminal, nembutal.) In larger doses than would be normally prescribed they can cause an intoxication similar to that caused by alcohol. Continued unsupervised use of barbiturates has been found to lead to addiction. Related to its misuse has been an increase in the incidence of barbiturate poisoning, which is a leading cause of death by poisoning. A person intoxicated with barbiturate drugs is irresponsible and capable of swallowing a handful of pills that will cause his death. Many such deaths are listed as suicides. It has also been discovered that barbiturates and alcohol make a dangerous combination. The taking of a moderate dose of barbiturates after a few alcoholic drinks may cause death. Because of the relatively easy access to these drugs, some authorities fear that barbiturate addiction may be more widespread than realized in our society. The number of barbiturate addicts that we have in this country is unknown. Estimates indicate that they may be in the many thousands.

Because barbiturates are dangerous drugs and since there are other drugs as effective but less dangerous, one must wonder why they are still being manufactured and medically used.

A number of authorities have concluded that people who tend to become addicted to barbiturates have a personality disorder. It is also generally agreed that this type of addiction presents a more severe problem than heroin addiction because it produces mental, neurological, and emotional problems of greater severity and because withdrawal is more dangerous.

The AMA has categorized abuses of barbiturates into four groups:

1. Those who deal with emotional stress by sedating themselves, sometimes right out of this world.
2. Those who have developed a tolerance for the drug and can tolerate large doses which produce feelings of excitation rather than depression. The reaction is similar to that experienced with amphetamines.
3. Those who use the drug to counteract the effects of other drugs such as LSD or amphetamines
4. Those who use the drug with other depressant drugs such as alcohol or heroin. The combined use of depressants produces a more instant "high." This combination of drugs is particularly dangerous. One must question the presence of the conscious or unconscious motivation to commit suicide or the influence of blatant ignorance.

The withdrawal illness associated with barbiturate addiction is more severe than with any of the opiate drugs. The sudden withdrawal of barbiturates from an addicted person will usually result in convulsions and a temporary psychosis. It may even result in death. The addicted person who attempts to withdraw from the drug on his own is risking his life. Withdrawal from the drug even under medical supervision is tricky and may take as long as two months.

Methaqualone

Methaqualone is the generic name of a drug that is a nonbarbiturate sedative-hypnotic; it also appears on the market under the brand names of Quaalude, Sopor, and Optimil, among others. Medically, methaqualone is prescribed for sleeplessness. The *Physicians' Desk Reference,* which publishes drug information provided by drug companies, described it as a drug which only occasionally caused psychological dependence with physical dependence rarely reported. Drug companies' advertising depicted the drug as nonaddicting and the fact that it is not a barbiturate caused thousands to use the drug for recreational purposes, resulting in a widespread faddish use. Abuse of the drug, however, soon demonstrated it to be a dangerous addicting drug. It is now described by pharmacologists to be chemically different from barbiturates but pharmacologically the equivalent.

The heavy abuser of methaqualone who abruptly stops the intake of the drug will go into convulsions. As stated by Dr. Craig Whitehead of the Haight-Ashbury Clinic, "If convulsions aren't treated, you risk status epilepticus developing. That means one grand mal seizure after another—and if they aren't broken, the body will expire of exhaustion."[11]

Methaqualone, like barbiturates, can be particularly dangerous when taken in combination with

[11] *Connection,* "Bigger than Marijuana Methaqualone: Dangerous New Abuse Fad Sweeping West?," Institute for Social Concerns, Oakland, Calif., p. 4.

alcohol. Many of the fatalities attributed to the abuse of this drug have occurred when the drug was used with alcoholic beverages. Research has also found the drug to cause skeletal abnormalities in the offspring of rats given the drug. Its use by pregnant women is therefore contraindicated.

More recently even the medicinal value of the drug has been questioned by physicians. Perhaps the legal medical use and the illegal faddish use of methaqualone was best summarized by Dr. Meyers, a pharmacologist. "Doctors and street people buy drugs the way old ladies buy detergents. They both get screwed—and both of them deserve it."[12]

Tranquilizers

Tranquilizers were first introduced about 20 years ago. Their initial use was for the treatment of the mental patient. The tranquilizing effect of the drugs made the patient more susceptible to psychotherapy, as well as blunting agitation caused by his emotional problem. In recent years there has been proliferate use of these substances with approximately a half million pounds of tranquilizers used each year in the United States. This is no doubt reflective of a great deal of self-doting, of the inability of people to "endure" normal nervousness. The hypochondriacal national attitude is often aided and abetted by the family physician too willing to prescribe such drugs.

To date, six tranquilizers have been found to be capable of addiction. The biggest problem related to these drugs is their strong habituating quality. The lethargic, tranquil attitudes and lack of coordination often induced by the drug have been responsible for many automobile accidents. The intake of large amounts of alcohol in combination with tranquilizing drugs can pose a serious threat to the health of the individual. In fact, it may precipitate an unplanned eternity of tranquility; this combination has in some instances caused death.

Tranquilizers provide the same dangers to the individual as do the barbiturates. They are addicting when abused, and withdrawal from them can prove deadly. Their massive use indicates the extent to which we have as a society attempted to avoid normal anxiety and stress. Where anxiety and stress are reflective of deep-seated problems, the drug merely masks the symptoms without resolving the causative factors. The physician who overprescribes the drug has also ducked the needed therapy. The busy harried physician does not have the time to discuss one's personal problems. It simply becomes easier to prescribe a "miracle drug."

Opiates

Opiates are obtained from the milky juice of the unripe seed pod of the opium poppy. All drugs derived from opium are addicting and tend to have a depressant effect on the central nervous system. Though they have no curative value, they can serve to relieve pain. *Morphine* is the opiate most commonly used medically for this purpose. Its administration must be under careful medical supervision.

[12]Ibid., p. 5.

Table 12-1. ***Common Drugs—Used and Abused***

	Drugs	General Information	Medical Use	Signs and Symptoms of Drug Abuse
Opiates	Morphine	Extracted from Opium. Used as a standard by which the other pain relievers are measured.	Pain relief	Drowsiness, restlessness, nausea and loss of weight accompany the effects of opiate abuse. Personal neglect, malnutrition and infection are signs that occur after extended use of opiates. Frequently you will find needle scars from repeated injections—particularly with heroin.
	Heroin	A derivative of morphine and a source of hard core drug addictions. Illegal in U.S.A. under all circumstances.	None in U.S.A.	
	Codeine	Extracted from Opium. An ingredient of some cough syrups.	Pain relief	
	Demerol	Synthetic. Used widely in medicine. Effective pain reliever.	Pain relief	
	Methadone	Synthetic. Used in the treatment of addicts.	Pain relief	
Stimulants	Amphetamines	Called pep pills, bennies and co-pilots. Can cause distorted images. Disguises fatigue. Methamphetamine (Methedrine) referred to as "Speed," often taken by injection.	Appetite suppressant	User will exhibit a great deal of nervous energy and will have difficulty sleeping. When effects of the drug wear off, the individual will have a feeling of depression which is referred to as "post amphetamine depression" or the Crash. Cocaine is an extremely strong stimulant but is not used very often by the drug dependent person because of its high cost.
	Cocaine	Very strong stimulant. Extracted chemically from the leaves of Coca bush in South America. Can cause excessive excitement and uncontrollable behavior.	Local anesthetic	
Depressants	Barbiturates	Referred to as "Goof Balls." Named for its color—"Yellow-Jackets," "Pinks," and "Rainbows" etc.	To induce sleep	The effect of depressants resemble alcoholic intoxication. Behavior is one of confusion and drowsiness and the thinking process is quite dull. Muscular control is uncoordinated; walking and reaching for objects becomes difficult. Staggering like a "punch drunk" person can become a permanent effect.
	Non-Barbiturate Sedatives	Doriden, Noludar, Methaqualone. Developed as substitutes for Barbiturates.	To induce sleep	
	Tranquilizers	Miltown, Valium, Librium, Thorazine.	Relieve nervous tension and treat mental illness	
	Glue and Others	Generally abused by young people. Brain damage likely with continued use.	None	
Hallucinogens	LSD	Lysergic acid diethylamide. Most potent hallucinogen. Made in the laboratory. Causes different reactions in different people. A very unpredictable substance. No known way of knowing who will react badly and who will not. Harmful effects can be prolonged and sometimes permanent.	None	Effects of the hallucinogens are unpredictable. Reaction to use of these drugs ranges from mild nausea and hallucinations to prolonged insanity.
	Mescaline	Derived from the Mexican cactus Peyote. Causes hallucinations.	None	
	Psilocybin	Derived from certain mushrooms found in Mexico. Causes hallucinations.	None	
	DMT	Dimethyltryptamine. A new hallucinogen made synthetically. Also found within certain plants.	None	
	Marijuana	Classified as a mild hallucinogen. Made from the flowering tops and leaves of the female plant. Main ingredient THC (tetrahydrocannabinol) synthesized recently. Much research is taking place concerning its effects. Resin extracted from the Marijuana plant (Cannabis) is called Hashish.	None	Effect of this drug depends on the individual, the parts of the plant used and climate in which it is grown; stronger varieties of marijuana can produce hallucinations.

Source: Copyright © 1970 by SCOPE. All rights reserved. Drug chart appears in *Decision* (Junior High Edition) and *The Drug Society* (Senior High Edition).

if addiction is not to take place. As with the other opiates, a tolerance can be developed for the drug, requiring larger and larger doses to obtain the same effect. Morphine is sometimes used by addicts; however, the more "popular" opiate used for this purpose is heroin.

Heroin is a white powder that is made from morphine. When first developed, heroin was thought to be nonaddicting. Actually, however, it is so powerful and addicting that it cannot be used even for medical purposes in the United States. One grain of the drug taken over a two-week period can cause addiction. The addict injects the heroin into a vein in order to produce its desired effects. The use of unsterilized needles by the addict often results in the transmission of such serious diseases as malaria, hepatitis, and syphilis. The strength of the adulterated heroin that reaches the addict cannot be predicted. The underworld dilutes the heroin with milk sugar to the extent of 95 per cent. If the drug reaching the addict is less dilute than usual and is too strong, the user's "normal" dose may kill him. If, on the other hand, it is too weak, it will not relieve the addict's developing symptoms of withdrawal illness. The addict is essentially at the mercy of the underworld in what has become his most important commodity. The physical dependence on the drug causes the body to react in its absence. The symptoms of the withdrawal illness that follow resemble those of the flu, with the person experiencing chills, tearing eyes, running nose, aching and twitching arms and legs, followed by diarrhea and vomiting. Severe cramps develop in the arms, legs, stomach, and back, which cause the person to assume a curled-up position. The peak of the withdrawal symptoms is reached in 24 to 30 hours. A dose of the drug is good for only 4 to 8 hours; the addict lives in constant fear of the withdrawal illness. He is therefore strongly motivated to steal or, in the case of women, to resort to prostitution for sources of income. Maintaining the heroin habit may cost as much as $50 to $100 a day. There is no doubt an elevated crime rate related to drug addiction, particularly in large cities like New York. It is estimated that New York City addicts steal from $500,000 to $700,000 a day to maintain their habits.

Poor social conditions appear to be a breeding ground for heroin addiction. They create the climate for anxiety, frustration, and broken homes. The social pathology produces underdeveloped personalities, lacking discipline and dreaming of unrealistic goals. The euphoric effects of heroin, therefore, become very attractive. Once hooked on heroin, the addict centers all his activities on getting his next needed supply.

Drug Traffic

Raw opium is gathered by Turkish farmers and is converted into a morphine base before being shipped to Italy and France. There it is converted to heroin and then smuggled into the United States. Approximately two pounds of raw opium can be bought for about $350 from Turkish farmers. After it has been converted into heroin and diluted, it is then sold to addicts for a half million dollars. It has been estimated that the price of heroin is over two hundred times that of gold. The Federal Bureau of Narcotics, which is a part of the United States Treasury Department, has stationed agents around the world in its attempts to reduce the heroin traffic into the United States. This country is the principal target of the illegal narcotics trade, with New York City being the largest addiction center. The United Nations has made attempts to establish a controlling agency for all opiate drugs in world trade. Small countries that produce opium, however, receive a large income from the illegal sale of these drugs. This vested interest has been an inhibiting factor in the development of an international control agency. More recently the United States has made attempts to work with individual countries to effect a reduction in heroin traffic. Farmers are being encouraged to substitute other crops for the poppy.

In this country, participation in illegal drug trade carries heavy penalties, particularly where sales to a minor are involved. The sentence may run from 10 to 40 years' imprisonment and up to $20,000 in fines. A special penalty for the sale of heroin to a minor may include life imprisonment or even death if a jury so decides.

A great deal of concern, rhetoric, and action has been precipitated by illegal drug traffic, with the greatest focus on heroin. At the same time comparatively little concern has been expressed about those drugs produced by the American pharmaceutical industry, such as amphetamines and barbiturates, that find their way into the illegal market. Some estimates indicate that only 10 per cent of the amphetamines produced in the United States is needed for medical reasons; the rest either finds its way into the illegal market or is overprescribed by physicians. Since amphetamines and barbiturates can be even more harmful than heroin, controlling their traffic becomes at least as important.

Approximately 8 billion amphetamine pills are manufactured in the United States each year. This is equal to 40 pills for every man, woman, and child. Senator Claude Pepper, Chairman of the Crime Committee, has suggested that the Attorney General with the advice and counsel of the Secretary of Health, Education and Welfare set production limits on this drug. In October of 1972, Senator Pepper managed to get his proposal through the Senate but it was killed in the House of Representatives. Senator Pepper blamed this on drug industry lobbying. He reported that the American Pharmaceutical Association has a 70-member staff in Washington and a budget of over $3.5 million.

The AMA Committee on Alcoholism and Addiction has reported that the current production of all sedatives far exceeds medical needs, with over 6 billion capsules a year being produced. These drugs are often prescribed to individuals in a weakened psychological state which makes them more vulnerable to abuse such drugs. Large amounts of both amphetamines and barbiturates are shipped out of the country only to return as part of the illegal drug market.

Committee hearings showed that a Chicago manufacturer shipped 1.2 million amphetamine pills to an unknown consignee in Mexico. Investigating the transaction, federal agents found the consignee's address was actually the eleventh hole of a Tijuana golf course. The pills had gone into the black market and are believed to have been widely distributed in Southern California.[13]

Though law enforcement is helpful in attempts to control drug traffic and use, society's greatest protection is still the individual who will shun the injudicious use of these substances.

Various Approaches to the Problem

A traditional approach to a health problem has been to wait for the person to become ill, then attempt to treat and rehabilitate him. The drug abuse area has been no different even though little is known about effective treatment. The rehabilitation of the heroin addict requires much more than merely detoxifying him (removing him from his physical dependence on the drug). The addict is a person who is often a product of social pathology and who has spent all his time "hustling" (stealing) and "shooting up" (injecting heroin). His rehabilitation therefore hinges on his acceptance and preparation for a new life-style. He must develop a marketable occupational skill and discipline himself to accept the regimen of a working society. His desire for a new way of life must be strong enough for him to view heroin addiction as a threat to a good thing. Effecting that kind of dramatic change is not easy. The success rates of treatment and rehabilitation programs have therefore been understandably poor.

[13] *FYI* (*For Your Information*), edited and published by Governor's Office of Drug Abuse, February 1971, Edition 11, Lansing, Michigan 48913.

Methadone Maintenance Programs

Methadone is an addicting, synthetic, narcotic drug. Its pharmacological properties are quite similar to those of heroin. Methadone has the ability to block the euphoric high the addict gets from heroin as well as to prevent withdrawal symptoms from heroin. Methadone thus blocks the physical need for heroin. With this as a crutch, time is provided to help the addict develop psychologically, socially, and vocationally. Where successful, the addict finds a steady job, supports his family, and becomes a productive member of society.

Since methadone is itself addictive, the addict is really switched from heroin addiction to addiction of a more manageable drug. He must, however, take a daily dose of methadone usually dissolved in orange juice or a similar beverage. Some people have compared the addict maintained on methadone to the diabetic who needs a dose of insulin daily to maintain his normal functioning.

While methadone maintenance is helpful to some addicts, there are some drawbacks and criticisms of this approach. The cost of the drug is inexpensive, but the cost of the overall rehabilitation program ranges from $1,500 to $2,000 per patient.

The long-term effects of methadone use is as yet undetermined. Evidence indicates that alcohol use in combination with methadone can cause liver damage as well as other toxic effects. Since many addicted to heroin also abuse alcohol, screening out such individuals from methadone programs is imperative. Some researchers report that studies of brain tissue of methadone users (whose causes of death have been attributed to drug overdose) have shown abnormalities indicating early senile changes characteristically found in much older people.

A problem on the increase is the rising incidence of methadone-addicted babies born to mothers on a methadone maintenance program. Indications are that withdrawing these infants from methadone is more difficult than withdrawal from heroin. This presents an additional facet to an already complex problem.

The addict is also tied down to the ritual of receiving his methadone dose at a local hospital or clinic. In some programs, the addict is given several days' supply to take with him. This has sometimes resulted in some of the doses being sold by the addict on the black market. The sale of methadone can thus serve as a source of extra income to the person in the methadone program. He usually sells the methadone to an addict on the street who does not have the money for heroin but can afford the less expensive methadone to hold him over.

It has also been noted that there has been an increase in the illegal sales of cocaine which some relate to the increased use of methadone. Addicts finding that methadone blocks the effect of heroin, turn to the use of cocaine to gain the desired results.

There has also been an increase in the number of deaths due to methadone overdose. The orange juice in the refrigerator may be serving as the solvent of a methadone dose. A child or adult may drink it without knowledge of its true contents and be the victim of an overdose.

The shifting of a person's addiction to what is considered a less harmful drug can be viewed as progress, but it certainly is an incomplete answer to the problem. The success rate for the treatment of drug addiction has been highly questionable, with a small percentage truly rehabilitated. Methadone maintenance may prove to be a shaky step forward in this area. It is hoped, of course, that continued research will bring more adequate answers to the problem. Prevention, however, still remains as the best *cure* to any problem.

Drug Abuse: A Social-Health Problem—Not a Legal-Moral One

In the United States we have viewed the drug abuse problem as a legal-moral problem rather than the social-health problem that it is.

> Illegal drug traffic is largely responsible for the prosperity of organized crime which capitalizes both on national policies and individual problems. Organized crime is able to flourish as it does because it provides wanted services: gambling, prostitution, and drugs. The high risks involved in marketing illegal drugs drive up the price so that the addict must resort to crime in order to support his dependency. (The syndicate converts stolen goods or prostitution pay into the cash the addict needs to pay it for expensive drugs.) According to the National Institute of

Mental Health, society's cost of supporting organized crime in narcotics abuse alone amounts to $541 million annually. This amounts to a tax-free, tacit conspiracy between our policies and crime, with the addict and the public caught in the squeeze.[14]

A young person (preferably bearded) in possession of marihuana may be legally incarcerated, whereas the person (preferably white, older, middle-class) becoming addicted to a legal drug such as a barbiturate is on the verge of self-destruction with no one about to intercede. The societal judgments in the drug field appear to be made on the basis of legality and the particular values and life-style of the person in question. The effect on the health of the person appears to be a most secondary consideration. Does the legal-moral approach, then, have the opposite effects than intended? Does it also produce a hysterical environment with people feeling that crime is rampant but not knowing what the crime is, who is performing it, and where it is being performed? It would seem important to define the problem carefully so that it is understood and can be reacted to objectively and constructively.

This means that schools and universities need to develop programs that focus in on the motivations for drug abuse and the psychosocial issues surrounding it. Communities need to become much more knowledgeable of the *real* issues in the drug abuse field and the individual and societal responsibilities each person has in helping to develop an environment in which constructive action *can* take place. This means recognizing the problems of legal drugs, and adult drug abuse, among others. It also means a more responsible news media who are interested in accurate reporting rather than sensationalism that sells newspapers and air time. It also means putting to eternal rest the political rhetoric that daily declares war on drugs as though these inert substances were "the enemy." It is time that each of us began to really understand the underlying causes of drug abuse and, more important, to recognize constructive alternatives for ourselves and others.

These alternatives could include learning how to communicate with others of all age groups; how to promote needed social changes (à la Ralph Nader); and how to promote political change (including drug legislation). They also could include enjoyment of the arts, finding true meaning in life, and learning how to influence the course of events around oneself and how to maintain one's personal integrity.

Despite the criticisms we may level at the mismanagements of the drug problem by government, by news media, by industrial self-interest, and by a variety of inept community groups, when all is said and done, Pogo, the comic strip character, probably summarized the situation best when he stated, "We have met the enemy, and they is us!"

Alcohol

Man has been using some form of alcoholic beverage since the beginning of history. The natural fermen-

[14] Andrew A. Sorenson, ed., *Confronting Drug Abuse*, (Philadelphia: Pilgrim Press, 1972), p. 82.

tation of fruit and vegetable juices and cereal mashes provided him with his first sources of such beverages. Brewed beers and fermented wines have been a part of Western culture for over two thousand years. Distilled beverages (whiskeys) were first introduced in Europe about A.D. 1500.

There is evidence that the Romans gave their victims wine before executing them as a way of dulling the agony and anticipation of death. This was referred to as the "wine of the condemned," and was considered a merciful use of the beverage. Its use has more often been related to important occasions such as weddings and births, and to religious ceremonies. For some people it is simply a beverage that is part of the family meal; for some others, however, it is a means of escaping life's problems.

The attitudes of people toward alcohol are as varied as the nature of its uses. Some view any use of alcohol as being highly immoral, whereas others see nothing wrong with its use in moderation. Inebriation is alternately viewed as something humorous, disgusting, or as a sign of illness (alcoholism). Our attitudes with regard to alcohol and its use become rather personal in nature and are dependent on our experiences, what others close to us think, and what we know about it.

Who Drinks and Why?

While millions of people can drink alcoholic beverages without apparent harm to themselves or others, there are approximately 19 million people in the United States (10 per cent of the American work force) who have serious drinking problems. Why some people get into difficulty with alcohol while others do not has been a source of conjecture, a stimulant for research, as well as the cause of some despair. A great deal of research in the alcohol area has centered around a biochemical approach when a scientist is attempting to determine the effects of alcohol on the finite structure of a nerve cell. Although this kind of research may prove helpful, perhaps we are in some ways overlooking the obvious. For example, most people who drink alcohol do not know that they are drinking a potentially addicting drug. The importance of this simple fact is underscored by sociological research that points out, "countries with a high overall consumption of alcohol have high rates of alcoholism and countries with a low overall consumption have low rates of alcoholism."[15]

The rate of alcoholism in France is ten times that of Finland, Norway, or the Netherlands. The consumption rates of alcohol are also comparable. If alcoholism were to be regarded as the result of emotional disturbance and personality disorder, then the incidence of these conditions should be ten times higher in France than in the other countries. It clearly is not.

A drinking pattern can be described on the basis of two dimensions; namely, the frequency of drinking occasions and the quantity of alcohol consumed at a given occasion. The outstanding difference between low and high consumption countries lies in the frequency of drinking

[15] Report on the Governor's Conference on Alcohol Problems (November 1971), p. 45.

occasions. In high ranking countries, we find the custom of drinking on many occasions throughout the day. As the per capita consumption and the rate of alcoholism decrease, the frequency of occasions decreases. For example, in Canada, only 9 percent of all drinkers consume alcohol daily. In countries that rank lowest as, for example, Finland and Norway, daily drinking is very rare indeed. With respect to quantities consumed at a given occasion, the relationship seems to be reversed. From available statistics, we would estimate that, as an average, a Finnish drinker would consume four to five times as much per drinking occasion as a French drinker.

It would appear, then, that the customary frequency of drinking occasions in a society, rather than the quantity consumed at a given occasion, is a crucial determinant of the magnitude of alcoholism in a population."[16]

It would seem important to view patterns of alcohol use in the United States from the point of view of frequency of use and amounts of alcohol consumed.

The United States is one of the world's chief consumers of alcoholic beverages. Beer, this nation's most popular alcoholic beverage, is consumed at a rate approximating 22 gallons per person annually. Distilled spirits, with a consumption rate of almost 2 gallons per person per year, makes wine the third choice of Americans. Here the rate is less than 1.51 gallons. The rate of consumption for absolute alcohol, regardless of the beverage in which it is contained, is a little over 2 gallons per year for each person over 15 years of age in the United States.[17]

[16]Ibid., pp. 46–47.

[17]Marvin A. Block, *Alcohol and Alcoholism*, Basic Concepts in Health Science Series (Belmont, Calif.: Wadsworth, 1970), p. 9.

In some cases many have concluded that the use of alcoholic beverages with meals is a wholesome practice. In accepting a dinner invitation it is not unusual to find oneself exposed to several predinner drinks, several wines during dinner, an after-dinner drink and as many after, after-dinner drinks as one cares to attempt to handle. It would seem appropriate at any social gathering where alcoholic beverages will be served that nonalcoholic beverages also be available. The person choosing the nonalcoholic beverage should not be made to feel defensive about his choice as though he were selecting the much less desirable kind of drink.

If one travels and flies first class, he will find himself treated to four ounces of liquor on each leg of his trip. If there are enough legs on the trip, one could very well arrive without one to stand on. An increasing cause of concern is whether the automobile ride home at the end of the plane trip isn't becoming the most dangerous part of the trip because of the degree of imbibement on the plane.

Additionally an increasing number of people have invested a significant amount of space and money to build a bar in the home. Some of these have been motivated by Hollywood films that depict a "bar in the home" as the possession of the wealthy, and therefore becomes a sought-after status symbol. In other instances people relate alcohol use to pleasure and bring it to closer proximity with all the fixings. And eventually some use the bar in the home as the vehicle for becoming the neighborhood pusher.

The drinking patterns of the United States seem to be a combination of those found in Europe and

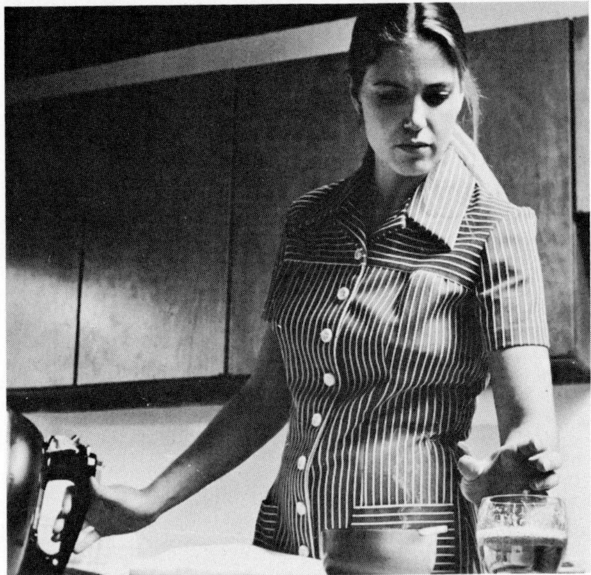

Fig. 12-2. If you drink while you do the ironing, send the ironing out. (National Institute on Alcohol Abuse and Alcoholism)

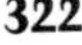

other parts of the world. Some Americans drink alcoholic beverages with their meals as do the French and Italian. Others seek intoxication as do the Irish and Finns. In addition, we have made drinking a part of a round of golf, the closing of a business deal, a way to pass an afternoon or evening, to celebrate an occasion, to mourn an occasion, to greet a friend, to say goodbye to a friend; in essence drinking has become a part of many of our everyday activities significantly increasing the number of occasions for alcohol use. As an extra added attraction, whiskey-flavored toothpaste and rum-flavored pipe tobacco are now available.

Despite the great amount of drinking in our society, it is estimated that approximately one-third of our adult population does not drink. The reasons for this abstinence usually include religious convictions, feelings that drinking will injure health, and also that alcohol can present many different kinds of personal problems these adults would just as soon avoid.

Because of the sedative effects of drug alcohol, it has often been used through the years as a means of dulling the sensation of pain and relieving some of the symptoms of various diseases. There was a time when alcohol was the only anesthetic used when surgery was performed. Alcoholic beverages are still used for supposed medicinal purposes. For instance, rum is taken for a cold, even though it cannot cure it. Whiskey is still used for snakebite, though it has no effect on the venom. Brandy is given to a person who has fainted, though it has no effect on the cause of the fainting. There are a few conditions for which physicians have found alcohol to be of some value. It does have the effect of dilating blood vessels. A drink for an elderly person suffering from hardening of the arteries, therefore, helps this condition. Its sedative effect also relieves aches and pains due to a developing arthritic state. The flush of warmth that a drink can cause helps older people overcome the feeling of chilliness that they often experience. It reduces their tension and irritability and helps to stimulate appetite. Those people below 60 years of age, however, who claim to use alcohol for medicinal purposes probably need to review *objectively* their reasons for drinking.

Another group includes the moderate drinkers whose drinking would range from an occasional drink for a family celebration to fairly frequent drinking with meals and at social occasions several times a week. The reasons given for drinking in this group include a desire for relaxation, the need for a mealtime beverage, and the belief that drinking acts as a social lubricant. Most are seeking the pleasant glow and release from tension that moderate amounts of alcohol intake can produce. How often, how persistently, and with what intensity some pursue the use of alcohol as a social relaxant determine their dependence on, or their independence from, this drug.

In an additional group is the drinker who feels he cannot have a good time without an alcoholic beverage. He also accords to drinking a certain status. It makes him feel important. He looks forward to the time when he can drink because of the satisfactions it brings him, whether the drinking be with friends or alone. This person is not an alcoholic and he may possibly never become one, but he could be identified as a type of prealcoholic. This person has woven some of his basic psychological needs around alcohol, which forms a rather unstable structure.

In general, research has shown that for groups that use alcohol to a significant degree, the lowest incidence of alcoholism is associated with certain habits and attitudes:

1. The children are exposed to alcohol early in life, within a strong family or religious group. Whatever the beverage, it is served in very diluted form and in small quantities, with consequent low blood-alcohol levels.
2. The beverages commonly although not invariably used by the groups are those containing relatively large amounts of non-alcoholic components, which also give low blood-alcohol levels.
3. The beverage is considered mainly as a food and usually consumed with meals, again with consequent low blood-alcohol levels.
4. Parents present a constant example of moderate drinking.
5. No moral importance is attached to drinking. It is considered neither a virtue nor a sin.
6. Drinking is not viewed as a proof of adulthood or virility.
7. Abstinence is socially acceptable. It is no more rude or ungracious to decline a drink than to decline a piece of bread.
8. Excessive drinking or intoxication is not socially acceptable. It is not considered stylish, comical or tolerable.
9. Finally, and perhaps most important, there is wide and usually complete agreement among members of the group on what might be called the ground rules of drinking.[18]

Alcohol as a Drug

Scientists classify drugs according to the effect they have on the body.

Sedative. This type of drug has a quieting effect, relieving tension.

Analgesic. Analgesics relieve pain without producing sleep (aspirin).

Anesthetic. This type of drug will bring about the loss of sensation to pain.

Alcohol can act as a sedative in small amounts and as an analgesic in even smaller quantities, with its most characteristic effect being that of an anesthetic. Describing a person who has had too much to drink as "feeling no pain" is apparently quite apt.

Alcoholic Beverages

Three basic types of alcoholic beverages are used, namely beers, wines, and distilled liquors.

Beer is made by boiling a broth of cereal grains such as barley, wheat, or corn. In these cereal grains, sugar is in the form of starch. Malt is first added to the broth, and this has the effect of changing the starch to sugar. Yeast is then added so that the sugar can be fermented into alcohol. The fermentation process in the making of beer is interrupted, with

[18] *Alcohol and Alcoholism*, National Institute of Mental Health Public Health Service Publication No. 1640, 1970, p. 28.

the result that beer has approximately a 4 per cent alcohol content in this country. Hops, which are a small bitter fruit, are added to the beer to add to its flavor.

Wine is made from the juices of vegetables, fruits, or berries whose taste and color vary to a great extent. Most wines, however, are made from grapes. Because fermentation usually stops at about 14 per cent, most wines will have about that level of alcohol in them. Some wines are referred to as fortified wines when additional alcohol is added to bring the alcoholic content up to 18 or 20 per cent. Those wines that contain no sugar are called "dry." Sparkling wines are those that contain CO_2 gas produced in the fermentation process. Producers permit some of the CO_2 to remain in order to produce this bubbling effect.

Distilled liquors are made through the process of distillation. It is known that various liquids have different boiling points; therefore, alcohol in solution with water can be separated out by heating the entire solution. Alcohol, having a lower boiling temperature, would evaporate off first. If this vapor is then passed through a cooling tube, the alcohol vapor is condensed back into a liquid that is pure alcohol. Whiskey is distilled from fermented cereals or grains such as rye, corn, and barley. Rum can be distilled from fermented molasses; brandy is distilled from wines. Gin is nothing more than alcohol flavored with berries, and vodka is plain, diluted alcohol. Distilled beverages contain from 40 to 50 per cent alcohol. This is usually expressed in terms of degrees of proof. In other words, a 90 proof beverage would contain 45 per cent alcohol. The type of alcohol found in beer, wine, and distilled spirits is ethyl alcohol. There are, of course, many other kinds of alcohol that are used for commercial and industrial purposes such as methyl, butyl, and propyl. These types of alcohol are poisonous to drink and if taken internally may result in death, blindness, or other tragic outcomes.

The Effects of Alcohol on the Body

The effects that alcohol will have on the body are variable and dependent on many factors. For example these will vary depending on whether the beverage is taken on an empty stomach or with food, or whether the individual is a light drinker or a heavy drinker. The same amount of alcohol will have differing effects on a person as compared to another and may even differ in the same individual from week to week. The absorption of alcohol takes place quickly from the stomach and continues mostly from the small intestine. The level of alcohol in the blood (or blood-alcohol concentrations) thus absorbed will depend on:

1. *Presence of food in the stomach.* The presence of protein and fat in the stomach, particularly, slow down the absorption of alcohol.
2. *Alcohol concentration.* The highest blood-alcohol levels are produced most rapidly by undiluted, distilled spirits (particularly vodka and gin), whereas the alcohol in wines and beers is ab-

sorbed more slowly. This is due to the fact that wines and beers contain additional chemicals or food substances. If a beverage is diluted with water or juice the rate of absorption is diminished. However, the presence of carbon dioxide in the stomach, such as in sparkling wines, champagnes, soda, or ginger ale, increases the rate of absorption.

3. *Speed of Drinking.* Sipping or drinking moderate amounts will keep blood-alcohol concentrations lower than if the beverage is consumed in one gulp.
4. *Body Weight.* If a standard amount of alcohol is consumed by two men, one weighing 200 lb and another weighing 140 lb, the blood-alcohol concentration in the heavier man will be less than that in the smaller man.

If a person of average height and weight were to quickly ingest three ounces of whiskey, this would result in a .06 per cent level of alcohol in the blood. This level of alcohol would begin to affect the judgment of the person, and signs of sedation, and tranquility would take place. The feeling of warmth that ensues is due to the dilation of the peripheral blood vessels. While this causes a feeling of warmth on the surface of the body it also results in a loss of body heat. Those who take alcoholic beverages to keep warm during outdoor, winter activities are actually causing the opposite effect than desired and will ultimately feel colder. If the person were to continue to drink, he would then reach the next level of impairment. This would include slurred speech and poor muscle control, and the person would probably stagger, possibly fall and have difficulty rising. If the alcohol level in the blood were then to reach a .40 per cent level, the person would lose consciousness and would be regarded as being "dead drunk." It takes more than a pint of whiskey for the average person to reach this stage. If the concentration of alcohol were to reach .50 per cent, the person would be in a deep coma and in serious danger of death. As the level of alcohol in the blood approached 1 per cent the breathing center of the brain would become paralyzed and death would follow.

Once the alcohol is absorbed by the blood, the rate at which the body metabolizes or gets rid of the alcohol will depend on the actions of the liver. For it is here that 85 per cent or more of the metabolism takes place. It can use up approximately one ounce of 80 proof whiskey in an hour or one-half ounce of pure alcohol in that period of time. If the alcohol intake is progressing at a faster rate than the liver can metabolize, then the level of alcohol in the blood would naturally rise.

The effects of alcohol on the liver are complex and not well defined. Cirrhosis of the liver occurs in about 10 per cent of alcoholic patients, or about eight times as frequently among alcoholics. Though it is a frequent consequence of excessive drinking, it does occur in nondrinkers, and is related to filterable viruses (i.e., hepatitis). It has been observed that heavy drinking causes the cells of the liver to become enlarged and unable to handle fat metabolism. This normally leads to a fatty degeneration of the liver, a forerunner of cirrhosis of the liver.

Table 12-2. ***Some Effects of Alcoholic Beverages***[*1]

Amount of Beverage	*Concentration of Alcohol Attained in the Blood*	*Effects*		*Time Required for All Alcohol to Leave the Body*
1 highball ($1\frac{1}{2}$ oz. whisky) or 1 cocktail ($1\frac{1}{2}$ oz. whisky) or $3\frac{1}{2}$ oz. fortified wine or $5\frac{1}{2}$ oz. ordinary wine or 2 bottles (24 oz.) beer	0.03%	Slight changes in feeling		2 hrs.
2 highballs or 2 cocktails or 7 oz. fortified wine or 11 oz. ordinary wine or 4 bottles beer	0.06%	Increasing effects with variation among individuals and in the same individual at different times	Feeling of warmth—mental relaxation, slight decrease of fine skills—less concern with minor irritations and restraints	4 hrs.
3 highballs or 3 cocktails or $10\frac{1}{2}$ oz. fortified wine or $16\frac{1}{2}$ oz. (1 pt.) ordinary wine or 6 bottles beer	0.09%		Buoyancy—exaggerated emotion and behavior—talkative, noisy or morose	6 hrs.
4 highballs or 4 cocktails or 14 oz. fortified wine or 22 oz. ordinary wine or 8 bottles (3 qts.) beer	0.12%		Impairment of fine coördination—clumsiness—slight to moderate unsteadiness in standing or walking	8 hrs.
5 highballs or 5 cocktails or $17\frac{1}{2}$ oz. fortified wine or $27\frac{1}{2}$ oz. ordinary wine or $\frac{1}{2}$ pt. whisky	0.15%	Intoxication—unmistakable abnormality of gross bodily functions and mental faculties		10 hrs.

*Source: Rutgers Center of Alcohol Studies.

[1]Based on a person of "average" size (150 pounds). For those weighing considerably more or less, the amount would have to be respondingly more or less to produce the same results. The effects indicated at each stage will diminish as the concentration of alcohol in the blood is reduced by being oxidized and eliminated.

Alcohol can have an irritating effect on those tissues of the body that it comes in direct contact with, those of the mouth, esophagus, and particularly the stomach. People who are heavy drinkers often have a chronic inflammation of the lining of the stomach. Those with ulcers, of course, would find the drinking of alcoholic beverages resulting in rather sharp irritations. Anyone who has experienced the application of strong antiseptic solution to a cut on the outside of the body can perhaps begin to imagine the effects of pouring an alcoholic solution on a sore found in the lining of the stomach. Moderate amounts of alcohol stimulate the flow of gastric juices which produce the sensation of hunger. This is why the predinner cocktail is used. When enough alcohol is consumed to cause intoxication, however, digestion is impaired.

It has long been known that alcoholics are less resistant to pneumonia and other infectious diseases and it is assumed that this is due to the usual malnutrition that becomes a part of the alcoholic syndrome. Recent research, however, demonstrated that lowered resistance may also occur in *well-nourished,* heavy drinkers. The blood-alcohol levels of .15 and .25 per cent inhibited the mobilization of white blood cells to the same extent found in states of severe shock.[19]

The hangover is the most common and infamous effect of alcohol on the body. The exact biochemical explanation for its occurrence is not known, nor is satisfactory treatment for its symptoms available. "There is no scientific evidence to support such popular remedies as coffee, raw egg, oysters, chili peppers, steak sauce, "alkalizers," vitamin preparations, or such drugs as barbiturates, thyroid, amphetamine, or insulin. For general treatment, physicians usually prescribe aspirin, bed rest, and ingestion of solid foods as soon as possible."[20]

The Problem of Alcoholism

Alcoholism, a progressive illness that is now epidemic in nature, affects men and women from both rural and urban areas. It has little regard for educational, religious, cultural, or financial status. One of the reasons for our slowness as a society in attacking problems like this is a lack of concern for the people affected. They are often not recognized as being "ill people" and to date the usual reaction has been to incarcerate them rather than to treat them. Broader understandings with respect to alcoholism must be universally accepted before progress can be made in its control through prevention and treatment.

As stated by Mark Keller, "Alcoholism is a chronic disease manifested by repeated implicative drinking so as to cause injury to the drinker's health or to his social or economic functioning."[21]

[19]Robert G. Brayton, Peter Stokes, and Donald B. Louria. Paper presented before American Federation for Clinical Research, New York, December 1964.

[20]*Alcohol and Alcoholism,* National Institute of Mental Health, Public Health Service Publication No. 1640, 1970, p. 23.

[21]Mark Keller, "Definitions of Alcoholism," *Quarterly Journal of Studies on Alcoholism,* 21:125–134 (1960), Center of Alcohol Studies, Rutgers, New Jersey.

ten terrific hangover cures.

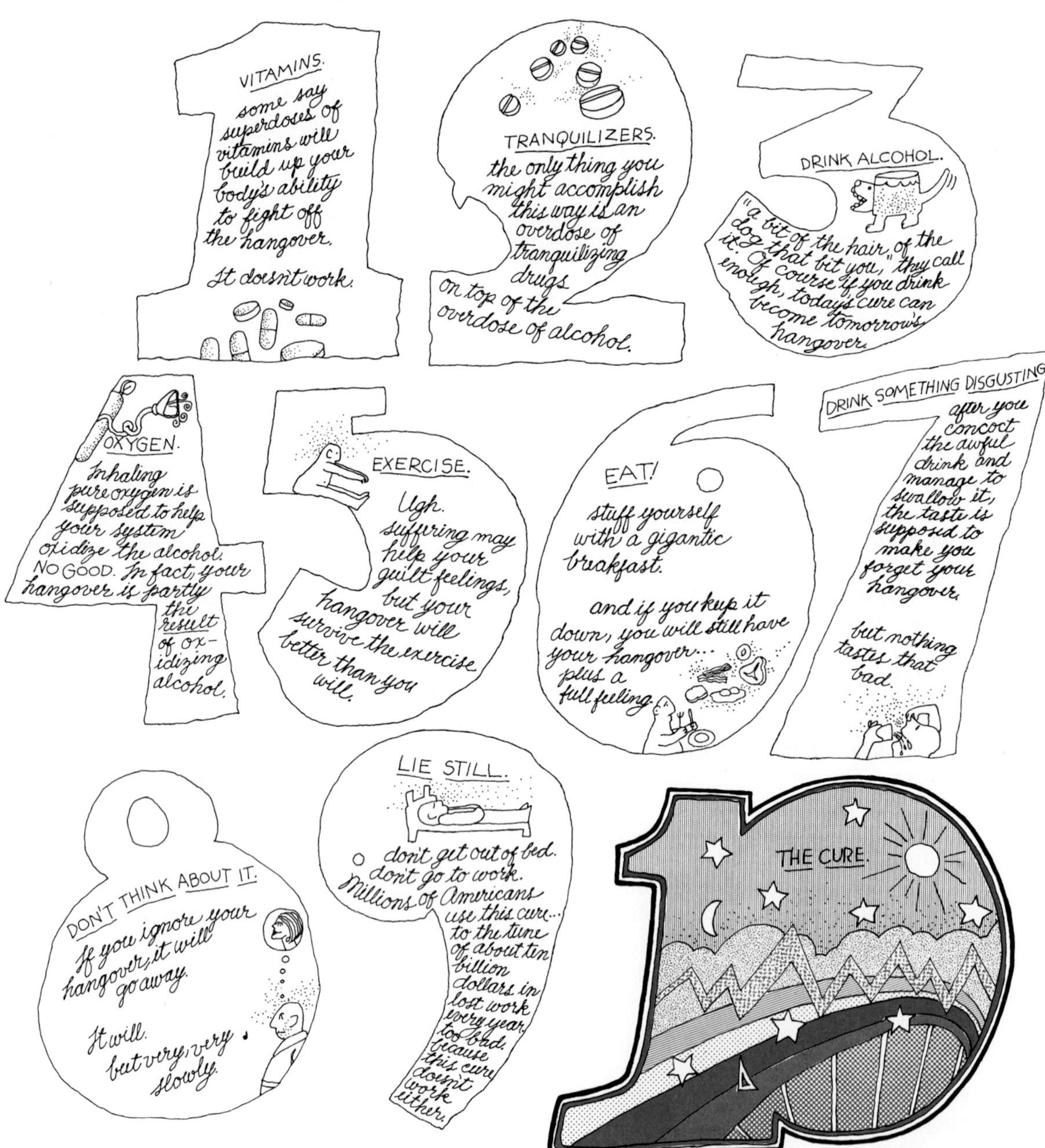

At last, modern medical science has found the perfect, fail proof, 100% effective cure. You guessed it: preventive medicine. The only way to cure a hangover is before it happens.

If you don't drink too much, you don't get a hangover.

Fig. 12-3. Ten Terrific Hangover Cures. (Adapted from National Institute on Alcohol Abuse and Alcoholism)

The specific causes of alcoholism are not well understood as yet. Research seems to support the multiple cause theory of disease in this case, and evidence suggests that there are physical or biological causes, psychological factors, as well as social considerations—all contributing in varying combinations to this illness. Typical of many alcoholics is a low frustration threshold and an inability to face everyday problems. They usually start out by relying on alcohol to get them over difficult aspects of life. More and more they need to fortify themselves with a drink before they can face their problems. They ultimately retreat from them completely, utilizing the alcohol as a crutch. It is rather ironic that the person who takes a drink because he feels it will help him to function more efficiently is actually using a substance that will undermine his ability to perform both professionally and socially. He also finds out too late that alcohol does not solve his problem; it merely irrigates as well as aggravates it.

Other alcoholics, when they feel overwhelmed by their problems, use alcohol as a means of reaching a state of oblivion. It represents a panicky flight from a responsibility they cannot face. Many alcoholics will complain that they have difficulty sleeping, although members of their families will indicate that they sleep as much as the average person. This desire for continual sleep is another indication of their need to escape.

Some alcoholics have a compulsion to drink. This is a form of compulsive behavior they cannot control and invariably results in their addiction to alcohol.

Many people feel that alcohol is the cause of all alcoholism. Actually, alcohol is a neutral agent that can be used or abused. The following case history gives an indication of how the escape agent can be transferred from one substance to another and how, in the absence of alcohol, other substances may often be used.

> . . . I was able to stay dry for several months at a time. But inevitably, after dry periods of from three to six months, I would wind up terribly drunk.
>
> Eventually I began to recognize the symptoms that preceded a drinking episode and realized that I needed help. I went to a neighborhood physician since the problem did not seem important enough for my family doctor. I explained that I was an alcoholic, that I was getting jittery and that I did not want to drink. I asked the doctor if he could give me something for my nerves.
>
> The doctor was sympathetic. Since I had not had a drink in six months, the doctor maintained that I was not an alcoholic. He also prescribed half-grain tablets of phenobarbital, three tablets to be taken during the day and two at bedtime.
>
> Needless to say, like so many alcoholics who attempt to prescribe sedatives for themselves, I found myself in a very short while taking fifteen pills a day.
>
> I had completely transferred my dependency from alcohol to barbiturates. I began to carry a supply of pills in my vest pocket. When something disturbing occurred at the office, I would make a trip to the water cooler and pop several pills into my mouth. After that, whatever had been disturbing me no longer would seem important.
>
> Because of the tolerance that I was developing to the drug, it is doubtful whether the phenobarbital had much effect on me physiologically. But I had definitely developed a psychological dependence that became more compulsive over a period of four years.

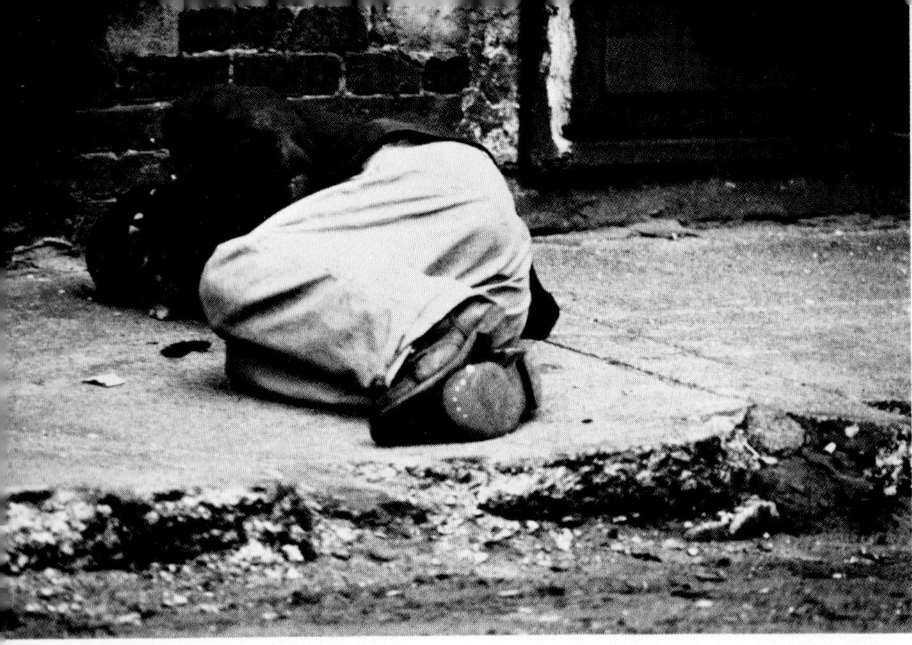

Fig. 12-4. Most people like to view the drunken vagrant as symbolic of the American alcoholic. The great majority of alcoholics actually come from the ranks of the professionals, housewives, blue-collar workers, and other walks of life. (George Mars Cassidy/VAN CLEVE)

There was one occasion when I remember taking three pills but actually took forty-five. I have absolutely no recollection of taking the other forty-two. By the time the doctor reached me I had virtually no pulse. My life hung in the balance for hours as my wife spooned hot, strong, black coffee into me throughout the night.

Both personal experience and observation have convinced me that an alcoholic cannot safely take "the first pill" any more than he can take "the first drink."[22]

Treatment of the Alcoholic

The first step in the treatment of the alcoholic is to detoxify him. It is helpful to give the alcoholic a tranquilizer during this phase, because withdrawal from alcohol will often cause the patient to go through an active phase. With a long-term or chronic alcoholic, the condition known as delirium tremens may occur as a result of alcohol withdrawal. Trembling and hallucinations of a terrifying nature characterize this disorder. With appropriate use of tranquilizers and other therapeutic aids, patients are helped to keep this activity under control, recover promptly, and are ready to start other forms of treatment.

Because the large intake of alcohol impairs the desire to eat, various nutritional problems must be corrected as part of the therapy. Nutritional deficiency diseases can be easily corrected with proper food intake and the addition of vitamins to the diet. After the alcoholic has been withdrawn from alcohol and is physically rehabilitated, the important job of preventing his future drinking begins.

Drugs such as disulfiram and calcium carbimide have been used in efforts to discourage the patient from drinking. An alcoholic on these drugs finds that any contact with alcohol produces nausea, vomiting, palpitations of the heart, and loss of breath. This method of treatment requires close medical supervision because of the severe physical reactions. The prescription of tranquilizers is another form of drug therapy requiring close medical supervision lest the alcoholic transfer his alcohol dependency to the tranquilizers. While drugs of this type may be helpful initially, ultimately the alcoholic must learn by himself to live without his dependence on alcohol.

Psychotherapy is often the method used to help the individual to self-examine his motivations for drinking, to counsel and guide him, and ultimately to change his feelings and behavior so that he may live effectively without his drug dependence. Psychotherapy may take many forms: it may be done in groups or alone; it may include hypnosis or role playing; it may include a conditioned-response[23] approach; or it may include the patient's family.

Supportive organizations, such as Alcoholics Anonymous, a voluntary organization made up of former or recovered alcoholics, stand ready to help.

[22] "Tranquilizers, Sedatives and the Alcoholic," Alcoholics Anonymous World Services, Inc., 1961.

[23] *"aversion,"* or *"conditioned response,"* is described by Marvin A. Block as a technique whereby in a controlled environment a patient is given whatever alcoholic beverage he wants. The beverage is modified, however, to make him ill. If the technique is repeated over an extended period, the patient will become ill when he even thinks of taking a drink.

Their sole purpose is to help the alcoholic to overcome his problem. Former alcoholics, having gone through the ordeal, understand the feelings and temptations that beset the individual with his alcohol dependence. People who seek help from Alcoholics Anonymous receive no preaching, are not asked to sign a pledge, and are not scolded for their past behavior. Other organizations offering special family aid are Al-Anon and Al-Ateen. Al-Anon was established to help wives and husbands, friends, and other relatives of alcoholics better understand the problem. An attempt to improve the environment to which a rehabilitated alcoholic must return would seem essential. Al-Ateen was established to help children of compulsive drinkers understand their parents' problems, to understand that alcoholism is not inherited, and to help develop in themselves better alternatives in coping with emotional and social stresses. They learn that their situation is not unique and try to find ways to adjust to them.

In determing what the alcoholic's chances for recovery are one must consider whether the patient is a *psychotic alcoholic*, a *Skid Row alcoholic*, or an *"average" alcoholic.*[24] The psychotic alcoholic, suffering from a severe chronic psychosis, is usually housed in a state mental hospital. The Skid Row alcoholic is usually a poor man, with no family, job, or accepted place in his community. The chance for recovery in these two groups is very limited, but it must be remembered that these groups comprise only a very small percentage of all alcoholics. The "average" alcoholic (70 per cent of all alcoholics) presents a different picture, however. This is either a man or woman, single or still married, employed and holding a respected position in his community. Their chances of recovery are good, depending on their motivation to get well, their intelligence, and the competence of the therapy employed. The earlier help is sought the better the chances for recovery.

"Recovery" from the disease means different things to different authorities. Some maintain that a rehabilitated alcoholic can learn to drink socially and moderately while functioning in his job and family. Other specialists maintain this is an impossibility and accuse those persons of making dangerous and unwise statements. These latter specialists endeavor to help their patients make complete abstinence from alcohol their goal.

A Giant Step Forward

In all the jails throughout our country, the number of prisoners with a drinking problem serious enough to result in arrest or imprisonment is very high. The jailing of people with an alcoholic dependence does not serve to solve the problem. The jailing represents nothing more than the setting up of a revolving door through which the alcoholic migrates from community to jail and back again. The jailing of a person for any crime or disorder represents on the part of society a kind of frustration. Being unable to prevent or cope with the situation, we seek correction through restraint. We have the knowledge and means for the correction of alcoholism; our continu-

[24] *Alcohol and Alcoholism*, p. 37.

 ing to jail the alcoholic renders us guilty of a kind of thinking that lacks logic.

The New York State Legislature recently introduced legislation[25] indicating that public intoxication is *not* a violation and that a person so indisposed should be directed to his home or to a facility suitable for the care and treatment of alcoholics. These could consist of a psychiatric facility, a ward, wing, or unit of a hospital or any other facility providing in-patient care or services for the alcoholic. Senator Harold Hughes of Iowa has introduced similar federal legislation. Such legislative efforts represent a milestone in that they will move a drug problem out of the legal-moral context into the social-health sphere where it can be dealt with constructively.

Man's Use of Tobacco

Contrary to popular opinion stimulated by current cigarette advertisements, cigarette smoking did not start with the cowboy, but with the Indian. Tobacco was used by the New World natives even before Columbus' voyage. The thought that the burning of the curious leaves and the inhalation of the smoke was to be the basis of a major industry apparently did not occur to the Indian. The Indian smoked not only for enjoyment and ceremonial purposes, but for the curative powers he believed tobacco possessed.

[25]State of New York, S. 9089–A; A. 10908–A; Cal. No. 860, Senate-Assembly, March 6, 1972.

Smoking, as well as the misconceived notion that tobacco had therapeutic powers, spread to Europe and there is evidence that in the seventeenth-century tobacco was used in attempts to cure cancer and to ward off the plague.

The early use of tobacco in Europe was in the form of pipe-smoking and snuff. It was during the mid-1800's that the cigarette was introduced in London by English soldiers. Cigarette smoking came into its own in Europe, and shortly thereafter the cigarette industry was born in the United States. In its infancy this industry did not flourish, but was, in fact, nearly wiped out by taxation. It was further threatened by temperance groups who succeeded in introducing anticigarette bills. During the 1920's and early thirties, all prohibitory laws with regard to cigarettes were repealed. The sale of cigarettes began to boom from this time on. The United States is now the world leader in tobacco production, exportation, and consumption. Americans spend approximately $8 billion dollars a year on tobacco products. This country, in addition, exports annually approximately 25 billion cigarettes.

Why People Smoke

The reasons why people smoke are as varied as the individuals themselves, with each person seeking satisfaction in one form or another. Much has been written on the subject of why young people start smoking. The reasons run the full gamut from the subconscious to the conscious. Some scholars state that the oral satisfactions derived from smoking are reminiscent of the suckling time in one's life, with all the security that went with the mother's breast. Whether the smoking habit stems from this subconscious motivation or from the very real pressures from one's own peers, it is obvious that this is a multifaceted problem.

One of the most important factors related to teenage smoking is whether or not the parents or older siblings smoked. If the family attitude toward smoking is one of acceptance, then smoking becomes a part of "growing up." There is also a higher incidence of smoking when the young adult does not enjoy peer group status. The smoking in these instances becomes a form of compensatory behavior. The smoking may therefore be symptomatic of emotional problems.

In further exploring why people smoke one cannot overlook the multimillion dollar advertising campaign of the tobacco industry as a causative factor in initiating cigarette smoking.

The reasons the veteran smoker offers for smoking are pleasure, sociability, relief of tension, self-assurance, stimulation, and nicotine craving. The question of whether smoking has addictive qualities is being less debated, as confirmed smokers experience definite withdrawal symptoms when they attempt to stop smoking. The term *addicted smoker* is being increasingly used by scientists who work in this field. The greatest reason, therefore, why people smoke is because they simply cannot stop. They are hooked on nicotine. As stated by former Surgeon General Luther Terry, "Ninety five per cent of smokers know the dangers of their habit and seventy five percent of them want to quit, but can't."[26] Research has been initiated to find ways of withdrawing people from addictive smoking. The medical record for reversing addictions, however, is not encouraging.

The Physiological Effects of Smoking

Many physiological changes take place when one lights up a cigarette. One of the offending substances resulting from cigarette combustion is nicotine, "a poisonous volatile alkaloid ($C_{10}H_{14}N_2$) derived from tobacco and responsible for many of the effects of tobacco."[27] In small amounts nicotine acts as a stimulant, but in larger doses it serves as a depressant. Hence, smoking will cause an increase in the heart rate of an individual, a temporary rise in the blood pressure, and a slight elevation of blood sugar level. Smoking reduces the blood flow in the coronary arteries, leaving an electrocardiographic picture similar to that in coronary artery diseases. Those individuals already suffering from narrowed coronary arteries as a result of atherosclerosis may often experience anginal pain pointing to the further narrowing of the arteries by nicotine-induced spasms. There is a constriction of the peripheral blood vessels, causing

[26] National Clearinghouse for Smoking and Health, *Newsweek*, September 27, 1971.

[27] Definition of nicotine in *Stedman's Medical Dictionary* (Williams and Wilkins Co., 1965).

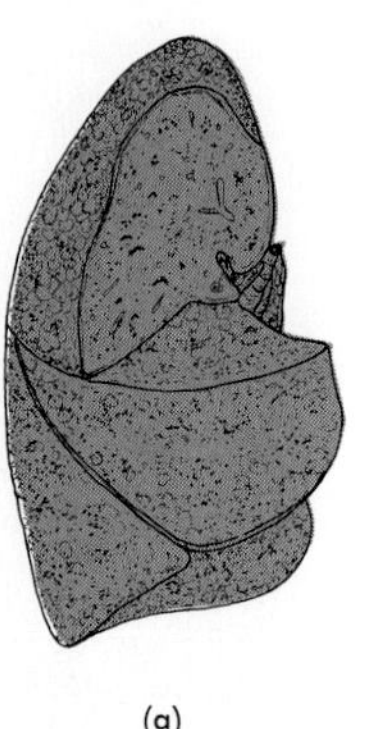
(a)

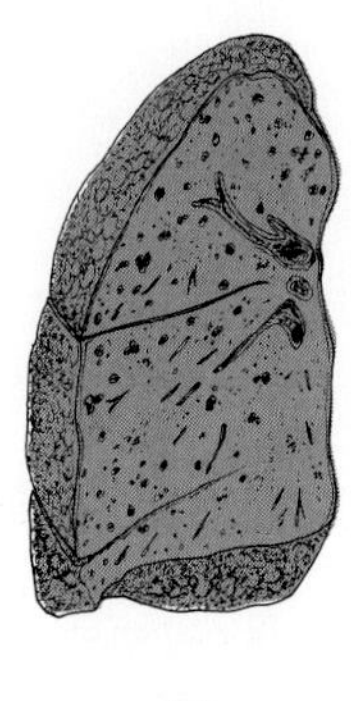
(b)

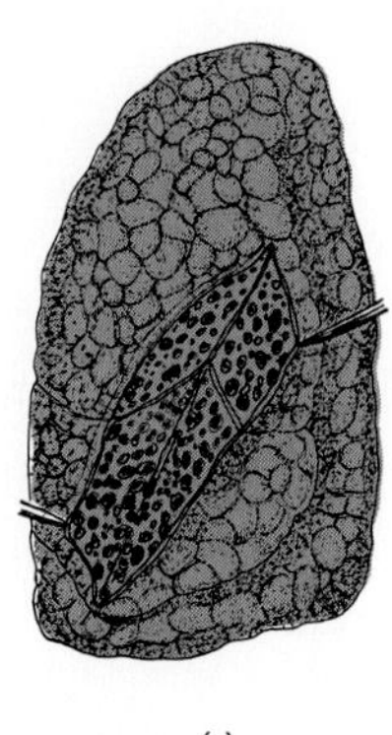
(c)

Fig. 12-5. (**A**) Normal Lung. *Gross specimen of normal lung with cut surface displaying typical appearance of adult lung.* (**B**) Bronchitis with Secondary Emphysema. *Lung in bronchitis with secondary emphysema showing inflammatory changes in bronchi filled with purulent sputum causing emphysematous damage.* (**C**) Panlobular Emphysema. *Gross specimen of large pale gray lung in panlobular emphysema. Distention of respiratory bronchioles, alveolar ducts, alveolar sacs and alveoli convert entire lung, including the peripheral parenchyma, to typical honeycomb appearance. (Knoll Pharmaceutical Company)*

a lowering of body temperature. In subzero temperatures, the possibility of frostbite of the fingers and toes is greater in the smoking individual.

In individuals with an *unusual* sensitivity to nicotine, severe spasms of the small arteries of the fingers, toes, cheeks, nose, and ears will result in a slowing down or stopping of the blood flow. Blood clots forming here will eventually result in gangrene of the extremity. This condition, Buerger's disease (thromboangiitis obliterans), is seldom fatal, but is most painful and handicapping because the amputation of fingers, toes, and other parts is usually necessitated. The disease is terminated when smoking stops; however, in the individual addicted to smoking a return to the habit precipitates a resumption of the disease. "It is a startling fact indeed that some patients who have already lost their toes, and who have been warned that they will lose their legs next, nevertheless have continued to smoke."[28]

Nicotine is only one of the many offending compounds found in smoke. Other substances include hydrocarbons, alcohols, esters, sterols, aldehydes, acids, phenols, arsenic, potassium, and some metals. Though these substances are found in minute amounts, several have been proved to be carcinogenic (cancer-producing) and some are co-carcinogenic (i.e., substances that increase the potency of the carcinogens). Upon the inhalation of smoke, the lining of the trachea and bronchial tubes are bathed with the smoke condensate or tar. In the lining of the trachea and bronchi, the production of mucus and the whiplike action of the cilia normally catch and then sweep upward any foreign particles that may be inhaled. However, the inhalation of cigarette smoke slows down and may completely paralyze the ciliary action while it stimulates an increase in the production of mucus. The result is a persistent cough which endeavors to expel the accumulated, excess mucus. This is referred to as a "cigarette cough" or more correctly a chronic bronchitis (inflammation of the bronchi). As the mucus accumulates in the bronchioles, there is a tendency for these tubes to close shut, often trapping air in the alveoli (air sacs). Over a period of years this trapped air can stretch the alveoli to large blisters, or bullae. When a person coughs, the increased pressure exerted on the delicate walls of the alveoli is enough to rupture them, thereby eventually cutting down the lung capacity of the individual. This is essentially what occurs in emphysema, with the person constantly short of breath because so much of his lung tissue has been destroyed in this fashion.

Emphysema can have a negative effect on the heart because it tends to cause a decrease in the amount of oxygen that may be taken in by the lungs. The effect is that it increases the work load of the heart to pick up the same amount of oxygen. A further strain on the heart is caused by the fact that emphysema reduces the number of channels through which blood can pass through the lungs. Cardiac failure is often associated with advanced cases of emphysema.

In discussing impairment of lung function, it then

[28] *The Consumers Union Report on Smoking and the Public Interest* (Mount Vernon, N.Y.: Consumers Union, 1963), p. 88.

Fig. 12-6. **A.** *This collection of tar can be analyzed and is used in biological experimentation.* **B.** *If tar is taken from just a few packages of cigarettes and a dilute solution is made, the application of this solution to the skin of small animals will cause 60% of these animals to have tumors of the skin within a year.* **C.** *This can be done repeatedly and consistently under laboratory conditions.* (*Roswell Park Memorial Institute*)

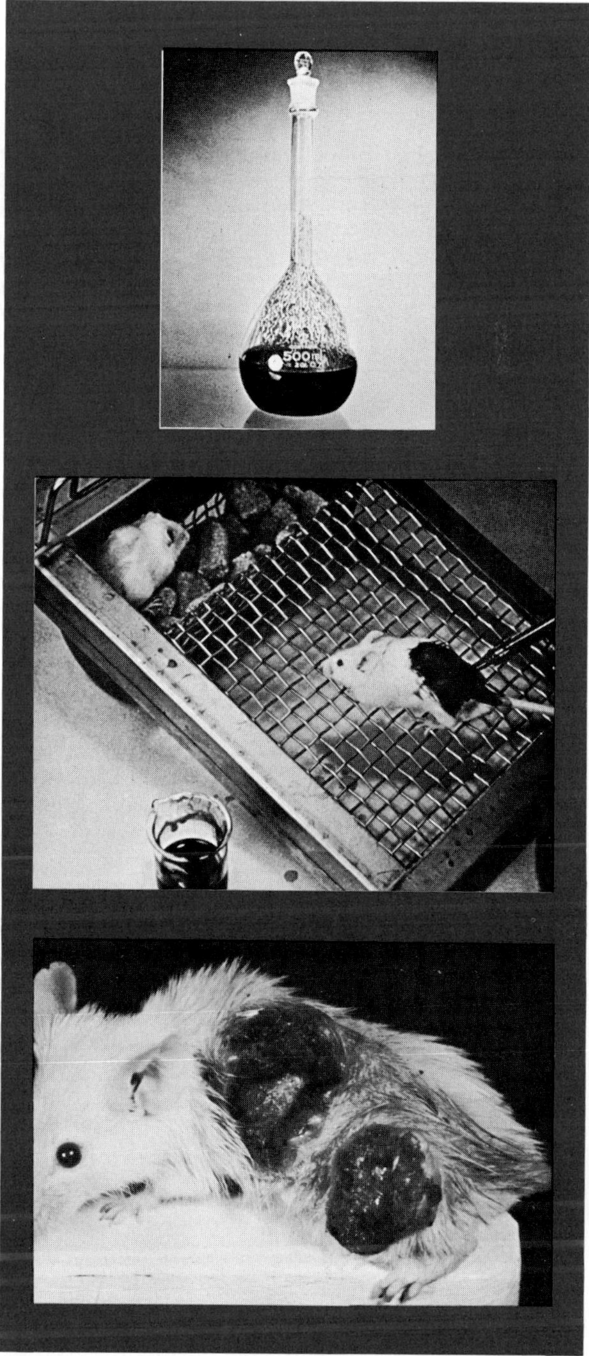

becomes obvious that we are discussing several problems. *Chronic obstructive bronchopulmonary disease* (COPD) is the inclusive term being used to refer to three common respiratory ailments. These include (1) chronic bronchitis, (2) pulmonary emphysema, and (3) bronchial asthma. The observable symptoms from these diseases may at times be similar, thereby making it difficult to determine if the patient is suffering from one disease or more, and if more than one is present, which one predominates. In the United States a major increase in deaths from COPD is evident:

1949 death rate from COPD was	2.1/100,000 resident population
1960	6.0/100,000
1967	12.9/100,000

It is thought the mortality rates are probably underestimated, since COPD is not listed as a contributing cause of death as would be the case in cardiac failure. The indictment of smoking is made clear in the statement of the Surgeon General: "Cigarette smoking is the most important cause of COPD in the United States."[29]

Perhaps the most dramatic indictment against cigarette smoking is the change that occurs in the epithelial lining of the bronchi, where most cases of lung cancer occur (see Fig. 12-7).

[29] *The Health Consequences of SMOKING,* A Report of the Surgeon General, U.S. Dept of Health, Education and Welfare, 1972, p. 3.

Fig. 12-7. Bronchial epithelium is the original site of almost all lung cancer. The progressive photomicrographs and diagrams show initially an increase in the number of basal cells. This is followed by the loss of ciliated columnar cells. The cells then develop atypical nuclei and become disordered. An early cancer is thus formed that could spread to the rest of the lungs and body. (Photos by Oscar Auerbach from "The Effects of Smoking," Scientific American, *July, 1962. Copyright © 1962 by Scientific American, Inc. All rights reserved.)*

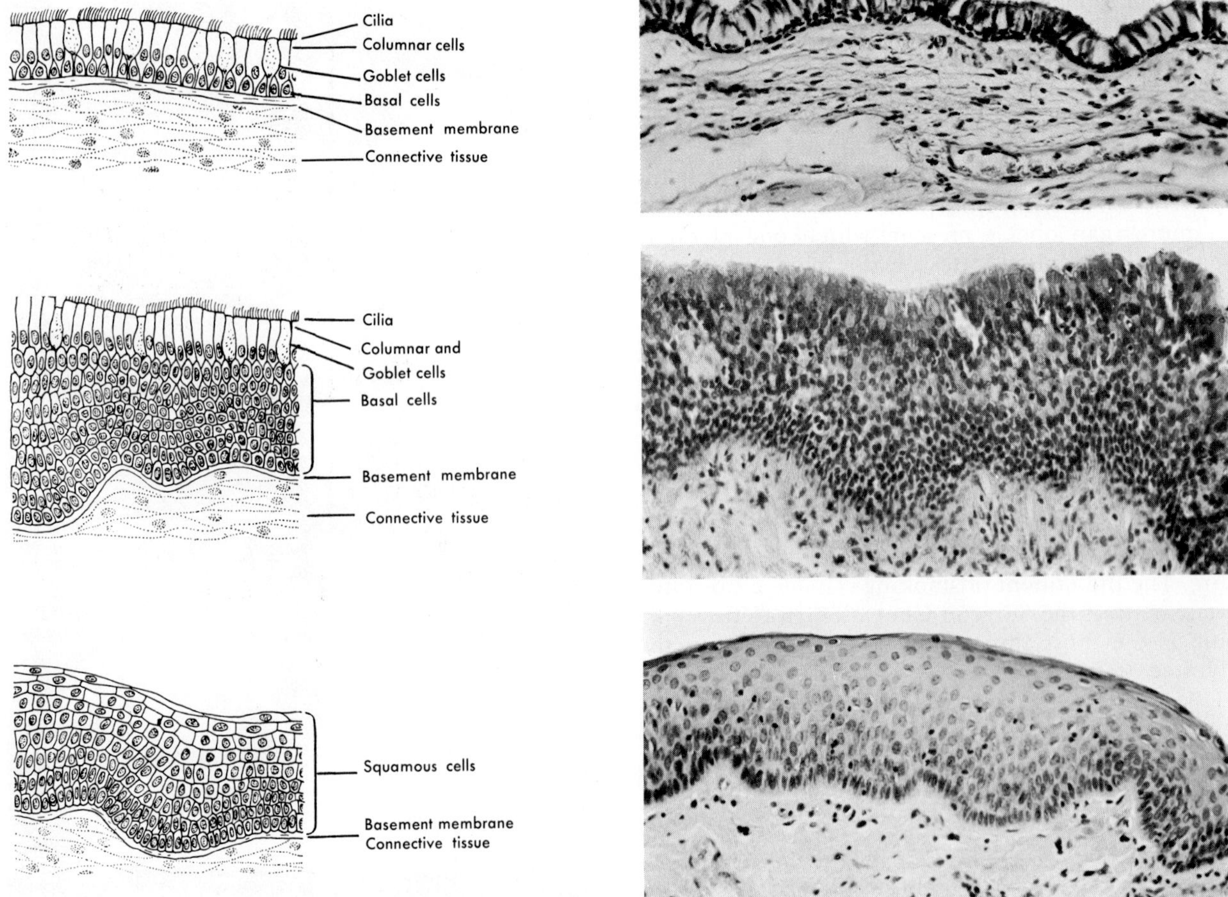

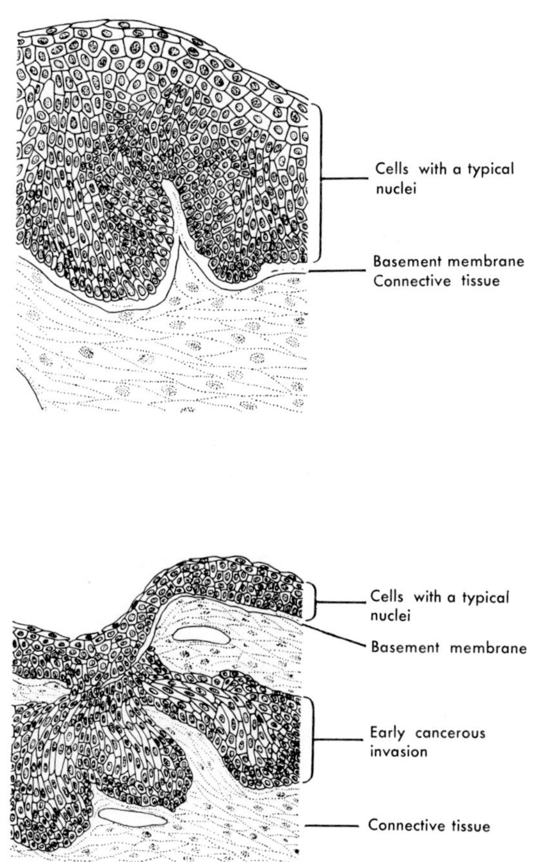
Cells with a typical nuclei
Basement membrane
Connective tissue
Cells with a typical nuclei
Basement membrane
Early cancerous invasion
Connective tissue

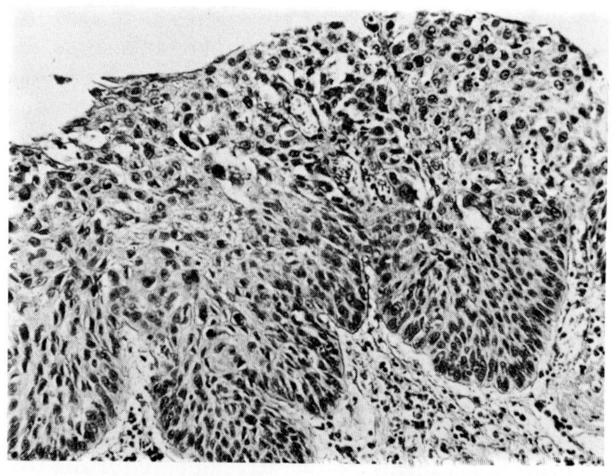

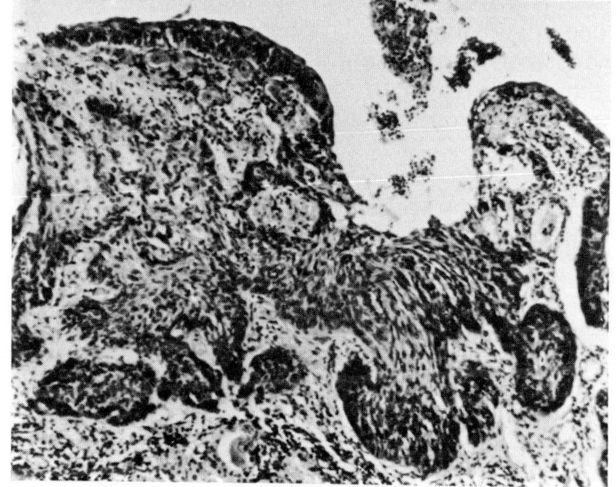

Polonium 210, a radioactive substance, is dispatched into the mainstream smoke, and some researchers believe that this substance is at least one of the causative agents of lung cancer. Several autopsy studies have shown that the bronchial epithelium of smokers contains significantly more Polonium 210 than that of nonsmokers. Though research with Polonium is inconclusive, study continues to pinpoint relationships between specific carcinogenic substances in cigarette smoke and the development of lung cancer.

Cigarette Advertising

From its early beginning, the tobacco industry in this country was a highly competitive one, requiring the use of varied promotional techniques and schemes. The advertising appeals were of a positive nature, with opera stars stating that certain brands of cigarettes would help to "save" their voices. Athletes were quoted on how a particular brand of cigarette helped them to "stay in shape."

In the early 1950's, the American Cancer Society presented a research report indicating a possible relationship between smoking and cancer. The immediate reaction to the report was a decline in the sale of cigarettes. The reaction of the tobacco industry was to increase advertising expenditures and to develop the filter-tip cigarette. The report also stimulated the "tar derby," in which each manufacturer made the attempt to convince the public that his cigarette was lowest in tar content. Though the filters that were placed on cigarettes were not very effective in filtering out tars, they did serve to satisfy the customer that he was now "safe from cancer." In 1953 regular cigarettes accounted for 80 per cent of the total sales. By 1963, however, they accounted for only 25 per cent of total sales, with filter cigarettes accounting for the rest. In 1954 the total cigarette sales in the United States had slumped to under 369 billion. By increasing its advertising costs by 134 per cent in the next six years, the industry caused an upswing in cigarette consumption so that by 1961 cigarette sales soared to 490 billion cigarettes. There were those who hailed this turnabout as one of the supreme achievements of marketing strategy! In 1964 the report of the Surgeon General's Advisory Committee indicting cigarette smoking as a cause of lung cancer and relating it to the high incidence of cardiovascular disease, emphysema, and a number of other conditions, again caused a dip in cigarette sales. In response to this challenge the tobacco industry once again increased its advertising expenditures. In 1965 this expenditure reached the total of 250 million dollars. This added effort reclaimed initial losses in sales due to the Surgeon General's report.

Since the publication of the report, advertising techniques have changed so that the mention of health factors in cigarette commercials is rare indeed. The tobacco industry has sensed that the average teenager has not been frightened by medical reports indicating the relationship between smoking and disease. It is difficult for a young person to be concerned about the possible developments of disease that might occur twenty or thirty years later. The result is that the teenager has been made an advertising target of the industry. Cigarette advertisements relate the use of cigarettes to athletic prowess, popularity, and datability.

Attempts to Control Cigarette Advertising

From 1955 to 1960 the Federal Trade Commission sought to control the many false claims made by manufacturers about the effectiveness of their filters, and the tar and nicotine content of their cigarettes. The FTC finally persuaded the tobacco industry to discontinue the tar derby because of this federal agency's inability to properly supervise claims being made in this area. In 1962, Italy banned all tobacco advertising. In Finland, as of July 1962, television advertising of cigarettes ended. In February of 1965, the British Labor Government said that it would ban all cigarette advertising from television and was considering a similar ban on newspaper and poster ads. The United States government, which had been slow to act in this area, finally approved a health hazard warning which began appearing on all cigarette packages in January 1966. Some people have implied that the United States government has not acted forcefully against the tobacco industry because it is one of the giant industries of this country, with an annual output worth approximately $4 billion. It is one that has large areas of agriculture dependent solely upon it. Because this country is also the largest exporter of tobacco products, the crippling of this industry would hurt the country financially.

On January 2, 1971, cigarette commercials were banned from television. While some viewed this action as a victory for the consumer over the tobacco industry, it has proven to be a reversal. A few years prior to the 1971 ban of the cigarette TV commercials, the Federal Communications Commission (FCC) declared that significant (if not equal) time could be given to anticigarette commercials. Health organizations such as the American Cancer Society, the American Heart Association, and the National TB and Respiratory Disease Association developed anticigarette commercials that began to have an effect on cigarette sales. As indicated in the *Wall Street Journal,*

> It now seems clear that the continuing falloff is attributable to the antismoking campaign, but the rate of year-to-year decline should begin to level off in 1971 for the somewhat ironic reason that Congress has banned all cigarette commercials on radio and TV after January 1, giving stations less incentive to run antismoking commercials.[30]

As the tobacco industry shifted its advertising to magazines, newspapers, and billboards, it moved into media that the health organizations could not follow without enormous sums of money (which they do not have). The health organizations could not receive "public service space" in these media as it did public service time on the airways. The tobacco industry thus shifted its advertising from media where their messages relating cigarette smoking to

[30] *Proceedings of the N.Y. State Conference, Smokeless 70's Independently or Interdependently?* N.Y. State Interagency Committee on Hazards of Smoking, April 1970.

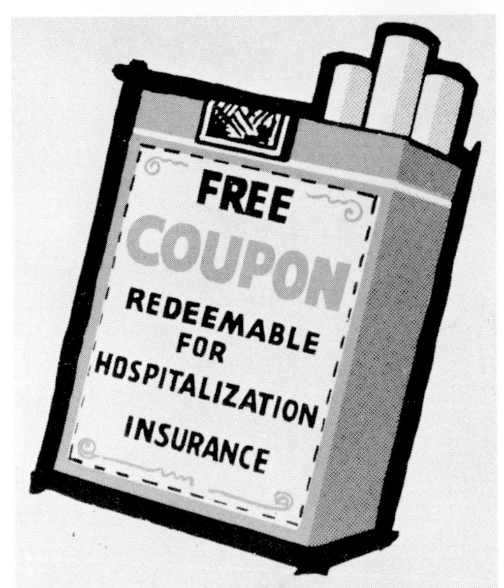

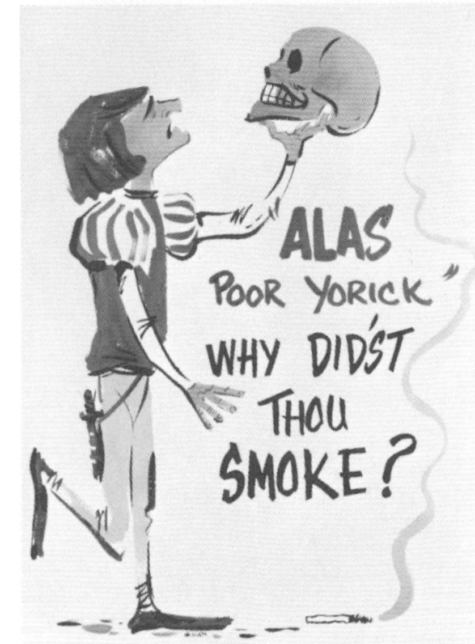

Fig. 12-8. A series of six posters developed by the Roswell Park Memorial Institute.

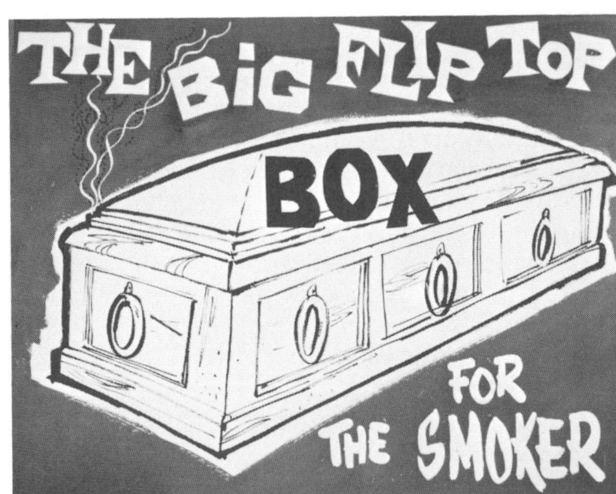

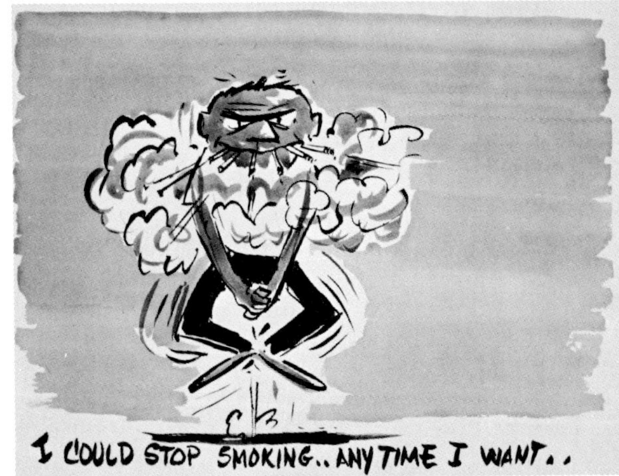

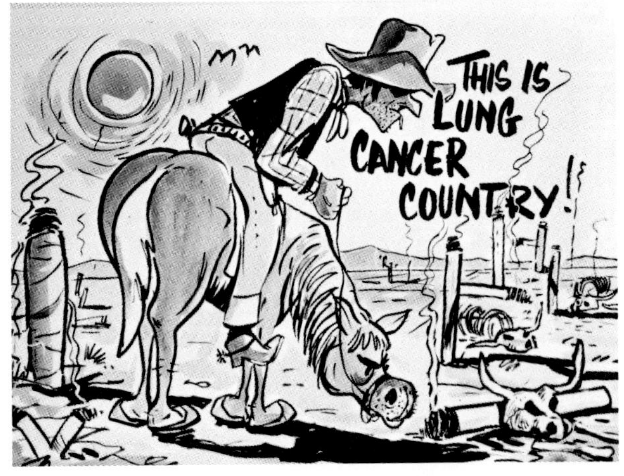

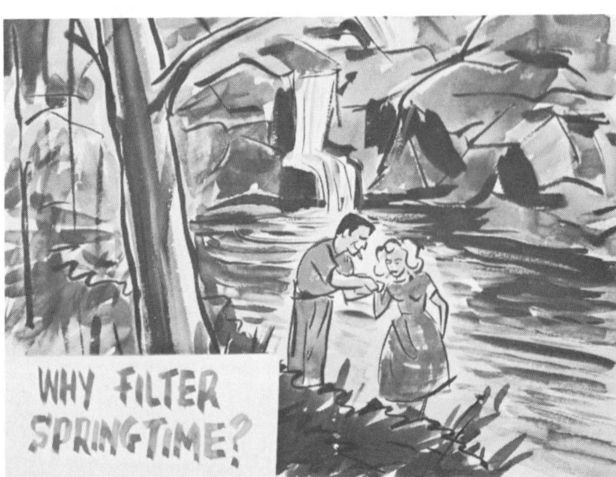

enhanced masculinity, femininity, Women's Liberation, spring, and independence could not be counteracted by messages relating cigarette smoking to lung cancer, emphysema, heart attacks, and premature death.

The Decade Since the Surgeon General's Report

In 1964 the ten members of the Surgeon General's Advisory Committee, all outstanding physicians and scientists of this country, evaluated three kinds of scientific evidence: (1) animal experiments, (2) clinical or autopsy studies, (3) population studies. In animal experimentation, animals were exposed to tobacco smoke, tars, and the various chemical compounds they contained. Seven of these compounds have been established as being cancer-producing (carcinogenic) in nature. Other substances in tobacco and smoke, although not carcinogenic, promote cancer production or lower the threshold to a known carcinogen. Toxic or irritant gases contained in tobacco smoke produced experimentally the kinds of noncancerous damage seen in the tissues and cells of heavy smokers. This included suppression of ciliary action, damage to lung air sacs, to mucous glands, and goblet glands, which produce mucus.

Clinical and autopsy studies among smokers showed that many kinds of damage to body functions and organs, cells, and tissues occurred more frequently and severely in smokers. Marked changes in the cells lining the trachea and bronchi have been observed with some of the advanced lesions noted in the bronchi of heavy smokers considered to be premalignant (or precancerous). Pathological changes in the air sacs and other functional tissues of the lung were noted to have a remarkably close association with cigarette smoking.

Population studies showed that cigarette smokers had a proportionately higher incidence of lung cancer than nonsmokers. The prevalence of specific signs and symptoms such as chronic cough, sputum production, breathlessness, chest illness, and decreased lung functioning were found consistently in much higher incidence among smokers.

After a careful review of studies and evidences in the area, the committee made the following judgments: "Cigarette smoking is a health hazard of sufficient importance in the United States to warrant appropriate remedial action."[31] The committee further concluded that cigarette smoking was causally related to lung cancer in men, and that the risk of developing lung cancer increases with the duration of smoking and the number of cigarettes smoked and is diminished by the discontinuation of the smoking habit. A study of the evidence led the committee to feel that there is a relationship between smoking and cancer of the larynx, esophagus, and the urinary bladder. It found a relationship exists between cigarette smoking and pulmonary emphysema and

[31] *Smoking and Health*, Report of the Advisory Committee to the Surgeon General of the Public Health Service, U.S. Department of Health, Education and Welfare.

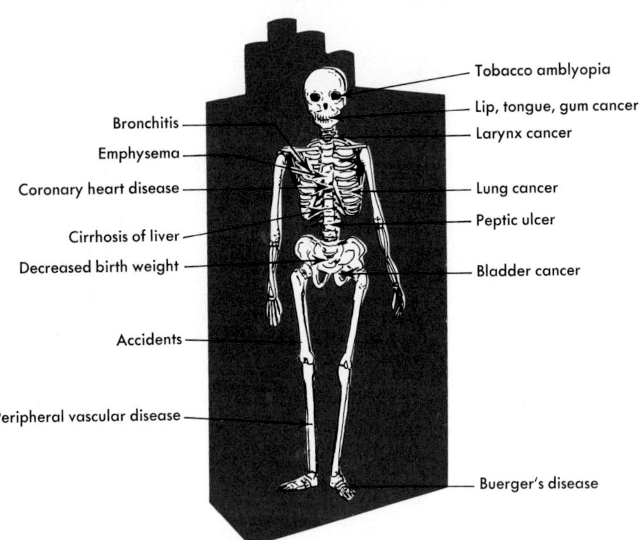

Fig. 12-9 Chart of distribution of diseases associated with smoking. (Roswell Park Memorial Institute)

chronic bronchitis. It found that male cigarette smokers have a higher death rate from coronary heart disease than nonsmokers. The cold facts are that in 1935, 4,000 deaths were attributed to lung cancer. In 1966 this death toll reached 50,000, and in 1970, 60,000. The American Cancer Society warns that if the current trend is not reversed, 1 million of our present-day school children will die prematurely from lung cancer.

In 1972 the Surgeon General's Report had been updated and further substantiated through the years by additional research studies. Recent findings not only confirmed a relationship between cigarette smoking and coronary heart disease but further indicated its relationship to the sudden, fatal form of heart attack. There is evidence that cigarette smoking accelerates the pathology of preexisting heart disease, thereby contributing to the individual's sudden and unexpected death. Further experimental studies on animals and autopsy studies have indicated that smoking contributes to the development of atherosclerosis of the aorta and coronary arteries.

Cigarette smoking has been established as the most important cause of chronic obstructive bronchopulmonary disease (COPD) and far outranks atmospheric pollution as a causative factor. Pulmonary dysfunctions as well as mortality is higher in smokers as compared to nonsmokers. The updated report further indicated that the hazards of cigarette smoking may fall on the smoker and *non-smoker* alike—though not in equal amounts. He stated, "We cannot overlook the fact that exposure to these concentrations of carbon monoxide may be especially hazardous for those who are suffering from heart disease or chronic bronchopulmonary disease."[32]

The new information relative to lung cancer was quite specific. Whereas the 1964 report said that cigarette smoking *was causally related to lung cancer,* the 1972 report, "confirms the conclusion that cigarette smoking is the main cause of lung cancer in men."[33] There no longer seems to be an honest disagreement among medical scientists concerning the hazards of cigarette smoking. The incidence of oral cancer, as well as cancer of the larynx and esophagus, is clearly greater in smokers than in nonsmokers. An alcohol and tobacco interaction has been indicated as a lethal combination associated with especially high rates of cancer of the esophagus.

In summing up developments concerning cigarette smoking since the original Surgeon General's report of 1964, Dr. Steinfeld said there would probably have been many more millions smoking cigarettes had the government not campaigned against the habit. With all this evidence one wonders how long the offering of a cigarette will continue to be viewed as a friendly, social grace instead of the threat it really is.

Prevention

Inevitably the question is being asked, what can be done to prevent or at least slow down this developing

[32] National Clearing House for Smoking and Health, January 18, 1972.

[33] *The Health Consequences of Smoking,* A Report of the Surgeon General, 1972, p. 11.

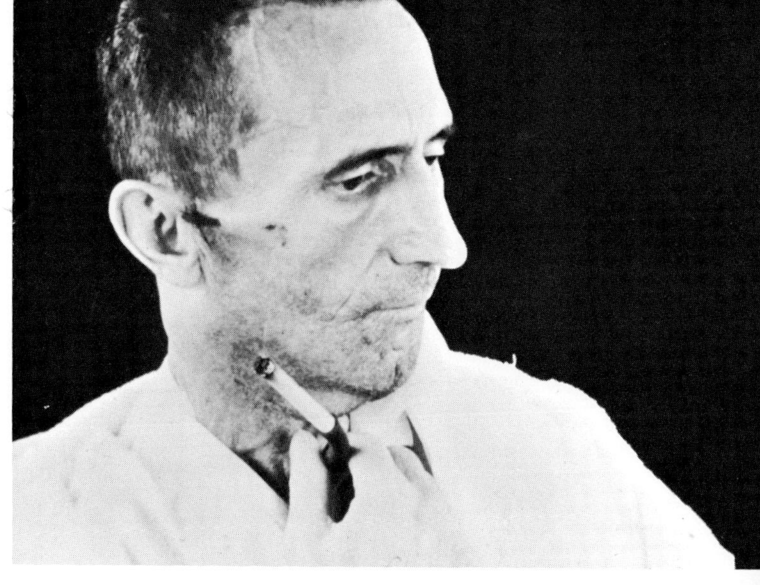

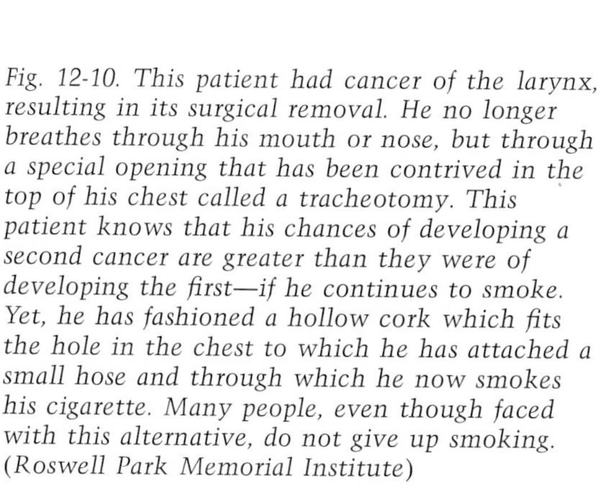
Fig. 12-10. This patient had cancer of the larynx, resulting in its surgical removal. He no longer breathes through his mouth or nose, but through a special opening that has been contrived in the top of his chest called a tracheotomy. This patient knows that his chances of developing a second cancer are greater than they were of developing the first—if he continues to smoke. Yet, he has fashioned a hollow cork which fits the hole in the chest to which he has attached a small hose and through which he now smokes his cigarette. Many people, even though faced with this alternative, do not give up smoking. (Roswell Park Memorial Institute)

catastrophic situation? A number of suggestions have been made and in many instances actions taken in an attempt to implement them.

Many feel that the development of an effective filter would significantly reduce tar and nicotine content in cigarette smoke. Current filters, however, are not highly effective. The most optimistic estimate is that current filters reduce the risk of lung cancer by 30 per cent over nonfiltered cigarettes. Other estimates are more pessimistic. A related factor is the tar and nicotine content of the tobacco in front of the filter. In some cigarettes, stronger tobacco is used to compensate for whatever filtering action the filter may effect. Dr. Ernest Wynder, President of the American Health Foundation, has suggested that we put "a maximum level (of tar and nicotine) on all American cigarettes and set it at 20 milligrams for tar and 1.2 milligrams of nicotine. I picked that level because 50 percent of all American cigarettes meet that level. That suggestion was violently opposed by the tobacco industry."[34] It is felt that it is easier for a smoker to break away from the cigarette habit if he is using cigarettes of low nicotine content. The University of Kentucky Agricultural Experiment Station is currently attempting to produce a low-nicotine burley tobacco breeding line in order that cigarettes with a low-nicotine content may be produced. In addition, of course, lowered tar content would protect the smoker to some extent from lung cancer and other tobacco related diseases. Other efforts to create a nontobacco cigarette has not yet been fruitful. Until such time as a safe cigarette can be produced, people who feel a need to smoke are still urged to switch to pipes and cigars.

As indicated by the Surgeon General, 75 per cent of those people who smoke would like to stop but cannot, and further do not know where to go for help. Smoking withdrawal clinics have been experimented with over the past ten years. It would seem that it is time to routinely establish such clinics in hospitals (for patients and staff), schools (for students, faculty and parents), and industrial plants. These clinics have had varying success in terms of the percentage of participants who can kick the nicotine habit. However, even those who fail can learn to smoke more safely by means of low-tar and low-nicotine cigarettes, switching to pipes or cigars, smoking a cigarette only halfway down the butt, and so forth. The constant availability of such clinics makes it possible for a person to try to break the habit a second and third time should he fail on the first attempt. Such clinics may also serve to comfort those who feel trapped in a dangerous habit. It has been suggested that smoking withdrawal clinics be subsidized by health insurance companies as a preventive activity. Since the treatment of tobacco-related diseases represents the greatest expenditure of health insurance monies, this kind of preventive activity would seem justified because it would save lives as well as money. It would also have the effect of shifting health professionals from a purely *treatment* context to one involving *prevention*—a long overdue shift!

[34] *Smoking and Health Newsletter,* National Interagency Council on Smoking and Health, Vol. 8, No. 1 (January–March 1972).

Increasing numbers of schools around the country have become involved in education programs in an effort to discourage people from taking up the smoking habit in the first place. Where schools have used knowledgeable teachers who know how to approach this kind of social health problem, the results have been laudatory. Too often, however, the educational program is attempted by teachers who are ill informed and convey the notion that it is all right for adults to smoke, but not for young people to do so. The latter does nothing more than to reinforce tobacco industry advertisements that have already planted the idea that smoking is associated with sophistication, adulthood, and independence. It amounts to throwing a gallon of gasoline on the fire while these teachers are saying to their communities, "Yes, we are teaching Tobacco Education." . . . indeed they are! The growing demands by high school students for smoking rooms reflect the failure of these programs. Certainly the demand for smoking rooms in our present state of knowledge cannot be classified as an informed one.

Instructional programs related to smoking and health have been most successful when they are started at the elementary level (before a decision on tobacco use has been made) with the students actively involved in the study of this health issue backed by well-informed teachers who see no place for propagandistic approaches in the classroom. Many of these programs have their students active in the community taking surveys of various kinds, assisting in the conduction of smoking withdrawal clinics, seeking out legislators to discuss possible legislation, and serving as a speaker's bureau to report the findings of their studies.

A fifth grade boy who was a part of an activist oriented education program pursued his studies at home by badgering his cigarette-smoking, psychiatrist father. He clearly outlined for his father the various health risks his smoking habit exposed him to and that he was in the process of shortening his life expectancy by some eight years. The fifth grader asked, "Who is going to take care of me? Who will provide for my college education? Are you trying to tell me you don't love me any more?" The father indicated that the only way he could avoid the badgering was to duck into the clothes closet everytime he felt the need to have a cigarette. He soon admitted that being a psychiatrist, he realized that hiding in the closet was rather peculiar behavior. He ultimately resolved the conflict by breaking his smoking habit. There was a time when children used to be afraid to smoke in front of their parents. Where good education programs are instituted in schools, it is the parent who smokes with trepidation in the presence of his children.

Following the pronouncement from the Surgeon General's Office with regard to the harmful effects of tobacco smoke on the nonsmoker, a new band of militants has arisen with a nonsmoker's Bill of Rights. Airlines, railroads, and bus lines began to take action by establishing nonsmoking sections in their vehicles. All the action was not due to the Surgeon General alone. Increasing numbers of nonsmokers have complained to transportation companies and to smokers who pollute the air. A number of airlines were threatened with lawsuits by nonsmokers who felt they were being forced to breathe polluted air that posed a danger to their health. Typical was an altercation that took place on a commuter train. Two men entered the train and sat next to each other. One lit up a cigarette and blew a ball of smoke. The other responded, "Would you mind not blowing your smoke over me?" The smoker retorted, "Where do you expect me to blow it?" The response of the nonsmoker was such that it precipitated a round of fisticuffs exemplifying how sensitive the issue has become. The 164 million Americans who do not smoke can no longer be classified as the *silent* majority!

Review Questions

1. How have drugs contributed to man's welfare?
2. A prescription drug is a personal thing. Explain.
3. Why are side effects in reaction to drugs a common response?
4. Why is it important to read the label on nonprescription drugs?
5. Describe briefly Dr. Lindesmith's views on addiction. What are the implications of the importance of the psychological aspects of addiction?
6. What is your definition of drug abuse?
7. What are the psychosocial implications of marihuana use?
8. What appear to be some of the limitations of methadone maintenance as a solution to heroin addiction?
9. Drug abuse is a social-health problem, not a moral-legal one. Explain.
10. Barbiturate addiction may be the most widespread form of addiction in this country. What have been the underlying reasons for the extensiveness of this problem?
11. What are the basic steps followed in the rehabilitation of the addict?
12. What procedures would you propose for the control of the drug abuse problem?
13. Discuss the relative dangers of the nonaddicting drugs as compared to the addictive drugs as societal problems.
14. Describe the various physiological effects of alcohol on the body.
15. Review the various reasons why people drink or do not drink alcoholic beverages. Support a point of view, pro or con.
16. What appear to be the underlying causes of alcoholism? Explain the susceptibility of alcoholics to habituation to other drugs.
17. What have been the contributions of Alcoholics Anonymous in the rehabilitation of the alcoholic?
18. Explain the futility of jailing the alcoholic.
19. One of every ten of the American work force have serious drinking problems. The United States Public Health Service describes the disorder as having reached epidemic proportions. To what extent do you feel remedial actions are in order?
20. How has cigarette advertising influenced the development of a gigantic tobacco industry?

21. To what extent has the Federal Trade Commission managed to control cigarette advertising?
22. What are the relationships of smoking and health as related in the Surgeon General's report?
23. Identify the offending substances in cigarette smoke. Explain the effects of these substances on the body tissues.
24. What are the preventive approaches that might be used to alleviate the numerous health problems related to cigarette smoking?

Chapter 13
Man's Self-Created Environment

Life is an adventure in a world where nothing is static; where unpredictable and ill-understood events constitute dangers that must be overcome, often blindly and at great cost; where man himself, like the sorcerer's apprentice, has set in motion forces that are potentially destructive and may someday escape his control. Every manifestation of existence is a response to stimuli and challenges, each of which constitutes a threat if not adequately dealt with. The very process of living is a continual interplay between the individual and his environment, often taking the form of a struggle resulting in injury or disease. The more creative the individual, the less he can hope to avoid danger, for the stuff of creation is made up of responses to the forces that impinge on his body and soul.[1]

Our environmental health problems of water and air pollution, pesticide and radiation control are reflective of man's progress. Paradoxically, they also represent obstacles to his future development if not properly dealt with. The increasingly sophisticated technology developed by man means not only a better way of life and perhaps the elimination of more primitive threats to health, but also the development of new health problems with shorter fuses. Our ability as a society to respond quickly and effectively to these newer problems will become determinants of our levels of well-being, in fact, of our survival as a species.

[1]René Dubos, *Mirage of Health* (Garden City, N.Y.: Doubleday Anchor Books, 1961), p. 13.

Air Pollution

While public health officials have been aware of air pollution problems for quite some time, it took a series of disasters before public awareness and interest in the problem was developed. The first of these to occur was in the 1930's in the Meuse Valley in Belgium. The valley is a highly industrialized area that is approximately 15 miles long and 1½ miles wide. An acute air pollution condition resulted in 63 deaths and the illness of many persons. In 1948 a combination of air pollution and adverse weather conditions precipitated a similar disaster in Donora, Pennsylvania. Within a few days this condition caused the death of 20 people and the illness of 6,000 more. In 1952 London underwent a similar experience. Air pollution plus fog and an inversion condition that lasted for about a week resulted in 4,000 deaths and untold illness. London has been the site of a number of such episodes, the last occurring in the summer of 1962. New York City has had a chronic air pollution problem for a number of years, with one of its episodes ironically occuring during the Thanksgiving Day weekend of 1966. According to a recent study a high concentration of sulfur dioxide during a ten-day period in 1953 was responsible for a rise in the average death rate per day in that city from 170 to 260. Although specific disasters have the effect of dramatizing the situation, we should perhaps be more concerned with the chronic air pollution problem faced by our society and with

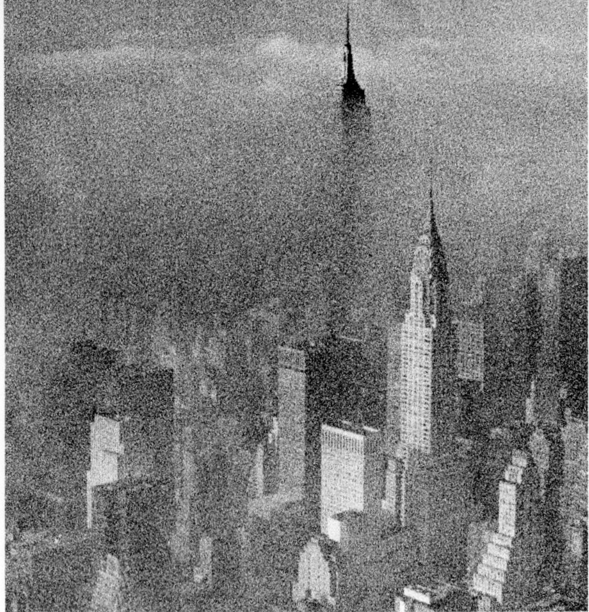

Fig. 13-1. New York City steeped in its own pollution. (New York Journal-American)

the daily toll that it takes not only in lives and illness, but in terms of its effects on crops, animals, and property as well.

The Pollutants

The impurities found in the air are essentially the waste products of a highly industrialized community. In the past, air pollution concern revolved around the amount of smoke that was produced by a busy factory. However, as a result of our technological advances, air pollutants are now many and varied. They are generally classified in two basic groups. The first group consists of gases which are usually the result of fuel combustion. In this grouping we find the nitrogen oxides, the sulfur oxides, carbon monoxide, hydrocarbons, aldehydes, acids, and ozone. The aerosols represent the second group, which are suspensions of solid or liquid particles. Examples of these would be smoke, dust, mist, gas, and fog.

The Gases

Nitrogen oxides are formed by the combination of nitrogen with one or two molecules of oxygen. The exhaust gases of engines and the effluents of furnaces will contain this pollutant. It has the effect of causing irritations to the eye besides reducing visibility and causing vegetation damage. *Ozone* is a gaseous pollutant that is poisonous as well as ill smelling. The action of the sun on nitrogen oxide causes it to lose a single atom of oxygen which unites then with an oxygen molecule to form ozone. *Sulfur oxides* are formed by burning fuels containing sulfur, such as coal, gas, or fuel oil. These fuels are used not only for industrial purposes but for home heating as well. *Carbon monoxide* is formed by the incomplete combustion of those materials containing carbon such as wood, charcoal, paper, coal, and oil. When it is present in high concentration in closed areas, it can prove to be fatal. The concentration level of carbon monoxide in a number of urban areas is being monitored and its effects on the population studied. *Hydrocarbons* are composed of hydrogen and carbon atoms. They are introduced into the atmosphere from many sources. The incompletely burned gasoline from the automobile exhaust represents a major source of hydrocarbon pollution. Hydrocarbons are known to react readily with other chemicals. *Aldehydes* are made up of hydrogen, carbon, and oxygen atoms, and they may be formed from the incomplete combustion of fuels or from the action of sunlight on hydrocarbons and nitrogen dioxide. The aldehydes are known to cause eye irritation. *Organic acids* are found in smoke coming from wood fires and from the incomplete combustion of fuels, while *inorganic acids* may be generated by the burning of coal or petroleum. The inorganic acids are known to be particularly damaging to vegetation.

The Aerosols

Smoke is a product resulting from incomplete combustion of a material. As a result, it will contain fine solid and liquid particles which will create dirt as

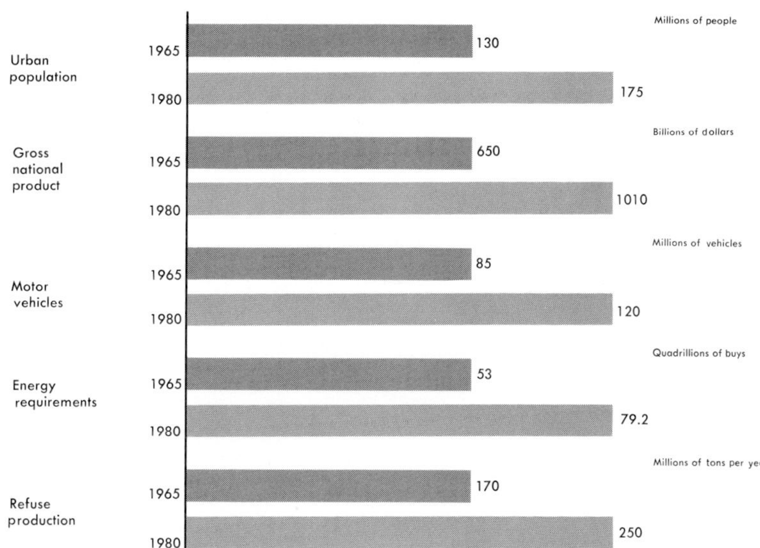

Fig. 13-2. Major growth trends affecting air pollution. (U.S. Public Health Service)

well as odor. *Fumes* are made up essentially of solid particles. These often are by-products of various industrial processes in which paint, rubber, metals, or chemicals are being manufactured. *Dusts*, which are, of course, solid particles, can be produced from various industrial processes that involve the making of cement, asphalt, soap, metals, rubber, and other products. They can be particularly damaging to vegetation. *Mists* are liquid particles that are oftentimes released by spraying, coating, or impregnating processes. An additional source of organic mists can be the automobile exhaust, with mist being produced by the reaction of nitrogen oxides and hydrocarbons to sunlight. *Natural pollutants* are supplied by nature in the form of ozone, bacteria, soil dust, water droplets that evaporate from the sea, nitrogen dioxide created by lightning, spores, pollen, volcanic dust, meteoric dust, sodium chloride from seawater, and ice or snow. These natural pollutants would exist in the atmosphere even without man.

Air Pollution and the Weather

An atmospheric condition known as temperature inversion is one that contributes to critical periods of air pollution. During an inversion, warm air makes up the upper level of the atmosphere, keeping the cold air closest to the ground. This combination results in atmospheric stability with air pollutants being held down by the cold air. Because of their inability to escape into the upper atmosphere, pollutants increase in concentration over a city. It was during inversion periods of this type that the disasters of Meuse Valley, London, and Donora occurred. While these inversion periods will not always cause a disaster, they do increase the level of pollution for

Fig. 13-3. An inversion system is formed when atmospheric conditions permit a cold air mass to form under the warmer air. Under these circumstances the pollutants given off in an urban area are trapped over a city by the inversion system.

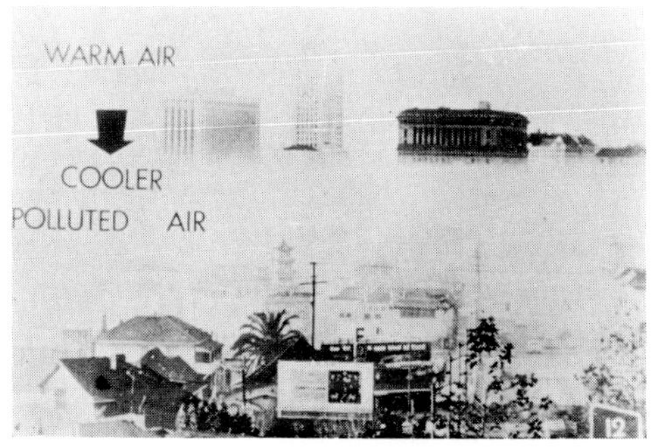

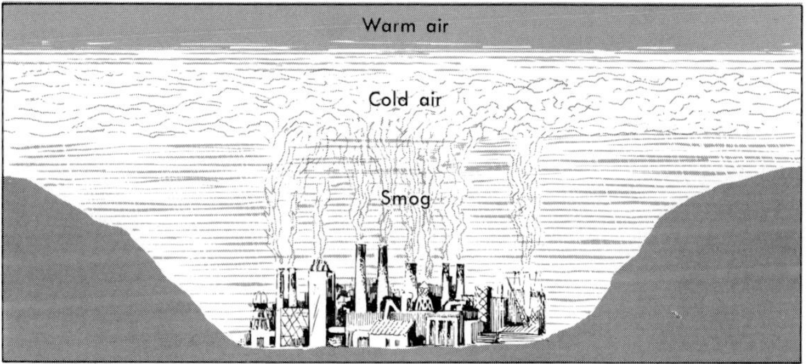

a given period of time, with ensuing deleterious effects. Where industrial areas are located in valleys with high hills on either side, they are particularly prone to periods of temperature inversion. It has been shown that inversion periods occur about one hundred days each year in Los Angeles. This city is particularly prone to this kind of condition because the cool sea air moves in under the warm desert air and an inversion layer is produced. It is only when the warm air rises high enough to permit the cool air to escape that the inversion period is broken.

Smog

It is interesting to note that there are really two types of smog, the London type and the Los Angeles type. The London type is made up of fog plus sulfur compounds developed from the burning of coal and fuel oil. The Los Angeles type is composed mainly of partially burned gasoline resulting from the extensive automobile use in that city. We also know that these hydrocarbons, when released into the atmosphere, can be converted by sunlight into more damaging and more reactive substances. Any city with a substantial amount of vehicular traffic will experience a certain amount of the Los Angeles smog.

The London-type fog, or famous "pea-souper," is almost something of the past. In 1956 the Clean Air Act was passed as a result of the 1952 smog catastrophe that killed thousands. This Act created smoke control areas where only authorized fuels could be burned (thus prohibiting the use of soft coal). In 1968 the Clean Air Act was amended to make its application even more effective. The results of these legislative measures is that the number of sunny days in London have increased by 80 per cent and the quality of the atmosphere has improved significantly. In addition, the number of deaths from chronic bronchitis in the large urban areas has decreased.

The Effects of Air Pollution

Numerous studies have demonstrated a relationship between air pollutants and various disease conditions in man. The specific extent to which air pollution affects the well-being of humans has not been completely ascertained. There is, however, no doubt that there is a relationship. Air pollution is a causal factor in the incidence of respiratory disease. Bronchitis-emphysema is found to be much more common among city dwellers, where air pollution rates are higher, than among their country cousins. The incidence of chronic bronchitis in Britain is found to be higher than in any other country in the world. This condition and its complications are now the leading cause of death in men over 45 years of age and the fourth leading cause of death for the entire population in that country. There has been a marked increase of chronic bronchitis-emphysema in the United States. Scientists studying this problem are having difficulty separating out the effects of cigarette smoking, which in essence is a form of self-pollution, as compared with environmental pollution. While both appear to be definite factors in the increased incidence of this disease, results so far

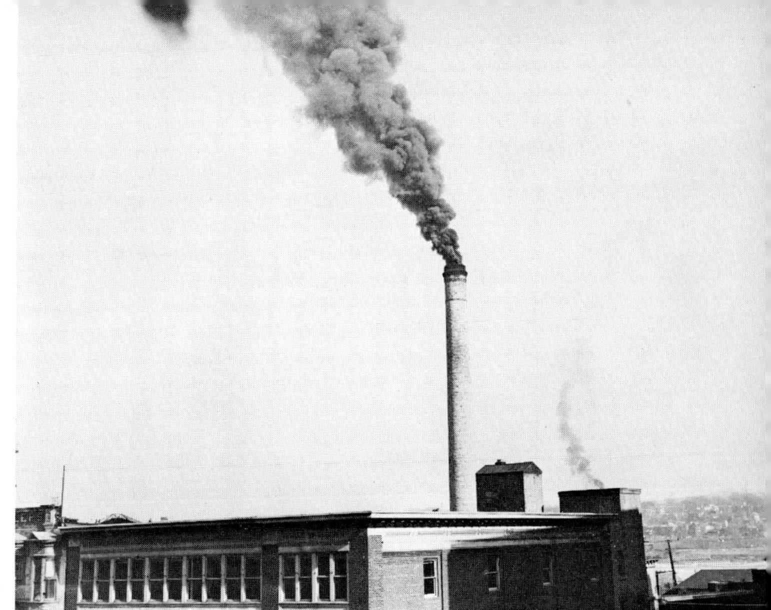

Fig. 13-4. What you see isn't all you get. Many air pollutants in gaseous form are invisible. (N.Y.S. Dept. of Health)

show that cigarette smoking probably has five times the effect of a polluted environmental area. Studies have also shown that there is a relationship between lung cancer and air pollution. The lung cancer death rate is approximately twice as high in cities, where air pollution is a problem, as compared to the death rates in rural areas. Prostatic cancer in men has also been found to increase because of high levels of particulate matter in the atmosphere.

Carbon monoxide poisoning of the driver in heavy traffic is a developing problem in this country. While the carbon monoxide level in heavy traffic conditions is not high enough to cause asphyxiation, it can affect one's driving ability and be a contributing cause of an accident. The number of urban areas approaching pollution levels which cause the above conditions is rapidly increasing joining the major cities who already have chronic pollution problems.

In addition to affecting man and his health, air pollution can also cause damage to crops and cattle. It has been found that it became impossible to grow vegetables commercially in certain areas because of high levels of air pollution. There have also been incidents in which cattle have become ill for the same reason. The pollutants found in air will oftentimes cause premature rusting of metals, and they have been known to discolor and deteriorate house paint. They have the effect of soiling clothes and can mar and even decompose public buildings and monuments. Current national estimates with regard to the widespread economic damage caused by air pollution range anywhere from 4 to 11 billion dollars annually.

Industry and Air Pollution

Industries all make their contributions to the state of air pollution in varying ways and amounts. The steel industries, chemical plants, oil refineries, and the power industry, to name a few, emit waste products into the air peculiar to their particular industrial activities. The clouds of orange dust, mainly iron oxide, are often found pouring out of the smoke stacks at steel industry sites. The switching from the open hearth to the oxygen furnace greatly reduces the steel industry's contribution to the pollution of air. This portion of American industry is spending a great deal on air pollution control equipment and it is hoped that most of the industry will have its air pollution factor under good control by the end of this decade. The chemical industry, with its thousands of products, usually makes its presence known not only because it is aromatic, but because its air pollutants are also dangerous to plant, animal, and human life. Work is being done to bring this condition under control. It is estimated that it may cost up to 500 million dollars in equipment to control the pollution factor related to the chemical industry.

Because of the rigid emission standards that have been applied to some areas of the West Coast, the petroleum refineries in that region have found means of sharply reducing air pollutants. Instead of expelling sulfur dioxide into the air, the petroleum refineries have developed devices to capture this gaseous material and convert it into sulfuric acid or sulfur. The electric power industry has been guilty of emitting into the air fly ash and sulfur dioxide.

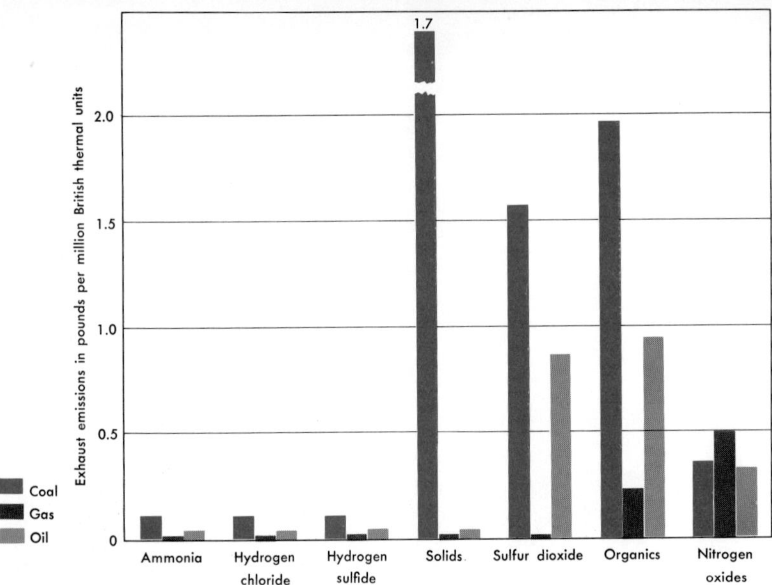

Fig. 13-5. The fuels we use—coal, natural gas, and oil —whether employed to provide transportation, heat, or industrial energy, or to generate electric power, also give forth in varying amounts a variety of air pollutants, the most significant of which are nitrogen and sulfur oxides, organics, and solid particles. (Troubled Air, *U.S. Public Health Service*)

Control devices have already been instituted for the fly ash control and literally millions of tons of fly ash are now prevented from entering the atmosphere. Electrostatic precipitators are being used to catch from 99 to 99.5 per cent of fly ash. The more troublesome pollutant in this industry is sulfur dioxide. It is estimated that somewhere near 23 million tons of this material is currently being sent into the air each year. It is not a toxic substance under ordinary circumstances, but in concentrated amounts it can prove fatal to some people, as evidenced by the disaster in Donora, Pennsylvania, in 1948. It has also been noted that sulfur dioxide can be easily transformed into sulfur trioxide, which is known to be particularly dangerous to lung tissue. A control measure being considered by the industry is the utilization of fuel oil that has a lower sulfur content. This type of oil, however, is more expensive and would inevitably cause a rise in the electric rates. Industry has already embarked on a program of air pollution control. While the program has a long way to go, it does reflect an awareness of a public health problem. New plants are now being constructed with air pollution control in mind, not only in terms of equipment, but also in terms of plant location. The geography of the area is considered as well as its topography. Old industrial plants are being retooled in order to minimize their pollution potential.

Air Pollution Control

At the present time, the automobile is the country's number one air polluter. In a study recently conducted in a Los Angeles area it was found that 1,000 operating automobiles contribute the following amounts and types of air pollutants a day:

1. 3.2 tons of carbon monoxide.
2. 400 to 800 pounds of organic vapors (hydrocarbons).
3. 100 to 200 pounds of nitrous oxides.
4. Plus added amounts of sulfur and other chemicals.

Additional studies are needed to determine to what extent pulverized rubber from automobile tires and particles of asphalt are further contributors to air pollution. It is estimated that the automobile contributes more than the four-fifths of the 85 million tons of pollutants given off by all forms of transportation vehicles that include trucks, buses, railroads, and airlines.

Attempts to control the emissions of the internal combustion engine have not proved to be overly successful. While emission-control devices reduce the amounts of some pollutants, the increases each year in the number of cars wipes out the gain. The emission-control devices actually increased the amounts of nitrogen oxides given off by pre-1973 cars. The effects of the nitrogen oxides were initially underestimated, but are now found to be a factor in the development of emphysema. In Los Angeles, on occasion, automobile-caused smog has even resulted in the cancellation of physical education classes at school to protect the respiratory health of the children.

Fig. 13-6. During the running of the marathon in the 1972 Olympics, the use of cars with internal-combustion engines was suspended to provide the athletes with a smog-free environment to run in. Pictured is the Olympic marathon champion, Frank Shorter, followed by a pollution-free electric car. (*United Press International*)

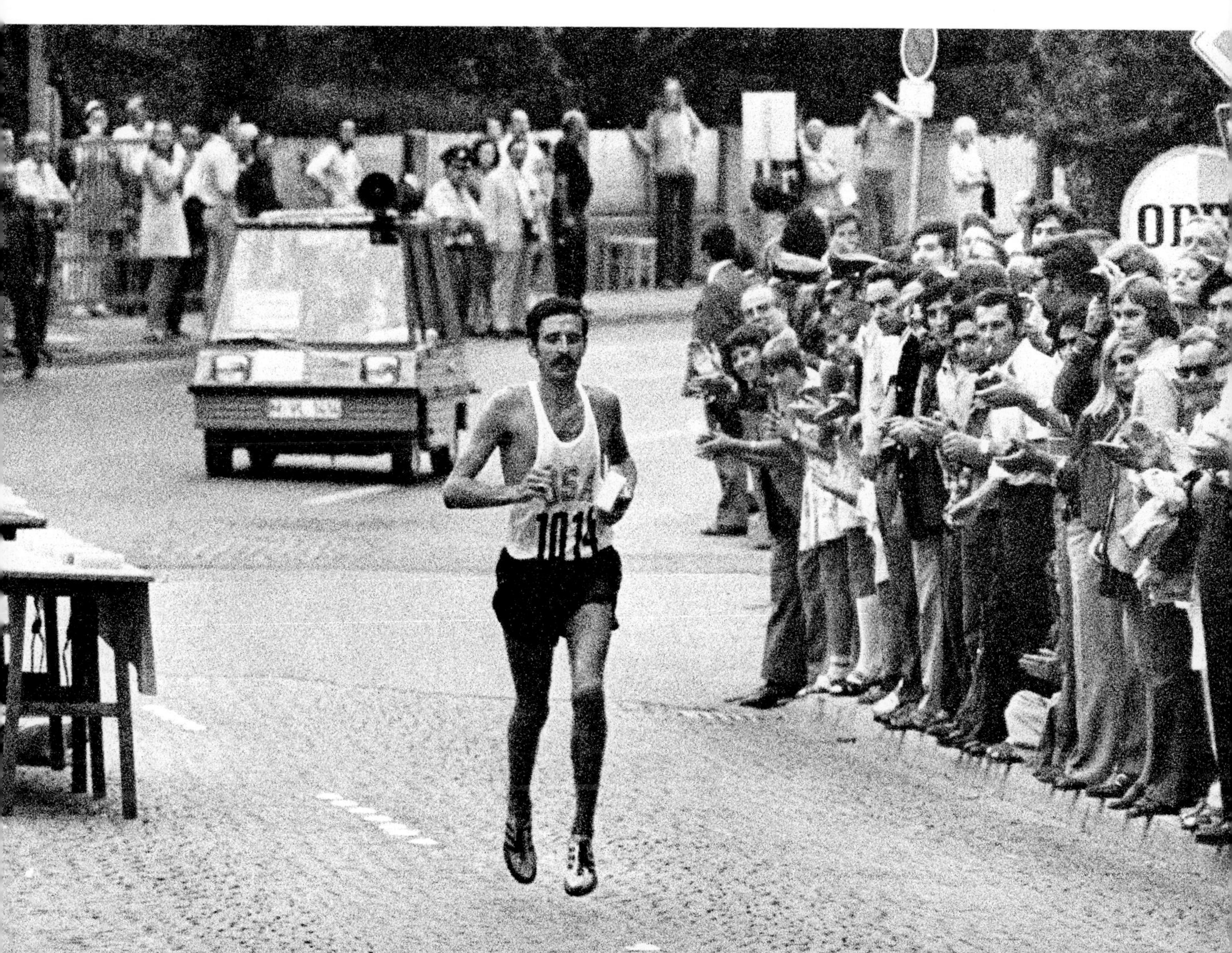

Urban areas are finding themselves blighted by the automobile and its smelly, dangerous exhausts. In addition, 60 per cent of urban land is given over to roadways, parking areas, and other facilities needed by the automobile. Anyone who has attempted to drive through the traffic of a major city comes away with frayed nerves as the least price paid. The overpopulation of the cities with cars is inversely related to the small amounts of money invested in badly needed mass transit systems. One or two persons in every car is hardly an efficient way of transporting large numbers of people in and out of a small geographic area, particularly during rush hours. The 1970 Urban Mass Transportation Assistance Act has made some federal money available to begin the improvement of now archaic mass transit systems. Some demonstration projects trying out new transit systems are under way. They include lightweight, rubber-tired vehicles that are computer controlled. They are propelled electrically and neither make noise nor pollute the atmosphere. Since they do not need operators, they can be run economically with continuous service at all hours.

Efficient mass transit systems will not only give life to our decaying cities, but will ban the illness-producing and death-dealing exhausts of the automobile from the congested environment of the city where it no longer belongs. The big question is when will we go from the pilot project stage to nationwide application? The infusion of large amounts of federal money is necessary to initiate the development of the needed change.

It has long been suggested that national standards be developed for permissible emission of pollutants of every industrial process. The uniform enforcement of such standards would then guarantee the country a strong measure of control over industrial pollutants. In 1970 President Nixon in a message to Congress proposed the inauguration of (Clean Air Act, 1970)

a program to marshal both government and private research with the goal of producing an unconventionally powered, virtually pollution-free automobile within five years.

—*I have ordered the start of an extensive Federal research and development program in unconventional vehicles, to be conducted under the general direction of the Council on Environmental Quality.*

—*As an incentive to private developers, I have ordered that the Federal Government should undertake the purchase of privately produced unconventional vehicles for testing and evaluation.*

He further proposed that

the Federal government establish national emissions standards for facilities that emit pollutants extremely hazardous to health, and for selected classes of new facilities which could be major contributors to air pollution.

. . . Federal authority to seek court action be extended to include both inter- and intrastate air pollution situations in which, because of local non-enforcement, air quality is below national standards, or in which emissions standards or implementation timetables are being violated.

. . . failure to meet established air quality standards or

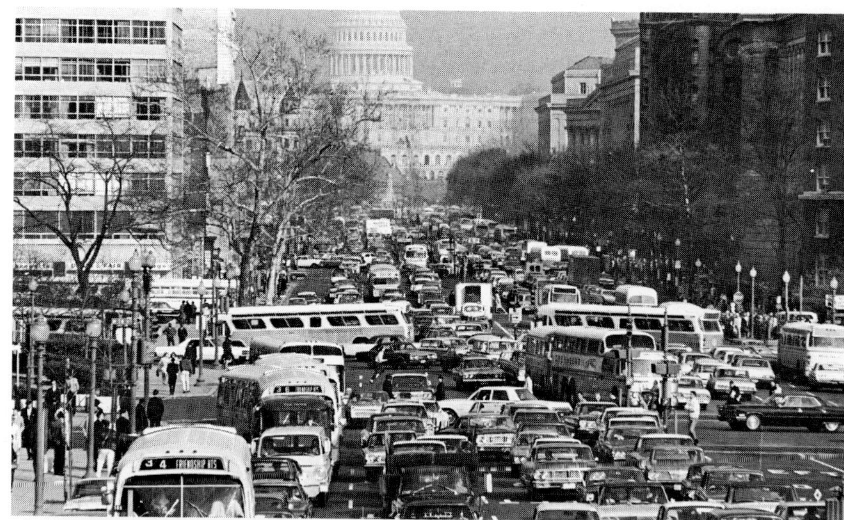

Fig. 13-7. *An ineffective transportation system that is becoming not only a blight on our cities but a danger to health as well. (United Press International)*

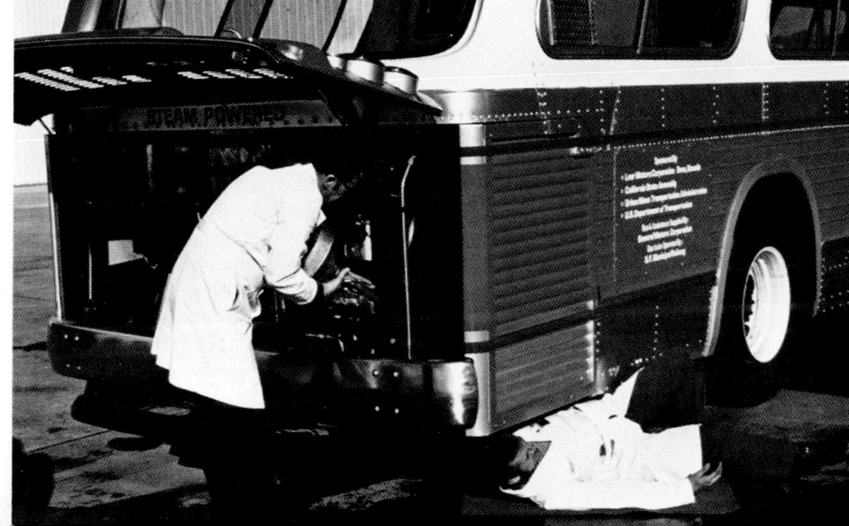

Fig. 13-8. *The Lear steam bus being checked by technicians who are preparing to add water. (Joseph S. Rychetnik/ VAN CLEVE)*

Air Pollution Alert

(*Ch. 12, Sec. 5.1 Air Pol. Contr. Code*)

1. Enforce Governor's order prohibiting open burning of tree wastes, vegetation, refuse or debris.
2. Enforce Governor's order limiting use of incinerators to 12 Noon to 4 p.m.
3. Enforce Governor's order limiting soot blowing from all large fuel-burning installations to 12 Noon to 4 p.m.
4. PLEASE NOTE: The State Department of Environmental Protection recommends that local governments contact industries indicated under "Recommended Actions" to activate the appropriate stand-by plan for the type emergency then existing.

Air Pollution Warning

(*Ch. 12, Sec. 5.2 Air Pol. Contr. Code*)

1. Enforce Governor's order prohibiting open burning of tree wastes, vegetation, refuse or debris.
2. Enforce Governor's order prohibiting the use of incinerators.
3. Enforce Governor's order limiting soot blowing from all large fuel-burning installations to 12 Noon to 4 p.m.
4. PLEASE NOTE: The State Department of Environmental Protection recommends that local governments contact industries indicated under "Recommended Actions" to activate the appropriate stand-by plan for the type emergency then existing.

Air Pollution Emergency

(*Ch. 12, Sec. 5.3 Air Pol. Contr. Code*)

1. Enforce Governor's order prohibiting open burning of tree wastes, vegetation, refuse or debris.
2. Enforce Governor's order prohibiting the use of incinerators.
3. Enforce Governor's order limiting soot blowing from all large fuel-burning installations to 12 Noon to 4 p.m.
4. Enforce Governor's order regulating operation of commerce, schools, amusements, industries and services, control of motor vehicles and other sources of air pollution indicated in the order. Local governments can anticipate special instructions regarding traffic control and the closing down of business establishments.
5. PLEASE NOTE: The State Department of Environmental Protection recommends that local governments contact industries indicated under "Recommended Actions" to activate the appropriate stand-by plan for the type emergency then existing.

Duration and Termination of Emergency

(*Air Pol. Emer. Contr. Act, 1967, N.J.S.A. 26:2C-31*)

The Governor's order will remain in effect for the duration of time set forth in the order. If no time limit is specified in the order, the order will remain in effect until the Governor declares by further proclamation that the emergency has terminated.

(*Courtesy of the New Jersey State Department of Environmental Protection*) *implementation schedules be made subject to court-imposed fines of up to $10,000 per day.*[2]

Alertness to local air pollution conditions is essential until such time as this problem is brought under control. The states of New York and New Jersey have developed a Regional Air Pollution Warning system to alert the populace when unfavorable weather conditions help to cause dangerous air pollution levels. These levels are continually monitored by automatic instruments that measure sulfur dioxide, carbon monoxide, and smoke shade. Should the air pollution index rise to a dangerous level because of a thermal inversion system, it would then be possible to alert the population to this fact and to take appropriate control measures. These might include the shutting down of factories, limited use of automobiles, and the prohibition of incinerator use.

Water Pollution

Our extensive problem of water pollution is no "Johnny come lately." We have been blithely looking the other way while this awesome problem reached such proportions that it could no longer be ignored. We now have the choice of cleaning up the mess or stagnating with it as a community.

In the past, we have used our waterways as open sewers and as reservoirs for industrial wastes. There was a time when this could be done without its having great impact on our civilization. However, with the growth in our population and our industrial complex, we find that the wastes are now almost six times what they were sixty years ago in our rivers, lakes, and streams. These conditions have had a number of unfortunate effects. There has been the outbreak of disease, particularly when shellfish were taken from polluted waters. Detergent foam has become a more and more familiar sight floating on the surface of rivers and streams and in the drinking water of some communities. Large areas for fishing and swimming have been rendered useless by industrial wastes and other pollutants. Each year more bathing beaches and boating areas have been closed down because the water is unsafe. Some of the newer chemical substances such as pesticides that are finding their way into our waterways in increasing quantities represent a new facet of the pollution problem. Probably the greatest danger presented by water pollution is that it contaminates our sources of water. Three-fourths of our water needed for industrial, agricultural, and municipal use comes from the rivers, lakes, and streams that we have been busy polluting. With our continued population growth as well as industrial and agricultural growth, the demands for water will surely increase. The challenge of producing enough usable water for the next few decades must be met. Water is without a doubt the number one raw material used by industry. It has been estimated that it takes 1400 gallons of water to produce a dollar's worth of steel and nearly 200 gallons to produce a dollar's worth of paper. Munici-

[2]"Environmental Quality," The President's Message to the Congress Recommending a 37-point Administrative and Legislative Program, February 10, 1970.

Fig. 13-9. Raw sewage outlet. "It has been said that what distinguishes Man from other animals is his ability to influence his environment. It could be said—with equal truth—that Man's distinguishing characteristic is that, unlike other animals, he fouls his own nest." From "O Dark Dark Dark, Amid the Blaze of Noon" by J. A. Scott, Abbottempo. (N.Y.S. Health Photo by McGaughan)

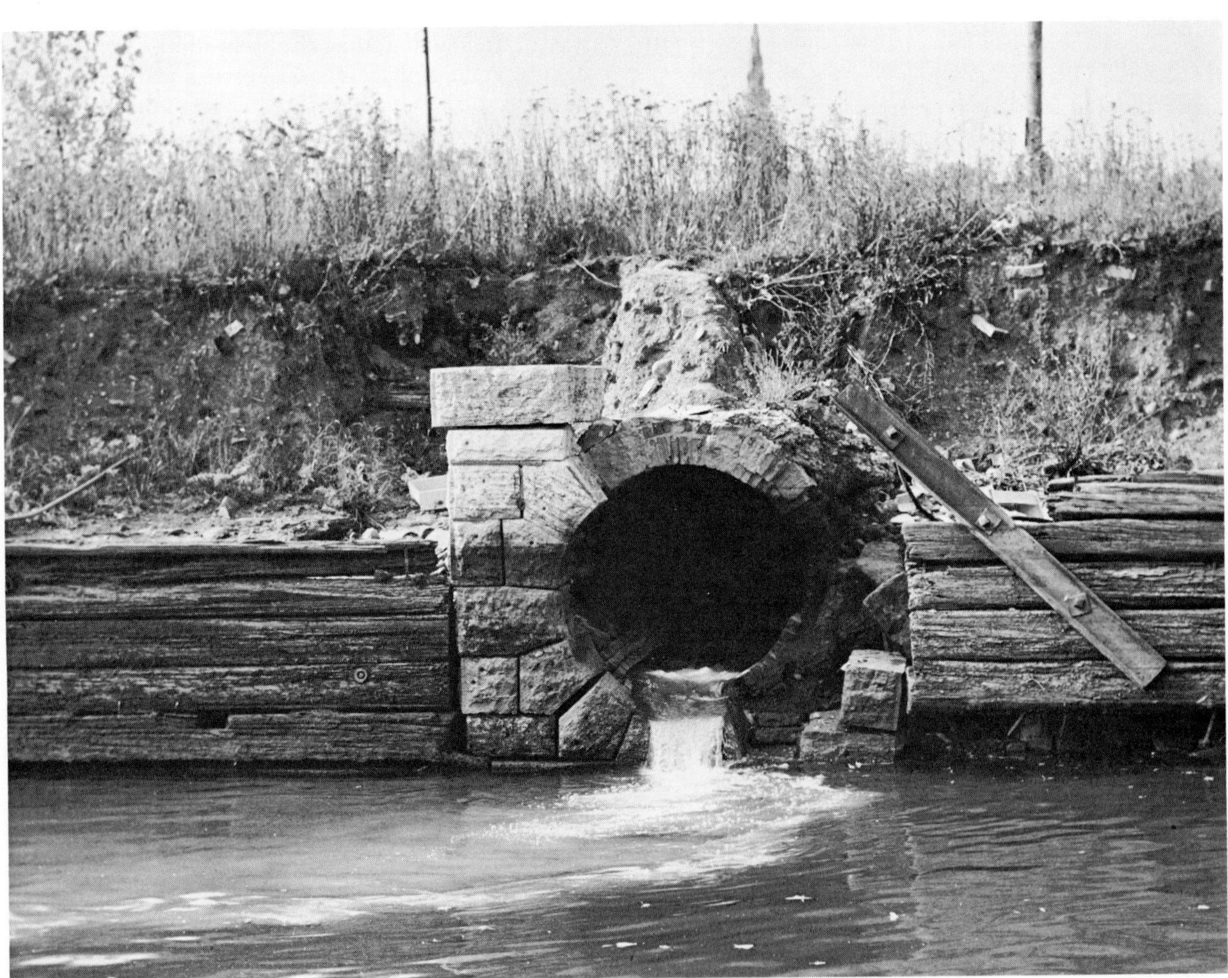

pal use of water has increased through the years as higher standards of living and sanitation have introduced swimming pools, home laundries, and multiple bathrooms. This has forced many cities to increase their water usage and to draw water from greater and greater distances.

Agriculture, because of increased use of irrigation, has many times multiplied the amount of water it uses. Fortunately, water is a material that can be cleaned and its impurities removed. There just will not be enough new water to meet the needs of our communities. The answer to the maintenance of an adequate water supply is to use water over and over again. This means that ways must be found to remove the impurities as well as preventing them from getting into the water in the first place.

Nuclear energy has begun to be used as a source of power. At the present time little more than 1 per cent of the country's power is developed by nuclear reactors. The great majority of the power plants burn fossil fuels (coal, oil, and natural gas). However, by 1980, 35 per cent of the country's power will be produced by nuclear reactors and by the year 2000, more than half the country's power needs are expected to come from this source. Nuclear plants are located by bodies of water because water is used as a coolant in the process. The heated waters emitted from the nuclear power plant can have detrimental effects on aquatic plants because of reduced levels of oxygen. When nuclear plants are placed by large bodies of water such as an ocean rather than a river or lake the thermal effects could have a positive effect by stimulating desirable biological growth. The pollutant potentials of nuclear plants need to be weighed against the kinds of pollution now being caused by power plants using fossil fuels.

Water Pollution Control

> The improper disposal of human exreta and sewage is one of the major factors threatening the health and comfort of individuals in areas where satisfactory sewerage systems are not available. This is so because very large numbers of different disease-producing organisms can be found in the fecal discharges of ill and apparently healthy persons. . . . Surveys show that 5 to 10 percent of the population are carriers of *Endamoeba histolytica,* causing amebic dysentery, and 25 percent of the population are carriers of ascarid, hookworm, or tapeworm. Studies in an American city showed that 9.1 percent of the local population harbored *Endamoeba histolyica* and that 23.1 percent harbored parasites. Knowing that other organisms causing various types of diarrhea, bacillary dysentery, infectious hepatitis, salmonella infection, and many other illnesses are found in exreta, it becomes obvious that all sewage should be considered presumptively contaminated, beyond any reasonable doubt, with disease-producing organisms.[3]

At the present time, many of our municipalities discharge their raw wastes into the most convenient waterways without giving them any treatment at all. Others give their sewage only primary treatment. This means that a large percentage of our munici-

[3]Joseph A. Salvato, Jr., *Environmental Engineering and Sanitation,* 2nd ed. (New York: Wiley, 1972).

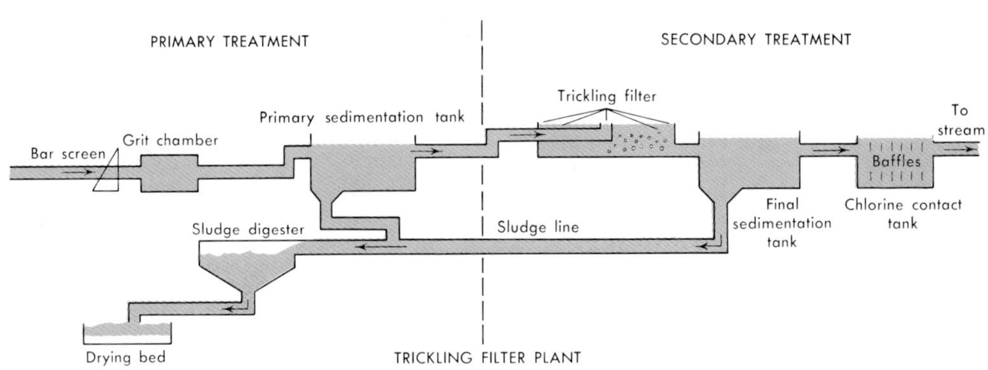

palities are giving completely inadequate treatment to sewage before dumping it into the nearest stream or body of water. There is a great need for modern sewage plants that would properly treat sewage and release it into the nearest waterway only when it is completely safe. In a modern sewage treatment plant both primary and secondary treatment is given. Sewage treatment plants have difficulty removing industrial waste materials, particularly some of the new substances such as plastics, detergents, pesticides, nylons, or radioactive materials. These are best prevented from entering the waterways at their source. The biggest difficulty with sewage treatment plants is that there are not enough of them. There is no question that these are expensive facilities, their costs ranging from $50,000 to several million, dependent on their size. However, no community is properly assuming its responsibilities if it does not adequately treat its sewage but merely sends it downstream for the next community to deal with.

The attitude that the treatment of water benefits only the next community downstream has prevented many a city father from taking appropriate action. What is being overlooked is that the same attitude is responsible for the influx of sewage from the community farther upstream. It is time for some concerted action.

Industry has a vital interest in conserving the country's water supply. Some industrial plants use more water than the entire city they are located in. By 1980 it is estimated that industry will be using two-thirds of the nation's water supply. Many industries have started water conservation programs. Changes in production procedure have curtailed the amount of water needed initially and have reduced the amount and nature of industrial wastes emitted. Most major industry is currently conducting research designed to curtail its waste output further. Industry has been reacting more quickly to the pollution problem, for while it is the major consumer of water it contributes less than half the pollution. The ability and the willingness of industry to move toward completely effective waste control programs will continue to be vital.

Federal Water Pollution Legislation

The Water Pollution Control Act of 1948 was enacted as temporary legislation so that it could be reviewed and revised after a five-year trial period. After a three-year renewal of the rather limited 1948 act, Congress in 1956 passed the Federal Water Pollution Control Act. This legislation was more extensive than its predecessor. It assisted 2,750 cities to build sewage treatment plants as well as to clean up some of our waterways. Before this legislation was passed, our municipalities and industries were spending less than half of what was needed to keep up with the enlarging pollution problem. Though the 1956 Act was a stimulant for increased pollution control, it was not strong enough to turn the tide. In 1961, in response to President Kennedy's appeal for stronger legislation, Congress amended the 1956 Act. The amendments made provision for the following:

Fig. 13-10. During primary treatment the water or sewage passes through a bar screen which catches large objects. The water next flows into a grit chamber that allows small objects like sand and gravel to settle out. It is then sent into a large settling tank where solid materials in the water will either settle to the bottom or rise to the top. The water between these two layers is drained off and sent to that part of the sewage plant that gives secondary treatment.

In secondary treatment water is sprinkled over a bed of stones and permitted to trickle through. Bacteria grow on these stones and their function is to dissolve organic matter from the water. The water then goes through a final sedimentation tank and from there to a chlorine tank. The treated water is then discharged into a river or a stream. The solid wastes that are removed from the sewage are deposited in a sludge digester and from there they move out to a sludge drying bed. This treated sludge can be used for land fill or fertilizer.

1. Increased Federal support for the construction of municipal waste treatment facilities.
2. Broadened and strengthened the Federal Government's enforcement powers.
3. Called for an intensified program of research looking toward more effective methods of pollution control, with special emphasis on regional variations.
4. Authorized increased federal support of state and interstate pollution control programs.
5. Established in law the principle of water storage in planning and building federal reservoirs to maintain water quality during periods of low flow.[4]

The Water Quality Act of 1965 called for water quality standards for interstate water and for satisfactory state plans to meet these objectives. This legislation was supplemented by the Clean Rivers Restoration Act of 1966 which authorized $3.4 billion for the building of sewage treatment plants. However, there are usually great gaps between the amounts of money authorized and those actually spent. In some areas states have come together as regional compacts such as the Ohio River Valley Water Sanitation Commission involving eight states. This has resulted in coordinated and more effective ways of dealing with the problems of water supply and the prevention of water pollution.

State laws will usually empower a control agency to make rules and regulations and to enforce them. They provide that a permit be sought from the control agency before any new or increased waste discharges are permitted. How effective a state's control agency is will be determined by the quality and number of its staff. By June 1973, 15 states and 54 cities banned the sale of detergents with levels of phosphates above 8.7 per cent. Some communities have banned the use of detergents containing *any* phosphates.

The federal government has enforcement powers provided through the Water Quality Act of 1965. Enforcement power was given the Secretary of the Interior who can bring suit against violators.

International Commissions

The International Joint Committee that involves the United States and Canada, and the International Boundary and Water Commission involving the United States and Mexico have been established to investigate water pollution as it affects the respective countries and to develop remedial procedures. The international implications of pollution are being increasingly recognized.

Research

Although the building of needed sewage treatment plants will significantly help the pollution problem, it will not furnish a complete answer. Sewage treatment plants are effective in removing sewage wastes from water, but they are not effective in filtering out the newer industrial and agricultural chemicals that are discharged or in other ways drain into our waterways. These include pesticides, deter-

[4]"Protecting Our Water Resources" (Washington, D.C.: U.S. Dept. of Health, Education, and Welfare, Public Health Service, 1962), p. 6.

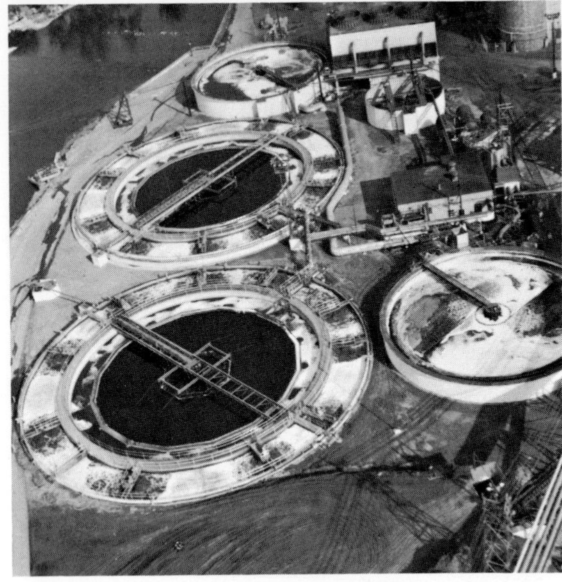

Fig. 13-11. One of the most advanced facilities treating industrial wastes in the paper industry. (West Virginia Pulp and Paper Company)

Fig. 13-12A. Lake Washington, 1958, before rehabilitation. (Metro, Seattle—Roy Montgomery photo)

Fig. 13-12B. Lake Washington, 1972, after rehabilitation. (Metro, Seattle—Roy Montgomery photo)

gents, and waste products of chemical and pharmaceutical manufacture. Relatively little is known of some of the newer and multiplying chemicals in terms of their composition and toxicity.

Research conducted by the United States Public Health Service as well as by industry is designed to find means of removing these materials at the source. It also seeks revision of the functioning of waste treatment plants so that they may effectively remove these kinds of materials as well. The design of present waste treatment plants is 50 years old and is no doubt in need of review in the light of the magnitude and changing nature of water pollution.

New regional laboratories are being set up in various parts of the country to study those pollution problems peculiar to a given region and to develop means of overcoming them. The federal government is also making research grants available to individuals and institutions to find all possible means for better pollution control.

Needed: Community Interest and Action

Increasingly, various groups are showing interest and concern for the conservation of the nation's water. They range from Junior Chambers of Commerce and Leagues of Women Voters, to the Outboard Boating Club of America and the National Wildlife Federation, among many others. As an interested and responsible citizen of your community, how many of the following questions can you answer?

Are Wastes Treated?

Does your community have a sewage plant?

What kind of treatment is provided—primary or secondary?

Do Wastes Escape?

In normal dry weather, is some sewage bypassed into the stream?

In wet weather, when pipes and plants may be taxed by stormflow, is some sewage bypassed? What percentage? How often does this occur?

Adequate Staff?

Does your waste treatment plant have enough employees to operate it efficiently on a 24-hour, 365-day basis?

Proper Training?

Does your State provide training programs for plant operators?

Does your plant (if it's large enough) provide in-plant training? If so, are the programs utilized?

Does your community pick up the tab for such training courses?

Staff Certified?

Does your State or other agency have certification requirements for plant operators?

Does your community live up to these requirements?

Adequate Plants and Sewers?

How many homes are not connected with sewer pipes?

How many sewer pipes are not connected with a waste treatment plant?

Is the plant itself modern and up to date?

Does your community prohibit connection with roof and other storm water drains?

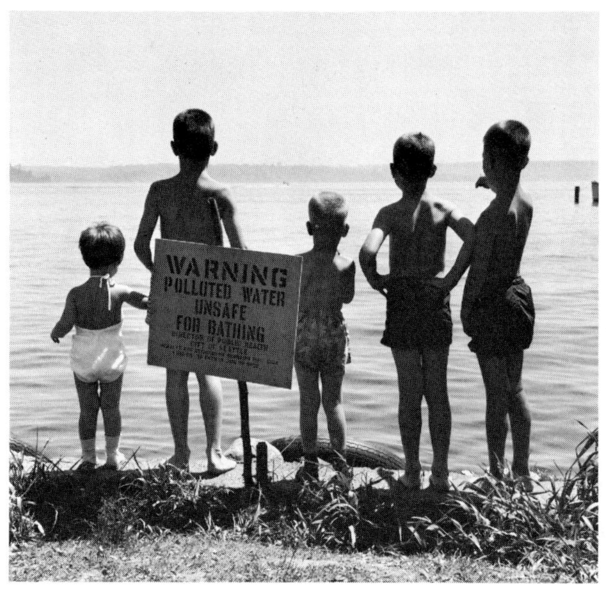

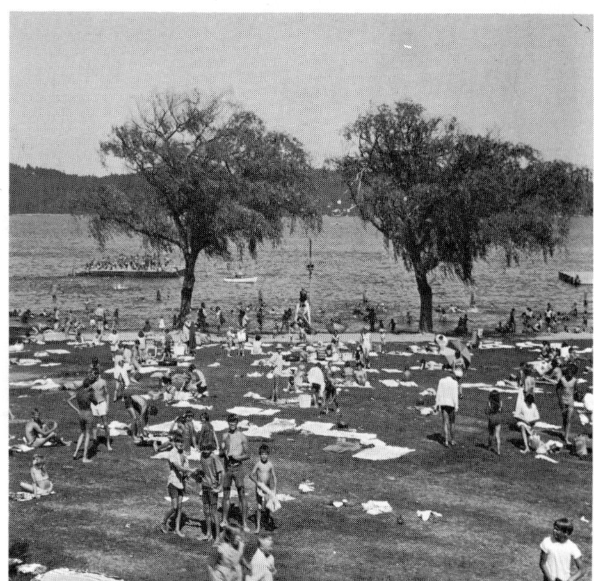

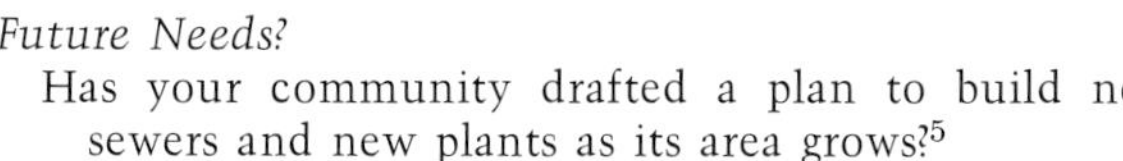
Future Needs?
Has your community drafted a plan to build new sewers and new plants as its area grows?[5]

THE RESTORATION OF LAKE WASHINGTON AND PUGET SOUND

The emergence of some isolated instances of success in the fight against pollution is now being seen. A remarkable example can be found in the greater Seattle area in the state of Washington. This metropolitan area is located between the salt waters of Puget Sound and the fresh waters of Lake Washington. The quality of water in the area was in the process of being destroyed by 70,000,000 gallons of raw sewage which was dumped into Puget Sound. Lake Washington suffered from bacterial pollution that closed down its beaches as well as from an overgrowth of algae. The latter's growth was stimulated by the effluents being discharged from existing sewage treatment plants. The effluents from these sewage treatment plants were serving as fertilizer for the algae. The lake was in essence being killed by overfertilization. The water transparency declined from 12 feet in 1950 to 2½ feet in 1962.

An enormous citizen effort then went into action. A municipal government was set up with the single function of sewage disposal for the city of Seattle and the surrounding counties. A comprehensive ten-year plan was developed for the rehabilitation of Puget Sound and Lake Washington. It required $125,000,000 worth of new sewage treatment facilities. The project progressed in many instances ahead of schedule. It was initiated in 1961 and by 1970 all effluent discharges into Lake Washington had ceased as well as the flow of raw sewage into Puget Sound. The waters were returned to their esthetic best as well as to varied recreational uses. Only 4 per cent of the cost of the project was subsidized by state or federal funds, an outstanding example of self-determination exemplifying what can be done when a community vigorously pursues a worthwhile objective.

[5]"Focus on Clean Water" (Washington, D.C.: U.S. Dept. of Health, Education and Welfare, Public Health Service Publication No. 1184), p. 8.

Land Pollution

The third phase of pollution which has been ignored far longer than either air or water pollution is land pollution. Through the years, the only progress made in garbage or trash removal was the hiring of persons to "take it away." Where they took it was of no concern to the suburban or urban dweller. With the establishment of air and water controls the elimination of many of the solid or semisolid wastes which were heretofore burned or dumped in riverways was prohibited.

The land, therefore, inherits not only the solid wastes of our urban society, but also the unwanted solid and liquid wastes resulting from water and air pollution control.

It is increasingly being recognized that the third dimension—the land, must be protected from pollution by

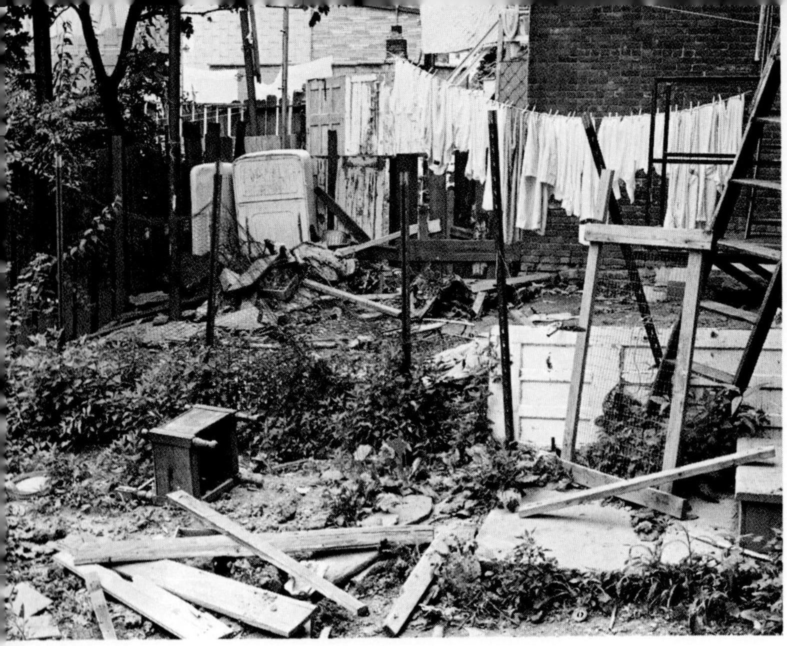

Fig. 13-13. Land pollution takes many forms. (N.Y.S. Dept. of Health)

urban, commercial, industrial and agricultural solid wastes. The land is the ultimate depository for the unwanted solid wastes from our society.[6]

Because of advanced technology and production we are now faced with the problem of getting rid of 500 billion pounds of solid waste each year, 4 billion pounds of which are plastic wrappings alone. For the most part, three-fourths of this solid waste is being delivered and periodically burned in open dumps. This primitive and unsatifactory method is being replaced in some forward-thinking communities by sanitary landfill operations. This is a controlled method of disposal whereby refuse dumped in a trench or lower valley area is covered by dirt at the end of each day. It is a carefully engineered project that eliminates the smoke, insects, rodents, odor, and ugliness of the open dump. When the sanitary landfill project is complete, the area can be salvaged for use as parks, golf courses, or structures not requiring excavation for basements.

With the increased awareness that the disposal of solid wastes is an important problem, cities and states have set up special agencies to arrive at a solution. The federal government has passed a Solid Waste Disposal Act which has been appropriating funds for demonstration projects. Though legislative mandates are by no means the complete solution to a problem—it is a start. Franklin, Ohio, is one community whose ingenuity, coupled with federal funds in the form of a grant, has come up with a promising solution to the problem.

Here's how the complex works: A disposal plant reclaims reusable fibers from waste paper and separates and salvages metals and glass through centrifuge action.

Adjacent to this plant is a sewage treatment facility. Sludge from this facility is mixed with the pulp residue from the disposal plant. This mixture is burned in a "fluid bed reactor"—a new kind of incinerator that burns trash more completely, thereby reducing the amount of residue.

The treated effluent from the sewage plant is used to supply the water requirements of the disposal plant paper-pulping process. The fine ash from the fluid bed incinerator is piped to the sewage treatment plant and used in *that* process.

After all this processing, there remains only about five percent of the original volume in the form of a clean, inorganic powder, which is placed in a nearby sanitary landfill.

But this favorable disposal ratio is only part of the story. Initial operations of the complex indicate that it will salvage daily nine tons of reusable paper fiber, with a market value of $25 a ton; three tons of glass cullet, worth $15 a ton; three tons of ferrous metals, worth $10 to $15 a ton; and one-half ton of aluminum, worth $175 a ton. Thus Franklin's new waste disposal facility will help to pay for itself.[7]

Two counties in Wisconsin and Florida are pulverizing garbage, and elsewhere a new method compresses waste into 4-foot-cubed bales which seem

[6]Joseph A. Salvato, "The Third Dimension: Land Pollution," *Health News,* Vol. 44, No. 2 (February 1967), p. 13. N.Y. State Dept. of Health.

[7]Richard D. Vaughan, "What to Do with Your Six Pounds of Garbage Every Day," *Today's Health* (June 1972), p. 47.

excellent for landfill projects. In California wastes are burned in a

high pressure incinerator to produce hot gases used to power a gas turbine. The turbine, in turn, drives a 15,000-watt electric generator. The projection is that not only will waste be burned up, but that the income from the production of electric power will offset the cost of operating the plant.[8]

The solutions of our land pollution problems will come from the creative professionals who can use the disposal process to fulfill other community needs and thus produce a constant productive cycle. The overenthusiastic, amateurish attempts at solid waste management that sporadically organizes community groups to collect bottles, cans, and newspapers are not effective in all instances. The collections are usually carried off to the town's open dump to add to the problem because arrangements were not made with recycling units (where they exist). Instead, community groups should arm themselves with knowledgeable professionals and evaluate their community's waste disposal system, then move to effect the changes needed.

Our Proliferate Pesticides

For the first time in the history of the world, every human being is now subjected to contact with dangerous chemicals, from the moment of conception until death. In the less than two decades of their use, the synthetic pesticides have been so thoroughly distributed throughout the animate and inanimate world that they occur virtually everywhere. They have been recovered from most of the major river systems and even from streams of groundwater flowing unseen through the earth. Residues of these chemicals linger in soil to which they may have been applied a dozen years before. They have entered and lodged in the bodies of fish, birds, reptiles and domestic and wild animals so universally that scientists carrying on animal experiments find it almost impossible to locate subjects free from such contamination. They have been found in fish in remote mountain lakes, in earthworms burrowing in soil, in the eggs of birds—and in man himself. For these chemicals are now stored in the bodies of the vast majority of human beings, regardless of age. They occur in the mother's milk, and probably in the tissues of the unborn child.[9]

When Rachel Carson's *Silent Spring* was first published, there were mixed reactions to the book. Some indicated that the writing was emotional and exaggerated. Others felt that the book was most timely and one that would stimulate public interest in the subject as well as better controls in pesticide use. In a paper on the subject, Dr. Kraybill stated:

The pesticide industry was most vociferous and unyielding in its criticism of *Silent Spring*. Some of the trade journals and the public press echoed the thoughts expressed by *Time* magazine which called the book an emotional and inaccurate outburst "that was likely to do harm by alarming the nontechnical public." *Consumer Reports* in its July 1963 issue on the other hand stated that the President's Science Advisory Committee in its

[8]Ibid.

[9]Rachel Carson, *Silent Spring* (New York: Fawcett, 1962), p. 24.

Fig. 13-14. **A.** *The initial step in a landfill operation, whereby a lower valley area is filled with solid wastes.* **B.** *The rubbish-filled area is covered over with dirt at the end of each day.* **C.** *This high school was built on a former landfill project.* (N.Y.S. Dept. of Health)

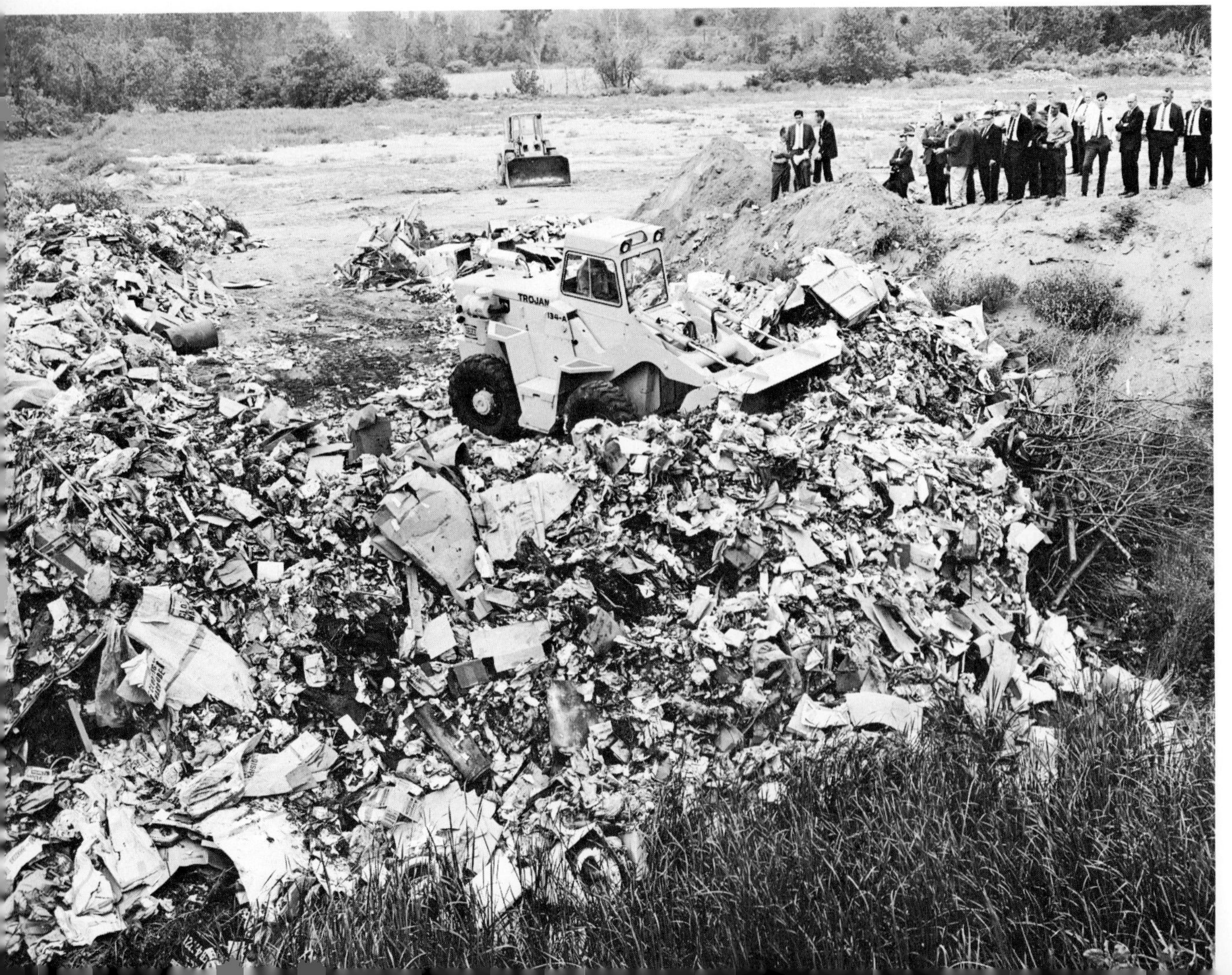

INTERNATIONAL
INTERNATIONAL

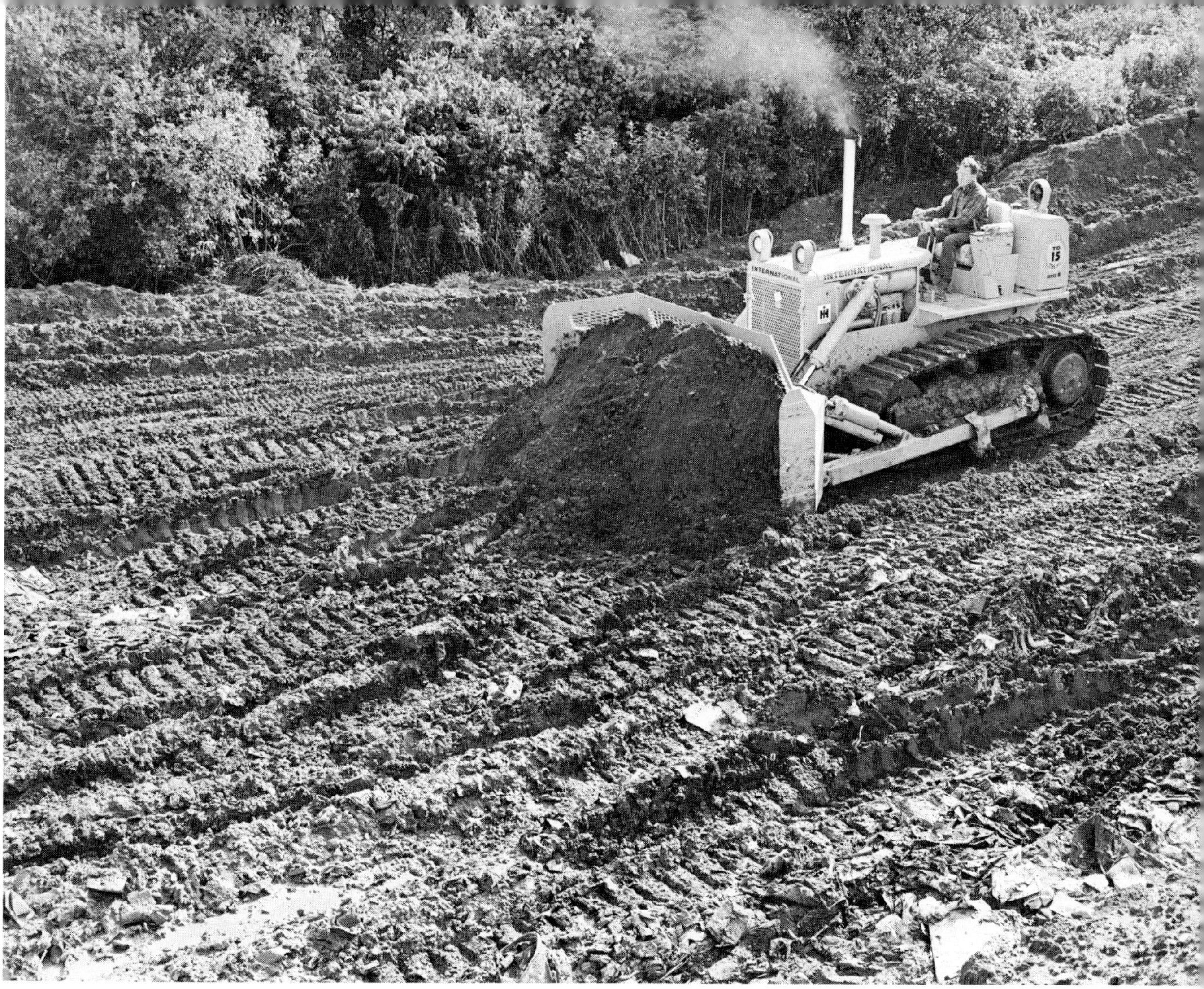

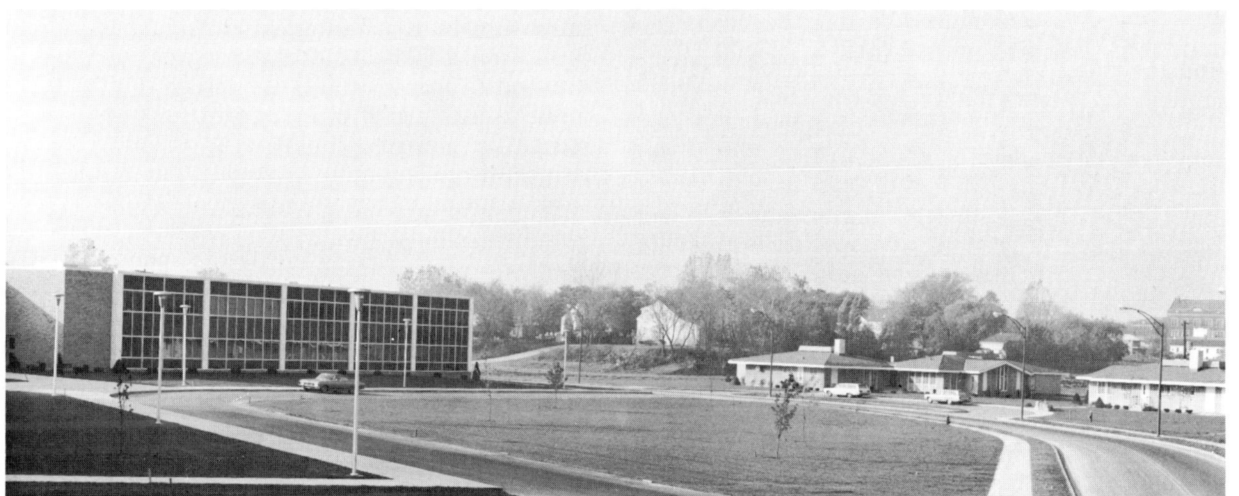

report on "Use of Pesticides" implied, the "nontechnical public needed to be alarmed." The outraged diatribes against *Silent Spring* have matched Rachel Carson's emotion with their own brand of emotion, and they have also unwittingly revealed their own bias.[10]

Perhaps Dr. W. B. Bean said it best in his editorial entitled "The Noise of Silent Spring," when he referred to the book as, "a call to attention rather than a call to arms."[11] Rachel Carson's publication set in motion a reexamination of legislation and public practices and some soul searching with regard to the manner and the extent to which pesticides had been used. In the minds of many, the objectives of the writing were thus achieved.

Pesticide Use and Exposure

The widespread use of these chemicals and how they find their way back to man are worth considering. Pesticides can enter the human body in three ways. They can be ingested as part of pesticide residue that may remain on food or contaminated dishes and utensils. They can also be inhaled when used as a spray, or they may be absorbed through the skin. The latter is a type of pesticide contact that is generally overlooked. Pesticides can be quite insidious, because we are often unaware that we have had contact with them. Pesticide poisoning frequently occurs without the persons' even considering pesticides as a source of his difficulty.

There has been an expanded use of pesticides in the last two decades. They are widely used in the protection of food crops. Carpet manufacturers use them in their products to discourage the presence of carpet beetles. In those areas where termites are a factor, termite poisoning is placed by the builder in the foundation of the home as well as in the soil around it. The dust from the soil could serve as a contaminant if inhaled. Some dry cleaning establishments impregnate clothes with pesticides, which can come in contact with the skin. When fields are sprayed to eliminate certain kinds of pests, the insecticides are eaten along with the grass by animals. The insecticide can then return to the dinner table via game shot by the hunter. Insect sprays of various types are used to get rid of mosquitoes and flies in the home. Many people use insect sprays in the home as gayly and as indiscriminately as demonstrated on television commercials, ignoring the fact that these are poisonous materials. The result is the subsequent contamination of utensils, dishes, table tops, food, and human bodies. Also to be considered is the greater ability to inhale the spray as well as absorb it through the skin in an enclosed area. A number of pesticides are used in the garden in the form of powders, liquids, and sprays. The gardener who stands downwind from an insecticide is giving the insects all the advantage.

About 150 deaths a year are attributed to pesticide poisoning. Most of these occur among young children who ingest the poisonous chemicals. The inci-

[10] H. F. Kraybill, "Pesticides in the Balance: Benefit or Risk," Paper presented at the Washington State Horticultural Association Meeting, Wenatchee, Washington, 1963.

[11] "The Noise of *Silent Spring*," Editorial, W. B. Bean, Archives of Internal Medicine, AMA Publication 112:62, 1963.

dence of pesticide poisoning that proves to be nonfatal can only be guessed at and some estimates run as high as 50,000. Some authorities believe it is probably even higher than this, because the symptoms produced by pesticide poisoning are similar to those of many common illnesses and are often not properly diagnosed. One of the real concerns in this whole area is the gap in our information with respect to the consequences of long-term exposure to pesticides. There just has not been enough research done in this area to give us clear-cut answers as to the significance of cumulative effects over periods of years. In one limited study, people who had a 35 milligram intake of DDT each day showed no ill effects from the exposure. However, it was found that there were 270 parts per million of DDT in their fatty tissues. This is more than twenty times the average level found in adults in the country. What continued exposure to DDT will mean to these people is unknown.

It has also been noted that there is an increased rate of pesticide poisoning among agricultural workers. What long-term exposure will mean to people in this occupation is yet to be determined. There is also little known about the effects of undue accumulation of more than one pesticide in the body.

Pesticide Effects on Wildlife

There is no question that there has been some injudicious use of pesticides. It has been noted that where these poisons have been used too casually there have been high fatalities among fish, birds, and other wildlife. Even when pesticide programs are carried out as planned, wildlife can be seriously affected. As reported by the President's Science Advisory Committee, mortality among birds approached 80 per cent in those areas where DDT was used for Dutch elm disease control. When DDT gets to bodies of water it can have a devastating effect on fish. In terms of sensitivity, it has been noted that fish are more sensitive to these substances than birds, and birds more so than mammals. One of the difficulties in controlling pesticide poisoning of animals is that wild animal populations roam freely and cannot be kept from treated areas. Birds, for instance, may fly into an area that has just been sprayed and eat worms that are now a source of poison and death to them.

Toxicity of Some Pesticides

A group of chemicals referred to as chlorinated hydrocarbons include such pesticides as DDT, dieldrine, chlordane, and heptachlor. These chemicals are known to cause liver damage in experimental animals. They seem to affect the central nervous system and can cause electroencephalographic changes as well as muscle tremors and convulsions. Experimental data show that these chemicals can also reduce the ability of animals to reproduce. Egg production is lowered in birds; dogs exposed to these chemicals produce fewer pups and suffer an increased mortality among their suckling young. Data also show that chronic effects can be produced by these chemicals. In some cases, humans have had

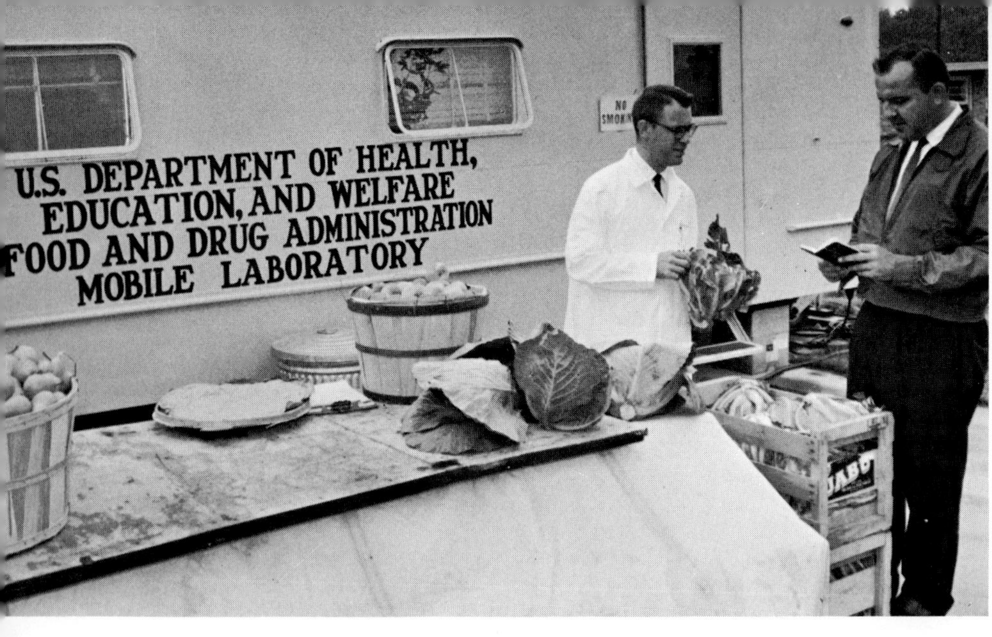

Fig. 13-15. An FDA inspector turns over samples of raw agricultural products taken from interstate shipment for analysis in a mobile laboratory. If analysis reveals excessive pesticide residues, action can be taken through Federal Courts to remove shipment from the market place. (FDA)

recurrences of symptoms after they have been free of the chemical for several weeks. Because these pesticides do not break down easily and persist in the soil for long periods of time, they should be used with caution.

Another group of pesticides known as organic phosphorus compounds seem to have the effect of interfering with the transmission of impulses from nerve to ganglion and from nerve to muscle. Poisonings with organic insecticides have produced a number of fatalities in man. Because these insecticides tend to deteriorate fairly rapidly, people exposed to them can recover if they are removed from the source of exposure. While there are some exceptions to how persistent some of these chemicals may be, the organic phosphorous compounds tend to break down more easily and are therefore considered safer to use than the chlorinated hydrocarbons.

Pesticide Control

The Federal Insecticide, Fungicide and Rodenticide Act is one of the federal laws controlling pesticide use. The administration and enforcement of this law is assigned to the United States Department of Agriculture (USDA). When new pesticides are developed by an industry, application must be made to the USDA requesting permission for its use. Recent legislation now requires that the FDA, the Public Health Service, and the Department of the Interior also review these applications to ensure the safety of the pesticide. When a pesticide is going to be used on food crops, the application must indicate which crop it is to be applied to, along with necessary data regarding its effectiveness and relative toxicity. If the pesticide leaves a residue and it is to be used on food crops, then a given residue tolerance (or a level of residue that may remain on the food when it reaches market) is tested for by the Food and Drug Administration.

Consumers Union, in its publication *Consumer Reports,* expressed some concern with regard to the permissiveness of current USDA pesticide labeling regulations. The USDA apparently classifies pesticides in four groups according to the danger presented by the chemical used. A mere taste of chemicals of the first group would prove fatal to a human. On the label of these appear a skull and crossbones and the words "POISON" and "WARNING." On all containers for these pesticides will appear a prescription for an antidote to be used in case of poisoning. In the second grouping the word "WARNING" must appear on the label. A mere teaspoon of these pesticides could kill a child, yet no antidote need appear on the label, nor need the word "POISON" be placed on the label, either. In the third grouping the word "CAUTION" must appear on the label, although this is not necessary for the fourth group. In fact, on the labels of the fourth group are occasionally found the words "SAFE and NON-TOXIC" even though it is a known fact that all pesticides, at least those presently known, are poisonous. The small print usually adds "if used as directed." Since some manufacturers are honest enough to put the word "CAUTION" on even their fourth grouping of pesticides, the result is a confused situation as far as the consumer is concerned.

The Federal Hazardous Substances Act under the jurisdiction of the FDA also plays a role in protecting the consumer from poisonous substances. The law requires that substances that are poisonous if swallowed be labeled "POISON" (with skull and crossbones). The label will also include instructions for special handling or storage, the chemical name of the hazardous substance, first-aid instructions, the statement "Call a physician immediately," and a warning statement, "Keep out of reach of children."

Research

Some research is currently being conducted by industry to find an insecticide that is not poisonous and yet effective. In the meantime, a good deal of research is going on in a quest for alternative means of controlling pests other than through the use of pesticides. Crop rotation is one age-old method that has long been practiced as a means of leaving pests behind. There has been some work done to find insect enemies as a way of controlling the insect population. These could include insect parasites, predators, or diseases. The introduction of insect parasites and predators can accomplish a great deal in controlling the numbers of a specific insect. These methods, while controlling the numbers, will not eliminate the insect. Means are being sought to supplement this approach with selective insecticide use. This would involve insecticides particularly effective against the insect pest. Broad-scale insecticide spraying of the past often did a better job of eliminating the insect predator than the insect itself.

Microorganisms that are disease-producing in the insect are also being investigated as an insect control measure. One bacillus was recently found to be effective with a variety of insects. Insect viruses have also been found to be effective against insects in the laboratory. Means are being studied to utilize them in the field. Several types of fungi and protozoa, too, have been found to be pathogenic to insects. The great advantage is that these microorganisms are disease-producing in the insect, but not in man. Other biological control methods have been devised through the breeding of crops resistant to plant diseases. A new approach that is being tried involves the development of sterile male insects. The sterility can be effected by gamma rays or by specific chemical sterilants needed only in small amounts. Other researchers have found that 160 decibels of sound will kill cockroaches and that male mosquitoes can be attracted to an electrified screen that imitates the noise of female mosquito wings. These various approaches that are being explored may provide some alternatives to the massive use of pesticides for pest control.

Benefits of Pesticides

It has been estimated that the production of apples, cotton, citrus fruits, and potatoes would be reduced by some 50 per cent without the use of pesticides, and the production of meat, milk, and wool would be reduced by 25 per cent. Many people feel that they have now become essential for the adequate production of food in this country. They unquestionably have contributed a great deal to the economic strength of the country and the nutritional well-being of the American people.

Insecticides also serve to control disease incidence. In an effort to control an outbreak of encephalitis in Dallas, Texas, in 1966, an insecticide was used to spray the city as a way of destroying mosquitoes and controlling the spread of this dread malady. Worldwide control of such diseases as malaria, yellow fever, bubonic plague, cholera, and typhus is being successfully pursued by the spraying of DDT. The incidence of malaria in India, for instance, has been reduced from 70 million cases a year to 5 million. Pesticides, like many other potentially dangerous aspects of our environment, need to be used properly so that we may reap the benefits they afford and avoid needless undesirable consequences.

Proper Personal Use of Pesticides

Where pesticides are to be used by the individual in the home or in the garden, the United States Public Health Service recommends that the following precautions be taken:

READ THE LABEL each time you use a pesticide—no matter how often you have used it and no matter how well you think you know the instructions—and FOLLOW THE LABEL DIRECTIONS EXACTLY. KEEP PESTICIDES AWAY FROM CHILDREN AND CHILDREN AWAY FROM PESTICIDES.

Other precautions are:

1. Use a pesticide only when you are sure it is needed. Use the one best suited to your needs. The label on the product explains the proper uses.
2. Keep the pesticide in a plainly labeled container, preferably the one in which it was bought. NEVER transfer pesticides to unlabeled or mislabeled containers.
3. Store pesticides under lock and key, away from food items and OUT OF THE REACH OF CHILDREN, pets, and people who might not be able to understand their danger.
4. When handling, mixing, or applying pesticides, avoid inhaling dust and fumes and avoid getting materials on the skin.
5. Check the label of the product BEFORE USING, so that you know what to do quickly if there is an accident. In case of an accident, call a doctor or get the patient to a hospital immediately.
6. The very few people who suspect they may have a special sensitivity to pesticides should consult an allergist, and if necessary, take steps to avoid any exposure to the offending agent.
7. Wash hands thoroughly after using pesticides and before eating or smoking.
8. Get rid of used pesticide containers in a way that will not leave the package of leftover contents as a hazard to people—particularly children—or to animals or plants.
9. Work in a well-ventilated area, to avoid inhalation of fumes.
10. Do not spray into the wind.

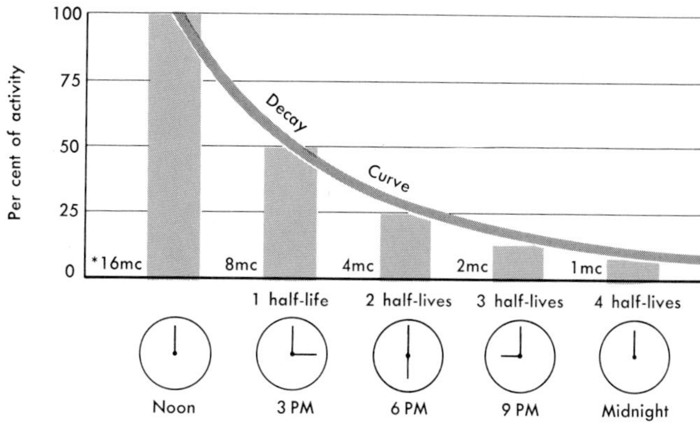

Fig. 13-16. Radioactive decay pattern. (*U.S. Atomic Energy Commission*)

11. When so directed by the label, wear protective clothing, such as goggles, gloves, aprons, respirators, and masks.
12. When mixing or using inflammable chemicals, be especially careful to avoid the fire hazards caused by smoking, defective wiring, and open flames.
13. Cover food and water containers when using pesticides around livestock and pet areas.
14. Do not spray or treat plants or animals or animal feeding areas with pesticides unless you are certain such treatment is safe for that use.[12]

Radiation

The atomic age has brought with it great hopes for the future as well as some concerns. The detonation of nuclear bombs and the ensuing fallouts have been watched and tested very carefully by scientists. We are seeing greater use of nuclear power in industry and consequently greater amounts of radiation wastes that need to be disposed of carefully. The question that must be answered is, What is the significance of this radiation exposure when added to the natural radiation that we receive from the sun and to that from medical and dental X rays?

The greatest source of natural radiation is, of course, cosmic radiation that originates in outer space with the sun as its source. The amount of cosmic radiation that one would be exposed to would multiply as the person left the surface of the earth and moved toward the upper atmosphere. It is estimated that cosmic radiation is three times as high at a level of 3,000 meters above the earth than it is at sea level. The amount of radiation on various parts of the earth will vary depending on different types of soil and rock, each having a varying ability to carry radioactivity. There will be certain deposits, of course, like uranium and thorium, whose radioactive content is quite high and can serve as a source of radiation. Man thus has been in contact with natural radiation from his very beginnings. What the effect of this natural low-level radiation has been on man is open to conjecture at this stage of our knowledge.

[12] *Pesticides* (Washington, D.C.: U.S. Dept. of Health, Education and Welfare, Public Health Service Publication #1081).

The Nature and Effects of Radiation

Radioactive chemicals have the tendency to disintegrate or decay. It is as a result of this disintegration that they give off various kinds of radiation, as exemplified by gamma rays or X rays. The rate at which this decay takes place varies considerably among these materials. Cesium 137, for instance, would require something like 250 years to decay to less than 1 per cent of its original level. Strontium 90 would require 150 years for a similar amount of decay or disintegration. The great majority of radioactive materials, however, decay within a few days or a few weeks. A basic characteristic of all radiation is that it serves to carry energy from one point to another.

Radiation is measured by a unit of measurement called a roentgen. A thirty-year exposure of fallouts amounts to .1 roentgen, more or less, with medical radiation amounting to 2 to 5 roentgens. A chest X ray is rated at about .3 roentgen.

What kind of bodily changes and reactions can be expected to take place in cases of undue radiation exposure? The following effects have been observed after short exposures to the following degree of radiation exposure.

0 to 25 roentgens	No observable effects produced directly.
25 to 50 roentgens	A dose of 25 r is the minimum known to produce a significant blood change as manifest by a blood count. No other body changes noted in this dose range.
50 to 100 roentgens	About 10% of people exposed would be exptected to exhibit symptoms of radiation sickness. Temporary blood changes. Full recovery of body function within a few days.
100 to 200 roentgens	A dose of 150 r produces radiation sickness in 25% of people. Probably no deaths attributable to radiation. Possible disability due to radiation effects.
200 roentgens	Fifty per cent radiation sickness. About 2% of cases may result in death.
300 roentgens	Over 90% radiation sickness and 25% radiation death. Radiation injury and disability very probable.
400 to 450 roentgens	Lethal dose to 50% of people exposed.
600 or more	Nearly all exposed people would be expected to die within 30 days.[13]

Studies have shown that radiologists and others occupationally exposed to increased doses of radiation are more likely to develop leukemia. Studies of the people of Hiroshima and Nagasaki exposed to radiation from the first atomic bombs confirm that a single high-dosage exposure produces a higher leukemia rate.

Another effect of radiation is that it tends to shorten the life expectancy of the exposed. Specifically why this occurs is not understood, but it has been noted.

Geneticists warn that doses of radiation considered to be below threshold level for somatic (bodily) effects can have potential for genetic harm. Early experiments by Dr. Muller with the drosophila (fruit fly) indicated that mutations increase with the amount of radiation received. Dr. Muller's studies and others also demonstrated that the vast majority of the mutations prove harmful to the species. Geneticists feel that the number of mutations that will occur in humans is in direct proportion to the amount of radiation reaching the reproductive cells. According to this principle, any amount of radiation is harmful, and therefore the less radiation we ex-

[13]Jack Schubert and Ralph E. Lapp, *Radiation* (New York: Viking, 1958), p. 181.

pose ourselves to, the better. The following statement by Schubert and Lapp illustrates the point:

> Of the next 100 million children born to the present population in the United States, 2 million will be burdened, either at birth or before adulthood, with obvious hereditary defects, including mental deficiency, congenital malformations, deafness, blindness, and many others. If the chances of producing these hereditary defects were permanently doubled, we would eventually have 2 million additional cases of mental and physical defects, of which 200,000 would probably appear in the first generation alone. Each dose of radiation, no matter how small, to which the reproductive cells of a future parent are exposed increases the chances of passing on additional hereditary defects to the descendants.[14]

Sources of Man-Made Radiation

Fallout from nuclear bomb testing has been a source of man-made radiation that has stirred up vehement controversy, with some outcries against it bordering on hysteria. When a "small" nuclear device is exploded, most of the radioactive debris falls to earth within a few days or a few weeks. With larger devices, the radioactive materials are sent up into the stratosphere and take longer periods of time to descend back onto the earth. It is estimated that in these instances it takes ten years for 50 per cent of the radioactive material to descend. During this interim, it becomes rather evenly distributed around the globe. Most of the radioactive particles will have disintegrated during this period, except for the more persistent ones like strontium 90 and cesium 137.

Radiation can enter the body by penetrating it directly. It can enter the body indirectly via radioactive materials taken in with food and water, or by inhalation. With fallout, the most common route of bodily entry would be by means of the food supply. The radioactive material may be deposited on food crops or may become a part of the soil and be absorbed by the plant. It may be deposited on grass that is eaten by the cow and thus is found in trace amounts in milk. Some estimates indicate that the amount of radiation we are exposed to via fallout is about 5 per cent of what we receive by natural radiation. It is difficult to make clear-cut assessments of this type, however, because different areas receive varying amounts of fallout. It has also been found that children will have larger amounts of strontium 90 in their bones because of its presence in milk and its ability to act like calcium in the body. Indications are that the amounts of these materials are minute and do not constitute dangers to health at these levels. The virtual elimination in recent years of atmospheric nuclear testing has brought this source of contamination under control.

Television sets give off what are referred to as soft X rays. They are not nearly as penetrating as radiation produced by X-ray machines and are shielded by the sides of the tube as well as the cabinet and outer glass covering on the set. Radiation exposure from this source is normally not considered significant.

Luminous radium-painted dials on watches and

[14]Ibid.

clocks give up small amounts of radiation. Their principal danger would be to young children who might remove the glass from the timpiece and either inhale or eat the flakes of paint. It is interesting to note that the sale of radium-dial pocket watches has been restricted in New York City. These watches are usually carried face inward below the waistline, and concern developed with regard to unnecessary exposure to radiation of the reproductive organs and the possible genetic effects.

Medical and Dental Radiation

The X ray and other forms of radiation are used for therapeutic purposes in cases of cancer. Cancer cells are more susceptible to the effects of radiation than normal cells and can thus be destroyed.

The utilization of X rays by physicians and dentists for diagnostic reasons has become more conservative in recent years. The principle adhered to is that X rays are unquestionably to be employed when necessary for a diagnosis—but only when necessary.

Some obstetricians at one time would X ray the unborn child to check its size and position. Studies have since shown that children X rayed prenatally suffered a higher incidence of leukemia. Mass chest X ray programs have also been reduced in number. Only specific groups with high tuberculosis incidence in the community are being screened. Broad-scale X raying of all groups in a community is now considered imprudent.

A good deal of progress has also been made in reducing the amount of radiation given off by X ray apparatus. Work along these lines continues to further reduce radiation exposure from this source.

Industry

Lack of experience or instruction, and carelessness have been the bases of those few industrial accidents that involved radioactive materials. However, with the increasing production of these materials, more complex problems related to their handling and transportation will arise. Where an accident such as a fire occurs in a plant producing radioactive materials, other problems present themselves. Firemen need to know how to handle the situation lest they unduly expose themselves to radiation or inadvertently contaminate other areas with the radioactive materials that they have been in contact with. Smoke from such a fire may also contain radioactive contaminants and serve to spread them in the adjoining community. A truck carrying radioactive cargo involved in an accident presents problems peculiar to its load, relating again to radiation and contamination dangers. Accidents such as these are covered by very carefully worked-out plans of assistance by federal and state agencies prepared to take immediate action.

The Grand Junction, Colorado, Incident

During the 1950's extensive mining of uranium took place, with Grand Junction, Colorado, being a primary mining site. A waste product of the mining process was a radioactive material referred to as "tailings," which looks like gray sand. The Atomic Energy Commission made no attempt to prevent people from trucking this mining waste material away to be used for a variety of purposes. It was later learned that the low-level radioactive tailings were used for construction fill for the foundations of 5,000 homes in Grand Junction.

As reported by Dr. H. Peter Metzger in his article "Dear Sir: Your House Is Built on Radioactive Uranium Waste": "In order to make comprehensible the doses of radiation that are involved, the health department has calculated that the lungs of the occupants in 10 per cent of those 5,000 houses are known to have been exposed to the equivalent of more than 553 chest X rays per year."[15]

Large enough doses of radiation can cause cancer in humans, with lower levels being capable of chromosomal changes that cause genetically damaged children. Uranium miners who were exposed to the kind of radiation given off by tailings have an abnormally high incidence of lung cancer. The level of radioactivity is apparently higher in some Grand Junction homes than was permitted in uranium mines. The tailings can produce a radioactive gas called radon that can seep through the basement floor and then allowed to accumulate with the enclosure of the house. Correction of the problem calls for the removal of tailings under and around the houses involved. The cost—20 million dollars. The alternative is X number of cases of cancer and genetic damage to future generations.

[15]Peter H. Metzger, "Dear Sir: Your House Is Built on Radioactive Uranium Waste," *New York Times Magazine Section*, October 31, 1971.

As radioactive materials are increasingly used for industry and as power sources, the problem of disposal of radioactive wastes becomes increasingly important.

When the materials are radioactive for short periods of time, they may be flushed into sewers, or disposed of via incinerators. However, where materials are radioactive for long periods of time, they are buried in vaults in certain areas underground, or disposed of at sea. When these materials are disposed of at sea, the recommended water depth is in excess of 1,000 fathoms. At the present time, an authority to control the dumping of radioactive materials at sea does not exist. The packaging and handling of these materials must conform, however, to regulations set by the United States Coast Guard and the United States Interstate Commerce Commission. As the production of these materials inevitably increases, the developing problem of waste disposal will rear its ugly head. The 1.5 million gallons of such waste material produced in 1965 is expected to increase to two billion gallons by 1995.

A source of concern and controversy has been the rapid increase in the number of nuclear-powered electric plants in the country. In 1972, 22 such plants were in operation, with 55 under construction and 49 more being planned. A major concern of some scientists is that the radiation released by these plants into the atmosphere could reach dangerous levels.

Target of much of the criticism is the Atomic Energy Commission (AEC), which is responsible for promoting the peaceful use of atomic energy and for protecting the public from atomic danger. Critics maintain that these responsibilities conflict; they accuse the AEC of working harder to promote atomic energy than to protect the nation from it. . . . Dr. Gofman and other scientists have been producing studies since 1963 which indicate that the incidence of radiation-caused cancer and genetic disorders is 20 times greater than the AEC claims. The AEC maintains these studies are not scientifically accurate, but the commission did set new standards in June 1971, which reduce by 100 times the level of permissible radiation emission.[16]

While controversy revolves around the relative safety of nuclear power plants, power companies are caught in the middle needing to construct additional plants as the electric power needs of the country doubles every ten years. They also recognize that the sources of coal, oil, and natural gas are rapidly being depleted.

Several concerned citizen groups have managed to delay the construction of some nuclear plants. One U.S. senator has proposed legislation making the electric companies rather than the federal government (AEC) liable for radiation damage caused by nuclear plants. This is aimed at dampening their enthusiasm for nuclear power. Some companies have begun to consider the possibility of solar (use of the sun's energy) plants or geothermal (use of the heat from the earth's core) plants which would be pollution free. Planned expansive use of nuclear power plants in the meanwhile persists. Continued public surveillance of this controversy is necessary so that future plans best represent the public interest.

[16]"Do Nuclear Plants Make Deadly Neighbors?" *Today's Health,* February 1972.

If the Great Pyramid at Giza had been a radioactive waste depository, if uranium tailings had been interred in the structure when it was built, about 15 per cent of the radium contained in those tailings would still be dangerous today. If that material were plutonium (the nastiest waste of them all), natural decay in almost 5,000 years would hardly have made a dent: 90 per cent of the radioactivity originally present would be with us now.

Our civilization in this nuclear age has a staggering responsibility to the future. The costs to coming generations of our mistakes are almost beyond the power to imagine. Our technologists must be nothing less than infallible. Accordingly, everything must be done to increase our chances of being right when we finally decide what to do.[17]

Review Questions

1. Why are our current environmental health problems actually reflective of man's progress?
2. What is the nature of the pollutants found in the air of our urban communities?
3. Describe a temperature inversion and its relationship to air pollution.
4. What have been the effects of air pollution on health and property?
5. What forms of air pollution control are being

[17]H. Peter Metzger, op. cit.

developed for the automobile, industry, and municipalities?

6. How extensive is our water pollution problem? What are the causes of this environmental problem?
7. Describe primary and secondary treatment of sewage. What are the limitations of modern sewage treatment plants in handling some of the newer chemical industrial wastes?
8. Why does industry have a vital interest in conserving the country's water supply?
9. What role has the federal government played in water pollution-control programs?
10. How can a community go about evaluating how well it is succeeding or failing in the area of water conservation?
11. What has been the contribution of Rachel Carson's book, *The Silent Spring*, to the more discriminate use of pesticides?
12. What are the means whereby pesticides can enter the human body? What can be their effects?
13. What effects can the careless use of pesticides have on wildlife?
14. How has recent legislation given greater protection to the consumer from the harmful effects of pesticides?
15. What are the sources of man-made radiation? To what extent have controls been developed to limit human exposure?
16. What are the potentials of radiation for somatic and genetic harm?

Chapter 14
Safety in Our Times

The National Research Council, an arm of the National Academy of Sciences, recently called attention to the public neglect of problems of injuries and death due to accidents. It referred to our accident problem as a "neglected epidemic of modern society," and considered it to be "the nation's most important environmental health problem." It further stated that the accident was "the leading cause of death in the first half of life's span."[1]

The dramatic decline in the death rate due to infectious disease has left the accidental death rate standing like a tall oak in a leveled forest. The death rate due to accidents has actually gone down in some age groups; however, as compared to other problems, we have not made significant progress in this field. It can now be said that the accident is the leading cause of death in the age group 1 to 37, and that in the age group 1 to 14, accidents claim more lives than the next five leading causes of death combined. In the 15 to 24 age group, accidents cause more deaths than *all* other causes combined, with the automobile accident as the predominant cause.

For too long we have accepted the accident as an unavoidable aspect of our environment. The result has been that as a society we have developed a tolerance for accidental death that we would not have for death caused by disease. If a plague were to hit this country and cause over 100,000 deaths, all kinds of emergency actions would be initiated and great concern would be evident. Yet we have this very situation caused by the accident with only a comparatively complacent reaction. Death, as we know, is not the only means of measuring the seriousness of a problem. Accidents result in a loss of approximately 18 billion dollars in medical and hospital expenses, wage loss, property destruction, and damage. They also cause over $10\frac{1}{2}$ million injuries, with 400,000 of these resulting in permanent, partial, or total disability.

While the accident represents an environmental problem that is not as well recognized by society as it should be, better-informed elements of the community have been at work. Increasingly, professionals from the areas of preventive medicine and public health are being involved in the study of safety problems. It is felt that the methods used by these groups to control the communicable diseases can have application in the field of accident prevention. Newer and more comprehensive research methodology is needed for more complete understanding of this environmental hazard. Even the definition of the accident has come under closer scrutiny. Generally, accidents have been described as unplanned or uncontrolled events that have resulted in injury or damage of some kind. A. G. Arbous defines an accident more broadly. "In a chain of events, each of which is planned or controlled, there occurs an unplanned event, which, being the result of some nonadjustive act on the part of the individual (variously caused) may, or may not result in injury. This is an accident."[2] Current

[1]National Research Council newspaper article.

[2]Maxwell N. Halsey, ed., *Accident Prevention*, The American Public Health Assn. (New York: McGraw-Hill, 1961), p. 19.

thinking is that for purposes of research broader definitions of the accident are more appropriate. This is based on the fact that a far greater number of unexpected events occur that do not result in injury or damage as compared to those that do.

The Use of Epidemiology in Safety Research

Epidemiology is the scientific study of those processes and factors that influence the health of people. The science of epidemiology started with Hippocrates back in the Golden Age of Greece. He recognized that disease outbreaks were not haphazard occurrences. Some diseases were seasonal, others affected certain groups such as children, adults, and so on. Through epidemiologic studies it has become possible to determine that people with certain characteristics are more susceptible to a given disease than people without those characteristics (e.g., people with high cholesterol levels in their blood are more susceptible to cardiac disease). Epidemiology has also helped to identify reasons for illness in certain groups (e.g., cigarette smoking is related to a higher incidence of lung cancer).

The epidemiological study of an accident involves the analysis of the interactions between the *host* (the person), the *agent* (those things that inflict injury—glass, fire, poison, explosives), and the *environment* (lack of visibility at night, nonskid rugs, highway design). Studying the accident from this rather broad approach usually leads to the conclusion that it takes a combination of factors to cause an accident.

An epidemiologic approach was used in the study of off-duty motor vehicle accidents in the armed services. The motor vehicle accident ranked ahead of diseases and other types of accidents as a cause of death and disability. Study revealed that the accidents were not related to long-distance weekend driving, but to driving short distances around the army base, usually during late evening or early morning hours. It was found that 70 per cent of the accidents occurred within 10 miles of the base, and 90 per cent within a 50-mile radius. The high-rate accident group was identified as the young, unmarried, enlisted man who was in search of recreational activity which usually included drinking. A high proportion of the accidents also occured on a few particular sections of the highway. As a result of the study recommendations, the military police patrolled the high-incident sections of the highway. They took into custody those who appeared excessively fatigued or under the influence of alchohol. Countermeasures that were put in effect resulted in a 42 per cent decrease in the accident rate.

Epidemiologic principles in accident prevention revolve around (1) *Making the "host" less susceptible to accidents.* This could involve such things as increasing the person's skill (driver education), or developing positive attitudes and safer practices. (2) *Making the "agent" less hazardous.* For example, safety lenses in eyeglasses, safety devices on machinery, shatter-proof glass on cars. (3) *Modifying the environment to make it more accident-free.* Dual highways, guard rails, proper lighting to prevent falls—these would be but a few examples of this principle.

In the study of the host or human being, researchers have become concerned with determining the keenness of the person's senses (vision, hearing, and others) and therefore the ability of the individual to react to his environment. In addition, motor ability as measured by reaction time, coordination, and habit patterns are considered important. The physical condition of the body is also noted, with age, sex, strength, body build, and general physical fitness taken into account. The person's social attitudes and feelings of responsibility for himself and others are also reviewed. The driver in the flow of traffic is essentially in a social situation. Driving that would reflect the individual's lack of regard for others invariably would be more conducive to a higher incidence of accidents. Nothing the person may do to affect his physical and mental abilities can be overlooked. The keenest of senses and the highest level of coordination can be blunted by the use of drugs and alcohol. Patterns of behavior that lead to the habitual misuse of these substances can quickly negate other positive qualities the person may have and reduce them to a level that would make the person accident-prone. Safety knowledge and intelligence are also considered in evaluating the "host."

The environmental approach in the prevention of accidents has been influenced most by safety engineering and related disciplines. Various types of safety equipment that have made contributions here include machine guards, safety belts, and better door locks. There has also been developed greater control of atmospheric pollutants through engineering, although we still have a long way to go in this field. In the past, studies of accidents have attempted to relate a single factor or "cause" to the accident. The practice of isolating one factor out of the complex of physical, psychological, and social characteristics of the individual in interaction with his environment is considered inappropriate. It is comparable to pulling a factor out of context. For example, suppose a driver is momentarily distracted by a bird that flies into his windshield. As a result, the car swerves enough to cause the two right wheels to leave the pavement. In many such instances the driver might slow down and then return to the road. If, however, the shoulders of the road are soft or muddy, we have an environmental factor that might complicate the situation. The driver might find that he does not have the strength to control his vehicle on the soft shoulder (a physical factor). He may also have been exceeding the speed limit (a judgment factor). If he was driving a car with the engine in the rear, when leaving the pavement the added weight in the back of the car might have caused the vehicle to fishtail, resulting in the car's overturning (a vehicular factor). The driver might also react to the situation by slamming on the brakes, resulting in a loss of control of the vehicle (driver skill factor). So although a misguided bird may have initiated a potential accident, a number of factors such as the environment, driver strength, obeying the speed laws, vehicular construction, and driving skill could all come into the picture for consideration.

The attempts to develop accident prevention programs by modifying human behavior, though helpful, are not as rapid as effecting environmental changes. Things in the environment can be modified, rearranged, and added to with relative ease. The rearrangement of human behavior, however, does not take place as easily. Nevertheless, a full program of accident prevention will aim at effecting changes in the human (host), the agent, and the environment.

Traffic Safety

The automobile has become an inherent part of American life. In addition to providing a major means of transportation, it has also become a status symbol, a living room on wheels, a major source of air pollution, and a means of committing suicide and murder. The automobile, in becoming a part of our culture, has made major social and economic contributions to it. At the same time, it is exacting a price that makes us pause to question why the automobile must kill approximately 50,000 Americans a year and injure millions. At the present rate, more than one out of every two Americans can be expected to be killed or injured in an automobile accident. Is the carnage on the American highways a necessary price for the "luxury" of a car?

The automobile manufacturers have responded to this question by supporting driver education courses, the implication being that the driver is basically at fault in the accident. Properly train the driver and you reduce the accident rate. The government has reponded to the situation by subsidizing the construction of new and safer highways. The publication of the book *Unsafe at Any Speed,* in 1966, by Ralph Nader, opened up a third facet, the heretofore untouched issue of the unsafe construction of the automobile.

The Automobile as an Accident Factor

Mr. Nader's thesis is that for too long we have focused on the driver as the basic cause of all accidents. Law-enforcement personnel, in investigating accidents, look first for the presence of alcohol and, failing to find that, generally place the accident in the realm of reckless driving. In essence, the philosophy has prevailed that the accident can result only from the violation of a law and if laws are obeyed you cannot possibly have accidents. This foolproof, if illogical viewpoint, does not take into account the accelerator that got stuck, the brakes that locked or failed, the tire that blew out, or the windshield wiper that reflected sunlight into the driver's eyes at the time of the accident.

Mr. Nader used the following example to make his point. He indicated that in order to make shaving safer, we progressed from a very crude cutting device to a straight razor, to the safety razor, and finally to the electric razor (or shaver). He pointed out that exhorting people to have a steady hand, not to be temperamental while they are shaving, and to keep their eye on the mirror would not significantly reduce slashed faces if they were using a crude razor. The redesigning of the instrument in the form of an electric razor, for instance, would permit the individual to make an operational slip without slashing his throat. The obvious conclusion drawn, then,

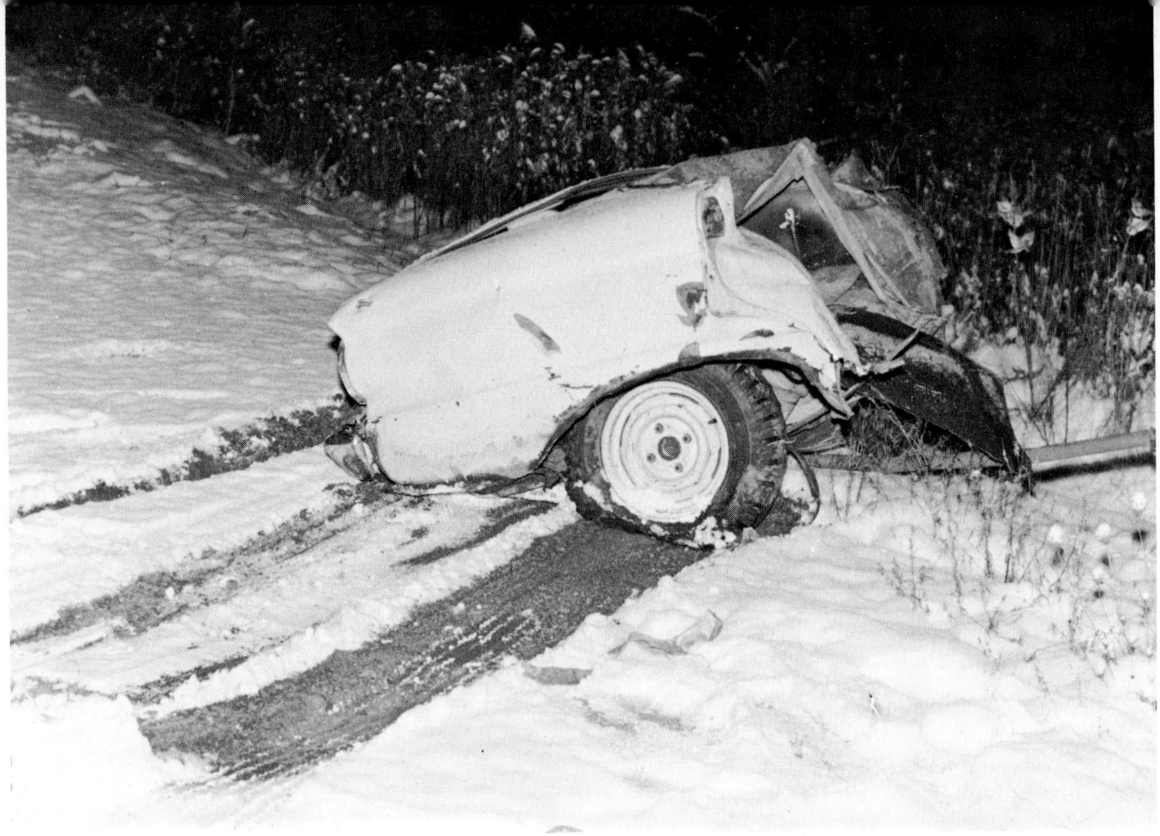

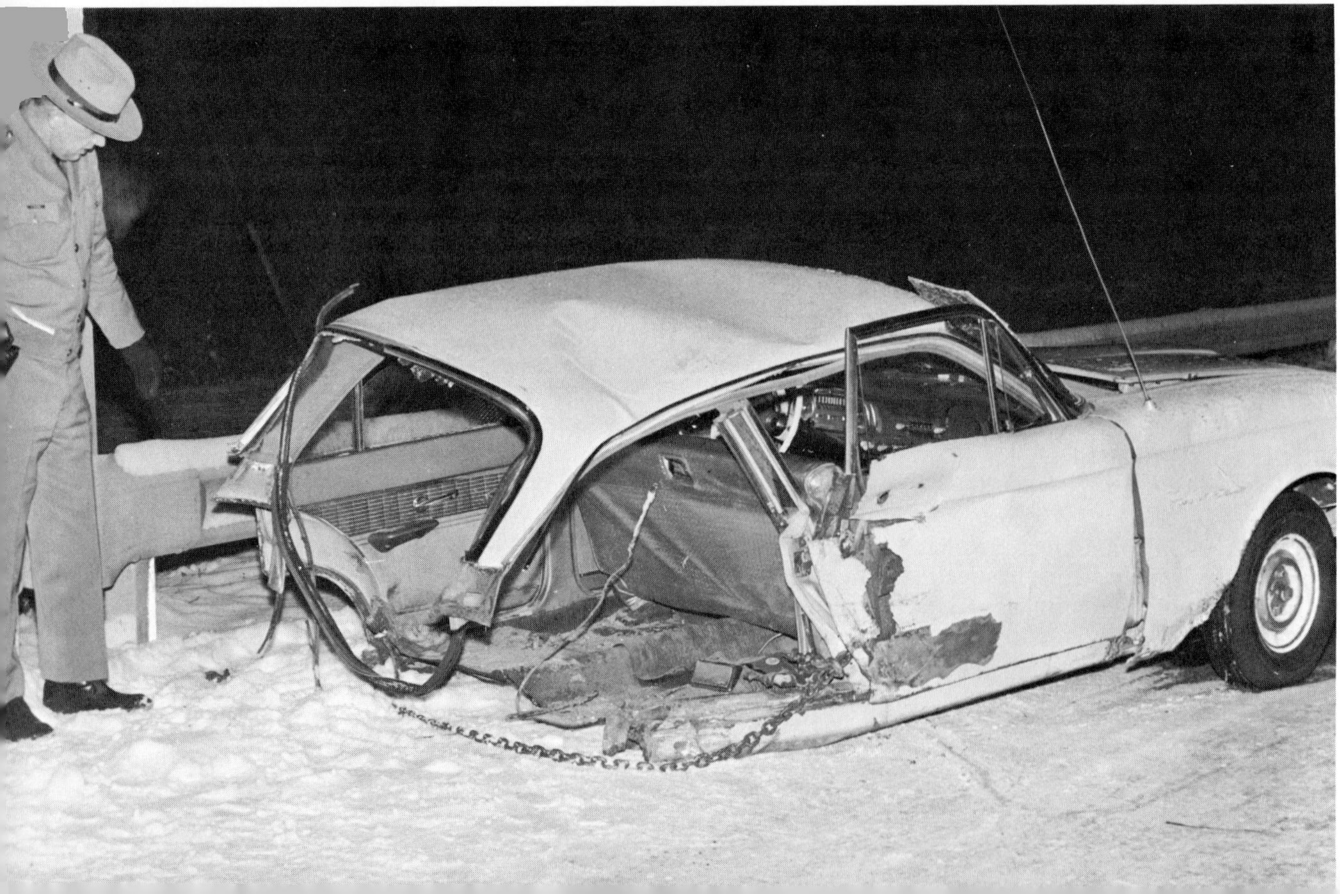

Fig. 14-1. Is this accident the result of poor construction (agent), poor driving conditions (environment), or the interaction of all three? (Ivan Kingsley)

is that we can significantly reduce injury and death by making the car safer. Because one out of every two cars produced will be involved in either a death or injury-producing accident, examination of the vehicle seems logical. Mr. Nader pointed out that General Motors had been spending approximately 1 million dollars a year on safety research for its vehicles. This is a company that grosses over 2 million dollars an *hour.* Therefore its commitment in the field of safety could hardly be considered excessive. Mr. Nader has further contended that the stylist for the automobile industry has been acting as a quack engineer, designing the car for its outward appearances rather than for its functional excellence or crashworthiness. The question has also been raised of whether the free enterprise system is actually functioning in the automobile industry, when its largest producer controls over 50 per cent of the market and its top three producers control 96 per cent of the market. Are there any relationships between these monopolistic-leaning figures and the fact that the automobile industry is taking 1 out of every 5 retail dollars in the country? Do these figures also explain the glaring reluctance of the car producers to invest in the safety of their consumers?

The publicity generated by Mr. Nader's attacks on the automobile industry and a Senate subcommittee hearing on the subject led to the conclusion that the imprudently built car, just like the imprudent driver, represents a social menace. It was generally concluded that the social responsibilities of a profit-motivated auto industry were somewhat anesthetized by its primary objectives.

In September 1966 the National Traffic and Motor Vehicle Safety Act was passed. This legislation provided for the establishment of a National Agency to carry out its provisions. One of the first actions of this agency was to recommend 23 safety features that would apply to 1968 automobiles, both domestic and imported.

Resistance and complaints by the automobile industry that the safety measures would require expensive retooling and additional time to implement resulted in three of the measures being dropped. Most of the remaining 20 standards were softened. One of the National Agency's top engineering consultants resigned in protest to this lowering of standards. The 20 safety requirements that went into effect on January 1, 1968, represented a start in the production of a safer automobile.

Recent research has sought to ascertain how well the structure of the average car will protect its occupants in a crash. Unfortunately, cars constructed with what must be described as *basic* safety features are still the exception rather than the rule. Tests conducted on the crashworthiness of the conventional car indicate the need for the following basic changes:

1. The frame of the automobile needs to be redesigned to increase its energy-absorbing capability for the front end and the sides of the car (see Fig. 14-2).
2. The engine of the car should be mounted in such a manner that in a head-on collision it is deflected

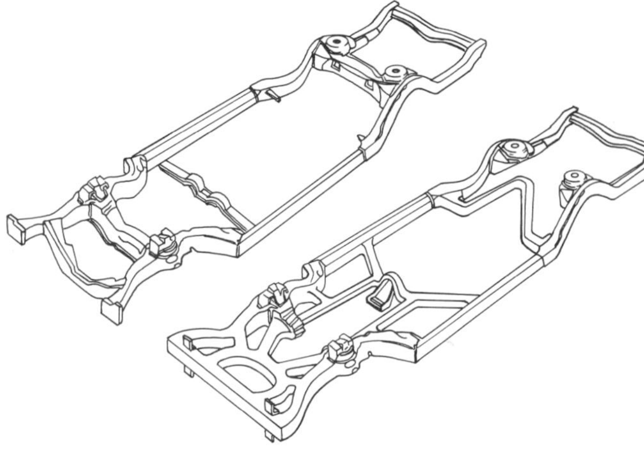

Fig. 14-2. The frame on the lower right has increased energy-absorbing capabilities for the front and sides of the car and provides for the engine to be deflected toward the ground in case of a frontal collision. (From "The Crashworthiness of Automobiles" by Patrick M. Miller. Copyright © 1973 by Scientific American, Inc. All rights reserved.)

toward the ground rather than into the passenger compartment (see Fig. 14-3).

3. All cars should have roll-bar construction to prevent the roof from caving in on its passengers in a roll-over accident (see Fig. 14-3).

The bumpers on cars have been completely inadequate. Starting with the 1973 models, cars had to be equipped with bumpers that would not result in damage to such equipment as headlights, cooling systems, trunk doors or tail lights in low-speed impacts (5 mph going forward, 2½ mph in reverse.) This will reduce repair costs for parking lot mishaps. What are now needed are bumpers that are effective where cars were intended to be used, namely, on the highway.

In recent years the recalling of cars by the automobile industry for the correction of structural defects has become a common practice. In the period between 1966 and 1971, 25 million American and foreign-made vehicles were recalled. This represents 40 per cent of all cars and trucks sold in this country. In 1971 General Motors set a new record by recalling 6.7 million cars and trucks for possible faulty engine mounts. It offered to install straps to hold possibly faulty engine mounts in place. While an official of General Motors described the failure of motor mounts as no more serious than a flat tire, motorists who went through the experience described it as terrifying.

In 1972 the Ford Motor Company recalled over 400,000 Torinos and Mercury Montegos to guard against bearing failures causing the rear end to fall to the pavement. Ford offered to place an extra set of retainer plates on the rear axles of the cars. In case of bearing failure these retainer plates would cause a loud screeching noise warning the motorist to head for his nearest Ford dealer before it was too late. How's that for a better idea! If the motorist made it to the Ford dealer, the bearings would be replaced without charge. The trauma is also free. Ultimately the Ford Company consented to replace the entire axle unit. The screeching that precipitated this action did not come from retainer plates but from consumer groups, including Ralph Nader.

Recalls generally come about when the National Highway Traffic Safety Administration (NHTSA) or an automobile manufacturer suspects that a safety defect may be present in a vehicle. The recall, however, can only be ordered by the company. The NHTSA can only recommend a recall. Ralph Nader has contended that in the interests of public safety the government should have the power to order such recalls and advocates the need for new legislation to effect this.

The Air Bag

At the present time approximately 30 per cent of the nation's motorists use the safety belts which were mandated for all cars. It is estimated that about 5,000 lives a year are saved as a result of the current level of use of safety belts. If all motorists could be convinced to use them, it is estimated that an additional 10,000 lives a year would be saved. An objective has been to get more motorists to wear their safety belts. Even with belt systems that are connected to the

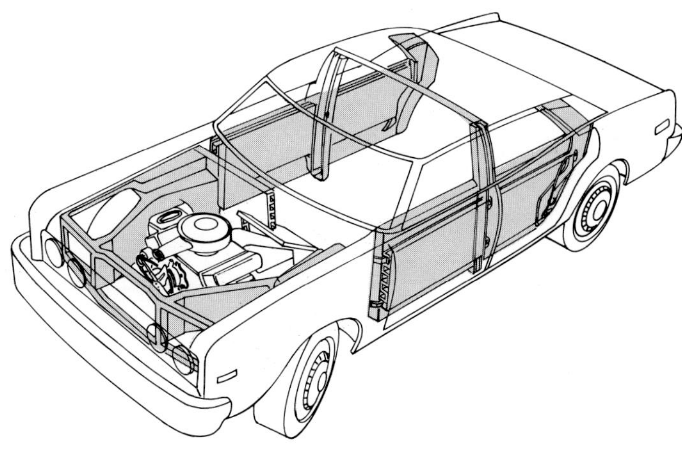

Fig. 14-3. Note the slanting structure at the rear of the engine to deflect it toward the ground rather than into the passenger compartment. Several inches of energy-absorbing material have been added to the interior panels of the passenger compartment. (From "The Crashworthiness of Automobiles" by Patrick M. Miller. Copyright © 1973 by Scientific American, Inc. All rights reserved.)

ignition system and require the motorist to buckle up in order to start the car can be circumvented. The person need only unbuckle the belt after the motor starts. The result of all this has been serious thought about a passive restraint that operates automatically. The air bag has been proposed as the solution. On impact, the air bag would inflate inside the car cushioning its passengers from the shock of impact. Standards call for the air bag to protect the occupants of a car when hitting a parked car at 60 mph.

Federal safety standards are requiring the installation of air bags for all cars sold in the United States as of 1976.

Some serious questions about air bags have been raised. Because the air bag inflates in a fraction of a second will it cause neck injuries? Since the air bag also deflates in one second, it gives little protection to the motorist in a roll-over accident in which he may be bounced about the vehicle. The bags would also not protect the occupants of a car against a second collision, as might happen in a chain series of accidents on a highway. They also provide little protection in side impacts. If the air bag is to be considered as a replacement for seat belts, these additional safety factors must be met in order for the air bag to be a suitable replacement for the seat belt.

The Life-Saving Interstate Highway System

Travel on the nation's developing interstate highway system is safer than on other kinds of roadways. The mileage death rate on the interstate system has been 2.2 per 100,000,000 miles of travel. This compares favorably with the 6.4 rate for all other roadways. The continued development of the interstate system will provide an extended environment for safer highway travel.

However, some controversy has arisen because the preponderance of transportation funds are going to the development of superhighways, with other means of transportation being ignored. Road builders and administrators are being charged with indifference to the other transportation needs of the people, to say nothing of their human and environmental needs.

> Pared down to its core, this final argument says, "The trust funds have paid for the superhighways, and also have kept the gas and rubber and truck weight and parts sales taxes from being used for any other purpose except building those highways." Agreed: The Trust Fund concept, thus described, has been a whopping success. Because of it the United States today can claim the most impressive system of superhighways the world has ever known—along with a collection of run-down railroads, limping urban transit services, and archaic local streets and roads that have been starved of public funding support by the Trust Fund's "new highways only" preoccupation.[3]

In order to cut down the accident rate on our highways further, a new international system of road signs is being implemented. The new symbol signs

[3]Ben Kelley, *The Pavers and the Paved* (New York: Donald W. Brown, 1971), p. 36.

DO NOT ENTER

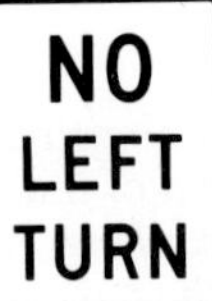

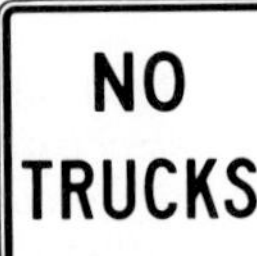

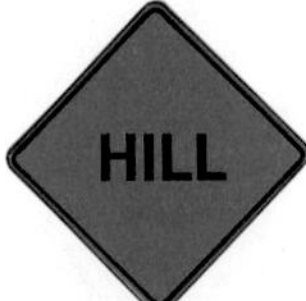

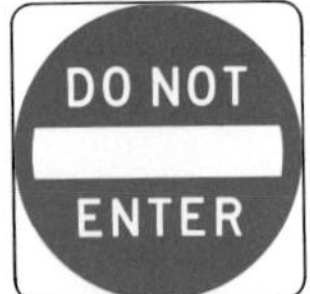

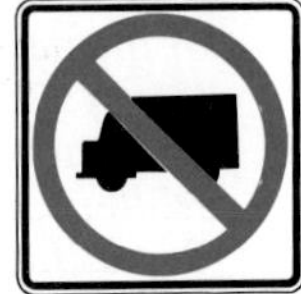

Fig. 14-4. The new international road signs at the bottom of the figure are compared to the old.

are more effective than words where reaction time and understanding are important. By adapting these signs on a nationwide level the differences in state-to-state travel signs will be minimized.

The Driver

The safest vehicle and the safest highways can be negated by the driver who for one reason or another cannot perform in a responsible manner. A study by the Department of Police Administration at Indiana University indicates that where the alcohol level in the blood of the driver reaches .15 per cent the chances of that driver's having an accident increase 25 times.

The increase in the use of drugs has also resulted in larger numbers of people driving while under drug influence. Prescription as well as self-prescribed proprietary drugs can have side effects that can seriously affect a driver's performance. A number of drugs produce drowsiness, some affect vision and equilibrium, while others produce a dangerous overconfidence.

It has been standard procedure for the Interstate Commerce Commission to require medical examinations of commercial drivers involved in interstate travel. Operators of private vehicles who do most of the nation's driving are not subjected to the same scrutiny. There is apparently a need to establish some national norms to be used as guidelines indicating kinds of physical conditions that would prevent a person from acquiring a drivers' license. Though some states have set standards, the nationwide picture is rather spotty. In many communities, people drive when they should not, simply because there is no other means of transportation readily available in the community. Some taxi companies have recognized this need and have offered monthly rates (that reduce the cost per ride) to senior citizens and the chronically ill. The savings in yearly depreciation and insurance costs of a car can take care of a good many taxi fares.

The relationship of emotional stress to accident causation is another matter of concern. A person's driving can be affected by his emotional state. Careful research studies in this area are unfortunately lacking. There are no data on the number of highway fatalities that were actually successful suicide attempts. Nor is there any real attempt made to determine if risk-taking drivers have unconscious motivations to commit suicide. When such drivers are "caught," they are usually fined and then released. "A study relating to accidents in California states that 61.9 per cent of the teenage drivers are at fault. Speeding was considered the prime factor, followed in order by failure to grant right-of-way, improper turning, and driving on the wrong side of the road. These are all violations of the type to be associated with risk-taking, or unsafe practices."[4] Physical performance being at a peak during these teen years, other reasons must be responsible for the high accident rate. Inexperience as well as attitudes

[4]Frank Freeman, Charles E. Goshen, and Barry G. King, *The Role of Human Factors in Accident Prevention* (Washington, D.C.: U.S. Dept. of Health, Education and Welfare, 1960), p. 39.

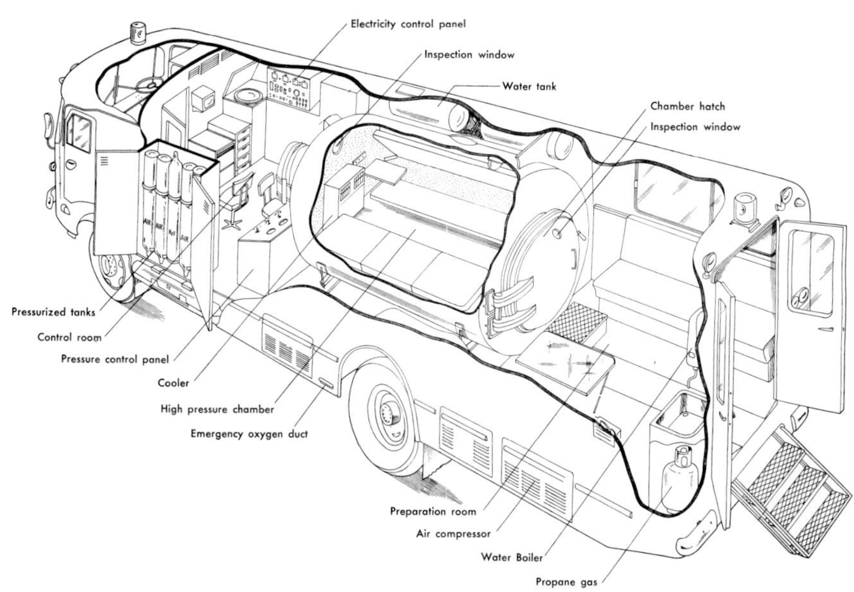

Fig. 14-5. The Japanese ambulance pictured here is equipped with surgical facilities and personnel. Its ability to get medical help to traffic accident victims has resulted in a 50 per cent reduction in fatalities. Major surgery that can be performed immediately saves patients who would not survive the trip to the hospital. (Medical World News)

reflecting emotional immaturity and risk-taking appear to be related factors.

The Expanded Use of the Motorbike and Snowmobile

The number of motorcycles (including motor scooters and motorized bicycles) has been increasing at a rapid rate in the United States since 1960. In the ten-year period between 1960 and 1970, there has been a marked increase in this type of vehicle. There has also been noted a sharp increase in the incidence of rider deaths associated with the motorcycle, out of all proportion to the increase in the number of these vehicles. The rider death rate for these vehicles during 1972 is estimated to be 17 deaths per 100,000,000 vehicle miles traveled. The death rate for all motor vehicles, including pedestrians and occupants, was 4.5 deaths (per 100,000,000 vehicle miles).

The reason for the increased death rate appears to be related to the increased number of inexperienced and improperly equipped riders. The most common cause of death to the cyclist is the head injury. Upon impact, the rider is projected forward, head first. The pavement, another vehicle, or a variety of other objects may be struck. An adequate helmet, then, is a must for the cyclist. Leather clothing also has a protective function in case of an accident. The cyclist riding with bare arms or legs is inviting serious injury.

The motorbike is also found to be a precarious vehicle when ridden on wet pavement. The more stable four-wheeled vehicles need to be driven with more care in wet conditions. The two-wheeled vehicles under these conditions can be outright menaces, particularly in the hands of the unskilled driver.

"If you can't beat 'em, join 'em." This has basically been the philosophy of the portion of our population who live where winter means snow. Instead of complaining about the weather, thousands have now joined in using the snowmobile as the vehicle for communing with nature or destroying it—depending on its use or abuse.

In order to ensure that snowmobiling is the fun it was intended to be, it is important to dress warmly for the occasion. Dress should include a one-piece insulated snowsuit, snowboots, goggles, heavy leather gloves, and helmet. On a cold night the wind-chill factor on a fast-moving snowmobile can cause frostbite for the inadequately dressed.

It is also important to snowmobile in familiar territory, preferably on well-marked trails. To scout out new trails, particularly at night, can be dangerous. The number of accidents involving snowmobiles running into barbed wire fences has been increasing. Permission to travel through someone's farmland is essential. It is only the abuses of the activity that have angered so many of the naturalists and farmers.

Avoid frozen bodies of water for it is impossible to judge the thickness of the ice. Should a person fall into icy water, it is important not to panic and reach out for pieces of ice that will only break off in one's hand. The person should extend the arms and by vigorously kicking the legs propel his body onto solid ice, then squirm and roll to safety.

Fig. 14-6. Proper equipment and dress can minimize motorcycle accidents. (N.Y.S. Dept. of Health)

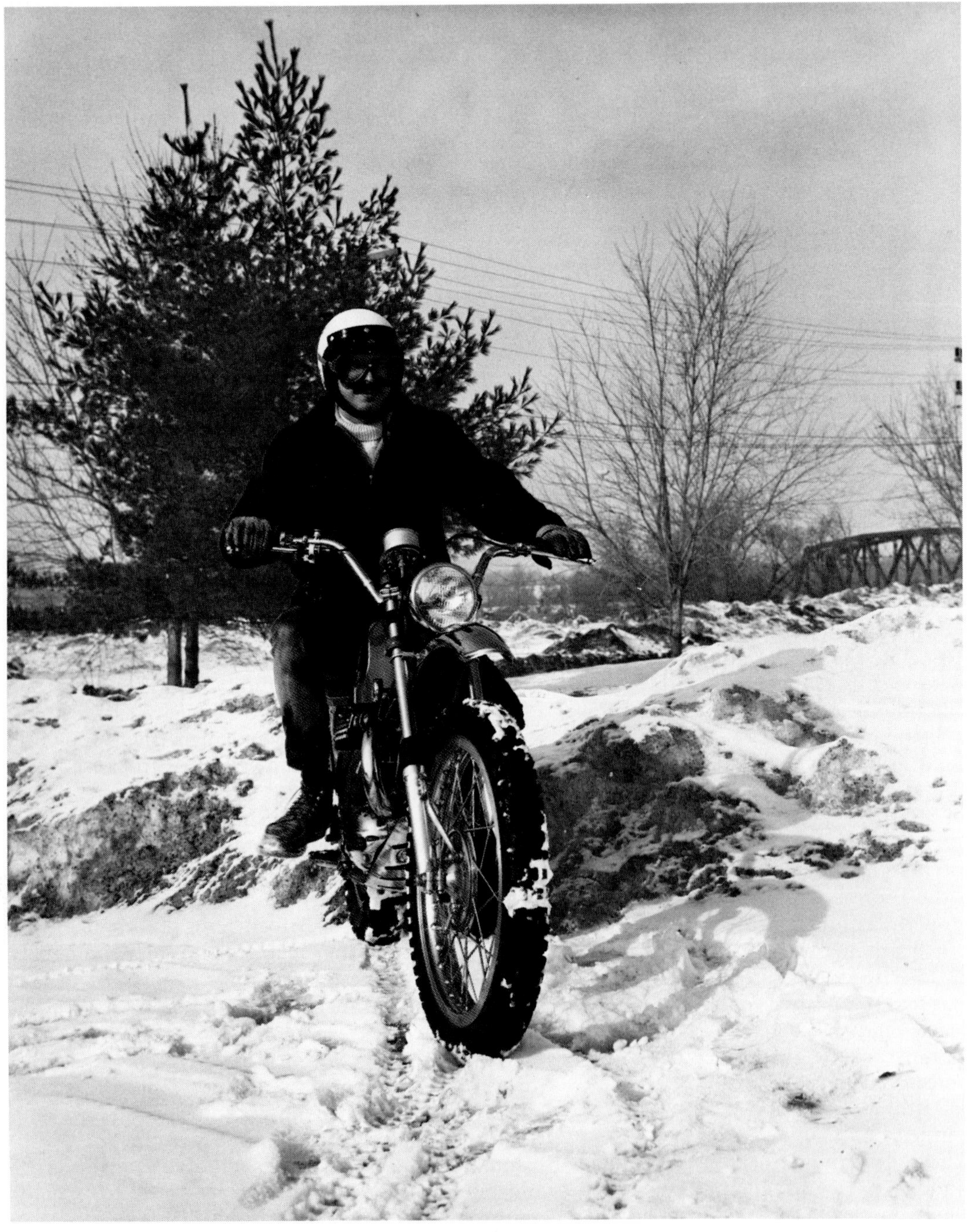

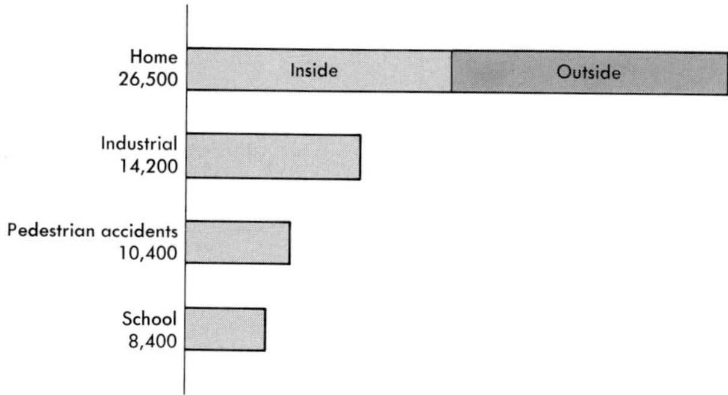

Fig. 14-7. Places of accidental deaths. (National Safety Council)

Because of the variety of injuries that can occur while snowmobiling, it is a good idea to carry a first-aid kit. It is also wise to snowmobile with another person or group so that in case of a serious accident there is someone to aid the injured or to seek needed help. Taking some basic precautions as well as learning how to skillfully handle the bucking bronco of the snowdrifts can make snowmobiling a pleasant recreational pursuit.

Home Safety

It is a well-established fact that the home is considered the place of security and refuge. Just witness a group of children playing a tag game and shouting "Home Safe!" In actuality, the home is far from being the safe place we judge it to be. From attic to cellar it affords us contact with many more hazards than we generally realize. There is a lack of drama and publicity involved in the home accident as compared with the traffic accident, even though the results may be the same. The complacency on the part of the public is due in part to the fact that people are simply not aware of the magnitude of death and injury resulting from home accidents. When accidents are classified by place, those in the home are the leading category.

Types of Home Accidents for Various Age Groups

Home accidents in 1972 accounted for 27,000 deaths and 4,200,000 disabling injuries. The data will indicate what kind and to what age group home accidents occur. Vulnerable age groups in home accidents are children from 0–4 years and adults over 65 years; special emphasis on accident prevention for these groups is necessary.

Accidents and the Child Under Five

The accident threat to the lives and limbs of our children under five is far greater than the threat of disease. The high accident rate stems basically from the child's lack of experience and knowledge, which leads to his inability to recognize danger. The infant starts out being completely protected from danger by his mother. In infancy, the human factors of the guardian, rather than the infant, are of greatest concern, for while the infant is this young, the guardian is clearly responsible for any accidents.

In a study done by Jacobziner,[5] the kind of accident is related to the child's capability for activity and locomotion. For example:

Age	*Type of Accident* (In order of frequency)
1st Year	Mechanical suffocation, burns, inhalation, ingestion
2nd Year	Falls, poisoning, burns
3rd Year	Poisoning and falls
4th Year	Poisoning and burns
5th Year	Burns, falls, and poisoning

When a child can only crawl, he has access to only

[5]Ibid., p. 36.

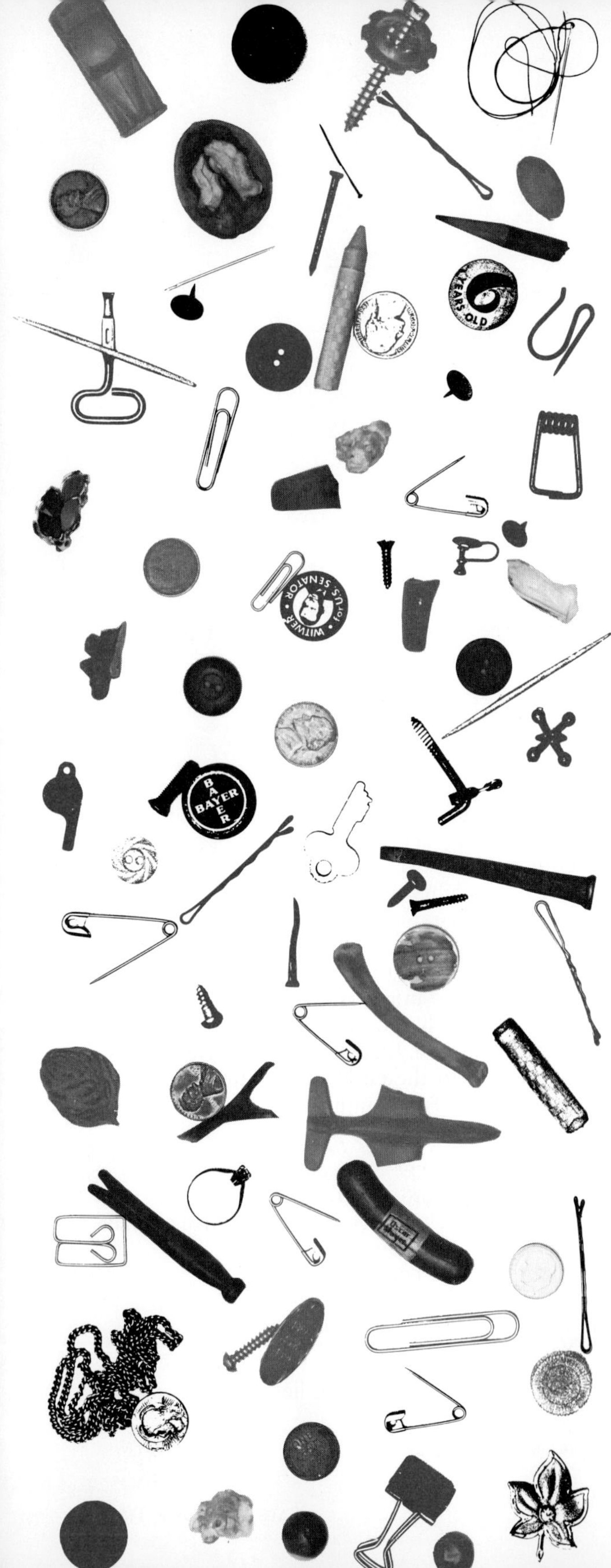

Fig. 14-8. Things children swallow. (N.Y.S. Health Dept.)

limited hazards; as he learns to walk and climb, the possibilities for trouble are limitless. Because safety must be learned, the parent must acknowledge that most of the learning of a preschooler is through imitation. The parents who are unconscious or careless of the need for safety spawn youngsters that are "accident-prone."

Fires and Burns. Our data indicate that fires cause the greatest number of preschool deaths. Children, whether awake or asleep, should never be left unattended at home for even short periods of time. Children trapped in a burning building are gripped with panic and do not even try to escape. More often than not they will attempt to hide under beds or in closets, waiting for rescue. The child who has been trained through fire drills is at a definite advantage here. Though the responsibility for the escape of the preschooler from a burning home is usually left with an older child or parent, the cooperation of the young child may be ensured if the child has been properly prepared for such an emergency.

Playing with matches should never be tolerated. However, matches are a source of fascination to the young child, and perhaps the parent might do well to permit a child under adult supervision to strike a match for an expressed purpose. In this way the child may not be overwhelmed with the desire to sneak away the matches when no one is around.

Scalding of the young child can be eliminated if the mother insists on children playing in areas away from the stove. With an 18-month-old, this may mean restricting the child with fences and gates. She can also use the back burners of the stove, or if the

Table 14-1. ***How People Were Killed in Home Accidents****

Type of Injury		*Number of People*
All Types	All deaths due to accidents in the home or on home premises.	27,000
Falls	Falls on the same level as well as falls from one level to another (down stairs, from roof, from ladder).	9,800
Fires	Burns and deaths associated with fires.	5,700
Suffocation (Ingested)	Deaths from accidental ingestion or inhalation of objects or foods resulting in obstruction of the respiratory passages.	2,600
Suffocation (Mechanical)	Deaths due to smothering by bed clothes, thin plastic materials, cave-ins, mechanical strangulation, or confinement in closed spaces.	800
Poisoning (Solids and Liquids)	Deaths from medicines, and commonly recognized poisons as well as mushroom and shellfish poisoning.	3,100
Firearms	Deaths due to firearms accidents, many of which occur while cleaning or playing with guns	1,400
Poisoning (Gases and Vapors)	Deaths caused principally by carbon monoxides due to incomplete combustion involving cooking stoves, heating equipment, and standing motor vehicles.	1,100
Others	The accidental deaths making up this group are caused principally by drowning, burns from hot substances, electric current, and blows by falling objects.	2,500

*Source: Adapted from *Accident Facts,* 1973 Edition, (Chicago, Ill.: National Safety Council), pp. 80–81.

front burners are used the pot handles should be parallel to the front of the stove.

Suffocation. (Mechanical and ingested). In 1972, death from suffocation claimed the lives of 1,250 children under the age of five. Though many of these deaths are due to respiratory infections, reports of babies smothering in bed coverings or clothing are still prevalent.

The child who finds an old refrigerator to "play" in, only to find the latch cannot be opened from the inside, is bound to be a victim of suffocation. The removal of doors or latches on any discarded refrigerator or freezer is essential.

Children playing "space man" with plastic bags over their heads are prime candidates to become accident statistics. Several years ago the dangers of

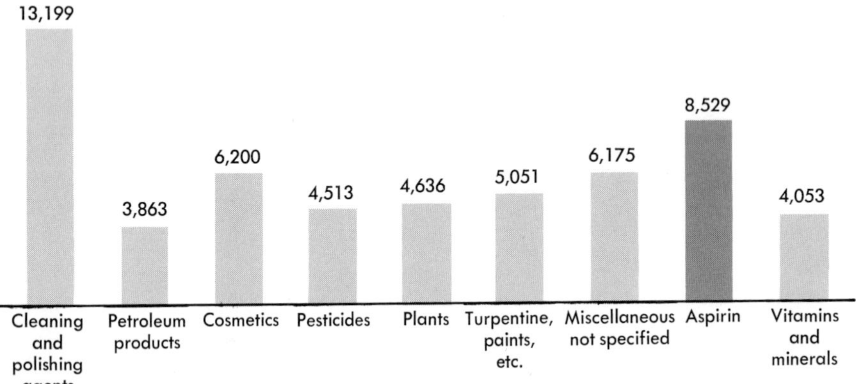

Fig. 14-9. Accidental ingestions among children under five years of age reported by the National Clearinghouse Poison Control Center, Bureau of Product Safety, FDA (1971).

plastic bags were demonstrated. Because of their extreme thinness, static electricity is generated through friction, causing the plastic to adhere to the skin. If brought in contact with the nose and mouth, the air is cut off and the struggling child will suffocate. Legislation has mandated that all thin plastic garment bags be labeled with regard to their potential danger.

Ingested suffocation refers to death resulting from some particles of food or other object the child has inhaled instead of swallowed. The parent or babysitter must know the level of development of a child and never offer hard candy or carrots to the young toddler incapable of handling these kinds of foods.

Poisoning. The ingestion of poisons and potential poisons has become a significant medical problem. There are a great variety of substances that a preschooler will experiment with. Medicines, cleaning agents, and pesticides, if left under the sink or in unlocked medicine cabinets, are fair game for the curious and imitative youngster. Authorities indicate that tranquilizers have dramatically increased as agents of juvenile death. In this age of increased drug use it is important that medicines be locked up or out of children's reach. This is particularly true of aspirin, which is the substance most frequently involved in children's poisonings. Parents must make a concerted effort to impress children with the fact that this is medicine, not candy, and that medicine must only be taken under parent's supervision. It is wise not to have children watch parents who must regularly take pills—the urge to imitate is strong in the preschooler.

It might be worth the time and effort to learn if your community hospital has a poison treatment center as part of its emergency room facilities. Since 1953 poison control centers and poison information centers have been established. The purpose of the information center is to collect and disseminate all information concerned with poisoning. Thus, in case of a poisoning, a physician may call for information about the poisoning agent and learn the level of toxicity as well as the specific toxic agent in the substance. If a nonmedical person seeks information, he is given first-aid instruction and advised to call a physician immediately. Poison information centers operate on a 24-hour basis and are usually located in large health departments or university medical or pharmacy schools.

The Poison control center is a unit combining a poison information center and a treatment center. It is usually located in a large hospital and is instrumental in aiding state and local health departments with their education programs aimed at prevention.

Certainly any accredited hospital will have facilities for a gastric lavage (stomach pumping), which is usually the emergency treatment prescribed by the physician when a toxic substance has been swallowed. It is wise to bring the container of the substance swallowed to the physician or hospital so that there is no question as to the identity of the poison.

Drowning. Most home pool drownings happen to children under 5, with the peak incidence being for 2-year olds (7 out of 10 are males). The chief causes of drowning are the temporary lack of qualified adult supervision and the absence of environ-

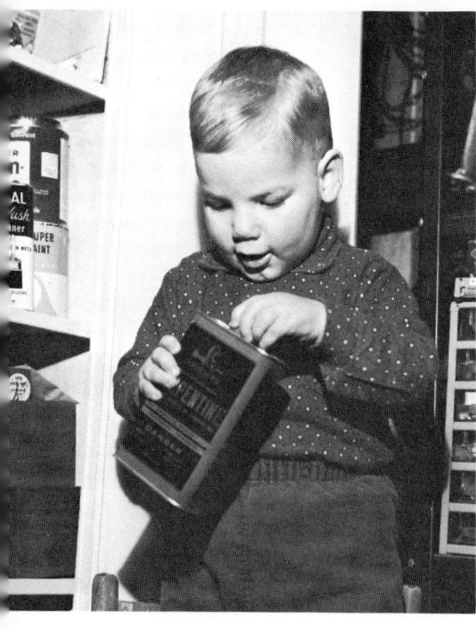

Fig. 14-10. Poisonous substances should be kept in locked containers and out of the reach of children. (N.Y.S. Dept. of Health)

Fig. 14-11. The accessible medicine cabinet can prove deadly. (N.Y.S. Health Dept. Photo by M. Dixson)

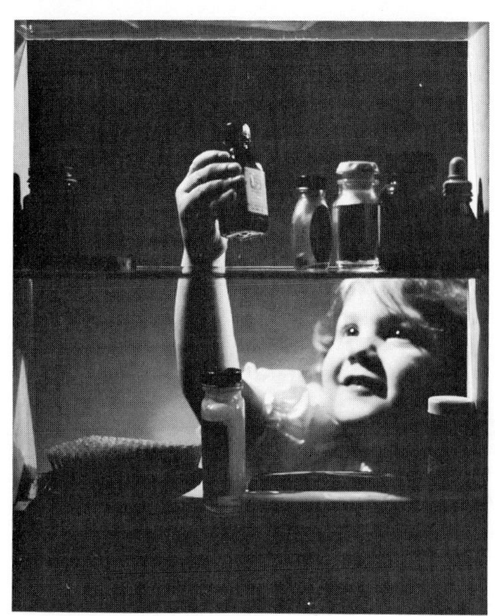

mental protection. Because most children under 5 are not able to float or swim, the bulk of the responsibility for accident prevention in this area rests primarily with the parent. Secondarily, prevention must rest upon the child-proofing of the backyard pool. This should include proper fencing that children cannot climb over or dig under.

Accidents and the Aging

Our most vulnerable group in home accident fatalities are the elderly, 65 years and over. The majority of these accidents are due to falls. In a study by Sheldon,[6] he indicates that about a third of the falls are due to vertigo and another third are associated with the greater tendency of older people to trip. The slower sensory-motor reactions tend to result in a slowness to recover when thrown off-balance, or in the inability to move quickly out of the path of a falling or moving object. Vision and hearing may become impaired at this age, lessening the acuteness of the individual's safety "alarm" system. With advancing age, the general brittleness of bones renders an individual most susceptible to fractures.

In order to prevent falling accidents among our elderly, it will be necessary to provide them with an environment that is free from hazards. This will include well-lighted stairways that are kept free of toys and other objects, and equipped with handrails; nonslippery floors and rugs that are well anchored; cellar stairs and porch steps that are kept in good repair. Housing specific for senior citizens includes,

[6] "The Role of Human Factors in Accident Prevention," op. cit., p. 50.

Table 14-2. ***Deaths from Home Accidents by Type and Age, 1972***

Type of Accident	*All Ages*	*0–4 Years*	*5–14 Years*	*15–24 Years*	*25–44 Years*	*45–64 Years*	*65–74 Years*	*75 Years and Over*
Total	**27,000**	**3,580**	**1,530**	**2,470**	**3,000**	**4,400**	**3,120**	**8,900**
Falls	9,800	250	100	50	300	1,000	1,400	6,700
Fires, burns, and deaths associated with fires	5,700	800	550	350	700	1,400	900	1,000
Suffocation—ingested object	2,600	800	120	180	250	500	300	450
Suffocation—mechanical	800	450	150	40	50	50	30	30
Poisoning by solids and liquids	3,100	180	50	1,000	850	650	170	200
Firearms	1,400	50	300	450	300	200	80	20
Poisoning by gases and vapors	1,100	50	60	250	250	300	90	100
Other	2,500	1,000	200	150	300	300	150	400

Source: Estimates by National Safety Council, based on data from National Center for Health Statistics and state health departments.

wherever feasible, ramps instead of steps, kitchen cabinets that are easily reached, and other facilities designed to prevent falls.

It will also be necessary to help the older person realize his physical limitations, the need to carry on former activities in a slower, more deliberate way, and the advisability of wearing properly fitted shoes to help avoid falls. This may be a difficult task after a lifetime of habit has already been established in the elderly.

Accidents and the 25 to 64 Age Group

A basic problem in home safety is that in the home the person deals with a wide variety of tools, appliances, and substances that he or she is only casually familar with. In industry, a worker is often responsible for one kind of job and one machine. He becomes thoroughly familiar with the one piece of equipment and the specific function he is to perform. In addition, a safety engineer on the premises is constantly seeking ways of making the work safer. These advantages are not to be found in the home. The housewife does not have a safety engineer assigned to her household. The worker, upon arriving at home, in his attempt to be a jack of all trades is often transformed from a skilled professional to an outrageously performing amateur.

Fire and Burns. The National Safety Council states that in the 25-to-64 age group 2,100 deaths represented the yearly death toll attributed to fires. In this age group, the frequent causes of fires are falling asleep while smoking, starting fires with inflammable liquids, using defective heating and cooking equipment, overloading electrical circuits, and using fuel oils, paints, or gasolines improperly. Becoming familiar with the materials and equipment one is using is an important first step. Inflammable materials are often well labelled and directions for their use described. Directions for the proper use and maintenance of the variety of appliances now found in households are usually available with the purchase of this equipment. The casual attitude that one does not need to read instructions or directions related to such items is fraught with danger.

The comparatively new idea of family fire drills is being urged by the National Safety Council. This is another example of preplanning for the emergency situation. The attitude is developing that surprises are best left for parties and that the realistic anticipation of accidents can save lives. The description of a family with six children (age $1\frac{1}{2}$ to 12) who evacuated their home in two minutes when an electrical outlet spurted fire and ignited a bedspread indicates the value in this kind of planning. Disorganization and panic at a time when precise and planned actions are imperative can only lead to tragedy and disaster.

The kitchen is often the place where fires start; the strategic placement of a fire blanket (preferably wool) in this room would seem logical. The installation of fire extinguishers throughout the home should be mandatory, along with the knowledge of their proper use.

Electrical Safety

Though prevention is the ideal way of solving a major health problem, knowing what to do if the problem presents itself is next best. The Lightning Protection Institute indicates that although most lightning accidents occur outdoors, one-fourth do occur in the home. Lightning enters houses via chimneys, plumbing, wiring, TV antennas, or directly through the roof. The safest place in the home is usually in the center of a room, away from walls, fireplace, plumbing lines, electrical equipment, and metal objects such as the stove, sink, or tub. If one is caught outside the home, one should stay away from utility poles, trees, and wire fences. The camping enthusiast should be sure that his "home away from home" is not pitched on rocky ground in the open, because lightning shows some affinity for this type of location. Groups of people in the open also seem to attract lightning, so that it might be wise for individuals to scatter. If a storm is hitting so close that the lightning and thunder seem almost simultaneous and a strong odor of ozone prevails, it is best to "hit the ground!"

Although over 100 deaths due to lightning electrocution occur each year, a far greater number (over 1,000) of accidental electrocutions take place. In this era of electric gadgetry, which enables us to open cans, sandpaper walls, brush teeth, trim hedges, and wash dishes, the need for electrical safety education has become critical.

We have all at one time or another experienced an electric shock that is sometimes described as an unpleasant sensation, as a tingling, throbbing, or hot feeling. The rate of flow of current through the body is measured in milliamperes (1/1000 of an ampere). The human body is very sensitive to electric current and some few individuals can feel a current of only 2/10 of a milliampere. Most people, however, can feel a current approaching 1 milliampere. An electrical shock at this level is not dangerous in and of itself; however, a startled reaction could lead one to drop a power tool or jump back into a hazard. When the current exceeds 5 milliamperes, muscular contractions stimulated by the electric current are so severe that the individual cannot let go of the object (such as a metal handle of an electric drill). This continual shock could lead to fatigue, collapse, and finally death. A shock of 50 to 100 milliamperes (or 110 volts or less) could kill a person outright.

When an electrical appliance comes off the assembly line with insufficient insulation or poor circuit design, you have the potential for a leakage of electric current from the live interior of the appliance to the outer metal covers. Though the outer casing of this product may be alive with current, by touching the appliance alone you will not feel a shock. However, if some other part of your body is simultaneously touching a ground (an electricity-conducting material that at some point enters the earth or touches a conductor that in turn, enters the earth, e.g., metal sink, radiator, faucet, cold water pipe, gas pipe, storm drain), you could receive a substantial electric shock. Most obvious grounds are moist earth, outside patios, and damp concrete basements. Persons may live with hazardous appliances for many

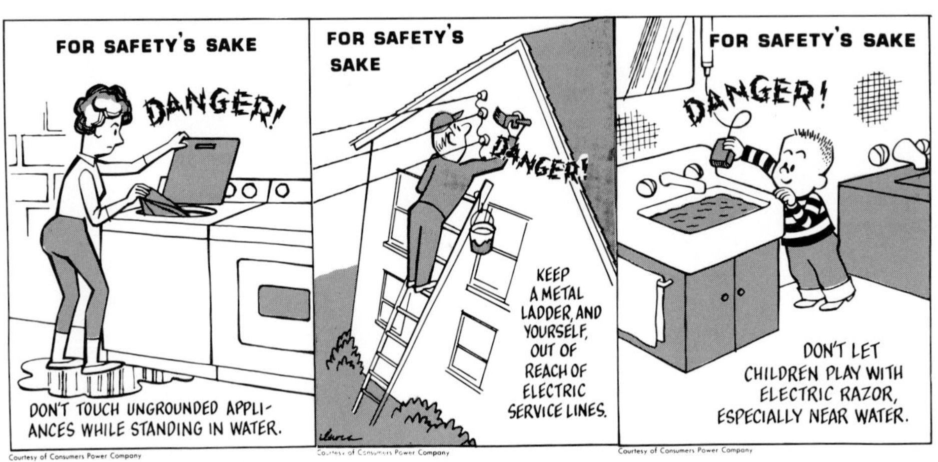
FOR SAFETY'S SAKE
DANGER!
DON'T TOUCH UNGROUNDED APPLI-ANCES WHILE STANDING IN WATER.
Courtesy of Consumers Power Company
FOR SAFETY'S SAKE
DANGER!
KEEP A METAL LADDER, AND YOURSELF, OUT OF REACH OF ELECTRIC SERVICE LINES.
Courtesy of Consumers Power Company
FOR SAFETY'S SAKE
DANGER!
DON'T LET CHILDREN PLAY WITH ELECTRIC RAZOR, ESPECIALLY NEAR WATER.
Courtesy of Consumers Power Company

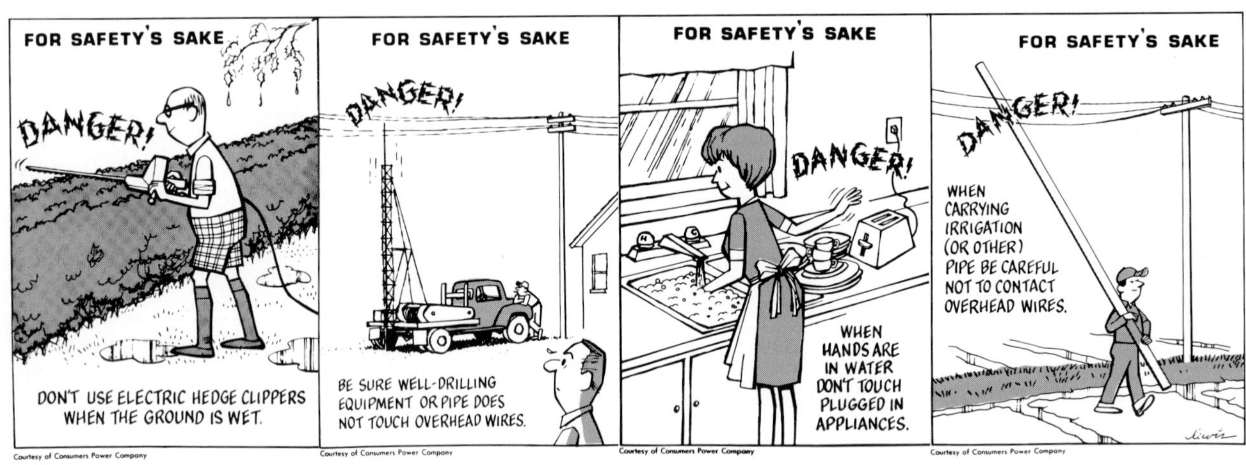
FOR SAFETY'S SAKE
DANGER!
DON'T USE ELECTRIC HEDGE CLIPPERS WHEN THE GROUND IS WET.
Courtesy of Consumers Power Company
FOR SAFETY'S SAKE
DANGER!
BE SURE WELL-DRILLING EQUIPMENT OR PIPE DOES NOT TOUCH OVERHEAD WIRES.
Courtesy of Consumers Power Company
FOR SAFETY'S SAKE
DANGER!
WHEN HANDS ARE IN WATER DON'T TOUCH PLUGGED IN APPLIANCES.
Courtesy of Consumers Power Company
FOR SAFETY'S SAKE
DANGER!
WHEN CARRYING IRRIGATION (OR OTHER) PIPE BE CAREFUL NOT TO CONTACT OVERHEAD WIRES.
Courtesy of Consumers Power Company

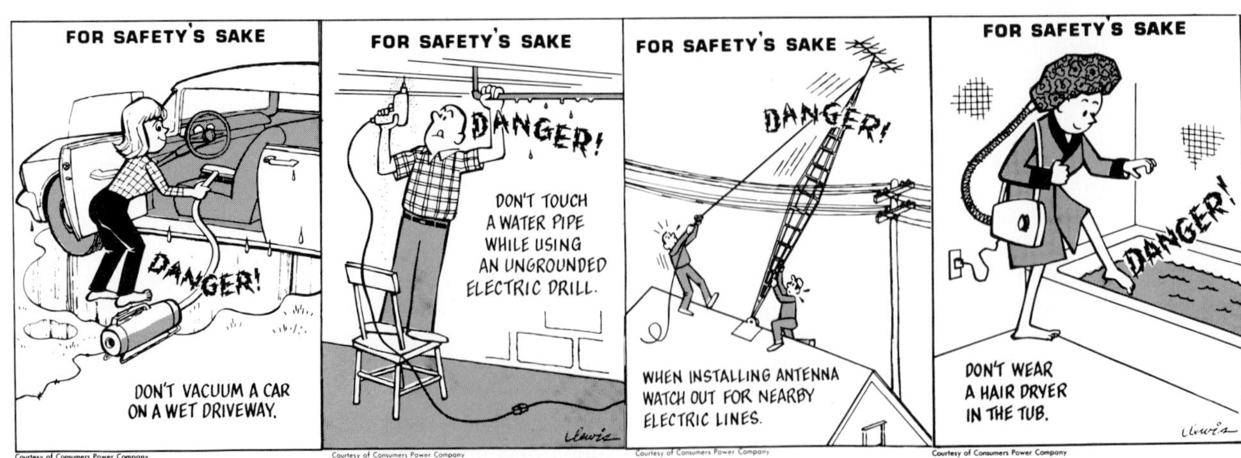
FOR SAFETY'S SAKE
DANGER!
DON'T VACUUM A CAR ON A WET DRIVEWAY.
Courtesy of Consumers Power Company
FOR SAFETY'S SAKE
DANGER!
DON'T TOUCH A WATER PIPE WHILE USING AN UNGROUNDED ELECTRIC DRILL.
Courtesy of Consumers Power Company
FOR SAFETY'S SAKE
DANGER!
WHEN INSTALLING ANTENNA WATCH OUT FOR NEARBY ELECTRIC LINES.
Courtesy of Consumers Power Company
FOR SAFETY'S SAKE
DANGER!
DON'T WEAR A HAIR DRYER IN THE TUB.
Courtesy of Consumers Power Company

Fig. 14-12. Composite of electric safety posters. (Consumers Power Co.)

years without experiencing any shocks, because they just never happened to touch a ground and the faulty appliance at the same time. This is a form of Russian roulette currently being played by thousands of people.

In order to minimize this possibility, electrical appliances and power tools should be properly grounded. This may involve the services of an electrician to convert outlet boxes to accept a three-prong receptacle and to be sure such boxes are correctly grounded. In some instances an adapter plug is utilized to enable one to use a three-prong plug into a two-prong receptacle. It is essential if an adapter plug is used that the small pigtail wire be secured by the screw holding the cover plate of the outlet. Using an adapter plug is considered a far less safe way to handle the situation, for very often adapter plugs are used without securing the pigtail wire to the outlet. Secondly, if the outlet is not properly grounded to begin with, even securing the wire of the adapter plug will not ground the appliance. It only gives one a false sense of security.

A safety device has been designed, which monitors the balance of current between the hot and neutral lines of a circuit. When the balance is off, as when current leaks to the ground because of a faulty electrical appliance, the device activates a circuit breaker which shuts the power down. This *ground-fault interrupter* works fast enough so that a nasty shock is the result instead of a person's electrocution. A ground-fault interrupter in this day and age of electrical appliance use should be installed in the fuse box of every home.

Most people are unaware that electric high voltage power lines are not insulated and that they pose a threat to the unsuspecting. The wet string of a kite can serve as a deadly conductor as can equipment such as a crane, or a well driller. In the summer, high school and college youths are often hired by tree-trimming companies and given little training with regard to the electrical dangers they may expose themselves to.

With the need for electrical power in our society doubling every ten years it would seem appropriate to either insulate power lines or to place them underground. The presence of bare power lines carrying thousands of volts of electricity currently stand as silent unrecognized killers in our environment. Legislation has been passed in a number of states to control this hazard. It is time for federal legislation to effect uniform safety measures nationally.

Poisoning. In this age group (25 to 64) poisoning is a common occurrence, and ironically it is most often caused by medication. Household preparations such as bleaches, lye, and pesticides also caused death in the adult group. Many of these tragedies could have been avoided if some precautions had been taken. Medicines that have been prescribed for a specific ailment should be discarded at the termination of the illness. Medicines may alter in composition while standing for months in the medicine cabinet and what was once a beneficial substance may now be harmful. Taking medicines in a dimly lit bathroom in the middle of the night may also be an invitation to disaster, particularly if medications for internal use are stored haphazardly with

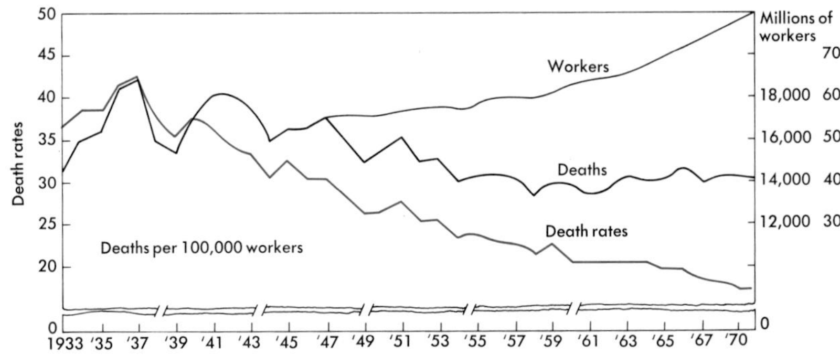

externally used compounds and disinfectants. To be sure, one must read and *reread* a label of the medication to be used, as well as clean out and organize the medicine cabinet. It is also recommended that medication not be left on the night table to be administered in the middle of the night; in addition to the hazard of poisoning oneself with an overdose, the medication on the night table is too accessible to the young child.

Poisons or possibly hazardous substances should never be placed in cups, glasses, soda bottles, or similar receptacles. The temporary pouring of caustic disinfectants into a soda bottle is bound to mean trouble.

Insect and rodent poison should always be used with great caution, particularly in or near the kitchen. Likewise, the use of pesticides in the garden must be done with care. Because certain toxic substances can be absorbed through the skin, the body should be well covered and upon completion of the spraying thorough washing should be encouraged.

The Spray-Can Menace. Hair sprays, shaving creams, toothpaste, deodorants, pesticides, paints, de-icers, and polishes are now all available in pressurized cans which spray or spurt their contents in a most convenient way. However, with their misuse have come many tragic accidents.

One most obvious problem is disposing of the empty can. Though the can no longer dispenses its product, the vapor left inside can reach explosive proportions when heated. It becomes important, then, to dispose of the can without exposing it to any form of heat. The inhalations of toxic fumes from spray cans can also be a hazard. Extensive spraying should be done in well-ventilated areas and not in the presence of a lighted cigarette or any other flammatory source.

Industrial Safety

The National Safety Council reports that since World War II the number of accidental deaths to workers on the job has *decreased* by 15 per cent. This, in spite of an increase in the number of workers. The rate of accidents resulting in death has actually been reduced by 13 per cent. It is also interesting to note that in 1972 three out of four deaths, and more than half the injuries suffered by workers, occurred *off the job.*

The reasons for the advances made in industrial safety revolve around the assumption by management of greater responsibility in this area. There are, of course, legal obligations that employers have had to meet that require reasonable standards of safety in the operation of their plants. They have also felt the social pressures of society reminding them of their obligations to their workers. Should management fail to meet these obligations, public opinion would then give support to increased government regulation in order to attain these goals. A key factor in the picture is that the employer has accepted responsibility for a portion of the financial loss involved in an accident. An accident invariably involves work stoppage and this in itself represents an economic loss to the company. In addition, accidents often involve expensive equipment or machinery

Fig. 14-13. Deaths and death rate trends. The above chart shows that although the number of workers has increased, the number of deaths has decreased resulting in a significantly reduced industrial death rate. (Accident Facts, *1971, Source: National Safety Council*)

that must be repaired or replaced. An accident often may result in machinery damage or loss without an employee's being hurt. The causes of these accidents are the same as those that produce employee injury or death. The point is that safety and production have become interwoven segments of the industrial pattern. Progressive managements have therefore recognized the need for accident prevention programs as part of the operation of a successful business.

Although the industrial safety problem has by no means been completely resolved, recent developments demonstrate the kinds of progress that can be made when some attention is given to the problem. It is at best ironic to note that death and injury rates run higher in the home than at places of work.

Review Questions

1. Why have we as a society tolerated for so long the thesis that the accident is an unavoidable aspect of our environment?
2. How does the human factor make its contribution to the accident picture? What are the effects of drugs, emotions, immaturity, disability, and old age on the driver?
3. How has the utilization of the epidemiological approach aided the study of accidents?
4. The development of accident prevention programs by modifying human behavior, while helpful, is not as rapid as effecting envionmental changes. Explain.
5. What have been the contributions of Mr. Ralph Nader in calling attention to the automobile as an accident factor?
6. What concerns have been expressed about the automobile tires as accident factors?
7. What are the functions of the National Traffic Agency?
8. To what extent has the expanded use of the motorbike aggravated the traffic safety problem?
9. Why does the home accident continue to reign as a leading cause of injury and death?
10. How can we better protect the preschool child from accidental injury and death?
11. What adaptations are being made to make homes safer for the aged?
12. What precautions should one take when caught in the open by a lightning storm? What are the safest places in the home during a storm?
13. How can the advances in industrial safety be explained?

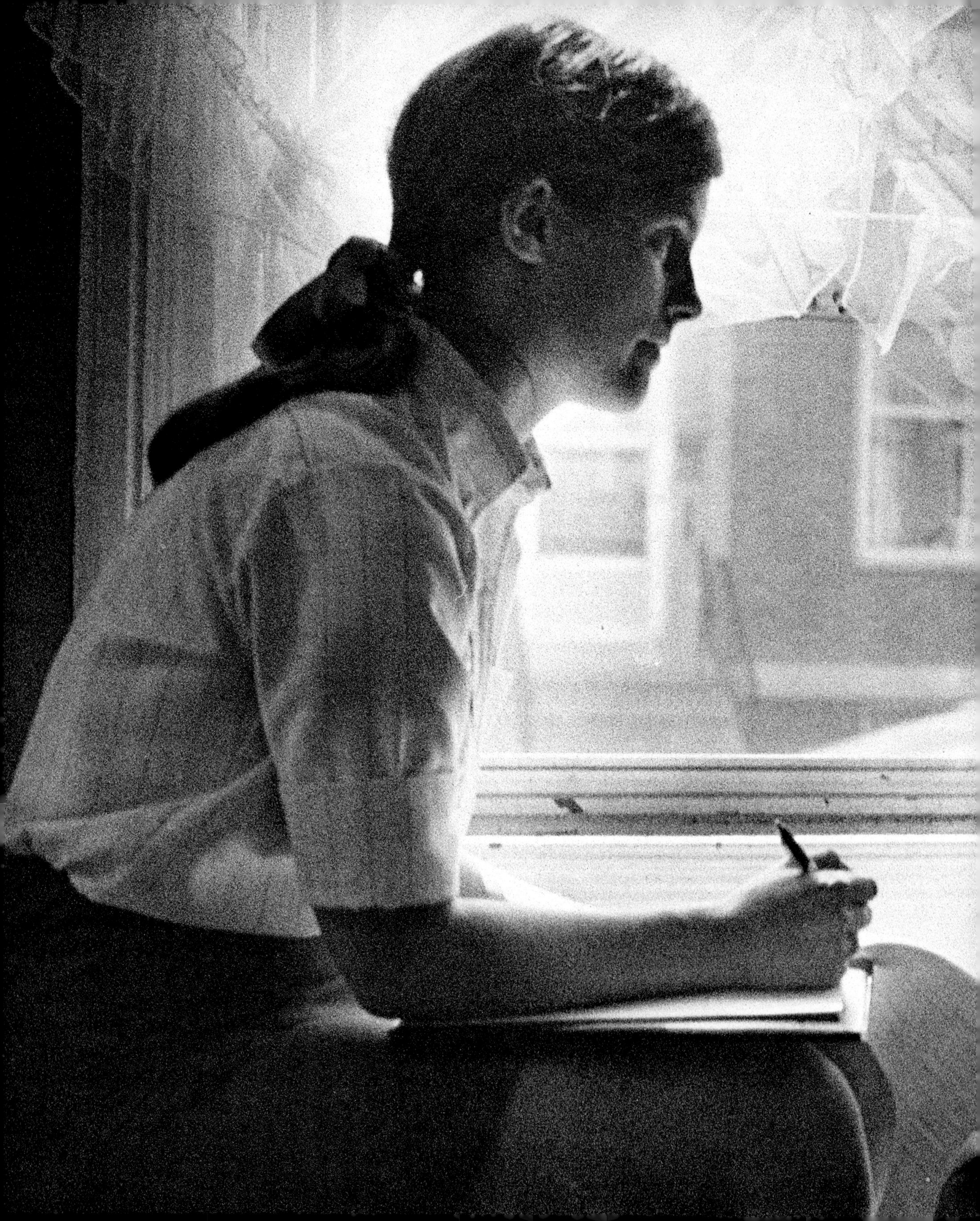

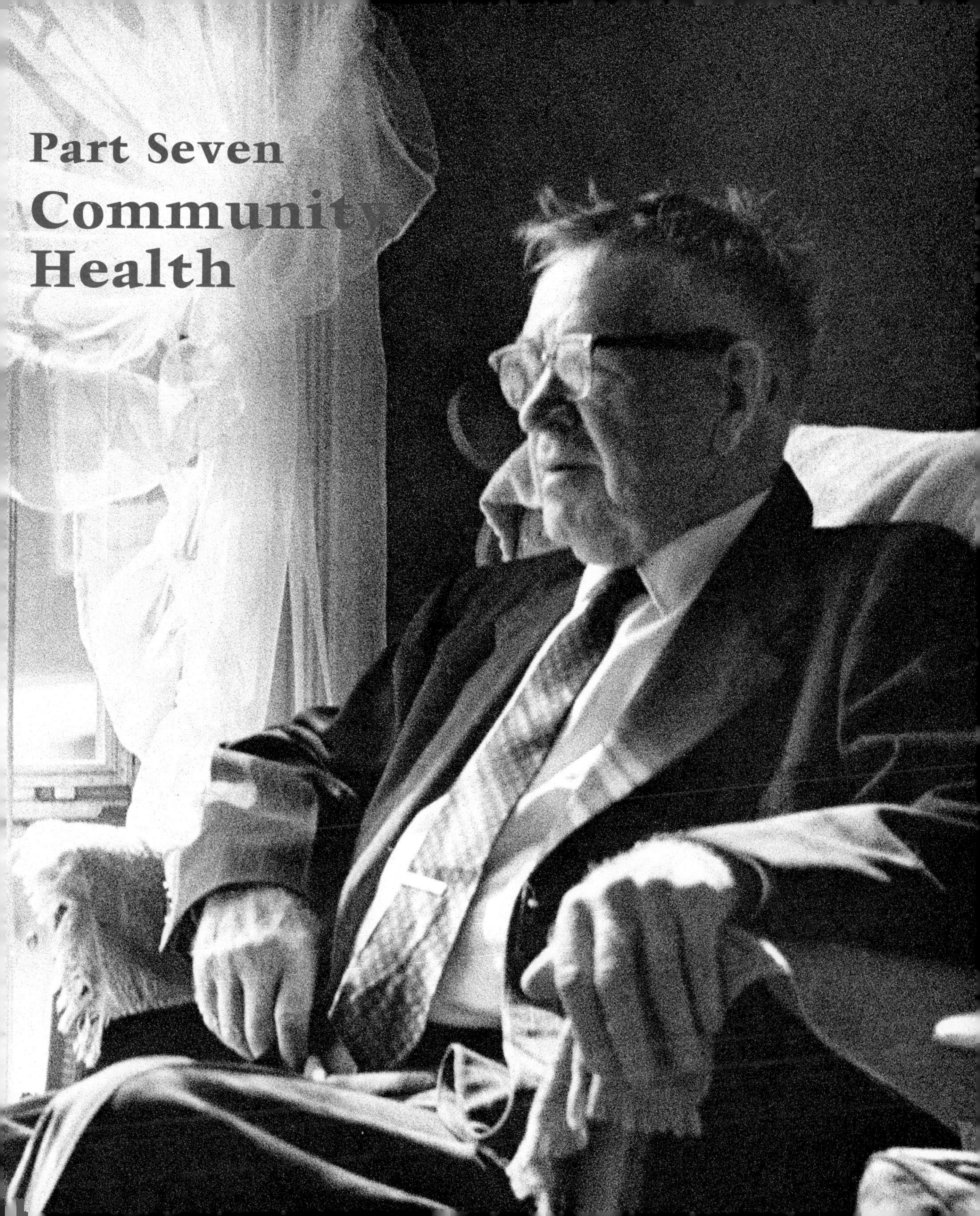

Part Seven
Community Health

Chapter 15
Public Health Organization for Community Action

The era of rugged individualism was probably best exemplified in this country by the heroes of the old Wild West. These heroes are still eulogized on the television serial—no doubt because the self-assertive spirit and the desire for personal independence still burn in the hearts of men. In our sophisticated culture rugged individualism has given way to intricate and complex group efforts. The Wright Brothers of today, our astronauts, would never get off the ground without the help of hundreds of scientists, engineers, and technicians. The Louis Pasteurs of our modern age are part of a research complex that discourages the glorification of the individual. The person is at best a part of a gigantic jigsaw puzzle. His absence can make the puzzle incomplete (if no one takes his place), but his presence will not represent the entire structure. While this arrangement may prove bruising to the egos of some, for most it represents a methodology leading to a better way of life.

In the area of public health there is an analagous situation. The individual finds himself virtually helpless in trying to combat or avoid the effects of a broad-scale environmental health problem such as air pollution. The quality of his water supply, food, environmental sanitation, and medical facilities, to name a few, is beyond the control of the individual. He must rely on others to help ensure that elements of his surroundings are designed to support rather than hamper his existence. The ability to maintain levels of health is more and more becoming community based. Increasingly, how a community is organized and the effort it puts into the health area will determine the levels of individual health more surely than anything the individual can do.

The implications of this developing situation are quite clear. The person must first of all be familiar with those organizations in the community designed to protect his health. He needs to know how effectively they are working and to determine what he, as part of a citizen group, can do to support the effective functioning of these organizations.

The Official Health Agency

The health department at the local level is a part of the community local government. The budget to support this organization comes from local tax moneys. Its basic purpose is the protection and further promotion of the community's health.

The health officer serves as the director of the local official health agency. He is usually an M.D. (medical doctor) who often possesses an M.P.H. (Masters Degree in Public Health). In some instances, the health officer is a nonmedical person with specific training in public health administration. This is similar to the definite trend of training nonmedical personnel to serve as hospital administrators. The latter degree would be obtained from one of the graduate schools of public health in the country and would specifically train a man for his responsibilities as a health officer. In this position he serves not only as the head of his department but as a coordinator for all community health activities that would involve a number of other community groups.

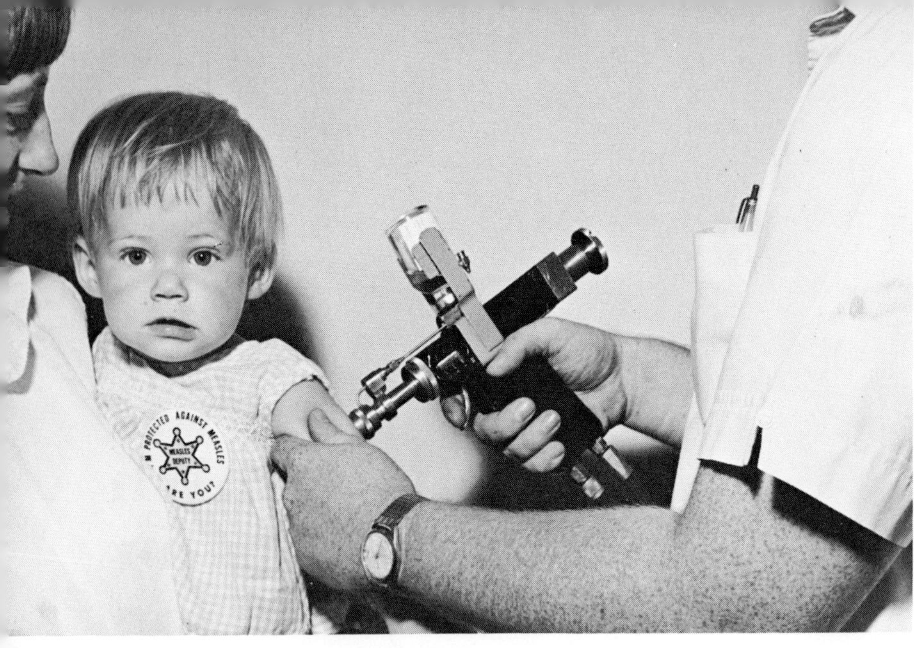

Fig. 15-1. Immunization clinics give protection against communicable diseases. (N.Y.S. Dept. of Health)

Functions of the Local Health Department

Vital Statistics. Keeping a tally of such things as births, deaths, marriages, divorces, and incidence of reportable illness serves a basic public health purpose. Vital statistics act as a community barometer indicating how things are going. Sudden increases of a given disease forewarn the health officer and ultimately the community of an impending epidemic or of a breakdown in one of the preventive disease measures. Appropriate action can then be taken to correct the condition at an early stage of its development.

Vital statistics from local health units are sent on to state health departments, which chart a statewide picture of what is occurring. From there they are sent to the National Office of Vital Statistics, where conclusions are drawn with regard to the health status of the nation.

Environmental Sanitation. The health department plays a major role in maintaining the health of the community through its activities in the area of environmental sanitation. It maintains a constant check on the fitness of community water supplies; impure water can serve as a primary means of transmitting disease. Health department sanitarians also serve to supervise the production and distribution of milk. Equipment used on dairy farms must meet optimum standards of cleanliness, with milk from diseased cows being barred from distribution. Sanitarians also supervise foods and food handlers in restaurants, and help set standards for cleanliness and food handling. They may, for instance, take bacterial counts from silverware and dishes in a restaurant as a check on the effectiveness of its dishwashing procedure. These health workers will often have bacterial counts taken of waters from public swimming pools and beaches to determine their level of safety. Occasionally, swimming pools are temporarily closed so that a dangerously high bacterial count can be corrected. Malfunction of the pool's filtration system may be one of several causes of the disorder. When beaches are closed down, it usually indicates that a dangerous level of water pollution is present. (This problem is discussed in detail in Chapter 13, "Man's Self-Created Environment.") Insect and rodent control is another key program in environmental health because these agents often serve to transmit disease.

Communicable Disease Control. While the activities of the health department in the area of environmental health make a number of important contributions to the control of communicable disease, the department engages in a number of other specific activities in this area. Health departments often conduct immunization drives as well as routine immunization clinics. The maintenance of high immunization levels in the community is considered a primary preventive objective. A number of health departments will operate special clinics, such as venereal disease or rabies clinics, where these particular communicable diseases pose special problems.

Maternal and Child Health. There is no other aspect of the public health program that is so broad and varied as that pertaining to mother and child.

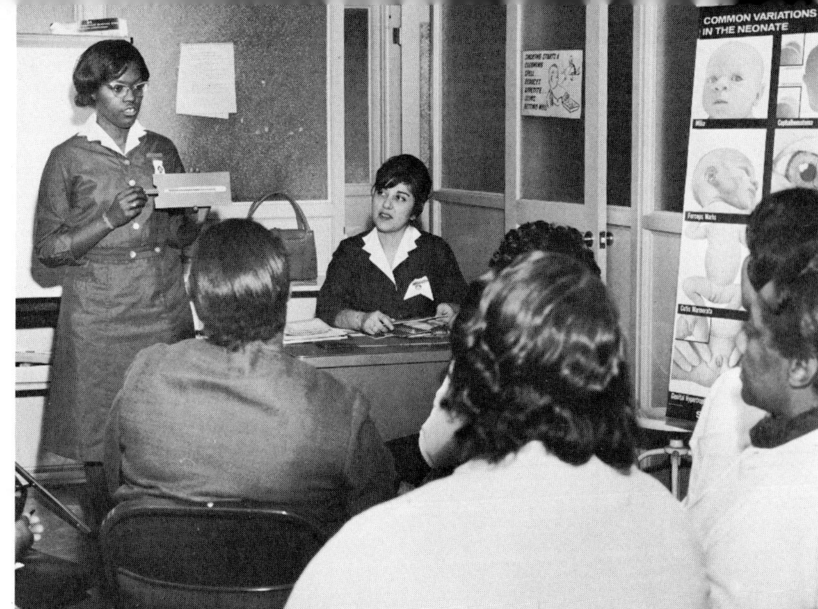

Fig. 15-2. Public health educators use the mass media as well as community meetings, classes and exhibits to get health information to the public. (N.Y.S. Dept. of Health)

Probably every facet of public health, with its many programs and numerous personnel, touches this population group.

Maternal health programs start before marriage or conception. Educational programs, often in cooperation with the school, are conducted to prepare the person for parenthood. For expectant mothers, nursing service and educational programs are conducted and are designed to prepare the woman for childbirth. Classes for expectant parents often include fathers so that they too may become acquainted with the varied tasks and adjustments that come with having a family. Health departments will also provide nursing service following childbirth. The nurse instructs the mother on proper infant care (the bathing of the infant, how to prepare formula, and so forth), as well as on alertness to any postbirth complications in the mother or illness in the infant. The nurse can also pave the way for pediatric care for the baby. This care may be given by private physicians or well-baby clinics sponsored by the health department.

The health department is also concerned with the identification of the ill or handicapped child. These children are sought out so that they may be recipients of needed care. Other community and state agencies are involved when it is determined that the child is in need of their services.

Increasingly health departments are conducting birth control clinics. These clinics are designed to inform women of the various means of contraception and their effective use. The goal is to prevent the unwanted pregnancy.

The health department works closely with schools, assisting them in their health instructional program and often serving as the schools' source of health services. The objective is to provide the child with meaningful information that will lead to the development of positive health attitudes and practices. The health services are not only designed to assure well-being, but to make sure that the child is physically and psychologically prepared to learn. The child with a vision, hearing, or emotional problem can be insensitive to the best teaching in the world.

Health departments are also represented on school health councils whose function it is to identify and resolve health problems in the school environment.

Public Health Education. Many of the activities of the health department rely upon community understanding, support, and cooperation for their success. Essentially, every member of the department staff has an educational responsibility in his contacts with various groups in the community. In addition, health departments have on their staffs public health educators who use the mass media as well as community meetings, classes, and exhibits to get health information to the public. Understanding of the principles of disease prevention and the maintenance of health precede meaningful health activity. The best-equipped and -staffed immunization clinic, for instance, will go unattended unless there is public acceptance of its need. Recognition that public education is pivotal in determining the success or failure of a particular health program has led more health departments to utilize health educators to prepare their communities for health programs.

Chronic Disease Control. Many public health programs are designed to facilitate the early detection of chronic diseases. Early detection invariably means a better prognosis. Increasingly, health departments have been developing rehabilitation programs in this area, helping people to return to useful and productive lives. Educational efforts in that area are also being accelerated. As stated by Hanlon: "In the final analysis, it may well be that increased public education in these matters would represent the single most important service that may be rendered by public health agencies."[1]

Other Functions

Some local health departments will, in addition, conduct programs related to public health nutrition, dentistry, accident prevention, mental health, rehabilitation, medical care, and research. The activities of health departments have been expanding, making more and better services available to local communities. Closer liaison with state health departments also appears to be developing, with local departments participating in area-wide and even statewide programs.

It has become apparent that health services demanded by the public go far beyond the "basic six" functions of the official health agency. Dr. Luther L. Terry proposed new guidelines for public health which take into account today's economic and political complexities in dealing with health affairs. His *new* "basic six" functions of an official health agency follow.

1. Health maintenance activities for the community and the people in it—against diseases or conditions caused by infectious agents, metabolic changes, genetic factors, emotional disorders, or environmental influences.
2. Continuous assessment of the ecology and resources of the community as they relate to health.
3. Leadership in planning for effective community health services, and participation in providing organized patient care services for both episodic and long-term illness.
4. Study of man's environment and appropriate action to reduce or eliminate hazards to health and to provide safe and pleasant surroundings.
5. Support and conduct research aimed at new health knowledge, and its efficient application to those who can benefit from it.
6. Partnership in policy determination and decision-making so that health is given rightful consideration in all activities of society.[2]

Health Organization at the State Level

The role of state health departments has become an increasingly important one. Their initial functions

[1]John J. Hanlon, *Principles of Public Health Administration* (St. Louis: Mosby, 1964), p. 603.

[2]Luther L. Terry, "The Complex World of Modern Public Health," *American Journal of Public Health* (February 1964), p. 195.

were quite limited, with primary concerns centered on the recording of births and deaths. Through the years the responsibilities of this organization have been considerably expanded. Its programs now include activity in the broad area of environmental health, medical and laboratory services, research, preventive services, supervision of hospitals, nursing homes, and other medical care facilities.

The state health department plays a leadership role as far as the official (local) health agencies in the state are concerned. It generally serves in an advisory capacity and leaves the administration of direct health services to the local health department. It also works to establish full-time local units where they are non-existent. Many times, it is instrumental in coordinating the efforts of several local health departments in the development of an area-wide program. Invariably, where broad-scale health problems (such as water and air pollution) occur the interactions of all the health agencies in a given region are required. The state health agency does in some instances act as a middleman between a Federal agency and a local one where federal assistance is given to local communities. The state health department will also coordinate its efforts with those of the voluntary state agencies when they share common health interests. This can be exemplified by interagency committees on smoking and health. The official agency at the state level can thus serve as the cohesive as well as the stimulating element of health activity in a given state. In addition, it provides financial assistance to supplement the resources of the local health department.

Health Organization at the Federal Level

The Department of Health, Education and Welfare

All of the agencies of the Department of Health, Education and Welfare (HEW) have some health-related responsibilities. The Social Security Administration manages the Old-Age and Survivors and Disability Insurance program as well as the Medicare program. The Office of Education has a division for Drug and Health Education that seeks to stimulate the development of such programs in the schools of the United States. It also provides supportive services for handicapped and deprived children. The Public Health Service has through the years represented *the* federal health agency headed by the Surgeon General. In a reorganization of the Public Health Service in the late 1960's three major components of the Service were developed which consisted of the Health Services and Mental Health Administration, the National Institutes of Health, and the Food and Drug Administration.

The Health Services and Mental Health Administration. This agency concerns itself with programs that involve comprehensive health planning and the development of comprehensive health services. It provides grants to states and to local recipients for these purposes. It also seeks to stimulate research designed to improve the quality and accessibility of health care for all segments of the population. Through the information provided by the National

Health Survey it continually evaluates the health status of the nation.

National Institutes of Health. The NIH supports, through its many thousands of grants, medical research and training for research in over 700 of the nation's schools of medicine, universities, and other research centers, and provides grants for construction and equipping of health research facilities; it carries out an extensive program of direct research in laboratories and clinics at Maryland, and in the field. An added responsibility of the National Institutes of Health is the Bureau of Health Manpower, which promotes the quality and number of professional health personnel. It does this by providing training grants, student assistance, and funding for the construction of educational facilities.

The National Library of Medicine is also a component of the National Institutes of Health. This library has the largest collection of publications of its kind in the world, containing over a million volumes of medical literature. It has combined a computerized storage and retrieval system with photoduplication services as a means of making this giant store of medical information available to other medical libraries.

The Food and Drug Administration is fully described in Chapter 11.

Other Federal Agencies

The *Veterans Administration* is responsible for a medical care program through the utilization of its VA Hospitals and outpatient clinics. The program is basically designed to provide for veterans with illness or disability associated with military service. The VA, however, will also provide medical care for veterans with nonservice illnesses who cannot afford to pay for medical care.

The *Department of Defense* furnishes comprehensive medical care for members of the armed forces and their dependents. The Corps of Engineers also is actively involved in ensuing environmental sanitation in and around military posts.

The *Office of Economic Opportunity* is directly and indirectly involved with matters of health, since poverty contributes to ill health, and vice versa. Many of its community action programs are aimed at meeting health needs.

The *Department of Housing and Urban Development* are responsible for the administration of grants for sewer and water facilities. In so doing, safeguards against the pollution of waterways is required. Grants are also made to finance health and recreation projects as well as other community services.

The *U.S. Department of Agriculture* has several health- (human) related programs. Its programs to eradicate tuberculosis, brucellosis, and other animal diseases also protects the human population. The department's meat inspection program is designed to protect the human population. It has also conducted a nutrition education program aimed at improving health and preventing nutritional deficiency diseases.

The *U.S. Department of the Interior* has within its structure several units with health-related functions. The Federal Water Pollution Control Administration has the powers to enforce federal water pollution laws. The Fish and Wildlife Service conducts programs related to animal-borne diseases. The Bureau of Mines conducts studies on accident prevention and the protection of the health of the miners.

The *Atomic Energy Commission* produces and distributes radioactive materials used in medical research. It has also supported and conducted such research itself.

The large number of federal agencies that have health responsibilities has caused the American Public Health Association to comment as follows:

> No important function of government has been more intentionally fragmented in recent years than has the health function. Federal fragmentation has made more and more difficult the maintenance of effective state and local health programs and departments. Each federal act should be, but rarely is, scrutinized for its effect on administration at the point of impact (usually state or local).

It then recommended,

> A unified health department, responsible and responsive to the entire population of a nation, a state, or a community, discharging agreed-upon governmental health functions, seems to be a reasonable, viable, and desirable proposition.[3]

[3] *The Nation's Health,* The Official Newspaper of the American Public Health Association, April 1972. Editorial by Thomas R. Hood.

The Voluntary Health Organization

The voluntary health agency is one that is supported by public donations raised in fund drives rather than by tax moneys. This kind of health organization is unique to the United States and not found in other countries. Its focus is usually delimited to a specific health problem, as exemplified by the American Cancer Society, the American Heart Association, or the United Cerebral Palsy Association. Voluntary agencies usually start with a few people who draw attention and interest to a particular health problem that might otherwise be overlooked. In the first organizations of this type, they were manned solely by volunteers. Though large numbers of volunteers are still used, these agencies now employ professionals as executive secretaries and in other key positions.

Education, service, and research are viewed as the major functions of voluntary health agencies. Many of their fund-raising activities revolve around making the public aware of a health problem, as well as community and personal actions that will help alleviate it. Year-round educational programs are usually constants with voluntary agencies.

These agencies often serve to supplement the efforts of the official health agencies of the community. Because they have greater flexibility with regard to their use of funds, they can pioneer in demonstration programs and try new approaches to old problems. Many times, when a voluntary organization demonstrates the worth of a new program, it will ask the official health agency to accept responsibility for its continuance. At times, the community's official health agency will lack funds to initiate a project alone. The voluntary health agency may then supplement the resources of the official health agency with its own funds and make the project possible.

These organizations are also active in the support of legislation that is in the interest of the public health. Increasingly, these organizations are becoming more broadly based in their concerns, not hesitating to support broadly-based community health programs in addition to their primary interests in a single area or small grouping of health problems.

Sizable portions of the voluntary agency's income are also contributed to needed research efforts. Noted researchers are often supported by funds from these organizations and serve to supplement the work done by the National Institutes of Health and other research organizations.

Voluntary health organizations, like the official health agencies, have a state organization that advises and coordinates the efforts of its local agencies. Each local agency passes on a percentage of the proceeds of its fund drives to support the operation of the state organization. Every state organization then passes on a percentage of its income to support a national office. Educational materials such as printed materials, films, and other things are developed or purchased by the state office of the voluntary agency and passed on to its local units for use. The state office also sends field consultants to local units to advise the executive-secretary on the development of the local agency's program.

Many of our voluntary health organizations are strong, nationally organized groups making a significant, unique public health contribution. Some examples of these organizations follow:

ALCOHOLICS ANONYMOUS, P. O. Box 459, Grand Central Station, New York, New York. 10017

ALLERGY FOUNDATION OF AMERICA, 801 Second Ave., New York, New York. 10017

AMERICAN ASSOCIATION FOR MATERNAL AND INFANT HEALTH, 116 S. Michigan Avenue, Chicago, Illinois.

AMERICAN CANCER SOCIETY, INC., 219 East 42 Street, New York, New York. 10017

AMERICAN DIABETES ASSOCIATION, INC., 1 East 45th Street, New York, New York.

AMERICAN HEARING SOCIETY, 919 Eighteenth Street, N.W., Washington, D.C.

AMERICAN HEART ASSOCIATION, 44 East 23rd Street, New York, New York. 10010

AMERICAN INSTITUTE OF FAMILY RELATIONS, INC., 5287 Sunset Blvd., Los Angeles, California.

ARTHRITIS AND RHEUMATISM FOUNDATION, 10 Columbus Circle, New York, New York. 10019

EPILEPSY FOUNDATION OF AMERICA, 733 15 Street N.W., Washington, D.C. 20005

MUSCULAR DYSTROPHY ASSOCIATION OF AMERICA, 1790 Broadway, New York, New York. 10019

NATIONAL ASSOCIATION FOR MENTAL HEALTH, 10 Columbus Circle, New York, New York. 10019

THE NATIONAL FOUNDATION, 1275 Mamaroneck Avenue, White Plains, New York. 10605

NATIONAL MULTIPLE SCLEROSIS SOCIETY, 257 Park Avenue South, New York, New York. 10010

NATIONAL SAFETY COUNCIL, 425 N. Michigan Avenue, Chicago, Illinois. 60611

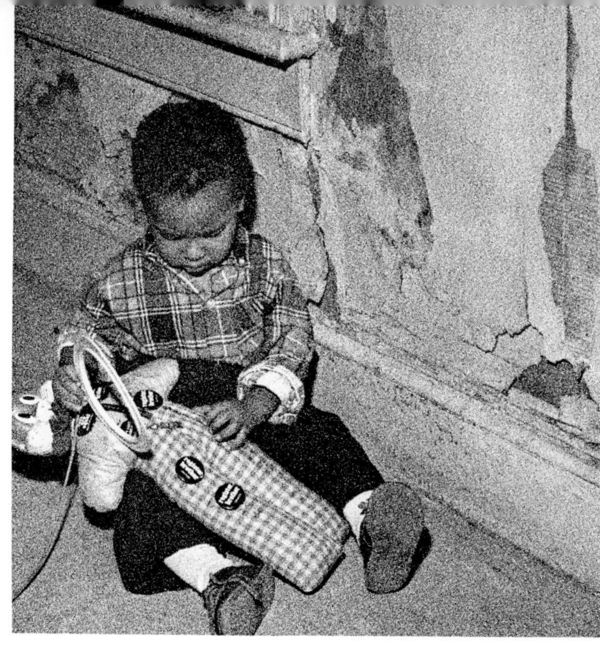

Fig. 15-3. Lead poisoning is an ever-present danger to this child. (N.Y.S. Dept. of Health)

PLANNED PARENTHOOD—WORLD POPULATION, 515 Madison Avenue, New York, New York. 10022

SEX INFORMATION AND EDUCATION COUNCIL OF THE UNITED STATES (SIECUS), 1855 Broadway, New York, New York. 10023

UNITED CEREBRAL PALSY ASSOCIATION, INC., 321 West 44th Street, New York, New York. 10017

The Hospital

The hospital is an integral part of the community's health organization. It has traditionally been viewed as a treatment center, though the activities of the hospital are to a greater extent becoming more concerned with services related to preventive medicine and the promotion of public health. Some hospitals have experimented with the use of the emergency ward as a springboard for preventive procedures. A person arriving with a badly cut hand may not only have the wound attended to, but have the readily available drops of blood tested for diabetes or anemia; the smoker may be advised to "kick the habit," and some vision testing may be thrown in for good measure before the patient is released. Two New York City hospitals routinely administered the Papanicolaou test (see Chap. 10) for cervical cancer to women admitted to the hospital for a variety of other reasons. In a matter of a few years, over 300 cases of cervical cancer were detected early enough to save the lives of the women involved.

A number of hospitals, as part of their new preventive role, are developing cooperative activities with school health education programs. The health professionals of the hospital participate in teacher training workshops. In addition, the hospitals have also provided field work experiences for the high school student. The student is involved in a variety of helpful roles, from reading to patients to conducting lead poisoning surveys in the community. These hospital-school interactions have not only added relevance to health education programs but have been helpful to the hospitals as well through the appropriate use of student manpower.

The United States Hospital and Medical Facilities Survey and Construction Act (Hill-Burton) of 1947 has stimulated construction toward the development of regional hospital systems. At the center of such a system is a hospital affiliated with a medical school. Smaller satellite hospitals service the outlying areas of the region. The purpose is to provide the most adequate medical care facilities possible in a given region.

This federal legislation is also subsidizing the remodernization of many of the older hospitals in the country located in the urban areas. Its initial efforts were directed toward the development of hospital facilities in rural areas where they were lacking. In addition, the Hill-Burton legislation provides funds for hospital research and demonstration programs. These activities are directed toward the development of improved patient care and more efficient hospital administration and operation.

The School

The school is not often thought of as a health organization. It can, however, make a substantial contri-

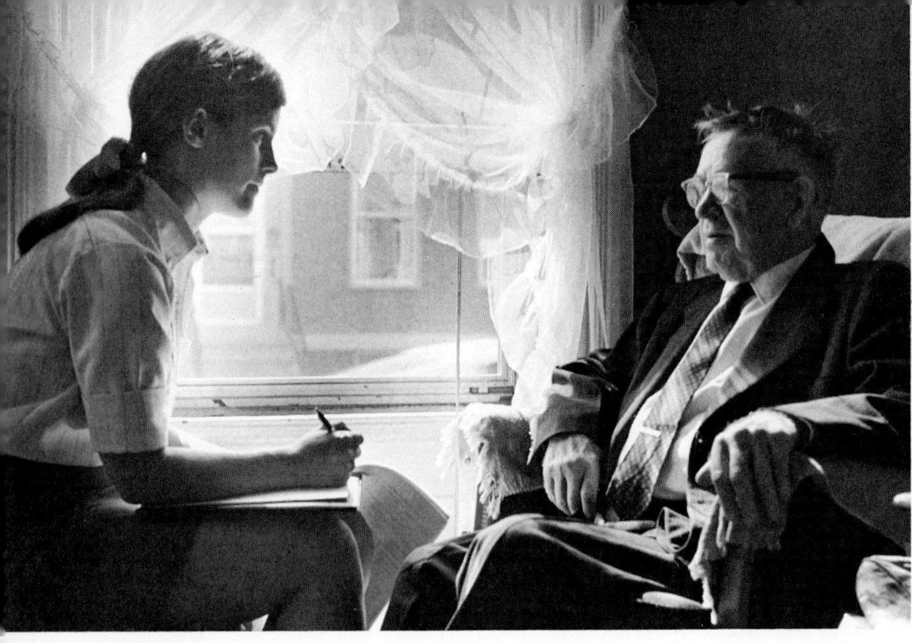

Fig. 15-4. A student conducting a survey as part of her public health field-work experience. (N.Y.S. Dept. of Health)

bution in this area with its programs of health education. Any educational institution concerned with the study of man, his environment, and his interactions with it would be remiss to exclude so vital an area as the health sciences from its curriculum.

Because many patterns of health behavior are best initiated at an early age, the school has unusual opportunities to influence young peoples' health values at a most receptive time. The quality of school health education programs can determine the levels of health information in a community and its willingness to undertake needed public health measures. Public health programs can be best initiated with the consent and support of the citizenry in a democratic society. In order that such decisions be properly based, a health-informed public is essential. A cultural lag in this area can be literally incapacitating to a community.

Health education is more than the more dissemination of knowledge. It also involves the development of values and even a life-style. Confining this kind of instruction within the four walls of a classroom immediately restricts its effectiveness. Intellectualizing about health information in a classroom accomplishes limited objectives. If we are to realize the real goals of health education we must increasingly make this form of education experientially based. Health education in schools ideally should become an inherent part of public health programs, with the student actively engaged in various field work experiences. If there is to be classroom discussion, let it consist of strategy meetings on what is to happen in the community and on how to effect the needed reforms in conducting our human health affairs.

Student involvement in the learning process should be all that phrase implies. Some high schools in the country are already planning public health field work experiences for their health education students instead of requiring a term paper. The reports they will be responsible for will be based on their actual experience. Students from a New York City school, for example, in cooperation with personnel from a local hospital, conducted a survey of 1,500 homes in an effort to detect cases of lead poisoning. The students *did* turn up 20 cases of lead poisoning, to the delight of their health colleagues at the hospital. The students in turn had the satisfaction of knowing that they helped to save 20 lives as well as to inform 1,500 families on the hazards of lead poisoning. (The latter is better than any letter grade a student can receive.) As part of their health education program in another high school, students are working in a program for mentally retarded patients in a nearby hospital. What better way for young people to understand the problems related to retardation and what better way of overcoming the unfortunate stigmas too often associated with these conditions. Many examples of school-community interaction are now evident as more complete approaches to our health problems and issues are sought. The community is the laboratory of the health sciences. If the education program of the school is to be effective, it needs to have access to that laboratory. It is also time that we ring an end to the "amateur hour" role of the school, by profes-

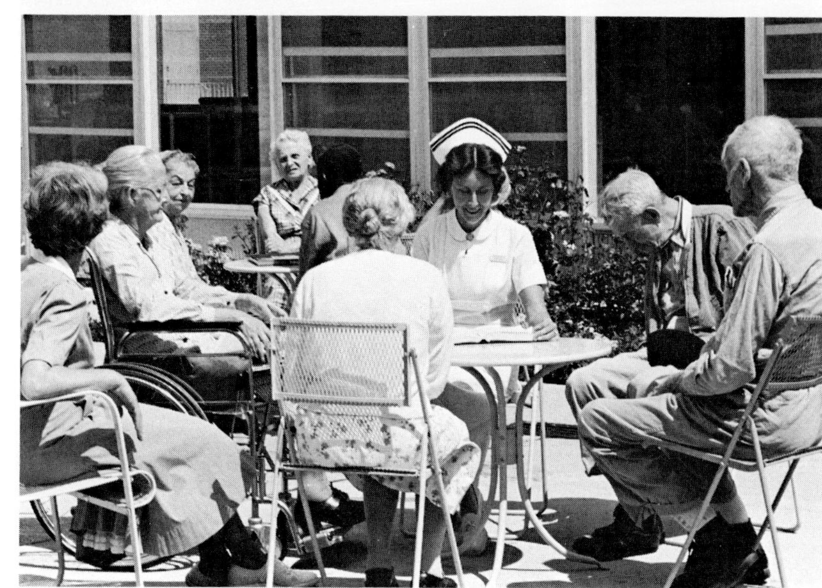

Fig. 15-5. Those in nursing homes do not need the elaborate care of a hospital. Here an elderly group spends a pleasant afternoon listening to a reading. (N.Y.S. Dept. of Mental Hygiene; Photo by Julian A. Belin)

sionalizing its role in conducting our societal health affairs. This means that boards of education need to provide appropriate curriculum time and trained teacher personnel to carry out meaningful programs.

One important objective of a health education program is to bring some objectivity into the health classroom. We need to get away from the traditional format of the teacher *telling* the students the do's and don'ts of how to be healthy and lead the good life. Rather, the students need to be involved in the learning process, not only for the purpose of coming to his own conclusions and making his own decisions, but also to add his own constructive efforts to the resolution of societal health problems.

Nursing Homes

The nursing home is rapidly becoming established as a necessary community health facility. It serves to care for people who do not need the elaborate services of the hospital, but are not quite ready to return home. These are often persons who have chronic diseases, are convalescing, or need long-term care for a variety of reasons. An advantage of the nursing home is that it provides the services needed for selected patients and is usually much less expensive than the hospital. Our nursing homes are populated mostly by the elderly, since the major chronic diseases affect them more heavily.

Though the caliber of the nursing home has been upgraded, the abuses, impatience, and despair prevalent in nursing homes has been well documented. The boom of the nursing home business brought with it many unscrupulous people. Privately owned, profit-making institutions were more often concerned with profit than the social, emotional, or physical welfare of its charges. In some cases they were being administered by businessmen whose training and qualifications were questionable. Legislation now requires the licensing of administrators of nursing homes, though owners of these institutions still need to meet no standards in education, training, or experience. The need for qualified personnel from the top administrator to the lowly aide has become critical. A beautiful new brick building "staffed by surly aides and minimally competent nurses is not much good."[4] An unprecedented effort to upgrade the services in some nursing homes must be attempted.

Initially the federal government became involved with nursing homes in 1960 when the Kerr-Mills Act went into effect allowing assistance payments for care in nursing homes. The federal government felt, however, that since Medicaid was to be administered by the states, it was their responsibility to establish standards of quality.

By 1967, however, following the hearings by the Senate Committee on Aging that revealed the inadequacy of state licensing standards, Congressional concern arose over the quality of nursing home care. Senators Frank Moss of Utah, Edward Kennedy of Massachusetts, and others, recognized the need for federal standards to up-

[4]The Nader Report, *Old Age—The Last Segregation*, Claire Townsend, Project Director (New York: Grossman Publishers, 1971).

grade the nursing homes receiving Federal funds under Medicaid.[5]

In July 1972, the Department of Health, Education and Welfare's Office of Nursing Home Affairs announced the de-certification of 579 Medicaid nursing homes and that federal funds would be withheld from these substandard institutions. In addition, of the "7,000 facilities, 4,766 were issued six-month certificates which will be renewed only after less serious deficiencies are corrected."[6] It was further declared that the National Council of Senior Citizens would set up ombudsman programs to assess complaints about nursing home care.[7] The development of these protective standards continue to guide many nursing homes to upgrade their services and facilities from recognized inadequate levels. It is unfortunate, however, that the governmental wheels of progress can only be set into motion *after* much suffering has been proven.

Humanizing Health Care

Some new concepts in medical care delivery have evolved in the last decade. The dire health needs of the indigent have heretofore been inadequately served by present health department and hospital facilities. The long lines at hospital clinics and the great distances the rural poor must travel in order to get medical care have been discouraging. The impersonal handling of patients oftentimes reflects a lack of "Establishment" acceptance of minority groups. In response, there has been a developing movement to establish health care facilities that are neighborhood or community oriented. They have involved people from the community as members of governing councils and boards. This has represented a "reaching-out"—in essence the provision of health services where the people are. In some instances, however, where militant neighborhood groups have decided to have a dominating voice in the management of the health care facilities without the professional expertise that is essential, programs have failed. Where health professionals *and* neighborhood groups have worked together in developing policy and program, the chances of success have been greatly increased. Where they have been successful, these health care facilities or clinics

have gained a wide popularity by respecting the needs and the imperfect humanity of their patients. They have revitalized the doctor-patient relationship and shown its relevance in modern, computerized medicine. They have demonstrated the desirability and practicality of minimizing red tape in dealing with people. They have pioneered the use of paramedical volunteers and staff workers in a country faced with a severe shortage of doctors and professional personnel.[8]

[5]Ibid., p. 51.

[6]Washington Report on Medicine and Health, July 24, 1972, No. 1308.

[7]National Council of Senior Citizens, 1627 K Street N.W., Washington, D.C. 20006.

[8]David E. Smith, M.D., and John Luce, *Love Needs Care* (Boston: Little, Brown, 1971), p. 370.

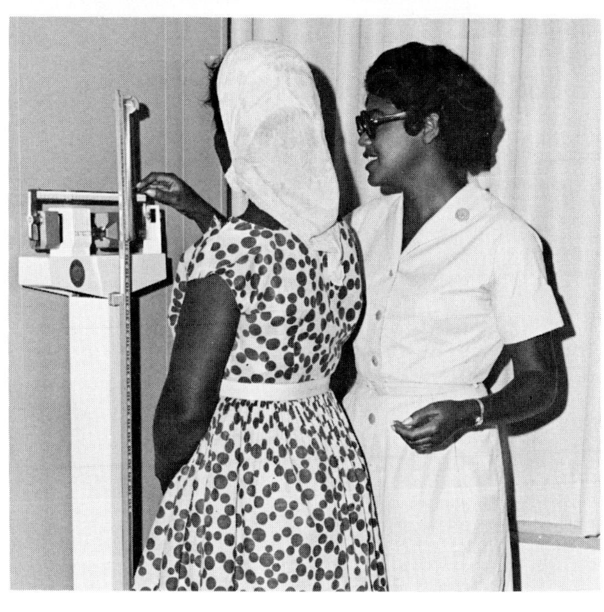

Fig. 15-6. The paraprofessional helping out in a neighborhood health center. (N.Y.S. Dept. of Health)

At the same time they can be expected to catch the wrath of those who abhor the imperfect humanity of their patients, who are threatened by changes in a paternalistic doctor-patient relationship, who are more obsessed with bureaucratic procedure than people, who see security in the shortage of doctors and health personnel, and who see paramedical volunteers as invaders of their professional turf.

The forms that these health care facilities have taken vary considerably, depending on the community being served. The Whitney M. Young, Jr., Community Health Center is funded by the United States Office of Economic Opportunity, and policy for the center is determined jointly with a nearby medical center and an advisory council. This neighborhood health center is able to offer continuous family-oriented care, which is often more personalized than clinic situations at hospitals. Patients seeking treatment are assigned a nurse who remains with that patient for the length of the treatment. The patient may also request the same physician at each of the health center visits. In this way, some physician-patient rapport may be established. Although the health care involves emergency treatment as well as health-related services, a concern for preventive medicine is also apparent. Lead poisoning and sickle-cell anemia detection, as well as nutrition education, obstetric, and pediatric care, are such preventive areas. Paraprofessionals from the community have been trained at the Center to follow up patients who have missed or canceled appointments or have no phone or other means of communicating with the Center. A listing of local pharmacists who agree to charge fixed fees for medications is available to the patient who must be medicaid-eligible in order to be a regular member of the Health Center.

Another neighborhood health center located on New York City's lower East side is the NENA (Northeast Neighborhood Association) Health Center. The structure of this center varies somewhat from the first in that it is a much larger operation employing over 100 persons and handling approximately 12,000 registered patients. Its community is an integrated one where economic levels vary and where many ethnic groups are represented. The large numbers of elderly people living alone and the young Spanish-speaking families with many children tend to require special consideration in this neighborhood, where the median income is the lowest in New York City. Policy for the center is determined by a Health Council whose members must be residents of the area served. The concept exemplified here is that the consumer must participate in determining health policy while he remains accountable to his "neighbors."

In the late 1960's, when the Haight-Ashbury drug scene was at its height, there was a critical need for an on-the-spot medical facility which was available 24 hours a day; a place where drug abusers could be treated for acute drug crises, detoxified, and counseled and where education about drugs, nutrition, and proper hygiene could take place. The emergence of the Free Clinic in this section of San Francisco was fashioned somewhat after the Watts Clinic, which began providing medical care for the poverty-stricken of that area after the riots of 1965. The infectious diseases ran rampant in the young people of the Haight-Ashbury district who were generally weakened from poor eating and hygienic habits. A variety of dental problems and parasitic infestations flourished, to say nothing of the incidence of venereal diseases, hepatitis, and skin disorders. Dr. David E. Smith, founder of the Haight-Ashbury Free Clinic, envisioned the clinic as a new medicine and health-care delivery system that was urgently needed in this country. During the year 1968, 20,000 people were treated at the Clinics Medical Section. For these many thousands, the clinic was their only source of medication, treatment and health education. As stated by Dr. Smith and John Luce:

> the free clinics have proven their ability to reach alienated economic, racial and philosophic minorities. They have advanced the goals of community medicine by seeking out patients in their own environment and by regarding the environment as an organism capable of being healed. They have provided an outlet for idealism and social frustration. And they have served as a conscience for the country.[9]

Presently there are over 200 free clinics in the United States with 1 to 2 million patient visits yearly, at an average cost of $2 per visit.

The health needs that free clinics meet are obvious. In a pluralistic society, facets of the health care delivery system must be flexible enough to meet the varying health care needs unique to a particular community.

[9]Ibid, p. 370.

Health Careers and the Expanding Health Industry

The expanding activities of the public health professions have been necessitated by a number of factors. They have been attempting to find applications for pyramiding research findings, as well as to disseminate health information developed from these sources. In addition, they have been responding to changes and dangers affecting our environment (pollution, radiation, proliferate use of drugs) in our advancing technology. They have also heard the public demand for more and better health services by a growing population. The entire field of public health is in an era of rapid change and advancement. The expansion and development of its programs are to a great extent being delimited by the numbers of available health personnel. The current critical shortage of health professionals represents a major stumbling block to the attainment of desired public health goals.

To ease this personnel shortage, the United States Public Health Service has made available traineeships through Schools of Public Health. These public health traineeships will not only cover the educational costs of recipients but will provide a sizable monthly subsistence allowance as well. The program has been effective in attracting people to the public health professions. These have included students who had not as yet decided on a career, and personnel from other professions. There are over 200 possible health careers for individuals interested in providing services that will promote the health of

Fig. 15-7. Health careers chart. (*U.S. Dept. of Labor*)

This calendar gives you a quick check on how many years of education, after high school, you should count on for the representative health occupations listed here: The lines and symbols show what is customary—some people take only minimum required training; many take more.

• *This kind of work requires no special training beyond what you can usually get in high school.*

•--- *After starting, you serve an apprenticeship or get similar organized on-the-job training.*

—— *Lines and symbols used with them indicate full years. To start requires special training either in college, in a hospital or special school, or in a professional school after 1–4 years of college.*

▬═ *Special training is required, but you have a choice, each type of training taking a different number of years.*

□ *First symbol means you can get beginner's job after college, but will usually need more study, as well as experience, for advancement. Graduate training ordinarily goes to or beyond master's or doctor's degree.*

⟶ *Your planning should look beyond minimum requirements; continuing study, after entering professional practice, is important to further advancement.*

○ *Though the line shows the minimum to qualify, more pre-professional years in college often lengthen the training time.*

(9m) *Special course or on-the-job training is shown in number of months.*

This calendar pictures training information in condensed timetable form. To get a more detailed picture . . . read *the Health Careers Guidebook Briefings . . .* consult *your school advisers for information and personal guidance on training.*

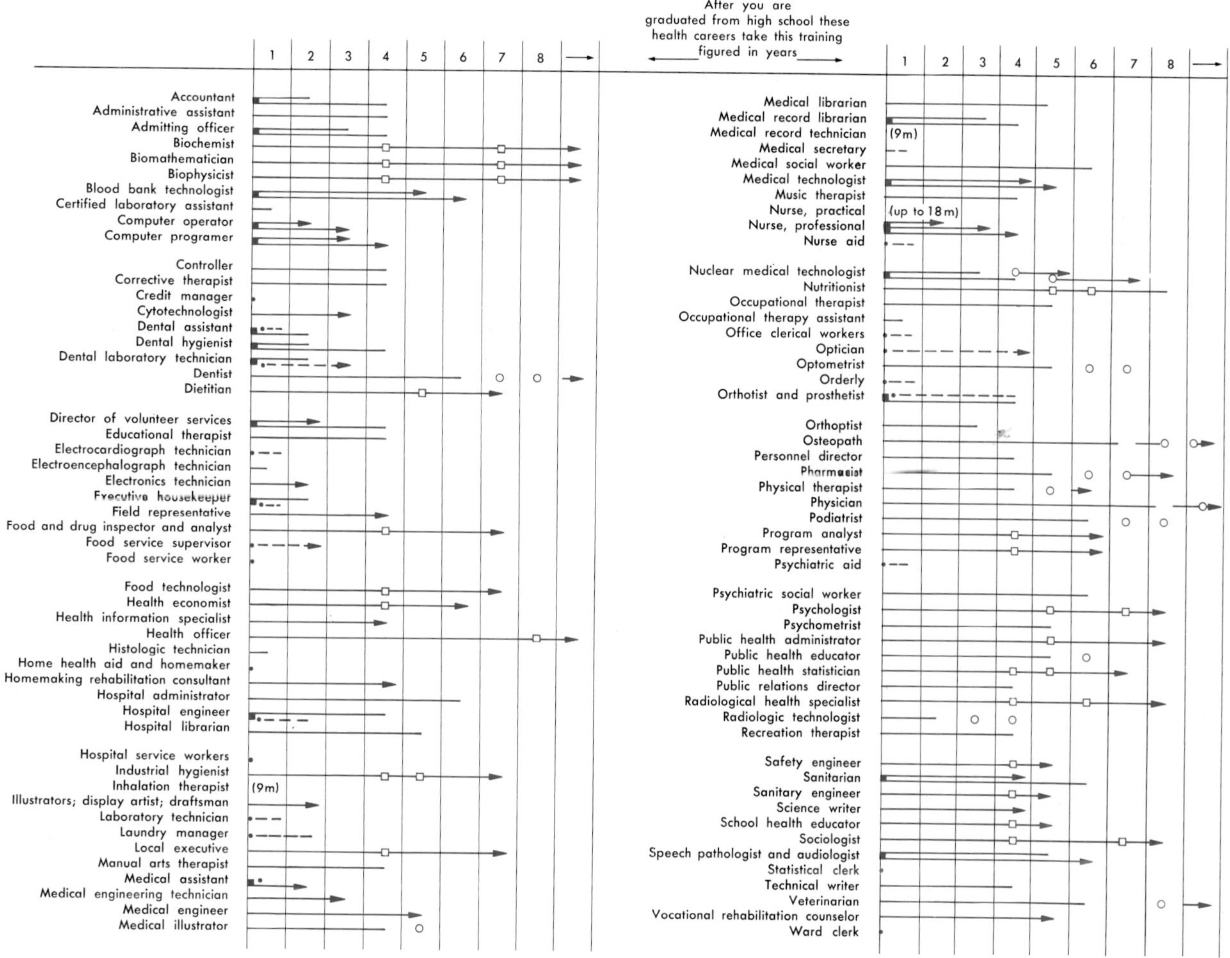

peoples and communities. Financial remuneration in this developing health industry is also competitive.

Review Questions

1. Why are public health organizations necessary to maintain acceptable levels of community health?
2. What are the major functions of the local health department? In what ways is redirection of these functions being suggested?
3. Why do voluntary health organizations have greater flexibility in their mode of operation? What has been the nature of their contribution?
4. How is the role of the hospital changing from that of serving solely as a treatment center?
5. What has been the contribution of the United States Hospital and Medical Facilities Survey and Construction Act (Hill-Burton)?
6. What are the medical care functions of the nursing home?
7. How are some of the early abuses occurring in nursing homes being overcome?
8. What is the role of the state health department?
9. What contributions can the school make in the health area?
10. What factors have contributed to the expanding activities of the health professions?
11. In order to relieve the critical shortage of health personnel, what program has been instituted by the Public Health Service?
12. How is the free clinic movement fulfilling unmet health needs?
13. How are the free clinics and some neighborhood health centers changing health care delivery?

Chapter 16
Global Health: Its Implications

We are living in a rapidly shrinking world where air travel has made all parts of the world accessible within a matter of hours. There are developing political, social, and economic ties with countries in "remote" regions of the world. It is also perceptibly clear that health is a basic factor in the political and economic climates of nations. When large percentages of people in some of the underdeveloped countries are incapacitated by disease, the productivity of those countries is seriously hampered. The startling fact that half the people of the world suffer from chronic diseases that modern medicine has the knowledge and skills to correct, gives an indication of the scope of the problem. Where there exist pockets of disease, such as smallpox and cholera, we now face the reality that these sources of infection are not in some inaccessible region of the world, but perhaps hours away.

Our interests in world health, while many times sparked by humanitarian motivations, are also stimulated by political and economic concerns, as well as by the need to safeguard our own health. The laudable spirit of an Albert Schweitzer will no doubt continue to influence our thinking and actions in this respect. However, being our "brother's keeper" in health matters will increasingly become a necessity rather than an altruistic nicety.

To illustrate the point, in the spring of 1972, a 36-year-old Moslem returned home to Yugoslavia from a pilgrimage to Mecca and Medina. On the way home he stopped off in Baghdad to buy gifts for his family. Two weeks later his 12-year-old daughter entered the hospital with what was thought to be chickenpox, since it had been 40 years since anyone in Yugoslavia had suffered smallpox. Later, a neighbor was admitted to a hospital with this rare disease. This patient was transferred to another hospital—infecting patients and hospital staff along the way. He died of smallpox in Belgrade. The next victim was a 19-year-old nurse who attended him. In short, a month after the Moslem returned from his pilgrimage, 75 cases of smallpox were recorded in Belgrade and 8 people had died. In a similar fashion the smallpox epidemic in Bangladesh was reportedly brought by Hindu refugees returning from India. The situation there was far more serious than in Belgrade and epidemiologists reported more than 2,500 cases of the disease and 700 deaths. Only swift preventive measures stopped these epidemics from being worse. The mass media issued public warnings to people to seek protection through vaccination. The eradication of smallpox became a possibility when Edward Jenner first developed his vaccine 150 years ago. Our shrinking world makes complete worldwide eradication of smallpox not an idealistic goal, but a necessary public health measure.

A further implication of global health is an economic one. Poverty-stricken areas of the world are caught in a kind of low-spiraling economic cycle. Their low production of goods and services result in sublevel incomes. This in turn causes the group to lack proper housing, education, and nutrition. These substandard living conditions produce a higher incidence of disease and decreased human energy, resulting in a low production of goods and services, whereupon the cycle starts all over again.

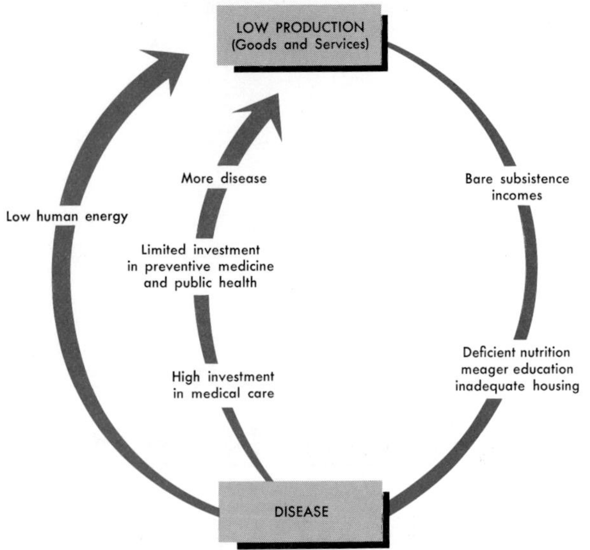

Fig. 16-1. The revolving door of poverty. (Pan American Health Organization)

Fig. 16-2. Comparison of health problems in highly developed and underdeveloped countries of the world. (Modified from WHO chart, "Health Teams Face Different Tasks")

The development of higher levels of health could do a great deal to break this cycle. Improved health status must be a part of a changed pattern of living if poverty is to be avoided and its revolving-door pattern broken.

Some World Health Problems

The health problems of the more developed countries of the world increasingly parallel those of the United States—heart disease, cancer, venereal diseases, problems of the aging, environmental pollution, automobile safety, and many others. It is not unusual to read of automobile pollution problems in Rome, or the traffic accident as a "man-made epidemic" in Buenos Aires. It is interesting to read of some solutions on aging from countries like England, Denmark, and Sweden. They are reportedly dealing with their aging population somewhat more successfully than we have done in the United States. These three countries emphasize preventive medicine and home care rather than institutionalizing or segregating old people in nursing homes.

"A backward nation to me is an area in which there are major sociological and cultural reasons which prevent the widest possible application of existing biological knowledge; New York City is a backward nation."[1] The failure to act because of ignorance is understandable. The failure to act in the health area in the presence of existing knowledge is tinged with immorality.

As political barriers began to fall in the early part of this decade, medical and health news from China and Russia began to be exchanged and explored. There developed widespread interest in acupuncture, a Chinese form of anesthesia. American physicians observed the technique of inserting long, sterile, stainless steel needles into parts of the body far removed from the site of surgery, and finally witnessed surgery under this method of acupuncture anesthesia. The increased interest in acupuncture precipitated a statement from the New York State Medical Board, which plays a key role in regulating (i.e. examining and licensing) the practice of medicine in New York. The statement read,

> The Board recognizes the need for, and desires to encourage, further research in the techniques, mechanisms of action, and uses of acupuncture. However, because acupuncture is considered at this time strictly as an investigational procedure, it should be performed only in medical centers and teaching hospitals having committees on human research, which will provide the necessary peer review of protocols and appropriate monitoring of such studies.[2]

Whether the use of needles will become a part of standard anesthetic practice in America remains to be seen. Considerable experimental data is being gathered so that a scientific judgment can be made. It is felt that if acupuncture is successful, it will be a panacea for those people in chronic pain who to date have no other means of treatment available. In addition, a great deal of surgery for older patients with cardiac and/or

[1] George James, M.D., M.P.H., *Human Potential in a Dynamic Environment*, School Health Education Study.

[2] "New York State Medical Board Adopts Position on Acupuncture," News Release, July 26, 1972.

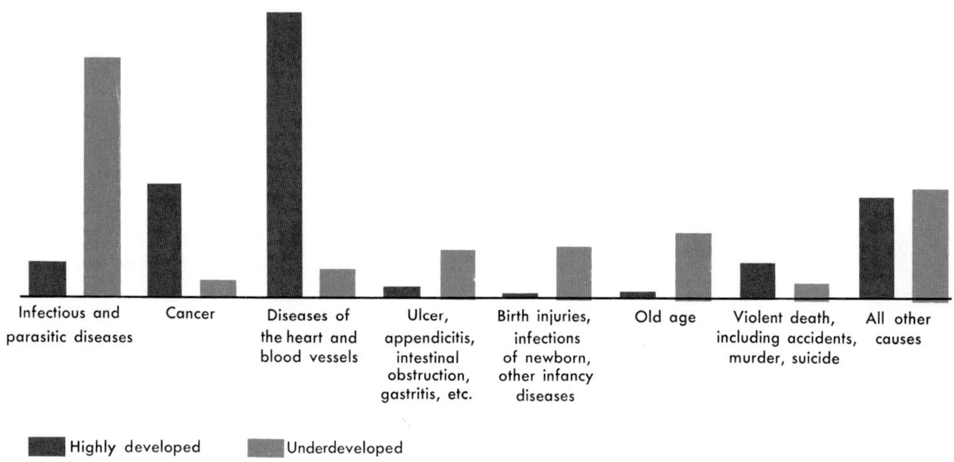

respiratory problems might be more safely carried out, since surgery for these patients presently is very risky with conventional anesthetic means.

The overall Chinese health care system has revealed that great strides have been made in some areas. For example:

- VD, which affected tens of millions, has been almost totally eliminated in most parts of China. In a few areas where sexual promiscuity is traditional, VD has been brought under control and is expected to disappear in the next generation;
- Drug addiction, rampant since the introduction of opium into China by foreign traders in the mid-19th century, has been wiped out. This was done in less than

Fig. 16-3. left: *Graph on reported syphilis;* right: *graph on reported gonorrhea.* (*World Health Organization*)

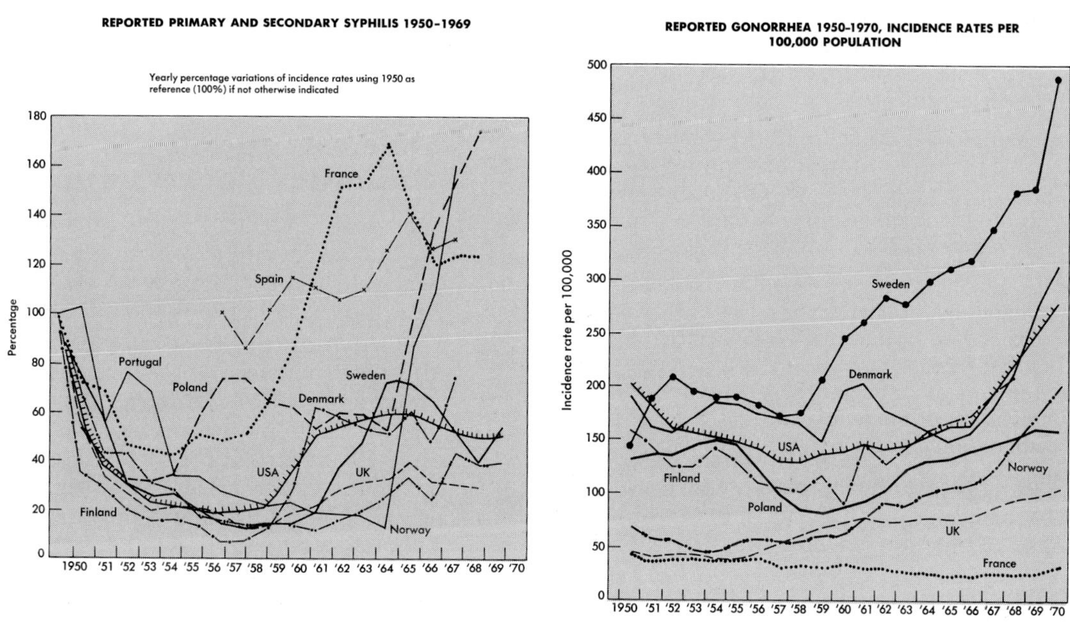

Fig. 16-4. *Severe malnutrition (shown in photo at left) of a two-year-old girl living in Venezuela's Trujillo State, Andes. At right, the same girl is shown ten months later, after supplementary feeding in the WHO rehabilitation center where nutrition education was given to the mother.* (World Health Organization)

five years, by public education, stiff legal penalties for those selling drugs (but not for users), and medical care for the addicted;

- Childhood diseases, such as diphtheria, have come under control through innoculation programs. Immunization against poliomyelitis and measles is also universal, and the number of cases has become insignificant;
- Public education in sanitation, its implementation in city neighborhoods and on agricultural communes by "health activist" residents, guided by sanitarians, has resulted in a very substantial reduction in parasitic diseases that were endemic in the past. Schistosomiasis, which as late as 1955 still afflicted many millions in river delta and swampy areas, has largely been brought under control;
- Emphasis has shifted from the curative aspect of medicine to the preventive. Checkups are on a regular basis, and people are urged to visit health clinics—located in the neighborhoods where they live, in factories, and on farms—as soon as they feel ill;
- Comprehensive care—medical, surgical, and dental, including hospitalization—has been instituted. It is either free or covered by cooperative plans that cost a few tenths of a per cent of an average income. Half the cost of drugs and hospitalization for nonworking members of the family must be paid, but it only costs about 50 cents a day.[3]

In Russia, cardiovascular disease research has been given high priority. At the S. L. Miasnikov Institute of Cardiology in Moscow, Russian scientists are exploring methods of prevention, diagnosis, and treatment of heart disease. The realization that education plays an important role in modifying the risk factors can be seen in Russia, where classes in exercise are encouraged; in Finland, where efforts to modify eating habits are in progress; and in England, where antismoking clinics are held. The risk factors have been identified, and the challenge to halt the coronary epidemic by modifying these factors is echoing the world over. The United States and Russia entered a Joint Agreement on Health Cooperation in 1972, which has resulted in a rich exchange of information, initially on heart disease and cancer but ultimately to extend to other areas of health as well.

Diseases Found in Underdeveloped Countries

The health problems of the underdeveloped nations of the world differ from those of the more highly technological societies. A review of the more prevalent disease conditions include the following.

Kwashiorkor (kwash-ee-or-kor) is the leading dietary deficiency disease in the world. The children in underdeveloped regions of the world are predominantly its victims because of a lack of protein in the diet. Characteristics of the disease include a swollen abdomen, thin arms and legs, stunted growth, streaks of patchy, reddish hair, and discolored patches of skin. General weakness and death often follow. The condition was studied in Africa by a group from the World Health Organization in 1949. Subsequent

[3] *The Nation's Health*, June–July 1972.

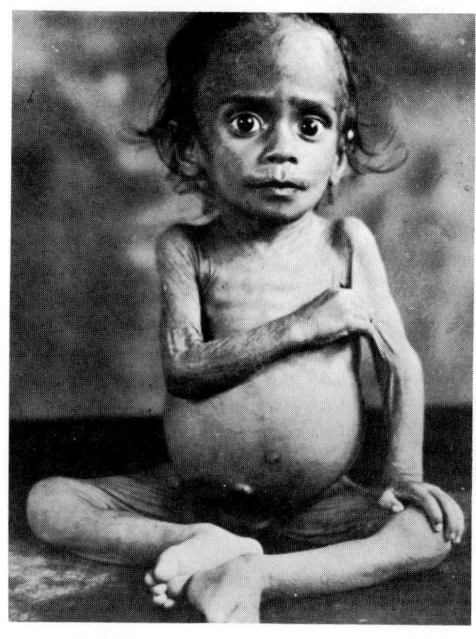
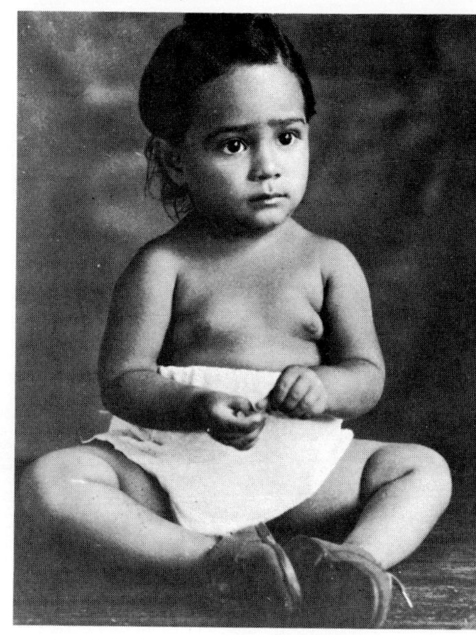

study showed the condition to be widespread in Asia and Central America as well.

Young children are particularly hard hit by the disease. They thrive well during their first year of life while they are being breast fed. Afterwards, they are given a diet rich in starch but deficient in protein. The child is particularly affected because he is in a period of rapid growth requiring a protein-rich diet. The adult is not as severely affected by the protein-poor diet because he has attained full growth. Kwashiorkor in the child ensues. It has been the cause of death of untold thousands of children around the world. A nutrition survey among a Zulu tribe in Africa showed that seven out of ten schoolboys lacked proteins. Any protein-rich food can quickly correct the deficiency. Skim milk and peanuts are commonly used for this purpose. It is interesting to note that a liquid dietetic food that is rich in protein has been successfully used in correcting kwashiorkor. As stated by Dr. John Miller, a missionary physician directing medical work in Africa: "I wish the people who make Metrecal could only see what their product does for starving babies with kwashiorkor. Children who have long since lost all interest in food beg for it."[4] Educational programs are now being conducted to make mothers aware of the cause of the condition. Attempts are being made to teach these people to grow protein-rich plant foods and to produce other sources of protein, such as cattle and milk. One of the real difficulties in reducing the incidence of kwashiorkor is that people like to cling to old, misconceived ideas about nutrition. In some areas, for instance, mothers refuse to give their children animal milk because they believe it is not good for them. In other places where fish, a good source of protein is plentiful, it is considered an acceptable adult food but unsuitable for children. The problem, therefore, is not always the lack of a source of proteins, but the difficult matter of changing old ways and ideas. In most instances, however, the gigantic job is that of increasing sources of protein foods to a level that will properly sustain a major portion of the world's population.

[4]Peter Wyden, *The Overweight Society* (New York: Pocket Books Cardinal Edition, 1966), p. 44.

Schistosomiasis (or Bilharziasis), or snail fever, has plagued man for thousands of years. Egyptian medical papyri refer to remedies for the disease as far back as 3000 B.C. It is recognized as the greatest unconquered parasitic disease afflicting more than 200 million people. In terms of its debilitating effects it ranks close to malaria. The disease is characterized by skin rash, headache, loss of appetite, nausea, fever, blood in the urine, and difficulty in breathing. In the chronic cases, there is liver damage, an enlarged spleen, a bloated abdomen, and an emaciated body. Treatment for the disease is far from satisfactory, since the drugs available are toxic and take several days or weeks to administer. The cause of the difficulty is a schistosome, a small worm whose life cycle involves both man and snail. To date, scientists have not found a weak link in the life cycle to effect a means of eradicating the schistosome. Scientists endeavoring to use chemical means to destroy the snail are discouraged by the high costs

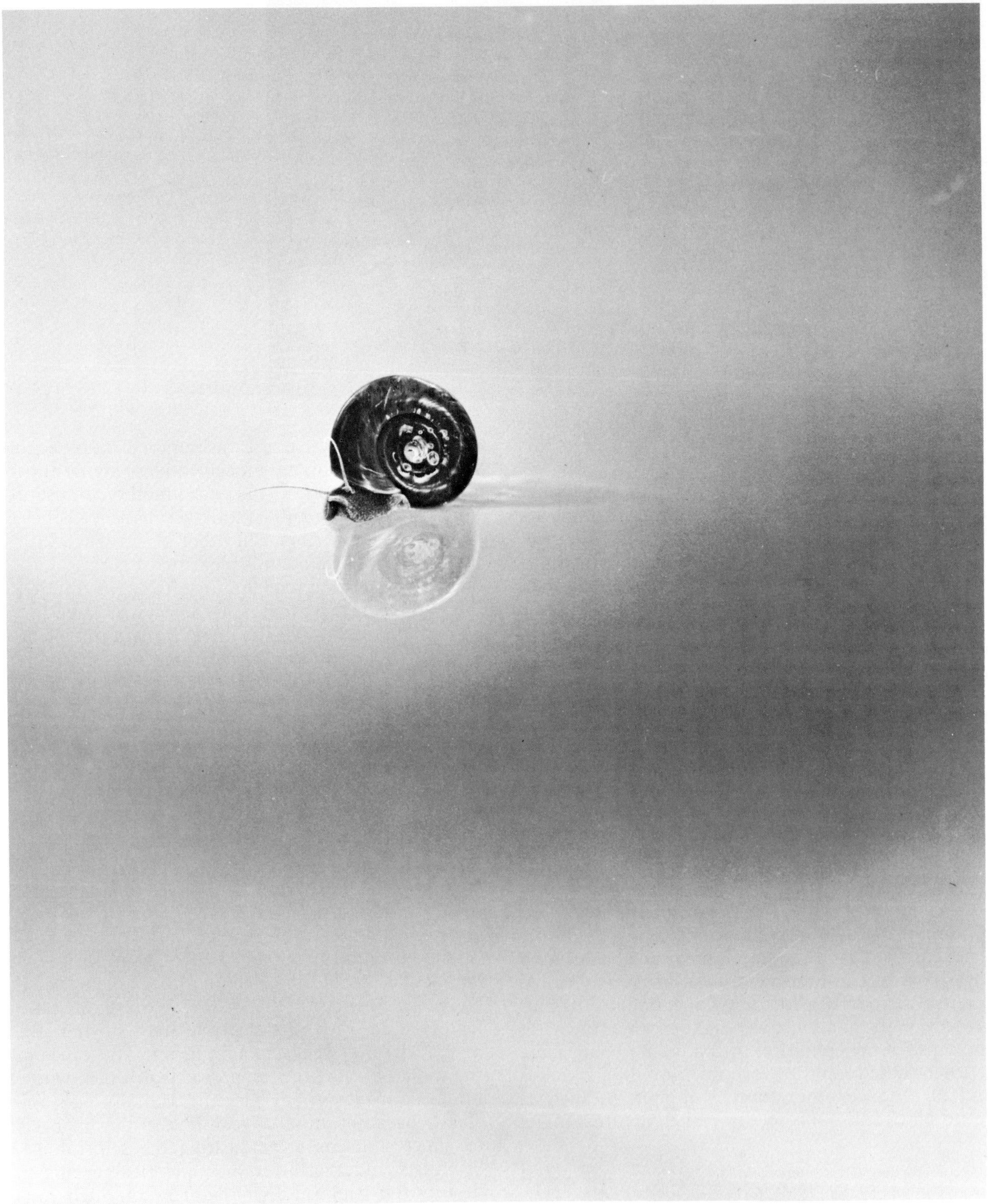

Fig. 16-5. This snail acts as the intermediate host for the tiny schistosome worm. Eggs of the worm given off in the wastes of the infected human hatch in water into embryo form and enter the snail's body. There they multiply and develop into swimming larvae forms. (Used by permission of Parke-Davis)

Fig. 16-6. The larvae forms of the schistosome worms swimming freely in water can infect man by penetrating his skin and migrating to his circulatory system. This farmer is thus exposing himself to the disease. (World Health Organization—Robert Miller)

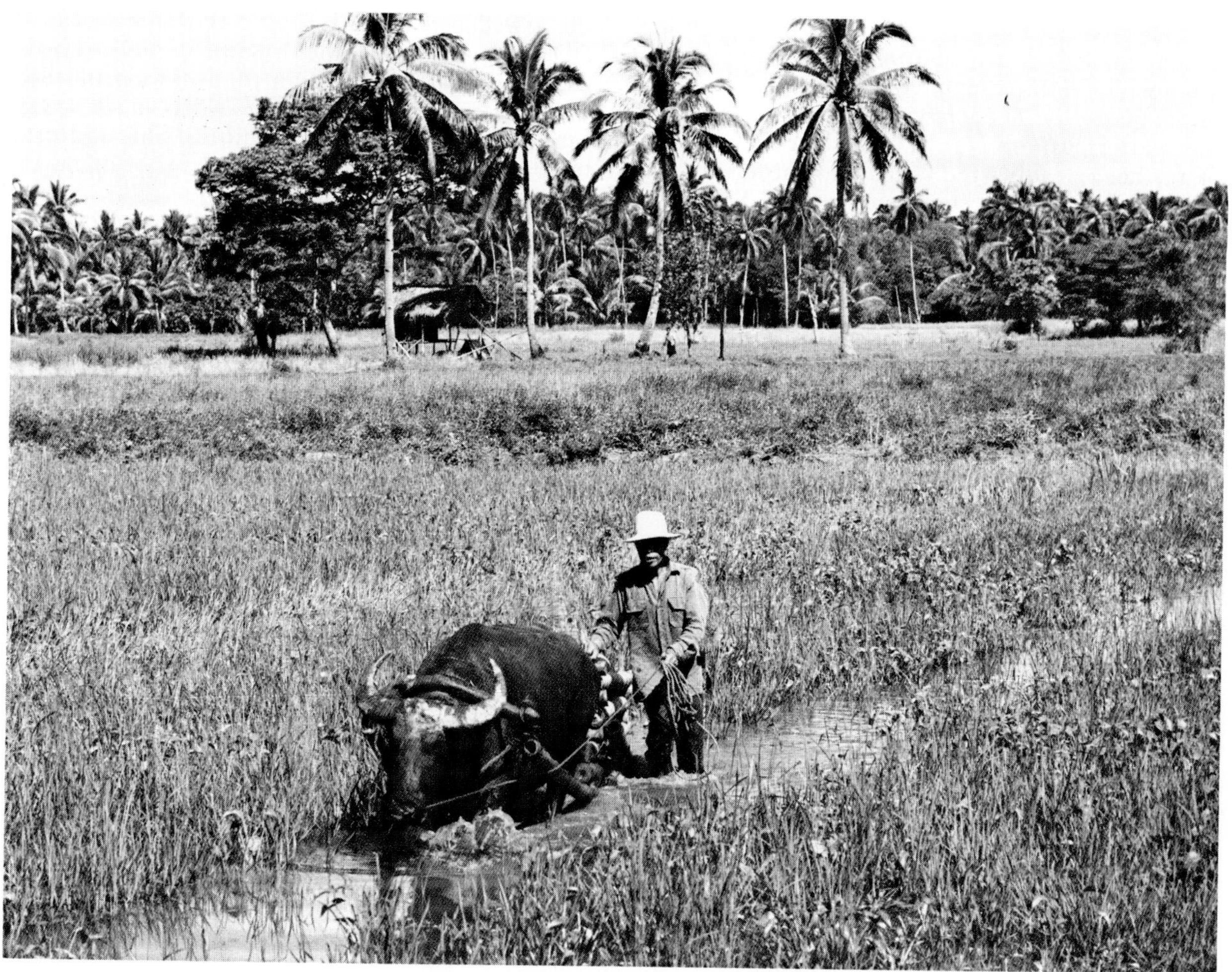

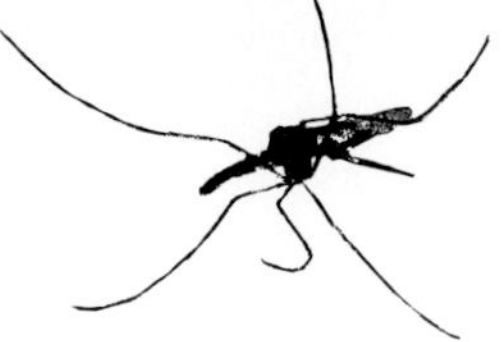
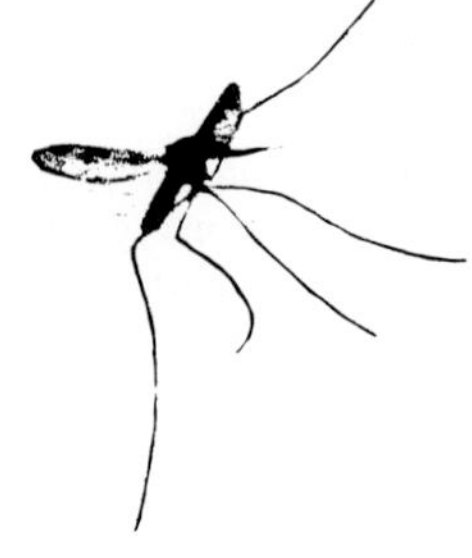
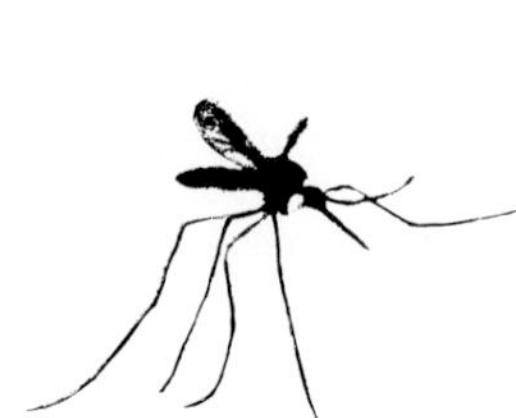

Fig. 16-7. Female anopheles mosquito. (National Institutes of Health—Vernon E. Taylor)

and loss of other forms of aquatic life resulting from this method. Biological control is also being investigated with the introduction of the snail-eating larvae of the marsh fly. These larvae seek and destroy only the snail. Irrigation projects have served as a means of further spreading the snails and the disease, so that the incidence is considered to be 50 per cent higher in areas where water improvement projects have taken place. Some authorities predict that the economic benefits of the Aswan Dam in Egypt will be canceled out by the further spread of this disease, since reinfection takes place easily with the first trip back to the rice field or other common sources of infection. Control of the disease, in addition to finding a suitable drug for its treatment, must include the elimination of the snail and careful control of irrigation systems as well as improved overall sanitation procedures.

Malaria has been one of the scourges of man. At one time it had an incidence of 300 million a year, with 3 million a year dying of this disease. It accounted for a staggering economic loss as well. The illness made people incapable of work, with the result that farms were not cultivated and other work projects went uncompleted. In 1955 the World Health Organization undertook the greatest public health venture of all time. It initiated an eradication program against malaria.

The disease is caused by a protozoan parasite that is transmitted by the anopheles mosquito. The mosquito spreads the disease by biting a person ill with malaria and thus picking up the infectious protozoans. It transmits these causative organisms by biting a well person. The campaign was started with DDT spraying to kill the mosquitoes, and with the use of antimalarial drugs for those already infected. The malaria eradication program has made significant progress, and 5 more countries and territories have been registered as malaria-free, bringing the total of malaria-free areas up to 18. The malaria eradication program consists of four phases:

1. Preparatory Phase: geographical reconnaissance and training of staff.
2. Attack Phase: house spraying or other attack methods are applied.
3. Consolidation Phase: attack measures are stopped and surveillance is carried out.
4. Maintenance Phase: vigilance operations aim at preventing the reestablishment of the disease.

In 1970 it was estimated that of the 1,802 million people who originally lived in malarious areas, 1,340 million (or 74 per cent) were in areas where malaria had now been eradicated or where programs were in progress. Of these 1,340 million people:

710 million (or 39%) lived in Maintenance Phase areas
296 million (or 16%) lived in Consolidation Phase areas
329 million (or 18%) lived in Attack Phase areas
5 million (or less than 1%) lived in Preparatory Phase areas
426 million (or 26%) lived where programs were not yet in operation.[5]

The cry against the use of DDT that has arisen from Western Europe and North America has re-

[5]Adapted from *World Health*, May 1971.

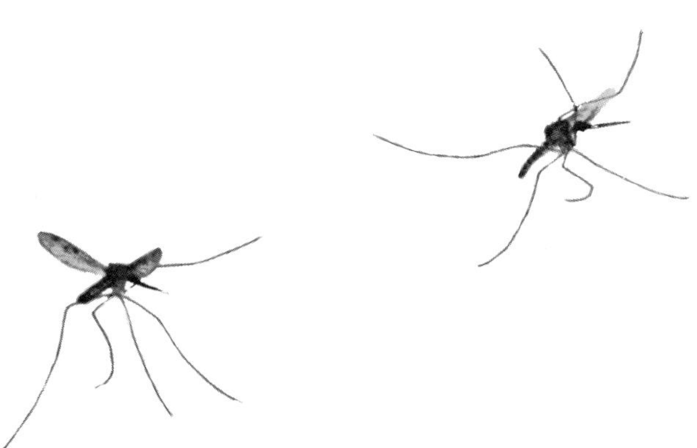
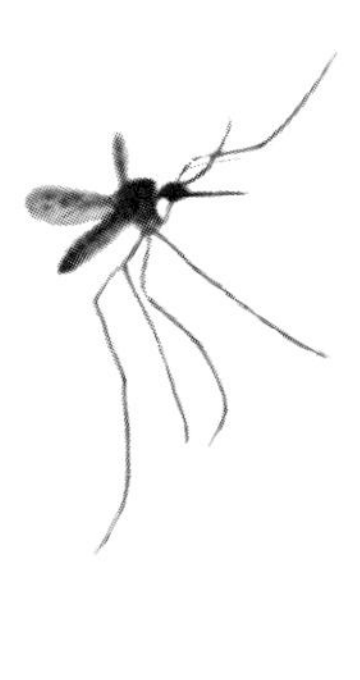
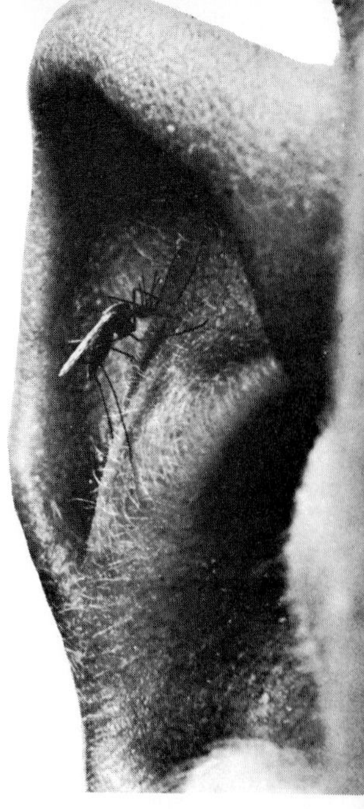

stricted its use in these areas. Fears from malarious areas is that this restriction will inhibit malaria eradication programs, as in fact it has. For example, as a result of premature cessation of spraying in Ceylon, their malaria rate went from 110 in 1961 (after a 15-year campaign against malaria) to 2.5 million in 1968–1969. The dilemma of DDT as an environmental threat on the one hand, and as the protector of human life on the other hand, will continue. This DDT controversy has made the research concerning the development of a vaccine against malaria increasingly significant. Biological means of controlling mosquitoes are being explored in Nigeria, for example, where a minnow-sized fish that feeds on mosquito larvae is being studied; and in India, genetically altering the male mosquito renders it sterile. Effective alternatives must be developed so that the relentless attack against malaria may continue.

Tuberculosis. There are still 15 million cases of tuberculosis, and 3 million deaths a year are caused by it. There has been a rapid decline in the death rate for tuberculosis in the economically developed countries. The development and use of effective drugs have been responsible in great part for the decline. The disease remains, however, a significant worldwide public health problem. In some countries 70 per cent of the children are infected before the age of 14. This does not mean that these children have active tuberculosis. It indicates that they have been in contact with the disease, as revealed by tuberculin testing and *could* become active cases. A committee on tuberculosis of the World Health Organization stated that tuberculosis could not be

Fig. 16-8. Efforts to eradicate malaria have given great emphasis to the elimination of the anopheles mosquito, by spraying the areas with DDT. (WHO Photo—Paul Almasy)

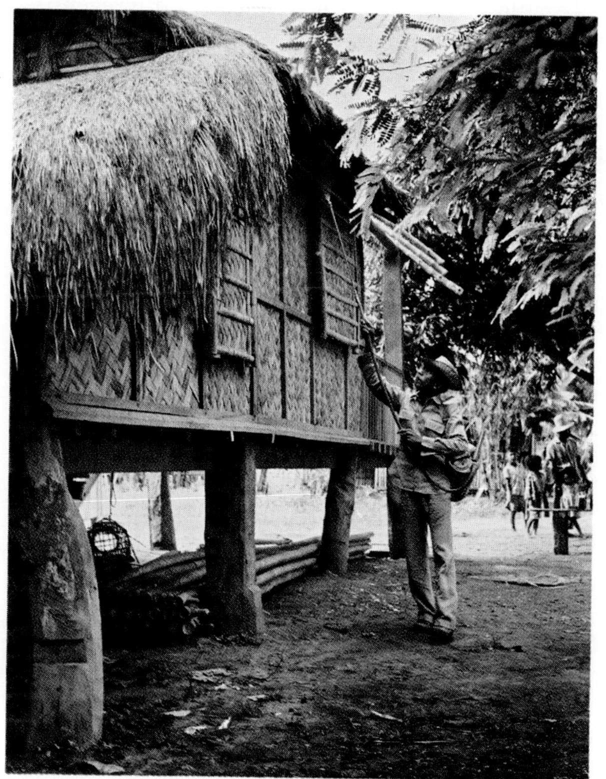

eliminated as a public health problem until less than 1 per cent of the children in a country became infected by age fourteen. No country of the world as yet can meet that criterion.

The BCG (bacillus Calmette-Guerin) vaccine is one of the major weapons in the effort to control tuberculosis. It is 80 per cent effective in preventing the disease in those who have been so vaccinated. In India, there are over 5 million cases of tuberculosis, and two-thirds of the population are carriers of the virulent tubercle bacillus. In a ten-year period, 50 million Indian children have been given BCG vaccine.

Another giant step forward was taken with the development of antituberculosis drugs, namely streptomycin, PAS (para-aminosalicylic acid), and isoniazid. These drugs are not only effective against the disease, but inexpensive as well, making their extensive use feasible. The drugs represent a major breakthrough in tuberculosis control.

With the BCG vaccine and the antituberculosis drugs, man now has the weapons to eliminate another disease. It is now a matter of producing them in sufficient quantities and getting them to the right places at the right times. Not an easy task! The BCG vaccine has seen very limited use in this country. Most American physicians feel that it is more appropriately used in countries where the tuberculosis incidence is higher. The vaccine masks the results of tuberculin tests designed to determine if a person has had contact with the tuberculosis germs. Anyone who has had the vaccine will automatically register a positive reaction on a tuberculin test. In this country it is felt that finding specific individuals who are serving as sources of infection through tuberculin testing is a more effective approach than mass BCG vaccinations. Some American physicians and public health authorities feel that the use of the BCG vaccine has value even in the United States. Some studies are being conducted in high-incidence areas (overly populated, low-income areas in cities) utilizing the vaccine. The results of these studies will shed some light on this controversy.

Cholera is an intestinal disease that is caused by bacteria and spread via food and water contaminated by human waste. Sanitation and personal cleanliness almost eliminate the transmission of this disease from man to man. In fact, the likelihood of the disease spreading is so rare in areas where hygiene is good that the United States no longer demands a certificate of cholera vaccination from international travelers. The cholera patient suffers from vomiting, diarrhea, dehydration, and collapse. Death from severe dehydration can occur with frightening suddenness. The fatality rates range anywhere from 10 to 80 per cent, depending on the availibility of early treatment, which includes the replacement of body fluids and antibiotics. Control measures that are taken include the boiling of water for drinking and dishwashing. Cholera vaccine is administered despite its uncertain value. The control of flies is also important in reducing the spread of the infection.

In the mid-nineteenth century, cholera raged throughout the world, killing tens of thousands of people. In Europe, it precipitated the development of the first public health measures that included a clean water supply and proper disposal of sewage to prevent the spread of the disease. There was an outbreak of cholera in the West Bengal in 1961, in which 1,422 people died during a six-month siege. Cholera moved north and westward and appeared in the Mediterranean area in 1965, and in 1970 reports of cholera came from Africa, Turkey, and Russia. *World Health* reported that "one of the outstanding events of 1970 was the extension of the seventh pandemic[6] of cholera, which began in 1961, to countries far from the traditional endemic areas in Asia."[7] The year 1970 was the worst year of the pandemic, with at least 46 countries reporting the disease. Though health officials of the United States have been warned that the disease will continue westward and ultimately reach this country, they see it as no immediate threat because of adequate water supplies and sanitation.

Trypanosomiasis is a disease found in most of Africa south of the Sahara Desert. Several types of protozoa are responsible for trypanosomiasis (sleeping sickness). The disease is transmitted by the tsetse fly, and animals as well as humans are susceptible to the illness. Some trypanosomes (protozoa causing the disease) are harmless to animals but dangerous to man. The animals in these cases act as reservoirs of infection. The tsetse fly, by first biting the animal and then man, transmits the disease. The opposite is sometimes found to be true where some trypanosomes are harmless to man but fatal to the animals. In these cases, the people are deprived of animals that are needed as a source of protein or to help cultivate the land for the growth of crops. Either directly or indirectly the disease is a source of hardship to man.

Insecticides are now used in many areas to eradicate the tsetse fly. Drugs are also used to treat people who have contracted the illness. In the past, sleeping sickness was invariably fatal, but it can now be cured if treated in the early stages. Programs of prevention and treatment of the disease need to be continued and further extended.

Onchocerciasis (ongko-sir-kiah-sis), or river blindness, is prevalent in tropical Africa as well as in the central portions of South America. Tiny black flies (simulium damnosum) transmit the disease by carrying microscopic young forms of parasitic worms. These are transmitted to the human bitten by an infected fly. In the human, when the worms reach the adult stage, they produce subcutaneous nodules in which they develop hundreds of thousands of young. These microscopic worms then invade the tissues of the skin and eyes, with blindness a frequent outcome. The disease is often referred to as river blindness because of its high incidence in river valleys. The fly that transmits the disease is known to thrive best in quick-running water.

New drugs developed for the treatment and control of the disease leave much to be desired. Some drugs are effective only on the adult worm and

[6]The end of the 6th pandemic came around 1923 when cholera retreated to its "homeland" in the deltas of the Ganges and Brahmaputra rivers.

[7]*World Health*, May 1971.

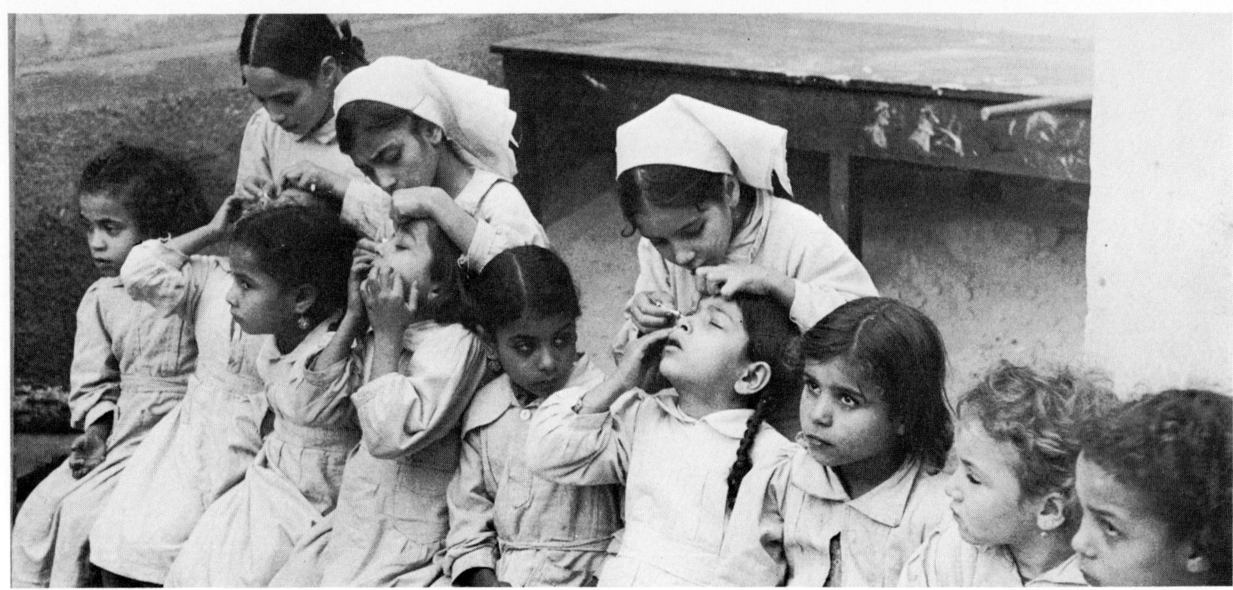

others only on the microfilariae (embryo form of the worm). In some areas, spraying with insecticides (DDT) has been effective in exterminating the *simulium damnosum* (the transmitting agent). More than 250 million people are still affected by onchocerciasis, and attempts are being made to organize mass programs for its eradication. In 1968 the Volta River basin on the west coast of Africa was singled out as a target area for a mass onchocerciasis control operation.

Trachoma and infectious conjunctivitis represent a leading cause of blindness in the world, affecting some 500 million people. It is particularly prevalent in North Africa, Asia, and parts of deeper Africa and South America, particularly in dry, arid regions. In certain areas, practically the entire adult population is infected. The rate of infection among preschool-age children runs between 70 and 90 per cent in areas where poor hygiene, poverty, and crowded living conditions exist. A study conducted in India revealed a 78 per cent infection rate among rural school children. A pilot project on Taiwan uncovered a 48 per cent incidence among its children. Sulfonamides, and particularly antibiotics, are effective in clearing up the condition. Mass campaigns on a national level are being encouraged to bring this disease under control.

Leprosy (Hansen's Disease). The inhuman segregation of patients in leprosaria is finally becoming a thing of the past. However, in some areas, getting lepers to register is still difficult because of the stigma long associated with the disease. In Africa, for example, only 50 per cent of the registered cases were under treatment, even though dapsone, one of the sulfone drugs taken orally, can cure the disease completely if it is detected early. It is estimated that there are approximately 10 million cases of leprosy in the world.

Leprosy, which is caused by a bacillus, has an incubation period of from one to several or many years. Its period of contagion is only that stage when the lesions on the skin are open and can discharge bacilli. This period of communicability can be shortened by the administration of drugs. In areas where it is common, leprosy is often contracted in childhood and may not appear until adulthood. Children appear to be more susceptible to the disease than adults. A study in Burma is under way to see what protection against leprosy BCG[8] may offer children up to 14 years of age. Educational efforts are being made to stress the greater risk of the disease when the individual is exposed early in life. As effective treatment for this condition is being recognized, the unreasoned fear that has been associated with it has been diminishing.

The World Health Organization

In 1945, when the United Nations was located in San Francisco, Brazil and China made the joint proposal that an international health organization be formed. This was followed by an international health conference in which the constitution for the

[8]Bacillus Calmette Guerin (BCG)—the vaccine used for the control of tuberculosis.

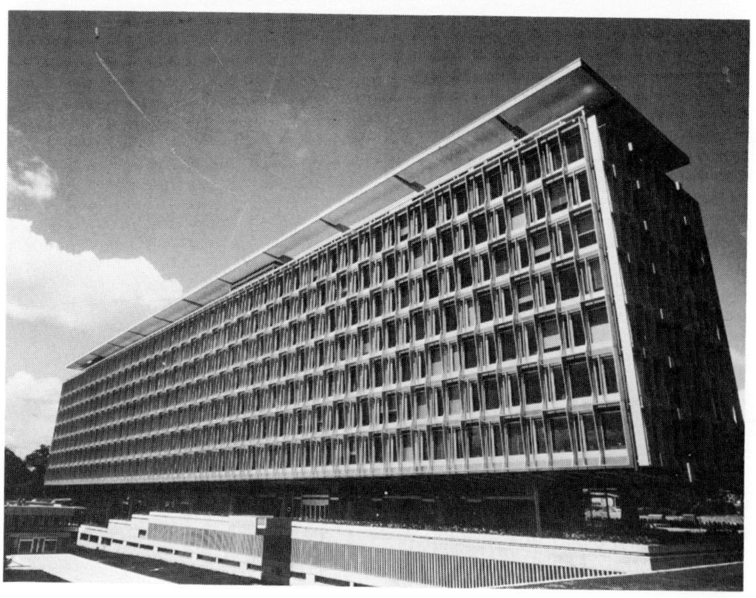

Fig. 16-9. The patient is a school girl. Her "doctor" is a classmate. In Egypt's fight against eye diseases the children themselves play a major part. (WHO Photo)

Fig. 16-10. The new WHO headquarters building in Geneva. (WHO Photo)

Fig. 16-11. Breakdown of the World Health Assembly. (Pan American Health Organization)

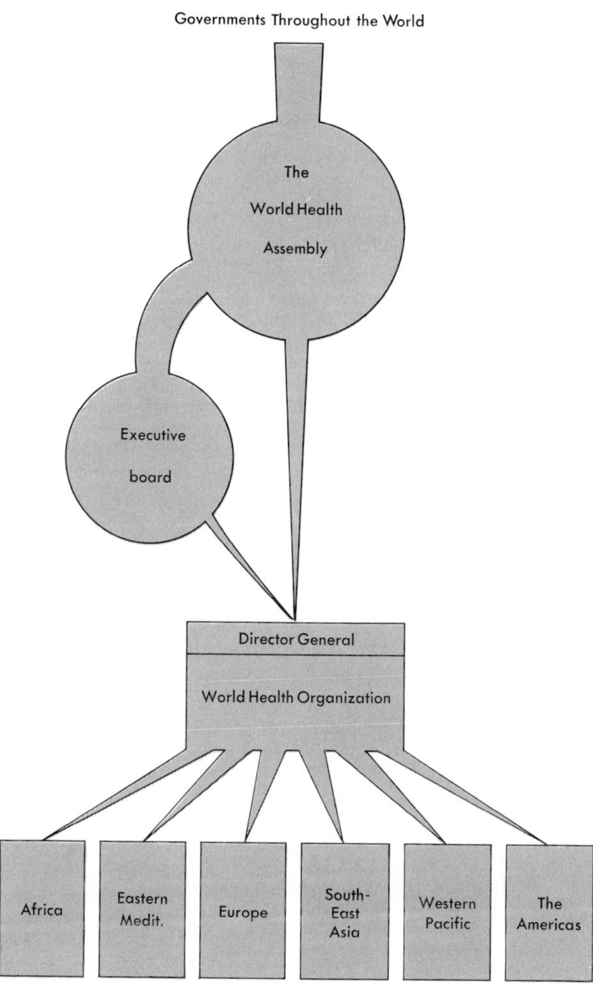

World Health Organization was drawn up. On April 7, 1948, the World Health Organization became one of eleven specialized agencies of the United Nations. Its stated objective is "the attainment by all peoples of the highest possible level of health." It operates as a fairly independent unit having its own constitution, budget, and administrative structure. Basic decisions for the World Health Organization (WHO) are made by the World Health Assembly. Delegates that represent each of the WHO member states make up the governing body. It is the World Health Assembly that determines policies, budget, and program. The Assembly meets annually, the meetings generally lasting three weeks.

The executive board of WHO is made up of 24 health specialists who serve three-year terms on this body. Eight are replaced each year, with the Health Assembly designating those countries entitled to choose persons to serve on this board. Members of the executive board are not there to represent their countries, but to make a contribution to the WHO.

In order to facilitate its operation, WHO has divided the world into six regions. The regional offices are located in Brazzaville (Republic of the Congo), for Africa; Washington, D.C., (United States), for the Americas; New Delhi (India), for Southeast Asia; Copenhagen (Denmark), for Europe; Alexandria (Egypt), for the Eastern Mediterranean; and Manila (Philippines), for the Western Pacific. Each of the regional offices is largely responsible for the development of projects within its area. In 1948, when the first World Health Assembly met, they chose Geneva, Switzerland, as the location for the organization's headquarters. The offices of the Director General of WHO and his staff are located there.

WHO Activities

International narcotics control is a responsibility the WHO inherited from the League of Nations. WHO has a committee, made up of international experts, that reviews various drugs considered likely to produce addiction. It then proceeds to place the addictive substances on the listing of controlled drugs. Biological standardization is another service rendered by WHO. WHO will provide samples of substances that have been internationally standardized such as vaccines, antibiotics, hormones, and other drugs. In this manner, laboratories have a standard of measurement and can compare the strength of their own products with that of WHO's standardized products. WHO also publishes the International Pharmacopoeia. It adopts internationally recognized names for pharmaceuticals which often have varying names in different countries. It also serves as a clearing house for new drugs and for information on dangerous side effects of drugs that may already be in use.

In order for it to obtain the best advice available on technical matters, WHO will many times set up expert panels made up of leading scientists and health administrators in the world. These experts are called together whenever a need arises. The services of these outstanding scientists are given free.

WHO maintains a watchdog service for the ever-present menace of epidemics of diseases like plague, cholera, smallpox, typhus, and yellow fever which still smoulder in our world environment. WHO also keeps nations informed about outbreaks of viral diseases like influenza. Before the WHO came into existence, there was little uniformity in quarantine regulations. There is now a uniform set of International Sanitary Regulations that give protection against the spread of disease. International health statistics have been made more accurate as the World Health Assembly makes provision for the uniform reporting of diseases and death.

The WHO also serves as a clearing house for health information. It has put out hundreds of technical publications on a variety of health topics and has stimulated and coordinated research activity, though it does not itself do research. Cooperative international research has obvious advantages in that it can focus the best talent and resources on a specific research problem.

The responsibilities of WHO will be rapidly increasing in the area of radiation control. The expanded industrial use of atomic energy will result in the need for international controls related to the transportation and use of radioactive products and the disposal of radioactive waste materials. It is assuring to know that WHO is anticipating these developments rather than waiting for them to mushroom into problems before taking remedial action.

Most of WHO's projects are initiated and developed through the regional offices. The health concerns of each region vary.

The Regional Office for Africa, which was set up in 1952, has been particularly concerned with the

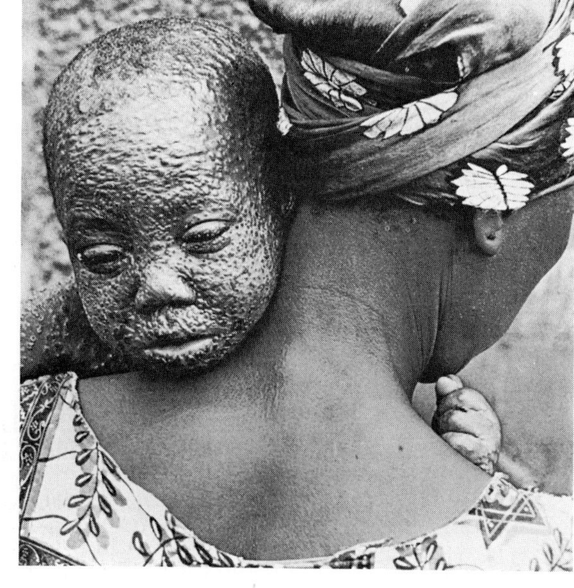

Fig. 16-12. Although we have had the ability to eradicate smallpox, the disease still persists. (WHO)

development of more public health personnel (doctors, nurses, laboratory technicians, sanitary engineers, and others). They have concentrated their activities in widespread campaigns against such diseases as leprosy, yaws, tuberculosis, and malaria. This region is also giving particular emphasis to mother and child health services, public health education, and environmental health.

The Regional Office for the Americas was initially the International World Health Organization. From this organization, in 1923, grew the Pan-American Sanitary Bureau. It developed an American sanitary code and had a wide range of functions. In 1947 the Bureau was reorganized and became a part of the Pan-American Sanitary Organization, which in 1949 agreed to become the WHO regional office for the Americas. In 1958 the name of the organization was changed to the Pan-American Health Organization (PAHO). PAHO has developed a very active program against malaria. It is also working to eradicate the aëdes Aegypti mosquito that transmits yellow fever. In order to reduce infectious hepatitis, typhoid, dysentery, and diarrhea in sixteen Latin American countries, PAHO has been working on the development of community water supplies by helping to construct water and sewage systems. PAHO now is an agency that employs over 1,000 persons and has a budget approaching 20 million dollars a year.

The Regional Office for Southeast Asia was created in 1948 and was actually the first of the WHO regional offices. Its major functions have been to support a member nation's actions against diseases such as malaria, tuberculosis, yaws, leprosy, bilharziasis, and smallpox. It has made rather remarkable progress with regard to malaria, protecting hundreds of millions from the disease. Burma, Indonesia, and Thailand have been supported in a campaign against leprosy. With the support of UNICEF (United Nations Children Fund), it has been conducting a broad-scale vaccination program against tuberculosis and has developed pilot projects for the home treatment of this disease. In this region, smallpox continues to be a pocket of infection. The Southeast Asia regional office has also been working to improve the environmental sanitary conditions in the area to help prevent the various parasitic diseases. This region has a rural population of 700 million people. It is a monumental task to attempt to develop health services and a preventive health program for this extensive population.

The Regional Office for Europe has within its area a large number (31 countries) of well-developed countries whose problems tend to reflect their economic development. As indicated by the Director of the European Regional office,

> Although Europe has more physicians than the rest of the world put together—about one million—and appears well protected against most traditional health hazards, there are problems old and new which require action at international level. Old scourges like cholera and smallpox still knock at our doors and their challenge can only be faced collectively. Looming larger ahead of us are gigantic problems brought about by technological progress and massive urbanization.[9]

[9]"31 Countries, One Health," by Dr. Leo Kaprio, Director, WHO regional Office for Europe.

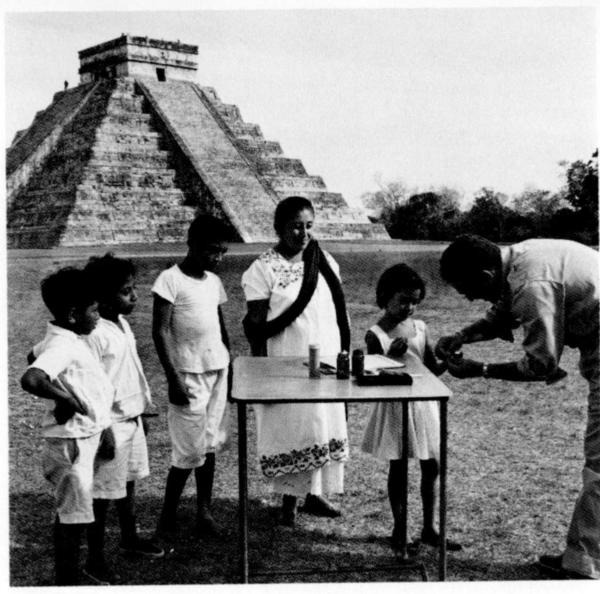

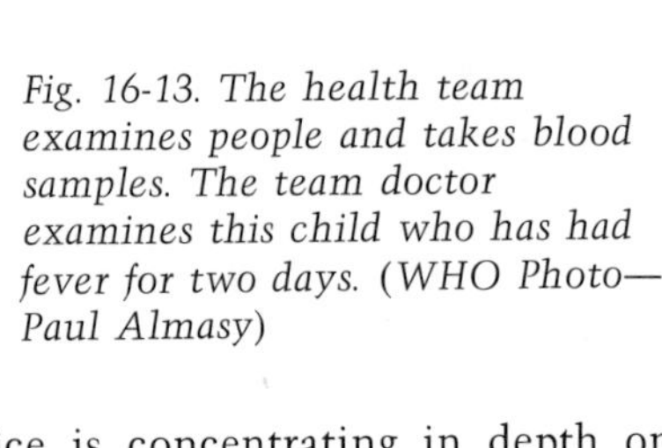

Fig. 16-13. The health team examines people and takes blood samples. The team doctor examines this child who has had fever for two days. (WHO Photo—Paul Almasy)

This regional office is concentrating in depth on several large health programs. Cardiovascular diseases, mental health (particularly that of adolescents and young people, and with alcoholism and drug dependence), environmental pollution, and the organization of medical care as a whole are some of the areas of concern in this region.

The Regional Office of the Eastern Mediterranean serves some of the most arid as well as the most fertile portions of the earth. Over 80 per cent of the people in this region live in rural areas. Some of the most basic health work needs to be done here. These countries have a high infant-mortality rate, with children under 5 years of age dying particularly of diarrheal disease. Major health problems exist here with regard to malnutrition, trachoma, and malaria, to which three out of four persons living in the area are exposed. One-half million people suffer from leprosy, and smallpox is endemic to the area. As water resources are developed in some of the more arid regions, bilharziasis will tend to spread. There is also an acute shortage of medical as well as auxiliary staff. A good portion of the budget for this regional office is devoted to the education and training of health personnel. As the area develops industrially and becomes more urbanized, this regional health office anticipates some of the new health problems that "progress" will bring with it.

The Regional Office for the Western Pacific started in that area with practically no health personnel available. In some countries, not a single nurse existed, and physicians were a rarity. In one country with a population of $1\frac{1}{2}$ million people, there was but one physician. The regional office has been busily at work in attempting to fill the needed positions with health personnel. As of 1968, health-related personnel totaled 147. In addition, a certain number of consultants on assignment for several months are associated with the Regional office. The major points of focus have been in the building up of health services, particularly in the rural areas, to fight the communicable diseases. Rather intensive work has been done to bring malaria under control, and it has been eradicated on Taiwan and the Ryukyu Islands. Tuberculosis has been fought with BCG vaccination programs, and successful efforts against yaws have been made in practically the entire region. Work also continues with regard to trachoma, leprosy, venereal diseases, nutrition, and environmental sanitation.

UNICEF (The United Nations Children Fund)

The United Nations Children Fund represents the only branch of the United Nations whose activities are devoted exclusively to the welfare of children. It was initially organized on December 11, 1946, as UNICEF (United Nations International Children's Emergency Fund). Its initial function was to help the children of war-torn countries. By 1950 UNICEF had completed its major tasks in Europe and in 1953 the General Assembly of the UN decided that UNICEF should continue under its changed name of United Nations Children Fund. Its purpose was designated as that of helping the millions of children, particularly in the underdeveloped countries, who were undergoing the hardships of hunger and illness. UNICEF has been working very closely with the WHO in its campaign against the major diseases of the world. UNICEF has provided various kinds of support for these campaigns. It has contributed supplies such as insecticides, sprayers, drugs, and health education materials. It has been busily at work helping to set up schools for the training of various health personnel. This organization has also made a major contribution by providing skim milk powder by the ton to alleviate nutritional problems. A drawback to the large-scale distribution of milk powder has been the discovery that some people cannot digest milk. They lack an enzyme (lactase) that is needed to break down milk sugar or lactose. The number of such people is more prevalent than has heretofore been realized. Even though lactase-deficient peoples can drink small to moderate amounts of milk and show no discomfort, there is a move toward supplying milk powder that is lactose-free so that intolerant populations can be provided milk—a major source of needed protein.

UNICEF has been at work with the FAO (Food and Agriculture Organization) and WHO in efforts to develop new high-protein foods. It has given assistance to communities in helping them increase their production of fruits, vegetables, and poultry. It has undertaken a program for the training of local workers to help overcome their many unscientific beliefs with regard to nutrition and health. At the same time it has instituted courses of study at the primary school level for the same purpose.

UNICEF is headed by an executive director who is appointed by the United Nations Secretary General. However, when it comes to budgetary matters, UNICEF is financed completely by voluntary contributions that come from governments and private groups of people from various countries. The United Nations does not provide money for the budget of UNICEF. Each year contributions that have been received from various governments have steadily increased, so that its budget now approaches that of the World Health Organization. Help from UNICEF is rendered only at the request of governments. Countries oftentimes will propose that various projects be carried out within their borders and make application to UNICEF for such programs. The requests are reviewed by UNICEF officers and upon approval are set into action. UNICEF activities are worked out very closely and cooperatively with the World Health Organization and other groups within the United Nations. The ultimate goal in any UNICEF program is the development within the country itself of *permanent* health, nutrition, education, and social welfare services that are supported entirely by the country's own efforts. Only in this way can the benefits to children be long-lasting.

Food and Agriculture Organization (FAO)

The Food and Agriculture Organization is one of the specialized agencies of the United Nations. Its major purpose has been to relieve the hunger and inadequate nutrition that afflict half the world's population. It tackled the twin problems of overproduction and undernourishment and sought the best possible use of food surpluses for economic development of struggling countries. In 1963, after much study, the World Food Program (WFP) was created. It was conceived by the United Nations and Food and Agriculture Organization, and was concerned with economic and social development as well as nutrition and the production and distribution of food.

One of the two largest projects of the World Food Program is in India where the development of a dairy industry is under way. This involves increasing capacity and output of dairy processing facilities, switching raw milk suppliers to modern dairies, and bringing the cattle from the cities to the rural areas. The social, nutritional, and economic benefits of this project will be widespread. The health hazards caused by cattle in the city will be eliminated. There will be increased availability of wholesome milk, which is the most important source of animal protein in the Indian diet since a large proportion in the country are vegetarians. In addition the price for pure milk will be cheaper.

The World Food Program had also been engaged in settling people on new land, for example, many of those who had to leave the Aswan Dam area. Reclaiming and improving the land is done by the laborers who are paid with food (or rations) as part of their wages. Food aid is given to families until their land can support them. In 1974 there were approximately 40,000 new settler families working with the program in this way. To meet the need for new and more abundant forests not only to provide timber but for erosion control and general soil conservation, projects in forestry are now under way. Livestock projects are also an essential phase of the agricultural scene. Rangelands that are turning into deserts because of overgrazing of sheep and goats are being renovated.

One interesting and highly successful operation of WFP is the watershed project in northern Turkey, where more than 85,000 goats and 17,000 native cattle constituted a liability rather than a source of income. The goats were progressively destroying the vegetation in the surrounding forest and hills, thus contributing to erosion. The cattle were yielding poor milk and the calves were fetching low prices on the market. But the most ominous element was that the rain was implacably washing away valuable topsoil into the Kirmir river and the silt carried downstream was clogging and damaging the reservoir situated below the village. In early 1964—when the project started—WFP began contributing rations as part payment to workers (and their families) who were occupied with the restoration of stripped forests, the afforestation of bare slopes, and the improvement of pasture and grazing lands. Rations were also distributed as an incentive to private farmers to carry out the watershed improvements. Later, it was agreed that WFP would also provide feed for the cattle, an improved high-yielding breed having been introduced. [In 1971] thanks to the success of this project, terraces and pine trees have prevented soil erosion and alfalfa is growing in the valleys as feed for almost 1,000 head of cattle of an improved breed. The net income of farmers has increased eightfold and people are no longer indebted to village moneylenders.[10]

[10] *World Food Programme, A Story of Multilateral Aid,* 2nd ed., rev., United Nations, Food and Agriculture Organization of the United Nations, 1971, p. 24.

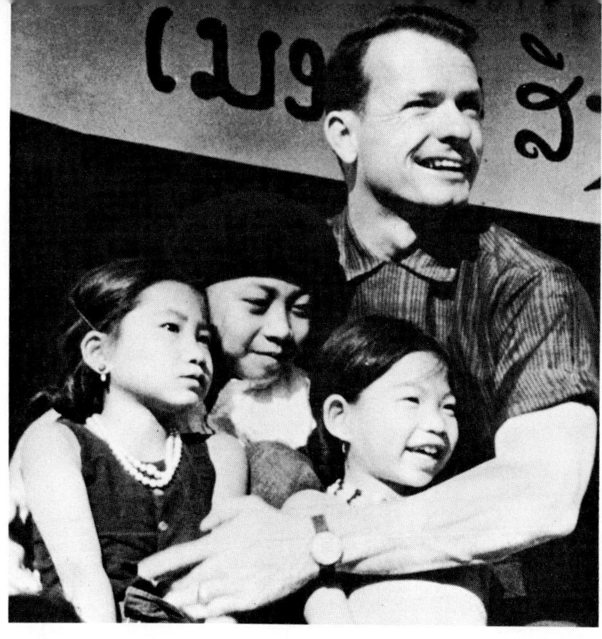

Fig. 16-14. Dr. Tom Dooley and friends. (The Thomas A. Dooley Foundation)

The many and varied activities of the FAO are often carried out in cooperation with WHO and UNICEF. These are exemplified by school feeding programs, responses to disaster needs due to earthquakes, floods, hurricanes, and other catastrophes, and stimulation of greater food production and use. The FAO, with its educational programs and agricultural demonstrations and projects, is continuing to make significant contributions to relieve hunger and promote health in the world.

The Helping Hands

Many Americans have shown great concern and empathy for the less fortunate people of the world. They have left their land of plenty to endure the hardships of underprivileged societies so they might help. Medical missionaries, the Peace Corps, The United States Public Health Service, and such organizations as Care/Medico, Project Hope, and others have gone forth to demonstrate man's humanity to man.

CARE/MEDICO

The humanitarian work of Tom Dooley in the northern Laotian village of Nam Tha had far-reaching effects. He not only treated the disease-ridden people of that area, but taught and trained those Laotians who would follow him in running "their" hospital. With Dr. Commanduras, Tom Dooley appealed to the International Rescue Committee for the establishment of six medical teams to be sent to critical areas throughout the world. On February 4, 1958, he announced the founding of a new organization called MEDICO, which stands for Medical International Cooperation Organization. MEDICO was in no way a religious or political organization. Tom Dooley envisioned it as a person-to-person, heart-to-heart program in which therapeutic medicine could be practiced for sick people in areas that had little or no chance of receiving medical aid. "It will aid those who are sick and by that simple act it will win friendship for America."[11] Dr. Dooley died of cancer in 1961 at the age of 34. In 1964, MEDICO and CARE merged. In this alliance, CARE supplies the money and logistical support, and MEDICO supplies the doctors. Tom Dooley's work in the form of CARE/MEDICO and The Thomas A. Dooley Foundation, Inc., goes on, and his spirit lives on in those dedicated to helping their fellow men.

SS Hope

In 1960 the Project Hope (*H*ealth *O*pportunity for *P*eople *E*verywhere) was launched when an unused Navy hospital ship was refitted and renamed the SS *Hope*. Under the direction of its founder and medical director, Dr. William B. Walsh, the SS *Hope* has traveled to South Viet Nam, Indonesia, Peru, Ecuador, Ceylon, and Nicaragua. Staffed by U.S. medical

[11] Thomas A. Dooley, *The Night They Burned the Mountain* (New York: Farrar, Straus and Giroux, 1960), p. 24.

Fig. 16-15. The SS Hope *spreading its medical care skills and reaffirming the dignity of man. (Project Hope)*

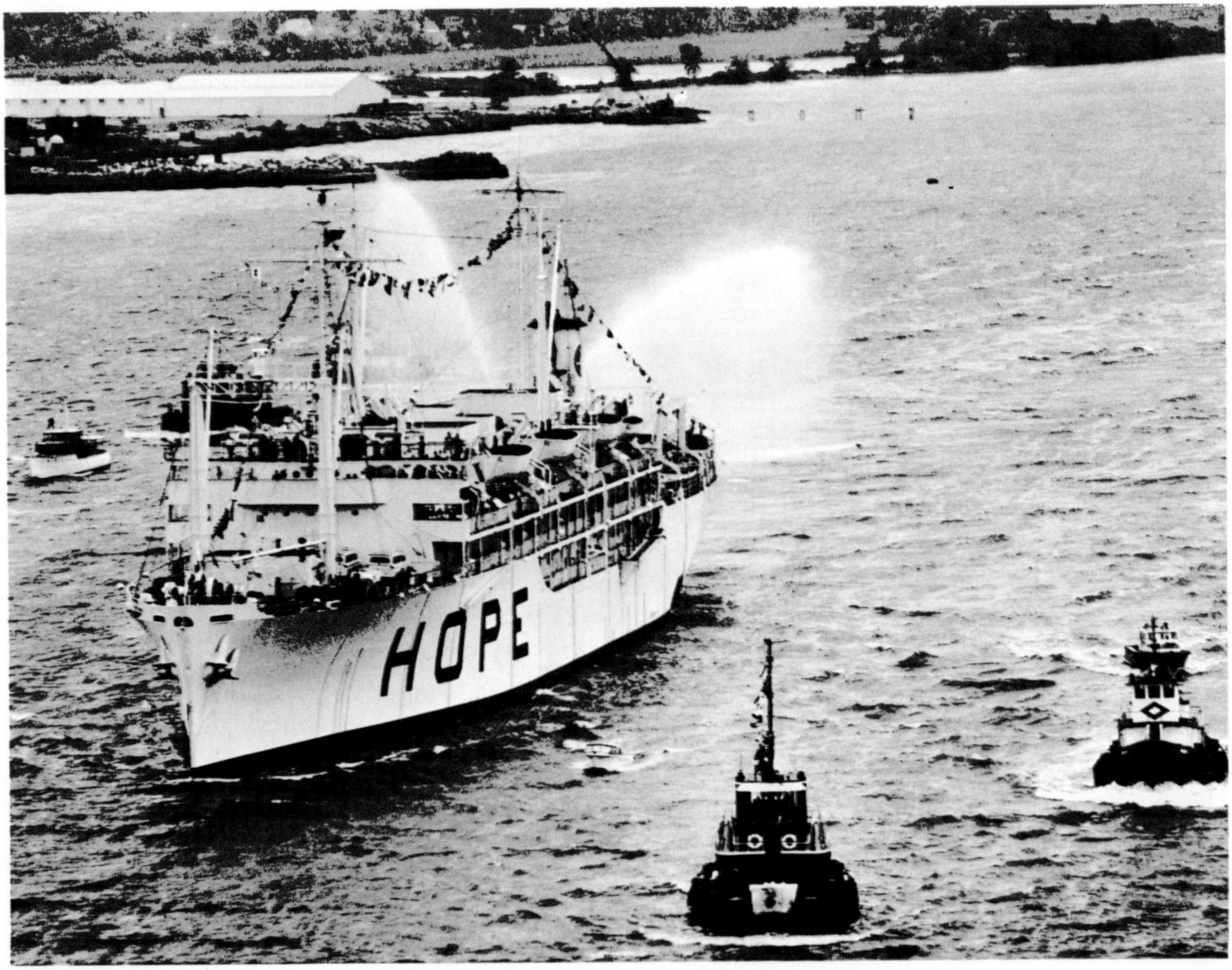

personnel, Hope participates in the development of emerging nations by elevating their health standards through education and by promoting international friendship and understanding. *Hope* operates on the principle of helping people who wish to help themselves and goes only where it is invited. Its professional staff has trained over 5,100 physicians, nurses, dentists, and paramedical personnel in those countries. More recently, *Hope* has expanded its people-to-people health project to within the United States. A program with Mexican Americans in Laredo, Texas, and another with the Indian Americans at Ganado, Arizona, have now been established. *Hope* has thus stimulated the development of medical services and facilities. Wherever the project travels it leaves some of its medical skills, texts, and dedicated zeal. In essence, it leaves a little hope.

Dr. Richard B. Stark, in his article "Medicine as a Force for Peace," stated:

> So, the Schweitzers, the Seagraves, the Dooleys, the Walshes, the Carlsons, the Commandurases, by reliving the parable of the Good Samaritan, have pointed the way. With planning and a continual supply of superbly trained humanitarian specialists, the medical export will grow. Administered with compassion as a gift of the giver, the parable of the samaritan need not be old hat, but may inject into our nervous, narcissistic, alcoholic, bored, rich, delinquent society, a sense of selflessness and indeed, of purpose itself.[12]

[12]Richard B. Stark, M.D., "Medicine as a Force for Peace," *The Journal of the American Medical Association*, Vol. 195, No. 1 (January 3, 1966), p. 108.

Review Questions

1. Why is interest in world health becoming a necessity rather than an altruistic nicety?
2. How are poverty and health status related?
3. What factors in addition to poverty contribute to the incidence of kwashiorkor in the world?
4. To what extent is schistosomiasis a threat in the underdeveloped regions of the world? Why are drugs that are effective in curing this disorder not a complete solution to the problem?
5. To what extent has the World Health Organization's program for the eradication of malaria progressed since its inception in 1955?
6. Why have American physicians had some reservation with regard to the use of the BCG vaccine for tuberculosis in the United States?
7. Since there is now effective treatment for leprosy, what problems must now be overcome in order to eradicate this disease?
8. Describe the structure of the World Health Organization.
9. Describe some of the far-flung activities of the World Health Organization. To what extent do the health problems differ for each of its regional offices?
10. What are the major functions of The United Nations Children Fund (UNICEF)? Why does this organization work very closely with WHO?
11. What are the purposes of the Food and Agriculture Organization (FAO)?
12. What was the contribution made by Dr. Thomas A. Dooley and MEDICO?

Chapter 17

Man's Moment of Decision

"Technology has elevated man-and there is no going back. "Natural man" is the cooperative creation of nature and man. Antitechnology is self-hatred."[1]

Man is in the process of experiencing all the discomforts of emerging from his adolescence and feeling the responsibilities of his developing adulthood. There was a time when man attributed all of life's happenings to God as a dependent child would to a parent. As man has learned more about himself and how to influence his environment he has discovered that his newly developed knowledge has awesome potentialities. He is now capable of self destruction, or conversely, achieving a quality of life heretofore unattainable. So long as he has a deep respect for his new found power and approaches his tasks with concern and humility, there is hope. Should he view his position of increasing influence with irresponsibility and a God-like posture he is surely lost. Thoughtful scientists in the process of discovering the new knowledges often express concern over man's ability to assume the added burden of responsibility their work will bring to bear. Let us review some of the research in the health and life sciences so that we may more clearly view the health, social, ethical, and legal issues they present.

Genetic Cloning

In the mid-sixties, Professor John Gurdon, a biologist from Oxford, found a way to destroy the nucleus of the egg cell of a frog. Through a complicated procedure he then managed to take a nucleus from a body cell of a frog (with the full number of 46 chromosomes) and placed it in the egg cell. The cell then behaved like a fertilized egg and began to grow. The cell grew into a tadpole and finally into a frog identical to the one that donated the nucleus. This process is known as *cloning*. It has been predicted that within ten to twenty years it will be possible to clone human beings. The implications are of course enormous. Through this procedure a man or woman could reproduce their identical selves since all of their chromosomes and therefore their characteristics would be passed on to the offspring. The procedure could find some practical application in the reproduction of prize cattle and therefore the production of fine meat. The ever ingenious football coach might want to use it to reproduce his finest athletes and ultimately field his personal all-star team. An elite of great minds could also be reproduced—for good or evil. It would even be possible for parents to replace their mortally injured child with an identical one—or *not* replace him if they were not pleased with him.

The era of genetic engineering is virtually upon us. It brings with it awesome responsibilities and should develop appropriate feelings of uneasiness and healthy concern in all of us. The issue raises some pertinent questions. Should human cloning be permitted? If so, who will determine what should be done and under what circumstances? When and who referees the issue of personal rights versus the public

[1] Willard Gaylin, "We Have the Awful Knowledge to Make Exact Copies of Human Beings," *New York Times Magazine*, March 5, 1972.

good? "Does an individual have a right to his uniqueness? What would be the psychological effects of seeing one's genetic blueprint played out in advance if, for example, the person one was cloned from developed muscular dystrophy at age 35"[2] We can add to the foregoing, research going on in the area of human reproduction indicating that surgically removed ovaries can be made to continue their production of egg cells. These cells can then be fertilized with donated sperm cells. Means are also being sought to separate out the sperm containing female-producing X chromosomes from those sperm containing X and Y male-producing chromosomes. As if the implications of all this were not strong enough, geneticists are attempting to pluck out undesirable genes from reproductive cells. Genes that would predispose an individual to diabetes or epilepsy, for instance, could be removed. Research in this area will soon make it possible to nourish a fertilized egg in an artificial placenta that will permit it to grow to full term—a development that will no doubt be cheered by the women's liberation since it will free women of what the liberationists consider an incapacitating (at least temporarily) biological function. With the developing advances in genetic engineering, approaching parenthood with order pad in hand to designate the kind of child one wants becomes not just a possibility but a probability. Needless to say the decisions will not come easy.

[2]Jane E. Brody and Edward B. Fiske, *Ethics Debate Set Off by Life Science Gains.* The Hastings Center—Institute of Society, Ethics and the Life Sciences, 623 Warburton Ave., Hastings-on-Hudson, N.Y. 10706.

A factor that must not be overlooked in all this is the environment in which one grows and lives. Anyone who has ever grown a plant knows that identical seeds can be planted in different environments with respect to soil, amount of moisture, and so forth, and produce a plant that will flourish and one that barely survives. The principle applies to human beings. How a person is sustained both physically and emotionally particularly in his early life is critical to his development. It is not always the "bad seed" that produces the inadequate and unfortunate. In most cases it is the improper nurturing of the young by parents or society who produce the crippling.

Randy's ordeal started in San Bernardino, California, twenty-three years ago, the day he was born. His father left town a week later. When he was eight years old, he moved with his alcoholic mother to Stockton, fifty miles east of San Francisco. When he was thirteen, they attended a party together where Randy took some of his mother's prescription diet pills for the first time. He enjoyed the drugs; they sped up his system and helped him forget his mother, a sexually starved and impulsive woman who apparently took out all her frustrations on him. One year later, he left home after learning to use amphetamines to heighten his courage and overcome his depression.

In Randy's own words, "I just couldn't take my old lady. She'd get loaded and start in on me and I'd be loaded too and pretty soon we'd really be at it. I was getting big then, big enough to hit her back when she started swinging. Finally she started coming on like some whore and it got so bad I just couldn't stay there anymore. So I cut out, made it to New York, got adopted by some junkies on the lower East Side and pretty soon I was hooked on heroin.[3]

Environment also refers to the human contact of the embryo in its attachment to the uterine wall of its mother. It grows and develops for nine months in a human environment. When a human-fertilized egg grows in an artificial placenta will it be deprived in any way by lack of its human contact? Will the laboratory produce infants who are genetically healthy but socially or emotionally impaired? Will they be less human?

Human Behavior Control

"Behavior control—*the modification of someone's behavior by means other than the motivational appeal of the desired behavior itself*—is as old as the caveman's club and admonitory stories of wrathful gods. It is as common today as parents who bribe, plead, threaten, or read stories to get a lively youngster to sleep. For better or for worse, behavior control has been exercised on men by themselves, by other men, by cultures, by institutions and by the necessities of nature."[4]

Efforts to control behavior are obviously not new and in fact are ongoing in increasing dimensions. Every advertisement and election campaign speech has little else in mind. Patients in mental institutions are given tranquilizers, children in schools being admonished for speaking to a colleague, and criminals confined to penal institutions have behavior control as a basic objective. Even the crudity of the male plying "his girl" with drinks has a similar goal. Behavior control has already been used for a variety of purposes, for good and evil. A cause for concern is the level of sophistication now being reached by research in this area with its implications, causing the invention of the wheel and the development of nuclear power to pale into insignificance by comparison.

For example, experimentation with animals and humans has demonstrated that electrodes planted in the brain can produce or halt emotional states. It has already been suggested that such a procedure could be used to pacify violent patients in institutions. The use of electricity to modify mood and/or behavior is being vigorously pursued by researchers who believe that electrical intervention has greater potential to alter mental states than drugs. Their continued success poses society with some complex legal and ethical problems. The inevitable questions that arise are under what circumstances, for what purposes, and under whose control should states of mind be altered?

A scientist has succesfully implanted electrodes in the "pleasure centers" of the brains of rats. He arranged for the rats to stimulate themselves by pressing a lever. The rats found this new sensation so pleasurable that they ignored food, water, and sex. Some pressed the lever thousands of times an hour for longer than a day until, when overcome by fa-

[3] David E. Smith, M.D., and John Luce, *Love Needs Care*, (Boston: Little, Brown, 1971), p. 42.

[4] *Program in the Ethical, Social and Legal Issues of Behavior Control*, Institute Program Series: Number Four. The Hastings Center—Institute of Society, Ethics and the Life Sciences, op, cit.

tigue, they fainted. Should this form of pleasure become available to man one could see the more hedonistically oriented becoming electric freaks. Pressing their levers for hours, they may have to be intravenously fed, while sitting in their excrement absorbing the wonders of electricity. Their only interruption would be a power failure. Then there would be those who would seek the ultimate experience—being struck by lightning! Aside from the bizarre there are practical positive applications of this new knowledge. It has been found that some people have damaged brain cells that make them prone to spells of violence. Electronic probing can locate such cells and in some cases surgery can remove the offending cells, restoring the person's behavior to normal. Some researchers see the possibility of using electrical stimulation of the brain for purposes of pleasure (in rational degrees) and see it as a routine form of pleasure. Others see electrical stimulation as a means of controlling violent people whose behavior cannot be corrected in any other way. This would involve a number of criminals in our penal institutions as well as some patients in mental institutions.

The ethical dilemma that presents itself is that we have always placed great value on human dignity and the freedom of the individual to make rational choices between alternatives. To what extent is the above-mentioned treatment imposed on those who see nothing wrong with their violent behavior? Is the person in question capable of making a rational or responsible decision? If we argue on behalf of individual freedom of choice, how do we respond to the need of the public to be protected from the violent?

One does not have to look into the future to find this kind of issue. It is estimated that approximately 4 to 8 million Americans are treated by doctors to relieve mental depression, probably the most common mental disorder. The number of patients treated by shock treatments is not known. Some hospitals consider it a basic therapy tool and use shock therapy more liberally than others. Consider the following case history:

Mrs. F., a quarrelsome and despondent matron in her midfifties, had admitted herself to the psychiatric ward of a private hospital in the depths of despair after a series of outpatient visits to a psychiatrist who prescribed medication. Her husband had died four months previously after an agonizing series of operations for cancer. She had refused an invitation to live with her son because she believed herself "unworthy to associate with such good people."

The diagnosis was acute involutional depression. Electroshock therapy was agreed upon by the two psychiatrists and the neurologist who had examined her. She was given a careful explanation of the treatment and told that a series of shocks would be necessary. She was aware that they would be very unpleasant, but she agreed to the treatment. She said she "really didn't care what happened to her any more. . . ."

On the morning of the first treatment she was given Sodium Amytal for sedation. At the instant of the shock there was a convulsion similar to a grand mal epileptic seizure.

Two days later she was scheduled for second treatment. That morning she was very anxious. She broke her fast, begging some food from another patient. The treatment had to be postponed until the next morning.

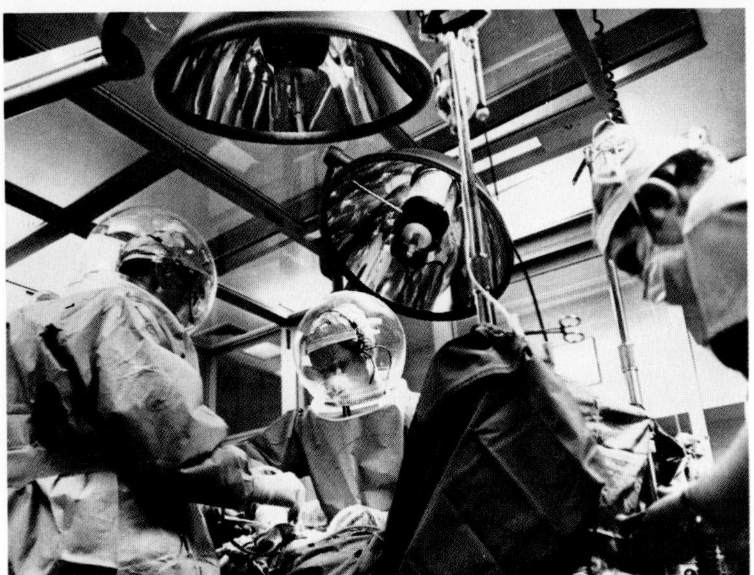

Fig. 17-1. The "space suits" above are a NASA spin-off and are now being experimented with in surgery. The suits reduce bacterial contamination and give the surgeon the freedom of working without a face mask. (Medical World News)

That morning she made her stand. In a fit of anxious and bizarre rage she screamed that she would have no further ECT.[5] "That machine was torture," she yelled. "I won't let you touch me again." She leaped for the door, but it was locked. She turned to flee from the staff who had gathered around her. The psychiatrist tried to explain to her that the treatment would make her well again; that even though they were unpleasant right now, they were really best for her. Every means of persuasion was used, but she was adamant.

In the staff meeting the debate was heated, but the decision was made. After explaining again the need for the treatment, the nursing staff, under the direction of the psychiatrist giving the treatment, restrained her and carried her to the treatment room.[6]

The Contributions of Space Medicine to Health

A major contribution of the space program is that it has stimulated the field of medicine to refocus from its traditional preoccupation with the ill to concerns for defining health and ways of maintaining it. It became important to know the physiological limitations of man and how to maintain normal body functioning under a variety of conditions and environments. Related to the basic objective of maintaining health is the area of nutrition. Initially low residue diets were developed for short space flights to keep digestive wastes to a minimum. As longer flights were planned, it became necessary to determine minimum food requirements and to recycle digestive wastes into reusable forms. Unusual forms of food such as algae and bacteria are being investigated for this purpose. The diets and foods developed for astronauts are already being used for patients confined to bed for long periods of time and are expected to make a contribution to artificial feeding techniques.

The use of communications science in the field of medicine has been given impetus by the space program. It is now possible to practice medicine at great distances as a result of the improved use of communications technology. This was graphically demonstrated when one of the astronauts became ill during a flight to the moon. The diagnosis and remedial action was effected by a physician many thousand miles away. Such technology is now being applied on earth, getting high-level medical care to areas where it would not normally be found. The potential for making medical expertise available to countries where medical personnel are in short supply is particularly great.

During takeoff and reentry the forces of acceleration and deceleration make it impossible for astronauts to move their arms or legs. It was found that the only parts of the body they could move were their eyeballs. To make it possible for the astronauts to operate switches during these periods of time, a device was developed that would respond to eyeball movement. This device is now seen as applicable to the disabled person. It would enable him to call a nurse, open a door, turn lights on or off solely

[5] ECT = electroconvulsive therapy.

[6] Robert M. Veatch, "Informed Consent: When Can It Be Withdrawn?" The Hastings Center Report, Institute of Society, Ethics and the Life Sciences, Vol. 2, No. 3 (June 1972).

Fig. 17-2. *Originally developed to measure the impact of very small meteorites on space craft, this device has been modified to detect muscle tremors and may be used to diagnose the early symptoms of Parkinson's disease and possibly serve as a monitor during neurosurgery. (USIS/WHO Photo)*

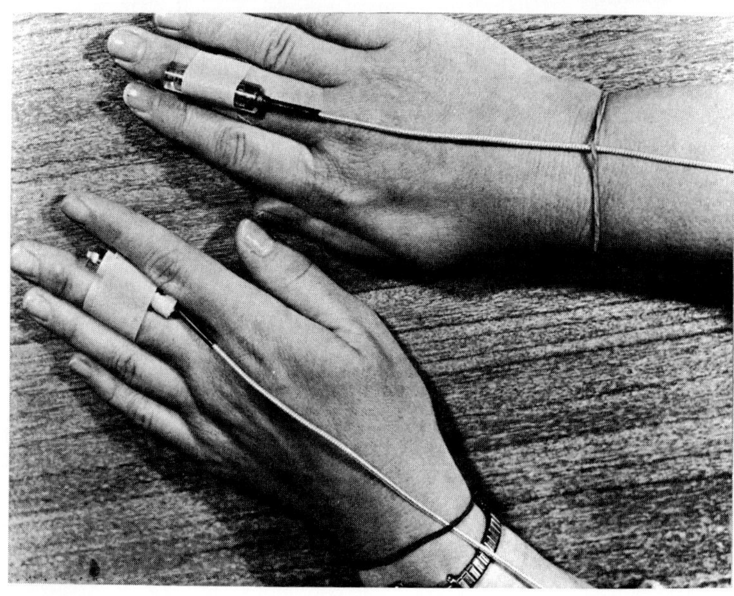

Fig. 17-3. *Space exploration has led to the invention of many devices that act like living sense organs. This cane emits light beams to detect obstacles. Here a blind man uses it to scan the area in front of him. (USIS/WHO Photo)*

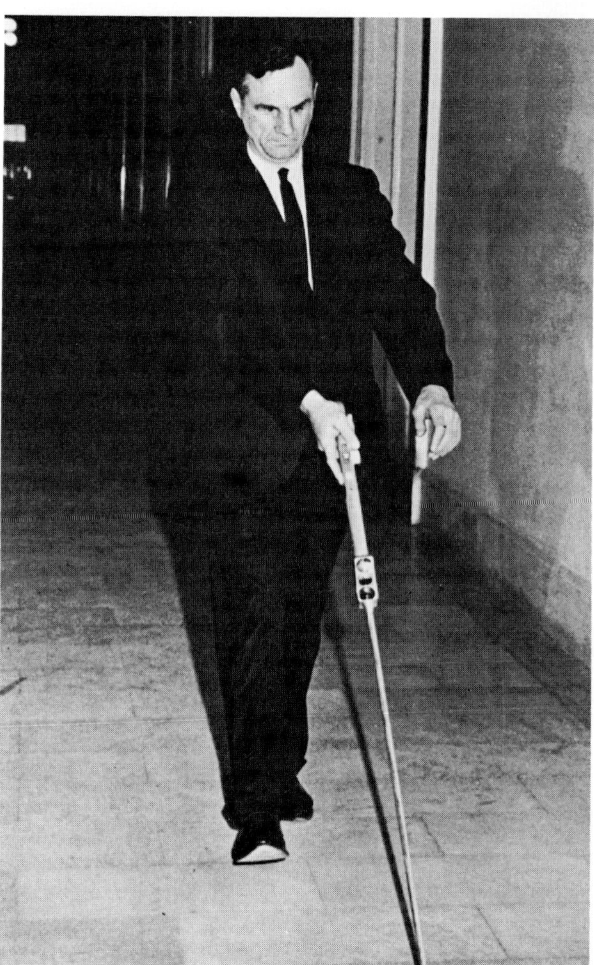

through the movement of his eyes. A motorized chair has even been developed that can be made to operate in this way.

The Spare Parts Department

"The inconceivable has become conceivable, and in the 20th century we find ourselves, indeed, patching human beings together out of parts. We sew on detached arms, and fix shattered hips in place with metal spikes; we patch arterial tubing with plastic; we borrow corneas from the dead, and kidneys from the living or dead; automatic, rechargeable pacemakers placed under the skin regulate the heartbeat, and radio receivers placed in the brain case may shortly control behavior; there are artificial limbs, artificial lungs, artificial kidneys and artificial hearts."[7]

Researchers working on the development of an artificial heart believe that the replacement of a diseased heart by a mechanical substitute will be routine in the future. Various models are currently in the animal experimentation phase and have maintained life in animals from 18 to 51 hours. Some are run on compressed air, others on fluid or electricity. Scientists are even thinking in terms of atomic-powered hearts.

[7] Willard Gaylin, "We Have the Awful Knowledge to Make Exact Copies of Human Beings," *New York Times Magazine*, March 5, 1972.

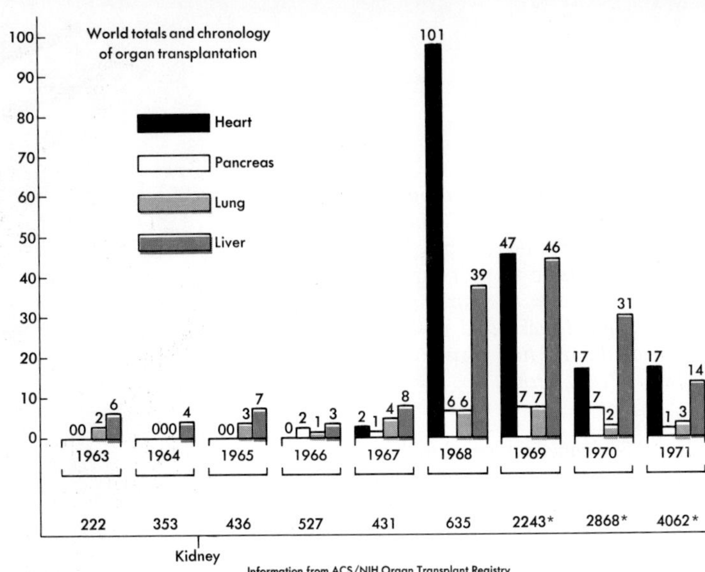

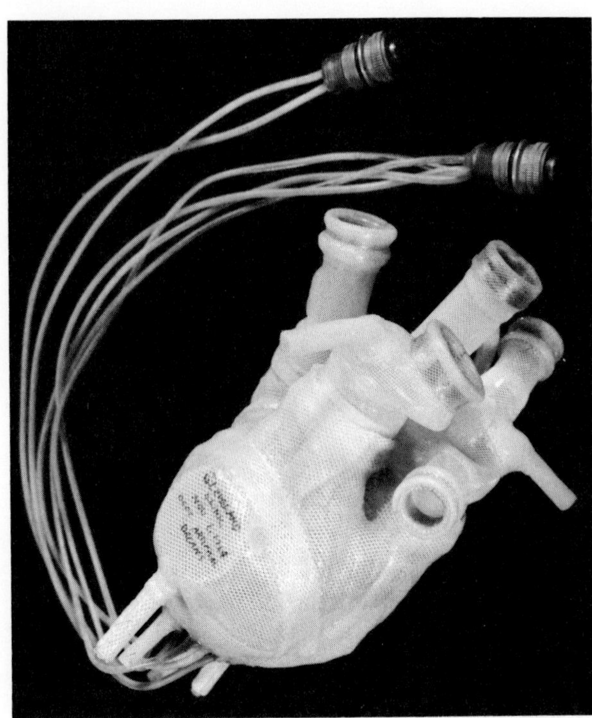

Fig. 17-5. By 1964, the two blood pumps of the Kolff air-driven sac-type artificial heart were constructed as a single unit, and experimental trials in calves had commenced. The latest version of this experimental total heart replacement undergoes continued developmental studies at the Cleveland Clinic Foundation, Cleveland, Ohio, with the aid of National Heart Institute research grant funds. (National Institutes of Health)

Already in use are heart boosters that aid in reducing the work load of diseased hearts. The heart-assist device, or booster, developed by Dr. Michael DeBakey and his associates at the Baylor University School of Medicine is designed to temporarily take over the function of the left ventricle during emergency periods such as heart surgery or a heart attack. The pump was used successfully to assist a patient for ten days following heart-valve surgery, after which she was successfully weaned from the device. Dr. Adrian Kantrowitz, has also developed a heart-assist device that works on a different principle from the DeBakey device. Work toward improvement of these devices continues so that clinical trials will not be as limited as they have been in the past. This work is laying the groundwork for the ultimate use of permanent heart-assist devices and ultimately a total mechanical heart replacement.

The years of 1968 to 1969 will go down in history as the era of the heart transplant. The startling news from South Africa that Dr. Christian Barnard had transplanted a human heart from a *dead*[8] man to the heart-diseased dentist Philip Blaiberg resounded around the world. The floodgates had been thrust open and in the year 1968, 102 heart transplants were

[8] "dead"—As a result of the era of heart and other organ transplants legislatures in more than 40 states developed laws establishing new definitions of death. The American Medical Association has also developed guidelines for physicians contemplating transplants. In June 1972 a jury in Richmond, Virginia, returned the verdict that death occurs with the cessation of brain function and not pulmonary or heart function. It gave legal sanction to the concept of brain death.

Fig. 17-4. *The chart shows the extent to which the number of kidney transplants exceeds all other organ transplants.* (National Institutes of Health)

performed. The happenings of this era bordered on the incredible. Heart-diseased patients encamped themselves in motels near a hospital that performed heart transplants. They constituted the waiting list for donor hearts. The wailing of an ambulance siren toward the hospital always raised the hopes of the heart-diseased patients. Perhaps this victim of a motorcycle accident or gunshot wound would die and be the donor of his needed heart. The initial enthusiasm for this procedure began to wane when it was realized that though the surgical techniques were sound and successful, physicians could not prevent the patient's rejection of the new "foreign" heart. It had been assumed that the heart would be initially struggled against, but with the aid of medications be tolerated and finally accepted, as had been demonstrated to a greater degree with kidney transplants. The year 1969 saw only 48 transplants and by 1970 the number dwindled down to 16. As of June 1973, of the 231 persons receiving donor hearts, there were 32 survivors, 5 of which will be celebrating their fifth anniversary. The physician who has had the most success with the heart transplant procedure is Dr. Norman Shumway of Stanford University, who has 23 survivors out of 60 cases. His success has been attributed more to his ability to control rejection of the heart by the body than to unusual surgical technique. One of the significant gains made from the transplant era was that for the first time in history fresh human heart tissue as well as newly removed diseased hearts were available for microscopic and biochemical examinations. In one study it was found that a chemical imbalance was

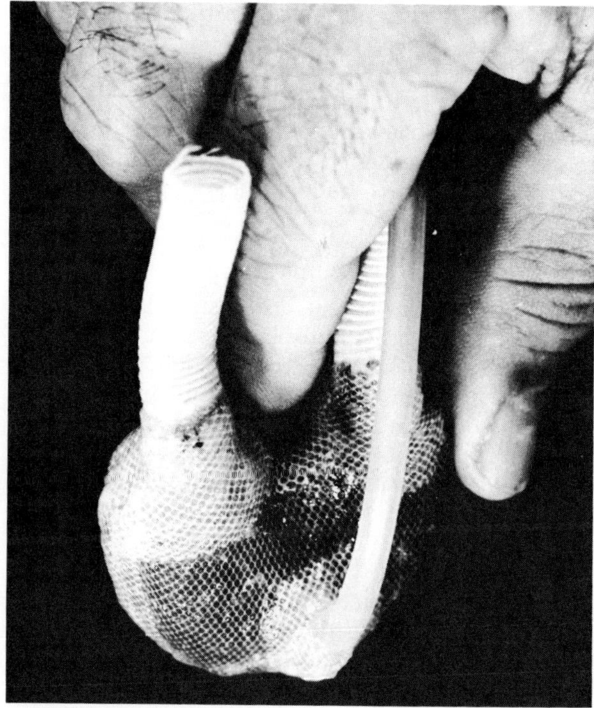

Fig. 17-6. *A heart-assist device (Kantrowitz Mechanical Auxiliary Ventricle—MAV) developed for use in humans by Dr. Adrian Kantrowitz, Adjunct Professor of Surgery, Wayne State University, Detroit. Within a hard outer shell of fabric mesh embedded in silicone rubber is an inner chamber of similar but flexible material which is compressed by air supplied through a plastic tube.* (National Institutes of Health)

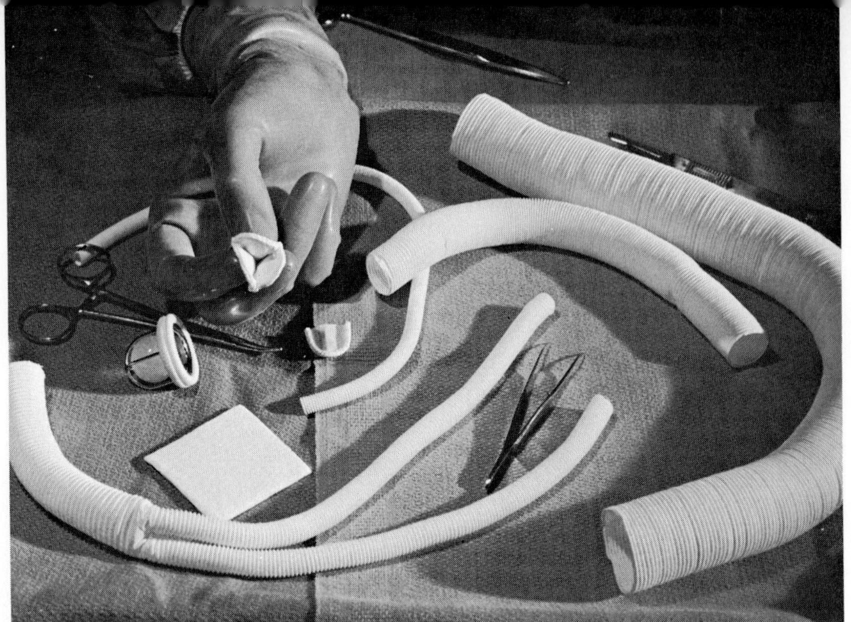

Fig. 17-7. National Heart Institute surgeons repair many once fatal or disabling defects in the heart and vascular system with modern artificial devices, including synthetic valves, vessels, and patches. In the picture a square of teflon patch material and varisized teflon blood vessels surround three artificial valves. (National Institutes of Health)

present in all diseased tissue. Further study of diseased hearts in dogs and rabbits revealed the same imbalance. The development of drugs or hormones to prevent this imbalance are now being studied. The moral, legal, sociological, and medical questions raised during this period will keep the philosophers, lawyers, sociologists, and physicians pondering for many a decade.

Traditionally the definition for death has been in terms of the absence of the heart beat and respiration. The redefinition of *death* stimulated by the introduction of heart transplants is now in terms of neurological death. A person can now be declared legally dead when brain injury results in the irreparable loss of brain function, even though the heart and lung function can be maintained by artificial means. Death is therefore being defined in terms of the loss of a vital organ that cannot be transplanted, namely the brain.

Transplants of the heart and lungs in tandem have already been attempted, while kidney transplants are rapidly becoming routine. Transplants of the cornea of the eye have of course been done for years. It thus is possible for a person to walk down the street with someone else's heart, lungs, kidney, and cornea, with synthetic tubing for blood vessels, and a questioning look on his face, asking "Who am I?" One can foresee the day when brain transplants become possible. The previous question would then have profound meaning. A quadriplegic (paralysis of all four limbs) could become the candidate for a new body—or a person whose brain was irreparably injured in an automobile accident could be a candidate for a new brain. The identity problem could stump even the surviving patient's psychiatrist. It might prove to be man's long-yearned-for dream of combining youth and maturity by placing a 40-year-old brain in a 20-year-old body.

As organ transplants become more routine the problems related to supply and demand inevitably begin to surface. Such has been the case with kidney transplants. The increased expertise in this transplant area has resulted in a shortage of kidney donors. A letter to the editor of *Today's Health* magazine offers a possible solution.

New Source of Kidney Donors?

In your December, 1972 issue Dr. Belding Scribner ("Health Criticism: An Action Plan to Help Kidney Patients,") mentioned that no country in the world gets more than 30 percent of the kidneys it needs for transplants.

Passing out donor cards for people to fill out and carry in their wallets apparently isn't working, probably due to the inertia we all have.

The best source for these donor organs would be the many thousands of healthy people who die every year in auto accidents. Why can't our state motor vehicle departments perform a public service by printing a donor agreement on the backs of all new drivers' licenses to be filled out by those people wishing to donate organs after their deaths?

Donald Lieberman, M.D.
Santa Clara, California[9]

The suggested plan may result in increased numbers

[9] *Today's Health* (March 1973), p. 72.

Fig. 17-8. *A fifty-year-old manager of a Paris photographic agency is one of the few people in the world with an atomic (plutonium 238) powered pacemaker. She leads a normal, active life.* (*WHO photo—Paul Almasy*)

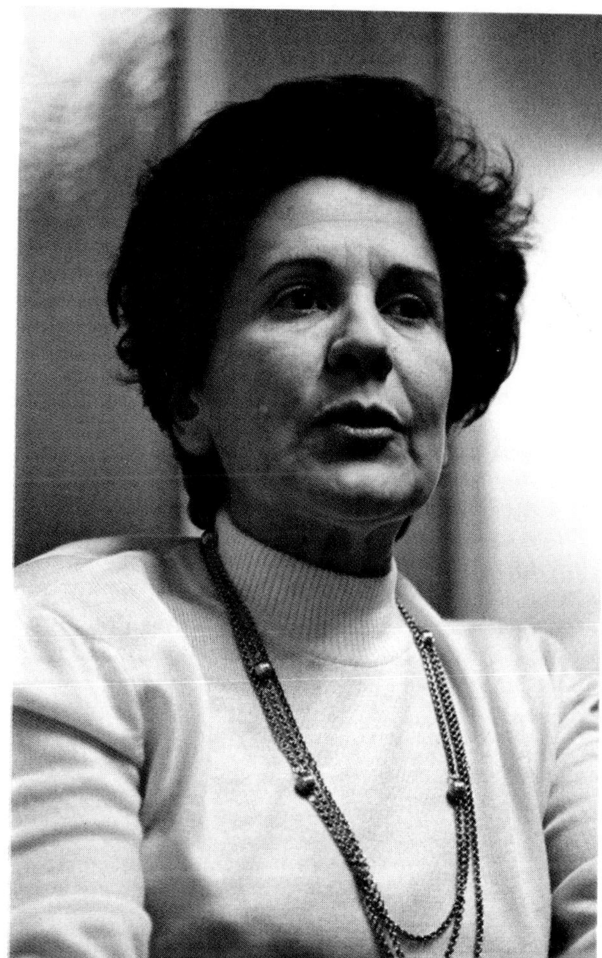

of donated kidneys as well as other needed organs. It might also result in more careful driving.

Synthetic tubing is now being used to replace diseased arteries. Where large aneuryisms (dilation of the blood vessel due to the weakening of the arterial wall) are found in major arteries such as the aorta, extensive Dacron or Teflon tubing is used to replace the damaged portion of the blood vessel. Artificial heart valves have been successfully implanted in thousands of people. There has also been the successful transplant of heart valves from cadavers to cardiac patients. The implantation of these valves has been made largely possible by the development of the remarkable heart-lung machine.

Artificial pacemakers have been successfully implanted to maintain a regular heart rhythm in those persons whose natural pacemaking mechanisms have been impaired. Many of these battery-powered electronic devices are implanted under the skin of the abdomen with the wiring connected internally to the heart. Before the two- to three-year life of the battery runs out, it can be replaced in a doctor's office under local anesthesia. Most pacemakers have a fixed-rate (usually 80 beats per minute); however, some of the newer, more sophisticated models make allowance for faster rates to meet the body's needs during exertion. These are highly reliable mechanisms; however, to date their failure has come from breaks in the stainless steel or platinum iridium wires that convey the pacing pulses to electrodes implanted in the heart. A new alloy developed (Elgiloy) may prove to withstand prolonged stresses better than any previously used. The need for wire electrodes is completely eliminated by a radio-frequency pacemaker developed at Yale University. A transmitter worn outside the body beams radio energy through the intact chest wall to a tiny receiver implanted in the pericardium, thus eliminating the need for minor surgery to replace worn-down batteries.

Scientists are currently in the process of developing artificial eyes. It has been known for years that the stimulation of the visual cortex of the brain can create the illusion of a point of light. Scientists have thus been working on a visual prosthesis (artificial eyes) that would make the points of light form a meaningful pattern—or sight. The visual prosthesis has to be connected directly to the brain of the blind person. A number of questions are being heatedly discussed by scientists involved. For example, is it ethically responsible to do research that involves possible brain damage? It is difficult to work with experimental animals in this case because animals cannot describe what they see. A danger is that the electrodes might cause heat damage to the brain as well as psychological trauma from hallucinatory effects that might be stimulated. A final question, what will be the effect of its availability on those blind persons who have made an acceptable adjustment to blindness?

In Conclusion

In 1971 the Italian Ministry of Health banned ovary transplants after an apparently successful operation. The action was taken because it raised the question of legal parentage. A child born after an ovary transplant would genetically be the child of the donor mother, while the woman who bore the child would also be the mother in another sense. When a woman donates an ovary, does she give up all legal rights to any offspring by the recipient mother? Or, in donating her ovary is she really asking another woman to serve as the bearer of her children, so her professional work would not be disturbed by childbirth? The father in the case would also have to examine his status with either or both women and/or motives in the situation. In the absence of legal studies or precedents in this area or societal preparedness for the implications of ovary transplants, the action of the Ministry of Health in this instance was to ban further transplants.

The above is perhaps symptomatic of a societal state of affairs where we wait until problem situations develop and then belatedly try to react to them. Our history is filled with such examples. The Federal Food, Drug and Cosmetic Act of 1938 was passed to protect the consumer only after an untested toxic drug was put on the market that killed 108 people. Alcoholism and drug abuse had to reach epidemic proportions before attention was paid to them. The responses in many instances were of the Keystone Cops variety with people running off in confused disorientation, so that it became difficult to tell who was drunk and drugged and who was confused and hysterical. When problems are not anticipated or given definition through early public discussion, inappropriate individual and societal reactions become highly predictable. As a society we have also permitted lung cancer and emphysema to reach epidemic proportions before reacting to them. We have allowed wanton destruction of large portions of our environment. We have been disease- and problem-oriented and too willing to pick up the pieces. We have permitted tragedy and disaster to serve as a roadmark for progress. It is time to recognize that it represents a bankrupt type of approach. The health problems of the future (near future) will become increasingly sophisticated—and potentially destructive. We can no longer afford the "luxury" of permitting problems to develop; rather, we need to begin to anticipate problems and prevent them in the first place. In applying this principle it would seem that before a new packaging material is allowed on the market, methods for recycling the material also must be developed. When the need for new public policy is predictable as a result of impending research results, public discussion should be initiated at the earliest possible moment.

The dramatic research developments that include the areas of genetic engineering, behavior control, organ transplants, and the production of synthetic body parts bring with them enormous implications for the future of man. The moral, social, psychological, and political impact of these developments make our present-day problematic decisions seem rather bland by comparison. It is time that earnest efforts were made to resolve our current health concerns. Concomittantly we need to call a public forum to initiate discussion so that the basis of public knowledge can be developed to prepare man to make the most difficult decisions he has ever been called upon to make—decisions that heretofore have been left with nature and God. At issue is who will make the ultimate decisions: a scientific elite, a prevailing political group, or an informed public? We have already delayed longer than is prudent to communicate publicly the nature of the knowledge and decision making that will shortly be needed. We dare delay no longer lest the tremendous advances in the health and life sciences leave us in stammering confusion. The moment of decision is at hand.

Review Questions

1. If genetic cloning were to become a possibility for humans, should its use be permitted? If so, under what circumstances?
2. Behavior control efforts are probably as old as man himself. Why, then, is the topic of behavior control now presenting ethical questions and dilemmas?
3. What are the implications of man's increasing ability to transplant organs and develop synthetic replacements for body parts?
4. In view of the remarkable and rapid development in the areas of the health and life sciences, why is public discussion so vital if disastrous results are to be avoided?

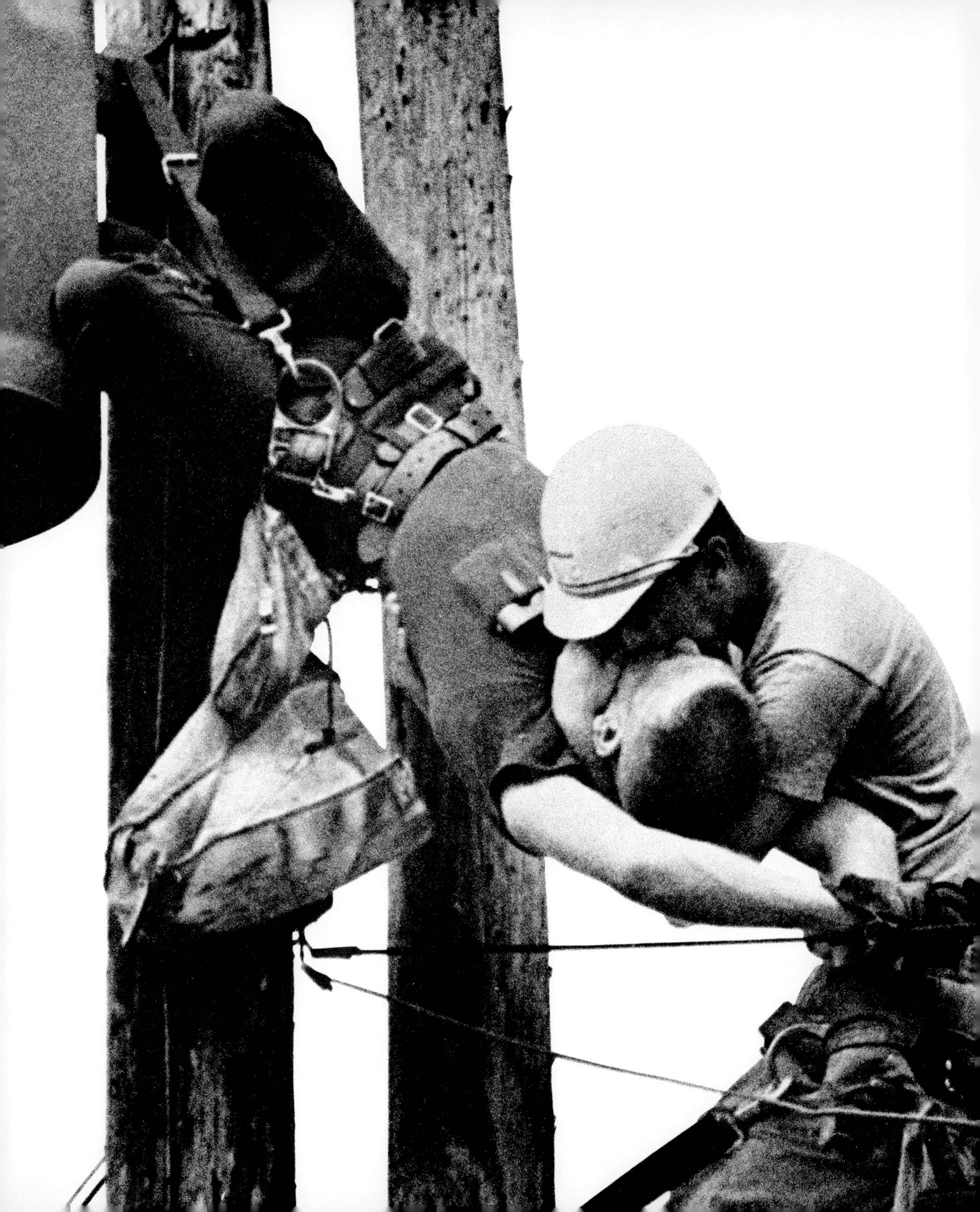

Appendix A
Emergency First Aid

Artificial Respiration

An adult at rest breathes about 18 times a minute, taking in about a pint of air with each breath.

Breathing may stop as a result of gas or drug poisoning, electric shock, choking, drowning, suffocation, injuries to the head, neck, or chest, poliomyelitis, or convulsions.

Most persons can live only about 6 minutes after breathing stops. Artificial respiration must begin as soon as possible after natural breathing has been interrupted or when natural breathing is so irregular or shallow as to be ineffective.

Artificial respiration is a method of getting air into and out of a person's lungs until he can breathe for himself. It is a lifesaving measure.

Mouth-to-Mouth Method

One of the simplest and most effective ways to give artificial respiration is by the mouth-to-mouth (or mouth-to-nose) method. This method is effective for both children and adults and can be used even when there are injuries to the chest and arms.

Here is how to do it:

1. Place the person who has stopped breathing on his back.
2. Open his mouth and clear out any foreign matter such as food or dirt, with your fingers or a cloth wrapped around your fingers. If the person has false teeth, remove them.
3. Tilt his head back so that his chin points upward and lift his lower jaw from beneath and behind so that it juts out. This moves the base of the tongue away from the back of the throat, so it does not block the air passage to the lungs. *Unless this air passage is open, no amount of effort will get air in.*

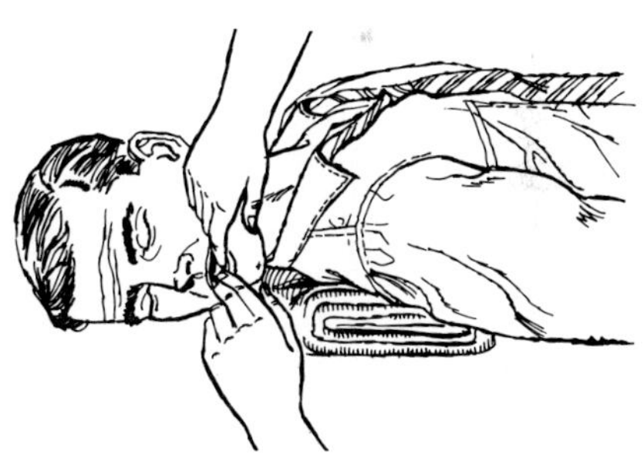

4. You can blow air into a person's lungs through either his mouth or nose. Open your mouth wide and place it tightly over the person's mouth. Pinch his nostrils shut. Or close the victim's mouth and place your mouth over his nose. *With an infant or small child, place your mouth over both his nose and mouth, making an airproof seal.* Air can be blown through an unconscious person's teeth even though they may be clenched.
5. Blow into the mouth or nose, continuing to hold the unconscious person's lower jaw so that it juts out to keep the air passage open.
6. Remove your mouth from the patient's mouth.

__A.__ Before starting any type of artificial respiration be sure that the mouth and throat are completely clear of mucus and foreign objects. Use your fingers to clean the mouth. You may cover fingers with a piece of cloth to help remove mucus and slippery objects. __B.__ The head must be tipped back to allow a free air passage with the jaw held in a jutting out position. The more you can achieve the "sword swallower" position the better. __C.__ Remember—Don't blow too hard. Your mouth and the mouth of the person receiving treatment should be wide open with a complete seal between them. Inhale more than usual before exhaling into person's mouth. In this way he will get more oxygen. __D.__ Pinching the nostrils prevents air from escaping through the nose. With your right hand be sure to hold the jaw in a jutting out position. __E.__ This is the mouth-to-nose type of respiration with lips being sealed by the two fingers of the right hand. This would be used when an obstruction is in the mouth that cannot be removed, or a severe mouth injury prevents proper contact.

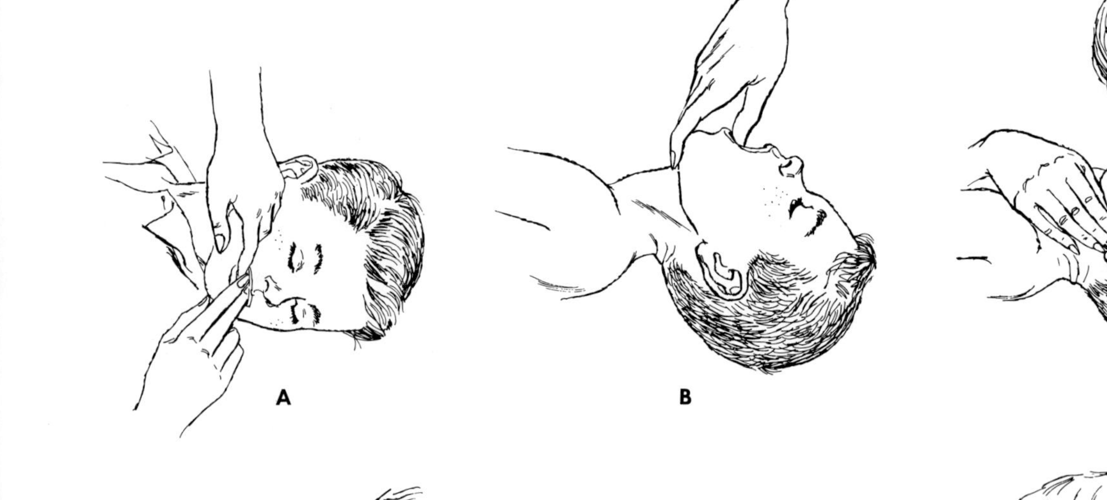

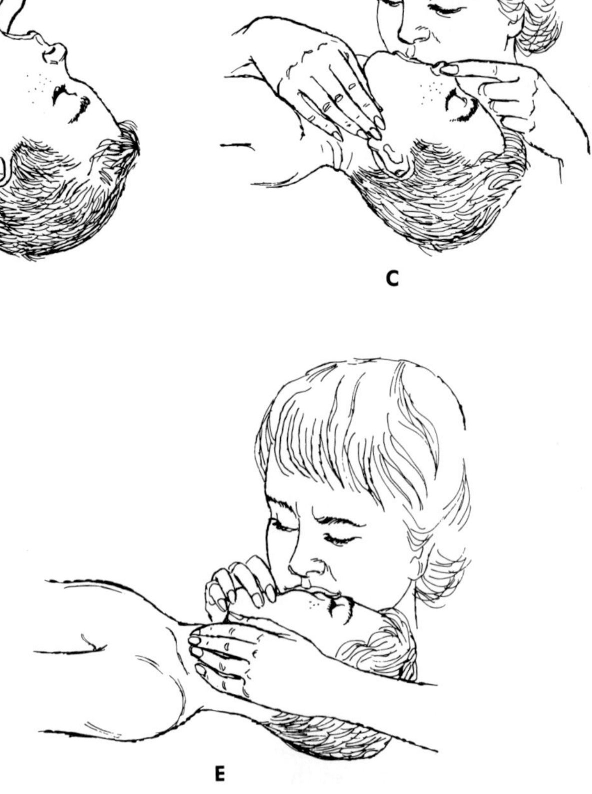

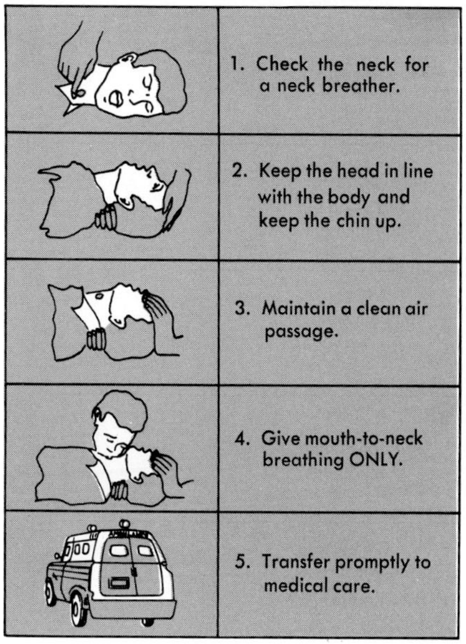

1. Check the neck for a neck breather.

2. Keep the head in line with the body and keep the chin up.

3. Maintain a clean air passage.

4. Give mouth-to-neck breathing ONLY.

5. Transfer promptly to medical care.

Mouth-to-Neck Respiration (reproduced by permission of the International Association of Laryngectomies, sponsored by: The American Cancer Society, Inc. Copyright issued to American Cancer Society, Inc.)

Turn your head to the side and listen for the return outflow of air coming from the patient's lungs. If you hear it, you will know that an exchange of air has occurred.

7. You can then continue your breathing for the patient. Blow vigorously into his mouth or nose about 12 times each minute. Remove your mouth after each breath and listen for the exchange of air. In the case of an infant or child, blow less vigorously, using shallower breaths about 20 times a minute.
8. If you are not getting an exchange of air, turn the person on his side and strike him several times between the shoulder blades, using considerable force. This will help dislodge any obstruction in the air passages. Check the position of the head and jaw. Again make sure there is no foreign matter in his mouth. If you wish to avoid direct contact, you may hold a cloth (piece of gauze, handkerchief, or other material) over the victims' mouth or nose, and breathe through it. The cloth does not greatly affect the exchange of air. However, do not waste precious seconds looking for a cloth if one is not handy.

Normal breathing may sometimes start up again after 15 seconds of artificial respiration. But if it doesn't, you should continue the procedure until you are positive life is gone. Alternate with other persons, if possible, so as to maintain maximum efficiency. Cases of electric shock, and drug or carbon monoxide poisoning may require artificial respiration for long periods.

The first signs of restored breathing may be a sigh. There may be irregular breathing at first. Artificial respiration should be continued until regular breathing occurs.

When normal breathing resumes, the person usually recovers rapidly. But he should rest for several hours. Then he may gradually return to normal activities unless other injuries exist.

Mouth-to-Neck Method

A laryngectomee or individual who has lost his larynx (voice box) requires some modification of the resuscitation technique. These individuals breathe through openings in their necks either completely or partially. The *total* laryngectomee does not breathe from his nose or mouth at all; all his air is drawn in from the neck opening (or stoma). In resuscitating this person, therefore, placing the mouth and lips tightly over the neck opening and blowing into the stoma should make the chest rise. If the chest fails to rise and the rescuer hears air escaping from the victim's nose or mouth, he can assume the victim is a *partial neck breather.* In this case the mouth must be closed and the nose pinched during the mouth-to-neck resuscitation.

Back-Pressure Arm-Lift Method

1. Place person who has stopped breathing in position shown on the following page.

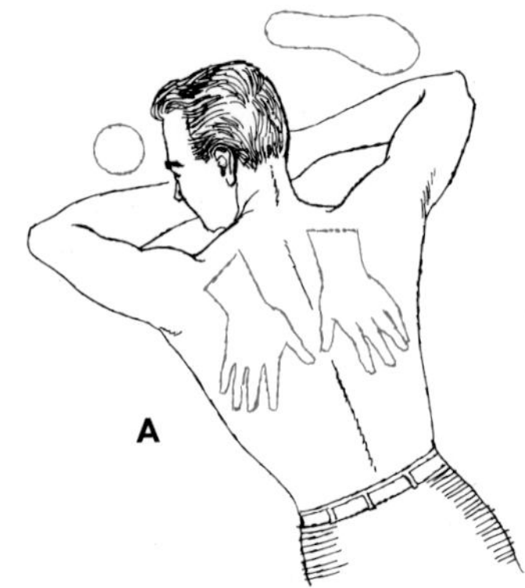

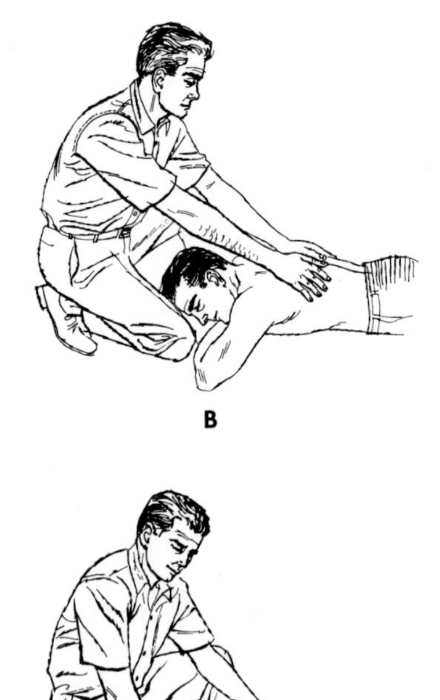

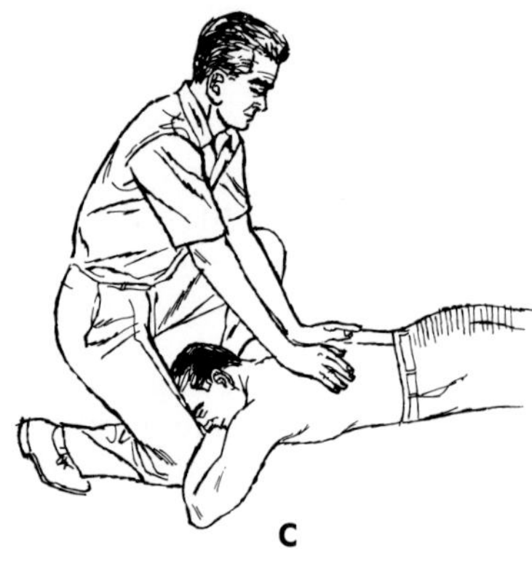

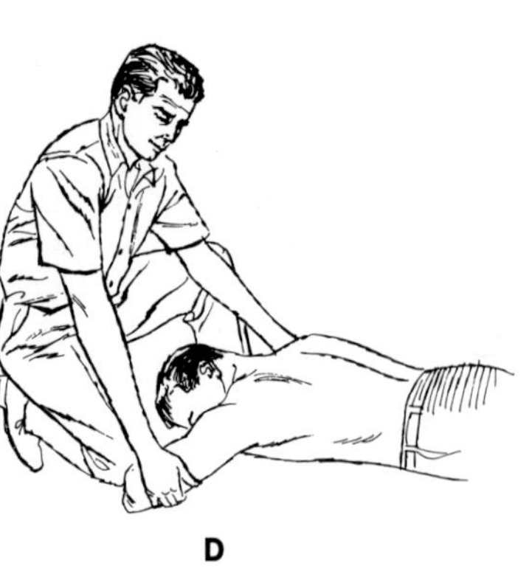

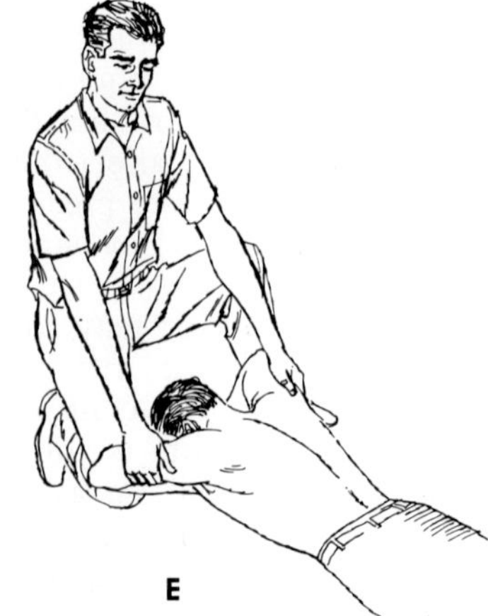

A. *This picture shows the correct position of the knee, foot, and hands in the first step of back pressure armlift method. The knee and foot may be alternated to make it less tiring for the person administering this type of artificial respiration.* ***B.*** *With hands in correct position the operator starts a rocking forward motion. Note that elbows are straight and stiff. This is when you start the timing. Chant: "Press—Release"—"Lift—Release." Say it in time to your own breathing.* ***C.*** *With arms almost vertical direct pressure is applied to the back.* Do not use quick, *jerking pressure. Use* Smooth even pressure. *Release the pressure in the same smooth way. Pull your hands away slowly.* ***D.*** *As the operator rocks back to his original position he grasps each arm just above the elbow. This is the next part of the timing. Chant: "Lift—Release." Slow—Regular—Even.* ***E.*** *The operator continues to rock back lifting the arms up and toward him. This is the end of one cycle. He will next place his hands in correct position on the back and start over again.*

TUBE WEARER

EMERGENCY!

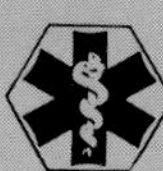

I am a Total Neck Breather
(Laryngectomee—No Vocal Cords)

I breathe ONLY through an opening in my neck, NOT through my nose or mouth.

If I have stopped breathing:

1. Expose my entire neck.
2. Give me **mouth to neck breathing only.**
3. Keep my head straight—chin up.
4. Keep neck opening clear with clean CLOTH (not tissue).
5. Use oxygen supply to neck opening, ONLY, when I start to breathe again.

BE PROMPT—SECONDS COUNT
I NEED AIR NOW!

(See other side)

2. Clear mouth and throat.
3. Start artificial respiration immediately.

The back-pressure, arm-lift method of artificial respiration is the second most desirable method. It should be used only when injuries to the head or face prevent the use of mouth-to-mouth or mouth-to-nose method.

Bleeding and Bandaging

What to Do

1. Apply dressing or pad directly over wound.
2. Apply direct even pressure—use your bare hand if necessary when bleeding is serious, and dressing not immediately available.
3. Leave dressing in place.
4. Continue pressure by applying bandage.
5. Secure bandage in place—check to be sure bandage is not too tight and cutting off circulation.
6. Elevate limb above heart level except where there is a possible broken bone.
7. Treat for shock.
8. IF BLOOD SOAKS THROUGH DRESSING DO NOT remove but apply more dressings.

ATTENTION!!

Do not use a tourniquet unless it is impossible to stop excessive life-threatening bleeding by any other method.

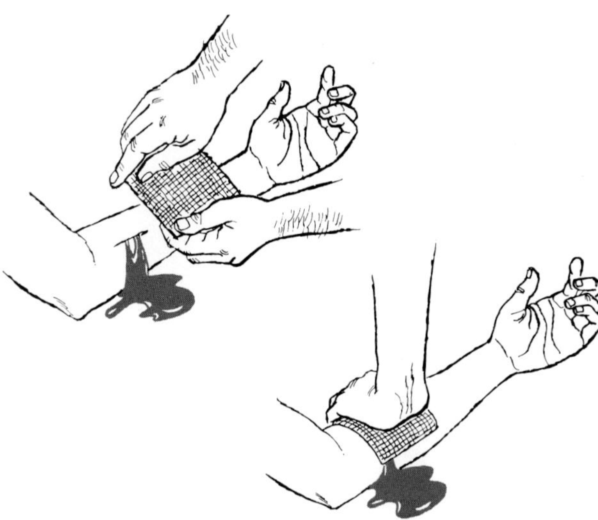

To stop bleeding apply dressing or pad directly over the wound and then apply pressure. Remember—immediate, direct pressure—even with the bare hand—is the important action to stop bleeding. Continue the pressure until the bleeding has stopped or slowed to the point that you will be able to apply a bandage. Don't be in a hurry to stop the pressure.

460 Excessive Bleeding

Bleeding needs immediate attention. Even the loss of small amounts of blood will produce weakness and can cause the condition known as shock. The loss of as much as a pint of blood by a child or a quart of blood by an adult may have disastrous results.

The first step in controlling bleeding is to exert direct pressure over the wound area. You can do this best by placing the cleanest material available (a pad of sterile gauze is best) against the bleeding point, and applying firm pressure with your hand until a bandage can be applied.

The cleaner the cloth, the better in preventing infection. But if sterile gauze is not handy, use a freshly laundered handkerchief, strip torn from a sheet, a shirt, slip, or a sanitary napkin.

The pad should be large enough to overlap the edges of the wound and, if possible, the pressure should be applied in a manner that brings the edges of the wound together.

When bleeding is serious you may have to use your bare hand while waiting for someone else to get material for a dressing. This can place dangerous germs in the wound and cause infection but it is obviously better to run the risk of infection than to let the person bleed to death.

Pressure should be applied evenly over the entire area of the wound. Properly applied, pressure squeezes broken blood vessels closed and helps clots to form; these block the blood vessels and prevent further loss of blood. However, if the pressure is unevenly applied, by bearing down with more force on one area of the wound, it may cause the bleeding to persist. Continue to apply pressure evenly until the bleeding stops.

After the bleeding has been controlled, do not remove the dressing from the wound, even though blood has saturated it. Simply apply additional layers

Apply the bandage firmly over the dressing to continue the pressure and thus continue to stop the bleeding. CAUTION—Check the bandage after you have tied the knot to be sure it is not too tight and is not cutting off circulation.

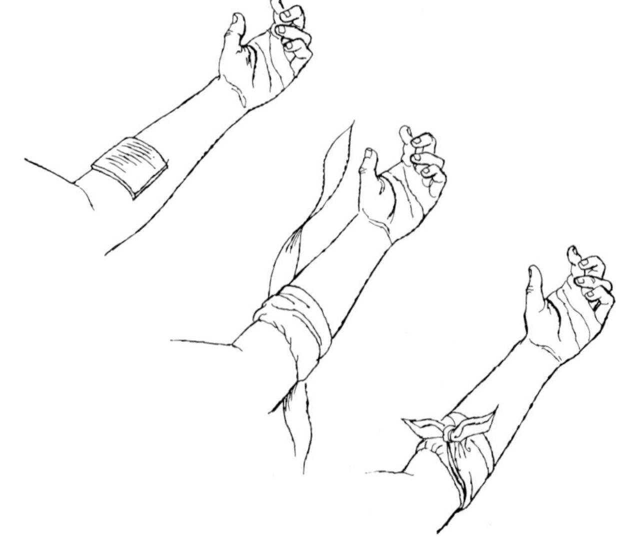

of cloth to form a good-sized covering and bandage snugly and firmly. The material you place directly over the wound (the dressing) should be sterile (if available), but the material to hold the dressing in place (the bandage) need not be sterile. If roller bandage is not available, strips from a sheet or shirt will do.

After a wound stops bleeding and the bandage is firmly in place, you can turn your attention to other important needs of the patient. Anyone who has lost much blood will need treatment for shock whether or not he shows signs of shock. (See "Shock.") In addition to this care, the wound area, if on an arm or leg, should be elevated on pillows.

A bandage that is too tight can cause further injury. Because of possible swelling around the wound, check the bandage periodically and loosen it if it seems to interfere with the circulation of the blood.

The patient should be kept warm and quiet. When his strength returns, allow him to resume normal activities gradually. At first, that means standing or walking for only 15 or 20 minutes in a morning or afternoon. Do not let him get tired.

Tourniquet Warning

The application of a tourniquet to control bleeding is mentioned here principally to discourage its use. It is dangerous to apply, dangerous to leave on, dangerous to remove. It will cause tissue injury and shut off the entire blood supply to the part below, causing gangrene and loss of the limb. A tourniquet is rarely required and should be used only for severe, life-threatening hemorrhage that cannot be controlled by other means.

Caring for Wounds

Injuries that break the skin are considered "wounds." In addition to damage to the tissues at the wound edge and possible blood loss, wounds are hazards to health since germs are always on the skin and can get in through a wound and cause serious infection.

If you take proper care of wounds as soon as they occur, you will cut down the possibility of serious infection.

You should wash the skin immediately around a wound gently with water and soap or detergent, using a piece of sterile gauze or clean cloth, wiping away from the wound. Do not touch the wound with your bare fingers.

After cleaning the wound area, cover it with a sterile dressing or folded clean cloth. Fix the dressing in place with a bandage or with strips of adhesive tape. For larger wounds where it is difficult to keep a dressing in place, a triangular bandage can be used.

If there is a possibility that the bone under the wound is broken, that part of the body should be kept completely still. This will reduce the possibility of delayed bleeding, prevent further injury, promote healing, and decrease pain and discomfort. (See "Broken Bones.")

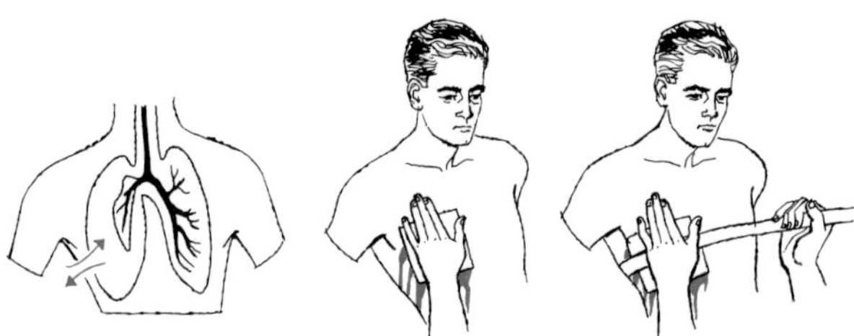

A sucking chest wound causes the lung to collapse. You must make the opening air-tight in order that the lung may continue to function properly. Place a dressing firmly over the wound and hold this pad or dressing securely in place. You must stop the air from passing through the wound.

462 Sucking Wounds in the Chest

"Sucking wounds" are chest wounds in which an opening may be created from the lungs to outside air. These wounds are caused by such injuries as crushing blows or penetrating objects. Air may enter and blow out of the wound with "sucking" or hissing sounds. Froth or bubbles may be seen. Cover this opening immediately. Put your hands at each side of the wound, push together, as victim breathes out, to cover the opening. Cover the wound with a sterile dressing, holding it firmly in place while bandaging to make it airtight. Have the patient lie down but keep his shoulders slightly raised, supported with pillows. Do not attempt to lessen shock by elevating his feet if doing so makes his breathing more difficult.

Infection in Wounds

Infection in a wound is easy to recognize. The wound will become red or discolored, swollen, painful, and at times pus will appear. The person may also appear sick and feverish. When the wound is on the arm or leg, red streaks may sometimes extend from the wound up the arm or leg and small tender lumps may appear in the armpit or groin, nearest the wound.

For the treatment of infected wounds, elevate the wound area on pillows. Keep the part at rest and apply warm packs to the wound area.

The warm packs are prepared by adding two teaspoonfuls of salt to a quart of water which has been boiled. Then cloths or towels are dipped in this solution and partially wrung out. The solution is kept warm but not so hot that it will burn the patient.

The warm packs are applied for 30 minutes and changed as often as is necessary during that time to maintain comfortable heat to the wound. These periods of warm packing are alternated with 30-minute free periods during which warm packs are not applied to the wound and it is allowed to dry.

This treatment is continued while the patient is awake and until the wound looks better. This may take several days.

The patient should be encouraged to take adequate food and fluid, eating and drinking as he wishes. Aspirin may be given for pain if necessary.

When the infection has subsided and the redness, swelling, and pus have decreased, you should still keep a sterile dressing over the wound. Dressings should be used until the would has healed.

Fractures and Splinting

What to Do

1. Look for bleeding and control it.
2. Whenever in doubt, treat as a fracture.
3. Apply the splint at the site of the accident.
4. Never move the person before splinting unless his life would be further in danger.
5. Prevent shock, further injury, and infection.
6. Splint securely enough to prevent any voluntary or involuntary motion at the point of fracture.

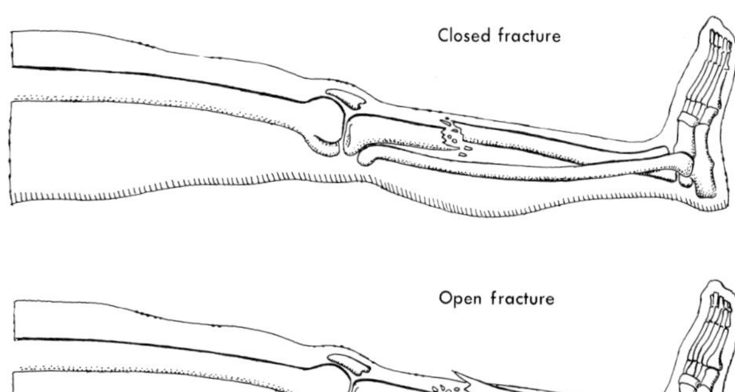

The top figure is a closed fracture but with improper handling it can very easily become a fracture such as you see in the bottom picture. All fractures or suspected fractures should be handled very carefully to avoid further injury.

7. Check splint ties frequently to be sure it does not interfere with circulation of blood.

In most cases of severe injury there is the possibility that the person may stop breathing. If this should occur stop all other lifesaving procedures and administer artificial respiration.

Broken Bones

Any break in a bone is called a fracture. If the ends of a broken bone do not come through the skin, the break is called a closed (or simple) fracture. If one or both ends of a broken bone come through the skin, the break is called an open (or compound) fracture. An open fracture is serious because germs can get in and cause infection.

In an open fracture, you will be able to see the wound where the bone breaks the skin. The bone itself may not be visible; it may slip back under the skin after breaking through.

In the case of a closed fracture, it is obviously more difficult to be sure that a break has occurred. One sign is pain at or near the break and tenderness and swelling around it. By running your finger gently along the bone, you may be able to feel an irregular piece of bone. A more obvious sign of a closed fracture may be the twisted or crooked unnatural position of an arm or leg or its appearance of being shorter than normal. The injured person may find it painful or impossible to move the limb.

Whenever there is any reason to believe that there may be a broken bone, treat the injury as though it actually is a fracture. Otherwise, you may cause further injury.

The important *first thing to do* is to prevent motion at the site of the break. This can be done by applying a splint to immobilize the broken bone ends. Do not move the injured person before this is done. Splint the break where he lies.

It may sometimes be necessary to straighten a limb slightly in order to apply a splint. To prevent movement of the broken bone ends while this is being done, one person should support the broken bone with his hands—one placed just above the break and one just below—while a *second person grasps the end of the limb and exerts a strong steady pull* to straighten it.

An exception to this preliminary immobilization of bone ends will be necessary in the case of an open fracture where a broken end of bone still sticks out of the wound. It cannot be left in that position. Allow it to slip back naturally under the skin when the limb is being straightened. Do not attempt to push it back in. Put on a sterile dressing to control bleeding and keep out germs. A clean sheet or towel can be used if necessary. Bandage the dressing in place with firm pressure. Then splint.

Splints can be made of almost any material that is rigid enough to give support to the fractured body part. They can be made of wood or metal, padded with cotton or cloth, or they can be improvised from umbrellas, tightly rolled newspapers, magazines, and blankets or pillows, if necessary. In applying splints see that they extend beyond the joint above and

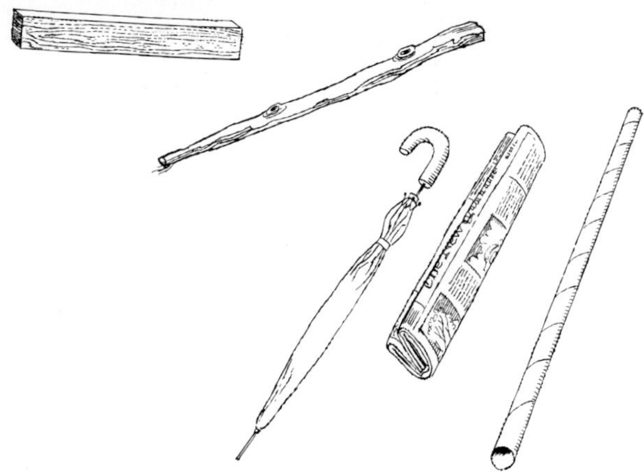

Here are just a few ideas of improvised materials to be used for splinting. Look around the room right now and see how many items you can find that could be used in the event of an emergency.

Apply splints so that they extend beyond the joints above and below the fracture.

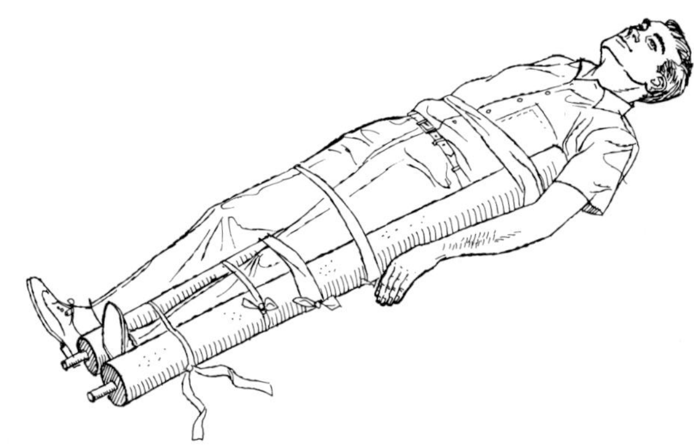

 below the fracture. Unless the joints are also immobilized in this way, they will move and disturb the broken bone.

Fasten a splint in place with bandages or strips of cloth, handkerchiefs, neckties, or belts. After splinting the limb, elevate it above the level of the heart with pillows.

Check bandage and splint fastenings at intervals to make sure that they are firm but not so tight that they cause swelling in the injured area or interfere with the circulation of blood. In doing this, do not remove the bandage from the wound because it might introduce infection or start bleeding. If the injured person complains that the arm or leg feels as though it is "asleep," this may be due to a splint that is too tight. Loosen the ties that hold the splint, or, if necessary, replace the splint. This will help the "asleep" feeling unless it is caused by internal damage other than the broken bone.

A broken collarbone can be immobilized by putting the arm on the side of the break in a sling (made with a triangular bandage) and then binding the arm close to the body.

If a triangular bandage is not available, you can make a sling by folding a large square cloth diagonally to make a triangle. Tie the ends around the neck. Let the fingers dangle outside the edge of the sling.

A broken rib should be suspected if a chest injury is accompanied by a sharp pain. The pain is usually located at the point of rib fracture and is increased markedly by the movements of the body, especially in breathing or coughing.

Swelling or deformity may sometimes be seen on thin individuals, but these signs are generally not visible.

Pain may be relieved by strapping the chest with long strips of two-inch adhesive tape. Start strapping from above the point of fracture and continue down the chest wall. Apply the strips so that they extend from a point on the unfractured side of the chest (about two inches beyond the midline in the back) over the fractured side of the chest to a point on the unfractured side in front (about two inches beyond the midline). When the strapping is finished, the adhesive strips should cover an area both above and below the tender spot.

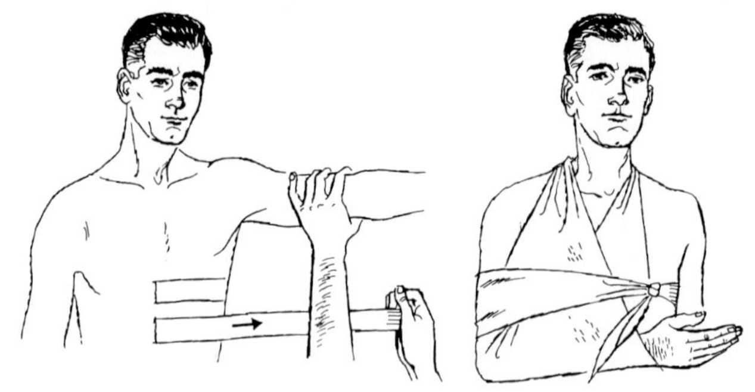

You will be able to strap the patient's chest properly if you have him blow the air out of his lungs before you apply the adhesive strips. If you can't finish strapping him before he needs to draw another breath, stop, let him take a small breath, and exhale again. Then complete your strapping.

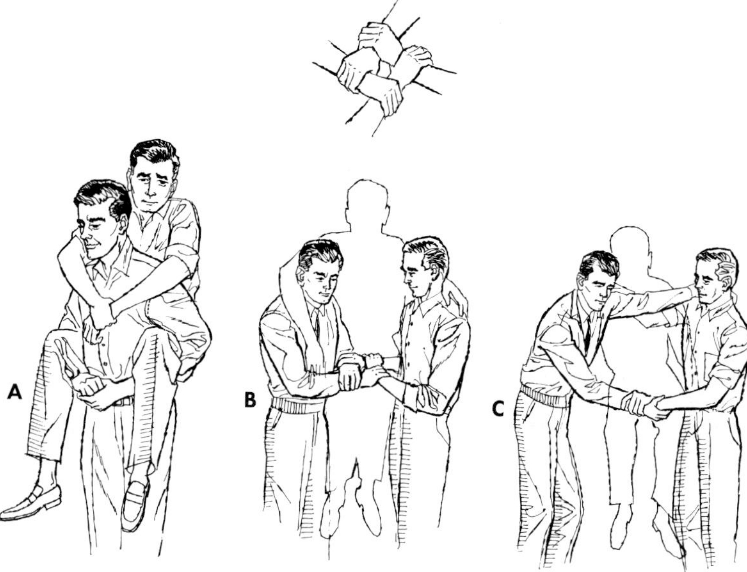

A. *This saddle-back carry is simple and effective for moving an injured person a short distance, when his injuries are not serious.* ***B.*** *The four-hand seat carry shown is an excellent method for carrying conscious, not too seriously injured persons a short distance.* ***C.*** *This is an effective method of carrying an unconscious injured person a short distance provided it is not necessary to keep him flat.*

Sprains

Sprains are injuries to the soft tissues surrounding the joints, usually occurring because of sudden movements beyond the normal range of a joint. Ligaments, muscle tendons, and blood vessels are stretched and occasionally torn. Ankles, fingers, wrists, and knees are most often affected.

A fracture of a bone may occur at the time of a sprain. Therefore, all severe sprains should be treated by splinting. First apply a bandage support, being careful not to make it so tight that it will interfere with the flow of blood (stop circulation). If possible, apply cold packs to the sprain during the first 30 minutes following injury. To retard swelling, all sprains should be elevated on pillows and the injured person kept quiet. Use of a sprained joint should not be allowed until such use can be carried out with little or no pain. Continue the bandage support of a sprained joint, such as the ankle, during the early period of walking or use.

Transportation of the Injured

What to Do

1. Before transporting any sick or injured person:
   Bleeding should be stopped.
   Breathing should be established.
   Fractures should be splinted.
   Shock should be treated.
   All other lifesaving methods completed.
2. Determine carefully the type and seriousness of the injuries and condition of the injured person.
3. Give complete emergency treatment *before moving* the injured.
4. Be gentle in moving the injured person; have enough help to assure safe moving.
5. Always carry a stretcher to an injured person, not the person to the stretcher.
6. Stretchers should be used for the more seriously injured persons and for transporting the injured over a long distance.
7. Be sure the person will not slip or fall from the stretcher while being carried. Belts or strong cloth bindings such as sheets may be used to secure the person to the stretcher.
8. Always use a two-man carry in preference to a one-man carry, if a hand carry is used. This helps to make the person being carried more comfortable, enables him to be carried farther, and is less likely to aggravate fractures or other serious injuries.
9. The various hand carries should not be used unless the person needs only slight support for short distances; or in case of emergencies where delay will endanger life. Examples—fire or explosion.

Transporting Injured Persons

Do not be in a hurry to move an injured person.

First aid authorities report that more harm is probably done through improper transportation of injured persons than through any other measure of

A. This is the first step in the correct method of using four people to load a seriously injured person on a stretcher. In this first step the fourth man does not touch the injured person. ***B.*** *The three persons now lift slowly and all together and roll the injured person gently toward them on injured side.* ***C.*** *The fourth man now places the stretcher into position and then assists in lowering the person into the stretcher. Even, slow motion assures greatest safety and comfort of the injured person.*

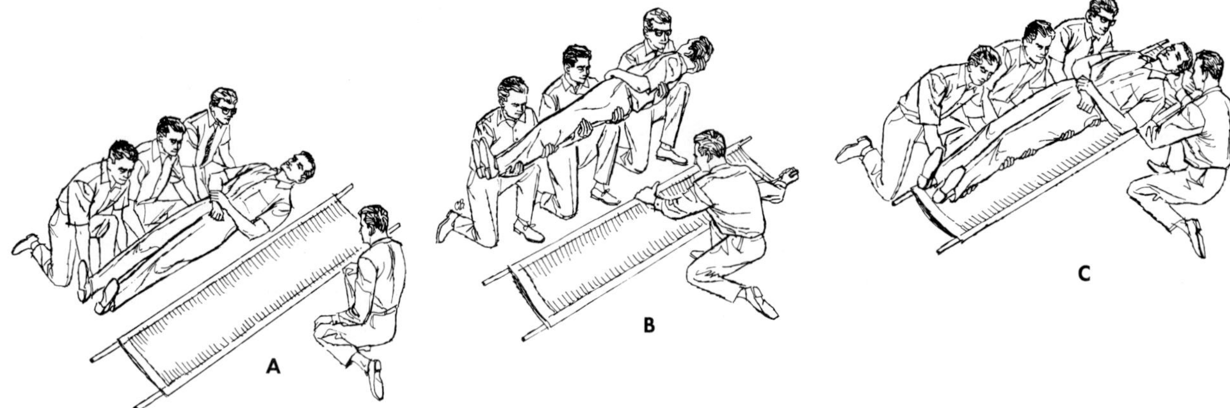

emergency assistance. The danger of causing paralysis or death in moving persons with head, back, or neck injuries has already been noted. Thus, before considering moving an injured person, except under the most urgent conditions, such as exposure to fire or fallout, you should make a careful check for all possible injuries so that you will know the right method of transporting him.

You should also make sure that bleeding is controlled, that the injured person is breathing satisfactorily, and that any possible broken bones have been splinted or, as in the case of neck or back fractures, are properly supported. Only then should you attempt to move him.

There are many ways of moving an injured person, depending upon the nature and location of injuries. Some of the most useful are illustrated. It is important to lift and carry a person gently, moving him slowly and carefully without jerky movements.

If it becomes absolutely necessary to move a person to safety *before* a thorough check of injuries can be made, you should try to *protect all parts of his body from the tension of lifting.* A body should never be jacknifed (lifted by head and heels only). Try to give adequate support to each extremity, to the head and the back, and to keep the entire body in a straight line.

If you are alone with an injured person who must be moved, and are unable to *carry* him, you may be able to *pull* him to safety. He should be pulled in the direction of the long axis of his body, not sideways. Danger of injuring him is less if a blanket (or similar object) can be placed under him, so that he can ride the blanket.

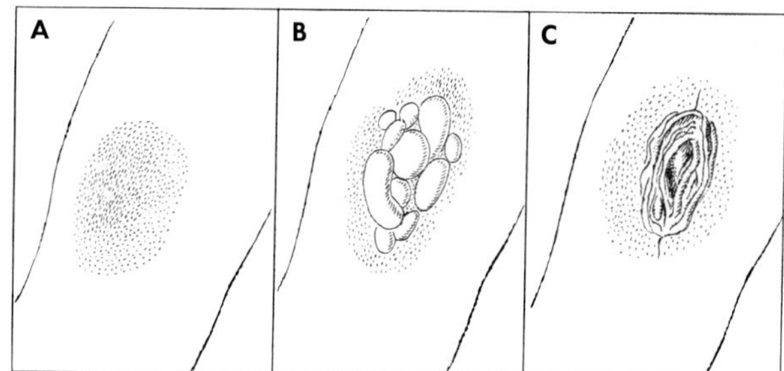

A. A first degree burn only reddens the skin and if it does not cover more than 25 per cent of the body, usually is not serious. ***B.*** *In second degree burns blisters develop and there is now the very real danger of infection. Extensive second degree burns will require giving additional fluids to the burned person. Do not apply grease or salve. Cover with sterile or clean dressing.* ***C.*** *Third degree burns even in a relatively small area are serious. The injury is deep and the underlying tissue has been destroyed. Keep this type of burn clean to avoid infection.*

Burns

What to Do

1. Treat for shock.
2. Relieve pain.
3. Prevent infection.
4. Cover burned area with dry sterile or clean cloth.
5. Encourage fluids to replace fluid loss from body.
6. Give water, salt, and soda solution: 1 teaspoonful salt and $\frac{1}{2}$ teaspoonful soda to 1 quart water.

What Not to Do

1. DO NOT pull clothes over burned area.
2. DO NOT remove pieces of cloth that stick to burn.
3. DO NOT try to clean the burn.
4. DO NOT break blisters.
5. DO NOT use grease—ointment—petroleum jelly or any type of medication on severe burns.
6. DO NOT use iodine or antiseptics on burns.
7. DO NOT touch burn with anything except sterile or clean dressing.
8. DO NOT change dressings that were initially applied until absolutely necessary. They may be left in place 5–7 days.

The seriousness of a burn depends upon its extent (amount of body surface involved) and "degree" (depth of destruction of tissues). There are three recognized degrees:

1. In first degree burns, the skin is merely reddened as by a slight sunburn.
2. In second degree burns, blisters develop.
3. In third degree burns, there is deeper destruction, and the burned area may appear either charred or white.

It is difficult or impossible to determine the degree of a burn at first. It often appears less deep than it actually is. The degree may differ in different parts of the affected area.

First aid objectives are to treat for shock, relieve pain, and prevent infection. In all extensive burns, shock and infection are major hazards. The danger of infection is greatest in second- and third-degree burns.

A burn should be covered with a sterile dressing and a bandage to hold the dressing firmly in place. Pain is common to almost all burns and is caused partly by contact with the air. The even pressure of a bandage will help reduce pain.

The area around the burn should be carefully washed with soap and water for a distance of several inches, wiping away from the burn. The gauze dressing will prevent surface washings from entering the burned area.

If a sterile dressing is not available, or is not big enough to cover a large burned area, use a clean towel or sheet. The dressing should be thick enough to keep air out of the burned area. Do not touch a burn or breathe directly on it. Do not attempt to open blisters or remove bits of dirt or debris from the burned surface. The blisters are not harmful and they protect the underlying tissues against entry of germs until the dressing is applied.

If adjoining surfaces of skin are burned, be sure they are separated by gauze—for example, between toes and fingers, between ears and head, between folds of the groin and genital region, and in the armpits. Otherwise they may stick together. The dressing on a serious burn should be left on as long as possible.

No ointments or salves should be used on burns. Never use iodine or any other antiseptic on burns. Dressings should be dry.

A person with an extensive burn needs a lot of liquid and salt. Give him a half glass of a salt and baking soda solution every 15 minutes. You can make this solution by mixing a teaspoon of salt and a half teaspoon of baking soda in a quart of water. If you have salt and soda tablets, use as directed on the packages.

Continue to give liquid every 15 minutes for 2 or 3 hours. If the burn is large and severe, give the person as much liquid as he can comfortably take. In the first 24 hours, he could well take 1 quart for every 20 pounds of his body weight. *Do not force him to drink. His own thirst is the best guide.*

For chemical burns, where the skin has been irritated by chemicals, the chemical should be washed away with generous amounts of water. Treatment can then be carried out as previously described for other burns.

Shock

What to Do

1. Keep the person lying down.
2. Keep head lower than legs and hips if no chest or head injury.
3. Have head and shoulders slightly raised with chest or head injury or difficulty in breathing.
4. Keep the person from chilling.
5. Encourage fluids by mouth if person is conscious. Use solution of 1 teaspoonful salt and ½ teaspoonful baking soda to a quart of water. Give ½ glassful every 15 minutes.

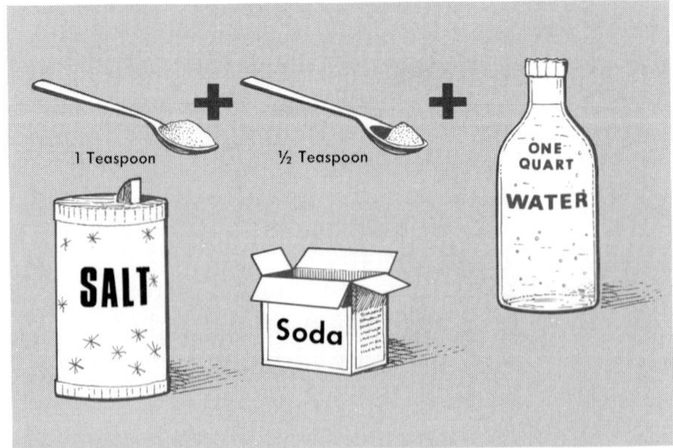

6. Never attempt to give fluids to an unconscious person.
7. Alcohol should not be used as a stimulant.

"Shock" as used in this section refers to a condition that frequently comes with serious injury such as severe wounds, burns, bleeding, and broken bones. It is due to a shortage of blood in various parts of the body. This causes the heart to beat faster in order

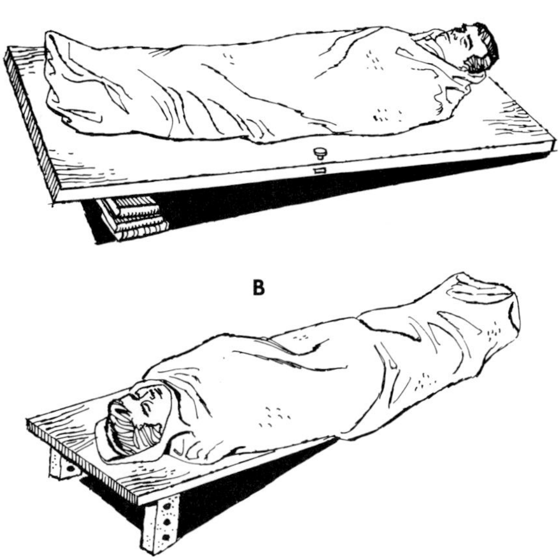

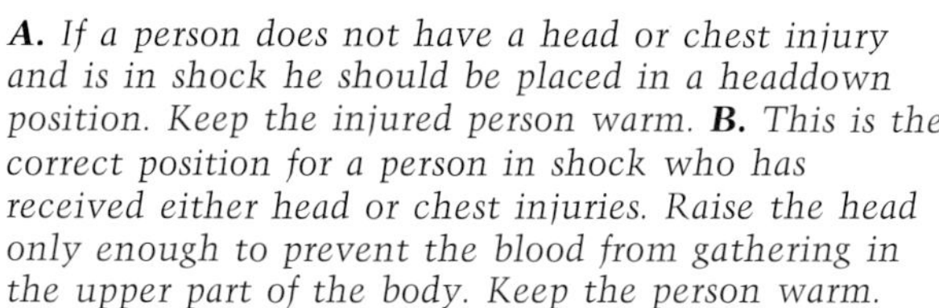

A. *If a person does not have a head or chest injury and is in shock he should be placed in a headdown position. Keep the injured person warm.* ***B.*** *This is the correct position for a person in shock who has received either head or chest injuries. Raise the head only enough to prevent the blood from gathering in the upper part of the body. Keep the person warm.*

to pump more blood, resulting in a rapid pulse. Lack of enough circulation through the brain causes unconsciousness.

Obviously a large amount of bleeding increases the danger of shock. In severe burns the oozing of blood fluids from the burned area increases the danger. *Shock may cause death if not treated promptly even though the injury which causes it may not itself be enough to cause death.*

Shock is easy to recognize. The skin gets pale and clammy, with small drops of sweat particularly around the lips and forehead. The person may complain of nausea and dizziness. His pulse may be fast and weak and his breathing shallow and irregular. His eyes may be dull with enlarged pupils, or he may be unconscious. A person may not be aware of the seriousness of his injury, then suddenly collapse.

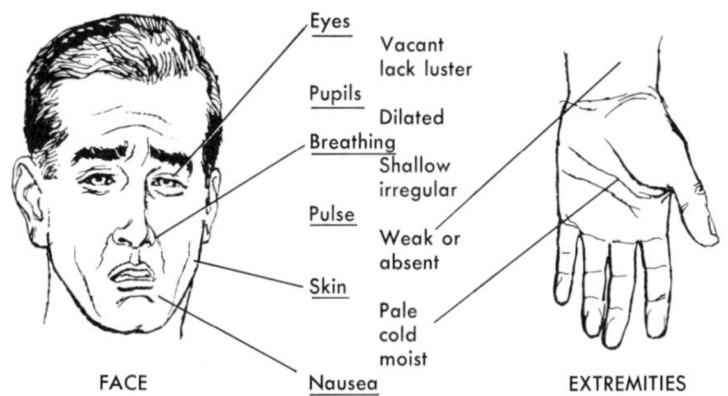

All seriously injured persons should be treated for shock even though all of these symptoms have not appeared and the person seems normal and alert. Treatment for shock may prevent its development.

Treatment for Shock

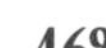

1. Have the injured person lie down.
2. Elevate his feet and legs 12 inches or more. This helps the flow of blood to his heart and head. *Exception:* If the person has received a head or chest injury, or if he has difficulty breathing, elevate his head and chest rather than his feet.
3. Keep the person warm, but not hot. Place a blanket under him. Depending on the weather, place a sheet or blanket over him. Avoid getting him so hot that he perspires, for this draws blood to the skin, and away from the interior of his body where it is needed. On warm days or in a hot room no covering will be necessary.
4. Give him liquid, about a glassful of salt and soda solution every 15 minutes if his condition permits. If he is unconscious, do not attempt to give anything to drink. If he vomits or is nauseated, delay giving liquid until the nausea disappears.
5. Keep the person quiet. See that bleeding is controlled and injured parts are kept still. Assure him that he will get the best care you can give. Reassurance is a potent medicine.
6. A person who has recovered from shock needs to be kept in bed. This is usually not difficult to accomplish as he will feel weak and exhausted. Sleep and rest will hasten his recovery.

Animal Bites

What to Do

1. Wash the wound thoroughly with soap and water.

2. Catch the animal and confine for 14 days (if practical).

Animal bites (those made by dogs and cats are most common) always involve the danger of infection since there are many germs on an animal's teeth and in its mouth, but in addition such bites may carry the greater risk of rabies, sometimes called hydrophobia. The virus or germ of this disease is present in the saliva of rabid animals. Rabies can attack humans as well as animals. Rabies is usually a fatal disease once it has developed; however, the incubation period is such that if the animal can be confined and watched for a period of 14 days and it is determined that the animal was rabid, the Pasteur treatment may be given to the person who has been bitten. This treatment consists of a series of injections usually given one a day for 14 days. The incubation period is rarely less than 15 days; therefore, if it is suspected that the person may have been bitten by a rabid animal, this person should be given early consideration to commence the Pasteur treatment after being seen by a physician.

It is unlikely that adequate laboratory facilities will be available to determine whether or not the animal was rabid; however, if the animal has been confined and has not died in 14 days the chances are excellent that it was not rabid. If it is rabid, it will, after several days, show what are called "furious" symptoms. Shortly thereafter the animal becomes paralyzed and dies.

Scratches caused by animals with other than their teeth should be washed thoroughly with soap and water and then treated as any other injury.

Blisters

What to Do

1. Wash blister area clean.
2. Sterilize a needle.
3. Open blister from edge.
4. Gently squeeze out fluid and cover with dressing.
5. Keep it clean.

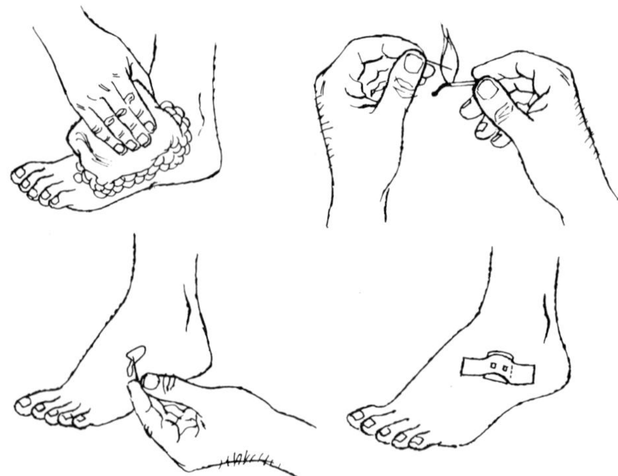

Blisters not caused by burns may result on the skin when it has been subjected to repeated pressures and excessive rubbing. They are not uncommon on the

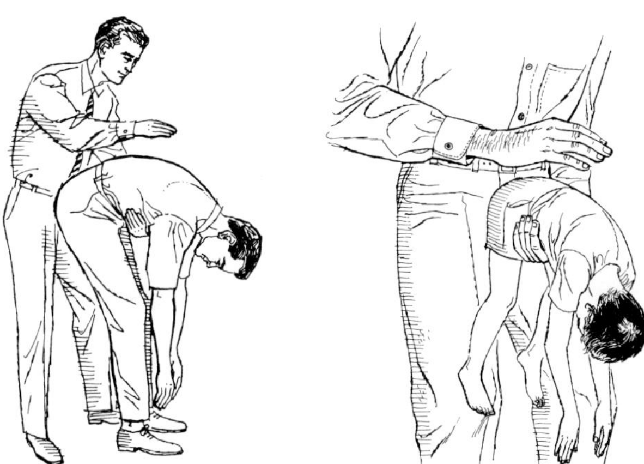

Hold as shown left—a vigorous slap on the back will help dislodge obstruction in throat. When objects are caught in the throats of children and cannot be reached with the fingers, they may be dislodged as shown at right. If breathing stops quickly try above methods of removing obstruction and start artificial respiration immediately.

feet from poorly fitting stockings or shoes, or on the hands from using unfamiliar equipment or doing unaccustomed work. They should be cared for to prevent serious infection from developing.

Do not attempt to remove the dead skin which formed the blister. Let it stay on as long as possible to provide protection to the tender underlying tissue and assist in the prevention of infection.

Choking

What to Do

When a person's windpipe becomes blocked, he chokes and becomes red in the face. If the windpipe is not cleared, he will suffocate.

Usually, a sharp blow on the back between the shoulder blades will remove the material blocking the air passage into the lungs. If not, bend him over and strike again. A small child should be held upside down and hit between the shoulder blades.

Convulsions

What to Do

1. Keep the person from hurting himself.
2. If you can without using force, slip something like a folded handkerchief or a piece of rubber (nothing hard) between his teeth to keep him from biting his tongue or cheek. Do not force the jaw open.

What Not to Do

DO NOT attempt to restrain the person having the attack, except to prevent his injuring himself.

No matter what the cause of the convulsion, little can be done to shorten the attack. *The most important thing is to prevent the person from hurting himself.*

If he has fallen to the floor, move objects that he might strike. Put a pillow or some rolled clothing under his head. If his teeth are clenched don't try to pry them loose. However, if you can without using force, slip something like a folded handkerchief or a piece of rubber (nothing hard) between his teeth to keep him from biting his tongue or cheek. A blanket wrapped loosely around his legs will tend to control their thrashing about. If due to epilepsy, the convulsion will soon end. When it does, the person will be sleepy and should be allowed to sleep as long as he wishes. He may be very irritable and have no memory of the convulsion.

In a child or infant, convulsions may occur with high fever. Efforts should be made to reduce the fever. Give aspirin, if the patient is able to swallow. Sponge his body with lukewarm water.

Diabetic Emergencies

What to Do

1. Put the victim to bed.
2. Prop him in a partial sitting up position.
3. Keep him warm.

4. *Remember:* There are two types of diabetic emergencies. One which results from LACK OF INSULIN, and one which results from TOO MUCH INSULIN.

Diabetic persons may become unconscious if they fail to take enough insulin or if they take too much.

If there is a *lack of insulin,* the person's face becomes flushed, his lips bright red, and he becomes sleepy and perhaps unconscious. This condition is known as diabetic coma. He breathes in gasps and his breath has an odor like nail polish remover. If insulin is available, give him his regular dose. If it is not available, make him as comfortable as possible.

To prevent diabetic coma, diabetics must make sure they have a sufficient supply of insulin on hand. As previously recommended, a diabetic person should maintain a 2-month emergency supply of insulin. If he sees his supply dwindling and fears that it will not be sufficient to maintain him until further insulin can be obtained, he should reduce his regular insulin dosage and also his need for it by cutting his food intake, particularly of carbohydrates.

A person who suffers from *too much insulin* will have an ashy white face with moist clammy skin. He will usually perspire a great deal and he may become unconscious. Such a person desperately needs sugar. If he is still conscious, give him a teaspoonful of sugar, a piece of chocolate, sips of a sugar and water solution, or orange juice, if available. If unconscious, place a teaspoonful of moistened sugar under his tongue. It will be absorbed into his blood. Recovery will usually be rapid.

Emotional Problems

SYMPTOMS: Apathy, blank expression, crying, nervous laughter, moodiness, irritability, untidiness, avoiding crowds, or overconfidence.

What to Do

1. First of all—STAY calm!
2. Be confident in your ability to handle the situation.
3. Use authority. Authority creates a feeling of security in the people.
4. Give the person hot coffee, warm soup, or food.
5. If bordering on hysterics, give maximum of four aspirin tablets and try to get him to lie down and sleep.
6. Assign specific duties when the person is able to do them.
7. Keep the person busy.
8. Encourage recreational activities.

What Not to Do

1. DO NOT scold or talk harshly.
2. DO NOT give alcohol or narcotics.
3. DO NOT slap or strike.

Emotional problems may increase in a time of disaster, particularly under conditions of confined living. They will vary with the mental and physical condition of individuals.

Some persons will remain remarkably calm in an emergency. They will accept the situation as it is and do everything possible to be helpful.

Others may temporarily show signs of weakness, trembling, nausea, vomiting, uncontrollable crying, and excessive sweating. Their thinking will be confused and they will be jittery. But in most cases these symptoms will disappear in a short time as the person gets used to the situation.

Another type of person will sit or stand alone and act unaware of what has happened. He will not speak or reply to questions. He will show no concern for his safety and may need to be protected.

Some people will react in an opposite manner. They will talk rapidly, joke, and show too much confidence in meeting the situation. They may not accept suggestions from others and may prevent desirable action.

Persons with panic reactions are the most difficult to control because it is so hard to get their attention, yet it may be necessary to restrain them for their own safety and that of others. Their blind, unreasoning efforts to escape from the situation can affect others around them. Panic, if uncontrolled, is contagious. If gentle firmness doesn't work with them, physical force may be necessary to isolate them as far as possible from other members of the group.

Some people in an emergency will show their great anxiety by insisting that a part of their body no longer functions. For example, a leg or arm may appear to be paralyzed though no injury is apparent.

Such symptoms are the body's attempt to relieve extreme anxiety. This reaction is beyond the control of the person involved. He is actually just as disabled as one who is physically paralyzed even though his injury is emotional rather than physical.

A person's emotional reaction may change rapidly. Intense activity may be followed by numbness and a "don't care" attitude. At other times, he may appear to be perfectly normal.

Do not blame or make fun of anyone for feeling the way he does. If a man has a broken leg, no one expects him to walk. Similarly if a man's ability to cope with his personal situation is lost, no one should expect him to resume normal behavior at once. Telling him to "snap out of it" will not help. He does not want to feel the way he does. Try to understand his feelings, not tell him how he should feel. Give him sympathy and encouragement but not obvious pity.

Let the disturbed person talk freely of his feelings. Even a few minutes of talk will relieve him remarkably. Try to suggest a job or two he can do to help despite his problem. By showing an interest in him and bypassing his temporary difficulty, you will help him back to normal. A cup of warm soup or tea is a physical help you might offer.

Frostbite

What to Do

1. Rapidly thaw frostbitten part of body.
   a. Place affected part next to warm part of your body or warm part of somebody else's body, or

b. Place frostbitten part of body in lukewarm water (about 108°F), or
c. Cover affected area with scarves, clothing, blankets, or other material.
2. Give hot coffee or hot tea.
3. Handle affected part with great care and gentleness.

What Not to Do

DO NOT rub the affected part.
DO NOT use *hot water.*
DO NOT use hot water bottle or heat lamps.
DO NOT disturb blisters if they develop.
DO NOT *rub with ice or snow.*

Exposure to dry cold causes the local injury known as frostbite. Parts of the body most likely to be frostbitten are the cheeks, nose, chin, ears, forehead, wrists, hands, and feet. Most cases of frostbite are caused by exposure to air below freezing temperatures.

The symptoms of frostbite vary depending on the severity of the injury. The frostbitten part is usually not painful, but is numb and stiff. The skin is first white or grayish white in color and then it beomes bright pink. If the exposure to cold continues the skin becomes white again.

When the frostbitten area is warmed it immediately becomes red and swollen and large blisters may develop. Severe frostbite causes the condition known as gangrene in which soft body tissue and sometimes even bone are permanently destroyed. In the course of healing, a gangrenous tissue is slipped off and leaves healthy tissue underneath, but if deep tissue has been destroyed, the injured part may require amputation.

Early detection of frostbite will permit early treatment. Persons in places which are improperly heated should not only frequently examine their own exposed parts but also those of other occupants for signs of frostbite. A grayish or white waxy appearance of the skin is an early sign of freezing. Whenever any part shows this sign start first aid at once. Distinct pain is usually not present as a warning that frostbite or freezing is occurring. Loss of feeling when the skin is touched is another important sign. In extremely cold weather stiffness caused by freezing can be detected by wrinkling of the face. *Contrary to popular belief rapid thawing of tissues frozen from relatively short exposures result in less loss of tissue than does slow thawing. Do not rub it with ice or snow.*

The correct treatment is directed toward the rapid thawing of the frozen tissue. To thaw a frostbitten part put it next to a warm part of your body or next to the warm part of someone else's body. For example, put your left hand under the right armpit. Extra cover with scarves, blankets, clothing, etc., will help in the rapid thawing process. Exposed parts, if possible, may also be placed in lukewarm water at about 108°F.

Caution: Rapid thawing with warmth is the correct care of this type of injury; however, *do not use hot water, hot water bottles or heat lamps. Do not place victim close to hot stove or furnace.* Extreme heats of the above type will cause greater tissue damage.

An arm or leg that has been frostbitten and then thawed should be placed in an elevated position and kept at rest.

Heat Illness

What to Do

1. Put the victim to bed or lay him down in a cool place.
2. Give him cool salted water to drink (1 teaspoonful of salt to 1 quart of water).

Caution: Do not give anything to an unconscious person.

Heat Exhaustion.—This condition may be mild or severe. In mild cases, the patient usually feels tired and may experience headache and nausea. In severe cases, perspiration is profuse, weakness extreme, and the skin is pale and clammy. *The temperature is usually normal or subnormal.* Vomiting may occur. Unconsciousness is rare, but often the patient will be unable to stand. Painful cramps in leg, or arm muscles may begin suddenly and continue for as long as 24 hours. *The patient's temperature is usually normal or subnormal.*

The excessive heat and high humidity which may exist in living quarters can affect your health. Preventive measures should be instituted in your quarters to avoid the onset of heat illness. Wear light, porous, loose-fitting clothing, and maintain adequate salt intake. Your salt intake can be increased by liberal use of salt on your food and can be further insured by salting your drinking water, using one level teaspon of salt to a gallon of water. This dilute solution is not unpleasant to taste.

Normally when the body is overheated, the excess heat is eliminated naturally through sweating and the cooling of the body surface by evaporation of sweat. In profuse sweating, however, large quantities of salt are lost and the essential salt balance of the body may be upset. Under conditions of high humidity and when tight or heavy clothing is worn, the cooling of the body surface by evaporation is sometimes interfered with. Under such circumstances, heat exhaustion, heat cramps, or heat stroke may occur.

Treatment for heat cramps should include giving the salt-water solution described in the treatment of heat exhaustion. Relief of cramps may also be obtained by massage of the cramping muscles, using firm pressure rather than vigorous kneading, and by applying warm, wet towels to the painful muscles.

Heat Stroke

What to Do

1. Undress the person and put him to bed in the coolest available area.
2. Sponge body freely with water or alcohol to reduce his temperature to 102°F. or less.
3. To hold temperature at 102°F. or less damp sheets or blankets may be placed over the victim.

4. Administer salt solution as soon as it can be tolerated. (One half teaspoonful of salt in a glassful of water every 15 minutes for 3 hours.)

What Not to Do

DO NOT give stimulants such as coffee or tea.

Heat Stroke. This is a serious condition. In contrast to heat exhaustion and heat cramps, a patient with heat stroke usually has a high fever (105 or higher), and no evident perspiration. His skin is hot and dry.

Symptoms include headache, dizziness, irritability, and seeing objects through a red or purplish haze. The patient may suddenly become unconscious, the pulse is full and strong, breathing is noisy like snoring, and there may be convulsions.

The first efforts in treatment of heat stroke should be to reduce the fever rapidly. Undress the patient and put him to bed in the coolest available area. Sponge his body freely with water or alcohol to reduce his temperature to 102°F. or less (by rectum). Vigorous efforts to reduce fever should be stopped when the body temperature reaches this point (102°F.), and the patient should then be observed for 10 minutes. The temperature may continue to decline or it may rise again. If it starts to rise, renew sponging cautiously.

Give no stimulants such as coffee or tea. Administer salt solution, as tolerated, and in the same way as described for heat exhaustion, provided the patient is fully conscious.

When the patient's temperature remains at relatively normal levels, cover him to the extent necessary and keep him in bed until fully recovered.

Insect Bites

What to Do

Bees, Wasps, Hornets

1. Remove the stinger.
2. Apply paste of baking soda (baking soda is available in medical kit).

Scorpions

1. Apply constricting band or tourniquet above the sting on the side toward the heart.
   Caution: Remove after it has been in place about 5 minutes.
2. Apply ice pack if available; otherwise, cold wet cloths.
3. Keep person warm.
4. Keep affected arm or leg *lower* than rest of body for about 2 hours.

Spiders (Black Widow and Brown Recluse)

1. Keep person quiet.
2. Elevate hips and legs in shock position.
3. Apply hot packs if abdominal cramps develop.

Only a few spiders are considered poisonous to human beings. The black widow and brown recluse are apparently the only spiders in the United States capable of causing death. The black widow is a glossy black covered with fine short hairs. The underside

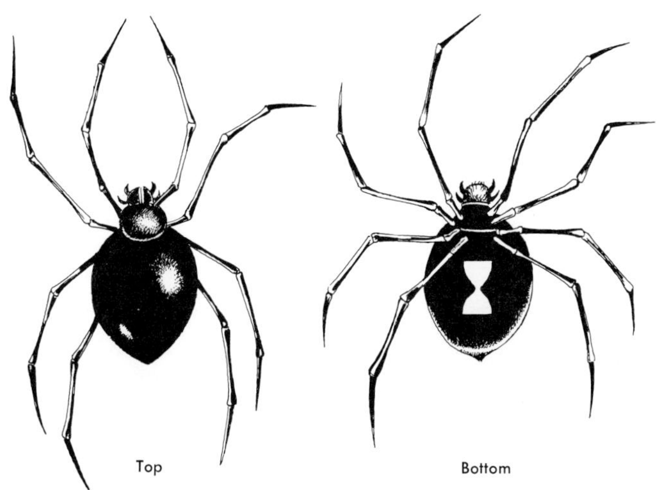

of the abdomen of the female has a characteristic red marking in the shape of an hourglass.

The female black widow spins her web in protective places such as dark corners of basement and between rocks. She stays near her web ready to bite if disturbed. The much smaller male black widow is harmless.

At the time of the bite there is usually a sharp pain. The severity of the reaction depends upon the amount of venom that has been injected. The greater the amount the more severe the reaction.

Usually redness and local swelling develop immediately with serious poisoning pain developing almost at once in the region of the bite and spreading to the back and shoulders, chest, abdomen, and limbs.

The person should be kept quiet and warm, and lying down with hips and legs elevated in the shock position. If severe abdominal cramps develop heat may give some relief, such as hot water bottles or hot compresses.

It is estimated that only about 5 per cent of black widow spider bites are fatal.

Nosebleed

What to Do

1. Place person in sitting position, head back *slightly,* and have him breathe through his mouth.
   Note: Most nosebleeds will stop spontaneously. If bleeding continues try the following measures:
   a. Gently grasp the lower end of the nose between the thumb and index finger, firmly press the sides of the nose against the center for 5 minutes.
   b. Release pressure gradually.
   c. Apply cold cloths to back of neck or over nose.
   Note: If bleeding persists, plug the bleeding nostrils with small strip of gauze rolled up loosely. Leave part of roll sticking out of nose so it can be easily removed later.

Nosebleeds occur both spontaneously and as a result of injury. There may be an underlying disease, such as high blood pressure, but in many cases there is no disease. Some people, particularly young people, develop nosebleed following strenuous activity, colds, or exposure to high altitude. The bleeding is usually more annoying than serious. Occasionally, where disease is involved there may be sufficient bleeding to be dangerous.

Anyone with a nosebleed should remain quiet. A sitting position with head thrown back, or a lying position with head and shoulders raised, is best. Walking about, talking, laughing, or blowing the nose may cause increased bleeding or start bleeding again after it has stopped.

Usually the bleeding area is near the tip of the nose. Pinching the nostrils together puts pressure upon this area and helps to stop the flow. It may be necessary to pack the bleeding nostril lightly with gauze and then pinch. Sometimes it is necessary to maintain pressure with a small amount of gauze for several minutes, occasionally considerably longer.

Poisoning

What to Do

For general poisoning: Dilute with water; induce vomiting.

Universal antidote: 2 parts scraped or powdered burnt toast, 1 part milk of magnesia, 1 part strong tea.

In acid or alkali poisoning, dilute and neutralize, but do not induce vomiting. Give milk, olive oil, or egg white.

First aid must be given immediately; minutes count. The general aim is to dilute and remove the poison, to neutralize it by an antidote, and to help the body fight the poison. These measures are effective regardless of the kind of poison.

Quickly administer fluids in large amounts—four glassfuls or more for adults. Water usually is the most readily available. Milk is good as it will slow the absorption of many poisons. Either or both may be given. *Do not attempt to give fluids to an unconscious patient.*

In all cases—*except those involving special poisons,* described below, try to remove the poison from the patient's stomach immediately by inducing vomiting.

The larger the amount of fluid given, the greater the tendency to vomit. A strong salt solution—two tablespoonfuls to a glass of warm water—is nauseating and may be given repeatedly. Vomiting may also be induced in a conscious person by touching the back of the throat with the fingers or handle of a spoon. The patient should be placed face down with his head lower than his hips to prevent the matter vomited from entering his lungs and causing further damage.

If you can find the package from which the poison came, its antidote may be given on the label. If available without delay, use the antidote as directed.

Unless the poison was a sedative (such as an overdose of sleeping tablets), have the patient lie down after he has vomited several times and keep him warm and quiet.

However, if the poison was a sedative, keep him awake by talking to him and encourage him to walk about. Give him several cups of black coffee every 2 hours until he gets better.

WASH AND DILUTE

- **MEDICINES**
- **INSECTICIDES**
- **DISINFECTANTS**
- **HOUSEHOLD CLEANERS**
- **RAT POISONS**

NEUTRALIZE

- **ACIDS**
- **ALKALIES**

Special Procedures for Special Poisons

Acids. Dilute quickly with a glass of water and then give milk of magnesia, or if it is not available, baking soda solution, to neutralize the acid. Several glassfuls may be given *but do not give enough to cause vomiting.* Then give milk, olive oil, or egg white to protect the digestive tract lining.

Alkalies. Give a glass of water quickly, then vinegar or lemon juice in the diluting fluid to neutralize the alkali. Follow with milk, olive oil, or egg white. *Do not cause vomiting.* The only reason for giving plain water first is that it is quickly available.

Kerosene Poisoning. Give a half cup of mineral oil, if available, to protect the digestive tract lining, and use strong coffee or tea as a stimulant. *Do not cause vomiting.* Keep the patient warm and combat shock. Be prepared to use artificial respiration if the patient stops breathing.

Carbon Monoxide Poisoning. The problem is inhalation of gas, so the instructions for inducing or not inducing vomiting and other procedures given above do not apply.

It takes a combination of two causes to bring about carbon monoxide poisoning—the improper burning of fuel, and insufficient ventilation. Prevention is the best "treatment," but it may be difficult when improvised methods for heating and ventilation are employed. If it is necessary to operate such things as furnace, fireplace, or space heater, be sure that the ventilation is adequate.

Carbon monoxide gives no warning. You cannot see, taste, or smell the gas. It does not tickle the throat, make your eyes smart, or make its presence known in any obvious way. First symptoms—headache, nausea, dizziness, or a feeling of great sleepiness—have so many other causes you may tend to ignore them.

If poisoning does occur, get the victim to fresh air if possible. If he is not breathing or is breathing irregularly, start artificial respiration at once. Keep him warm and aid his circulation by rubbing his arms and legs. Avoid use of such stimulants as coffee or tea, and see that the patient has sufficient rest and time to recover in order to avoid strain on the heart.

Unconsciousness

What to Do

When Person Is Flushed—Red Faced—With Strong Slow Pulse

1. Lay person down with head *slightly raised* above level of rest of body.
2. Apply cold wet cloth to head.
3. If breathing stops start artificial respiration.

When Person Is Pale—Cold—Clammy to Touch —With Weak Pulse

1. Lay person down with head *slightly lower* than rest of body.
2. Keep him warm.
3. If available hold aromatic spirit of ammonia under nose (except where head injury is suspected).

4. If breathing stops start artificial respiration.

When Person Has Bluish-Face, Weak Pulse, Irregular Breathing

1. Lay person down.
2. Keep him warm.
3. Start artificial respiration immediately if breathing stops.

What Not to Do

1. DO NOT give stimulant.
2. DO NOT give food or drink.
3. DO NOT move (except to remove from danger).

Unconsciousness may occur in such conditions as fainting, apoplexy (sometimes called a stroke), shock, and diabetes. (See treatment of shock, and discussion of diabetes.)

Simple fainting occurs when not enough blood reaches the brain. This may be due to hunger, fatigue, emotional distress, or severe injury.

Warnings of faintness are blurring of the vision, weakness, paleness, and giddiness. If you should have these symptoms, lie down immediately if possible. If not, sit or kneel and bend forward at the waist, putting your head down to get it lower than your heart.

A person who has fainted should be kept flat with no pillow under his head. His feet should be elevated. Be sure he is breathing without difficulty. (If not, use the same measures as described below for the stroke patient.) Usually he will recover in a few minutes without any further care. He should rest for some time after recovery.

Apoplexy (or stroke) should be suspected whenever an elderly person faints. Apoplexy is caused by interference with the blood supply to the brain. It may occur when a blood vessel in the brain bursts or becomes blocked.

Sometimes a person with apoplexy will collapse but not completely lose consciousness. His face may become red and congested. One side of his body or parts of one side may become paralyzed. His speech may be affected, blurred, and stumbly. He may have difficulty swallowing.

Where stroke is suspected, the sick person should be kept in bed but he does not need to lie flat. He can be propped comfortably with pillows. However, if he is unconscious, he should be placed flat in bed on his back or either side. To avoid bed sores, his position in bed should be changed every four hours. Remove any loose dental bridges or false teeth from his mouth. If secretions collect in the back of his mouth and interfere with breathing, he should be placed on his side and the secretion allowed to drain from his mouth.

Most persons recover from a slight stroke. If the stroke is severe, unconsciousness sometimes continues for days and days and death may result.

Emergency Childbirth

What to Do

1. Let nature be your best helper. Childbirth is a very natural act.

2. At first signs of labor assign the best-qualified person to remain with mother.
3. Be calm; reassure mother.
4. Place mother and attendant in a most protected place.
5. Keep children and others away.
6. Have hands as clean as possible.
7. Keep hands away from birth canal.
8. See that baby breathes well.
9. Place baby face down across mother's abdomen.
10. Keep baby warm.
11. Wrap afterbirth with baby.
12. Keep baby with mother constantly.
13. Make mother as comfortable as possible.
14. Identify baby.

What Not to Do

1. DO NOT hurry.
2. DO NOT pull on baby; let baby be born naturally.
3. DO NOT pull on cord; let the placenta (afterbirth) come naturally.
4. DO NOT cut and tie the cord until baby *AND* afterbirth have been delivered.
5. DO NOT give medication.
   DO NOT HURRY—LET NATURE TAKE HER COURSE.

Preparations

Usually there is plenty of time after the beginning of first labor pains to get ready for the delivery. Signs of labor are low-back ache, bloody-tinged mucous strings passing from the birth canal, or a gush of water from the birth canal.

The mother will need a clean surface to lie on. Her bed should be so arranged that the mattress is well protected by waterproof sheeting or pads made from several thicknesses of paper covered with cloth. Cover these protective materials with a regular bed sheet.

A warm bed should be made ready in advance for the baby. It may be a clothes basket, a box lined with a blanket, or a bureau drawer placed on firm chairs or on a table. If possible, warm the baby's blanket, shirt, and diapers with a hot water bottle. Warm bricks or a bag of table salt that has been heated can be used if a hot water bottle is not available.

A knife, a pair of scissors, or a razor should be thoroughly cleansed and sterilized in preparation for cutting the umbilical cord. If there is no way to boil water to sterilize them (the preferred method of sterilization), sterilize them by submersion in 70 per cent isopropyl alcohol solution for at least 20 minutes or up to 3 hours, if possible. Sterile tapes for tying the umbilical cord will be needed. (Do not remove them from their sterile wrappings until you are ready to use them.) If no tapes are available, a clean shoestring or a strip of sheeting (folded into a narrow tie) can be boiled and used wet as a cord tie substitute.

Change of Feeling

Gradually the time between the labor pains grows shorter and the pains increase in severity until they are coming every 2 to 3 minutes.

At this stage the mother will notice a change. Instead of the tightness in the lower abdomen and pain across the back, she will feel a bearing down sensation almost as if she were having a bowel movement. This means the baby is moving down.

When this happens, she should lie down and get ready for the birth of the child. The tightening and bearing down feelings will come more frequently and be harder.

She will have an uncontrollable urge to push down, which she may do. But she should not work too hard at it because the baby will be brought down without her straining too hard. There will probably be more blood showing at this point.

The person attending the delivery should thoroughly scrub hands with soap and water. Never touch the vagina or put fingers inside for any reason. The mother also should keep her hands away from the vagina.

As soon as a bulge begins to appear in the vaginal area and part of the baby is visible, the mother should stop pushing down. She should try to breath like a panting dog with her mouth open in order not to push the baby out too rapidly with consequent tearing of her tissue.

She should keep her knees up and legs separated so that the person helping her can get at the baby more easily.

Moment of Birth

The person helping the mother should always let the baby be born by itself. No attempt should be made to pull the baby out in any way.

Usually the baby's head appears first, the top of the head presenting and the face downward. Infrequently the baby will be born in a different position, sometimes buttocks first, occasionally foot or arm first. In these infrequent situations, patience without interference in the birth process is most important. The natural process of delivery, although sometimes slower, will give the child and the mother the best chance of a safe and successful birth.

The baby does not need to be born in a hurry, but usually about a minute after the head appears the mother will have another bearing down feeling and push the shoulders and the rest of the baby out.

As the baby is being expelled, the person helping the mother should support the baby on her hands and arms so that the baby will avoid contact with any blood or waste material on the bed.

If there is still a membrane from the water sac over the baby's head and face at delivery, it should immediately be taken between the fingers and torn so that the water inside will run out and the baby can breathe.

If, as sometimes happens, the cord, which attaches the child from its navel to the placenta in the mother's womb, should be wrapped around the baby's neck when his head and neck appear, try to slip it quickly over his head so that he will not strangle.

After the baby is born, wrap a fold of towel around his ankles to prevent slipping and hold him up by the heels with one hand, taking care that the cord is slack. To get a good safe grip, insert one finger between the baby's ankles. Do not swing or spank the baby. Hold him over the bed so that he cannot fall far if he should slip from your grasp. The baby's body will be very slippery. Place your other hand under the baby's forehead and bend its head back slightly so that the fluid and mucus can run out of its mouth. When the baby begins to cry, lay him on his side on the bed close enough to the mother to keep the cord slack.

The baby will usually cry within the first minute. If he does not cry or breathe within 2 or 3 minutes, use mouth-to-mouth artificial respiration.

Very little force should be used in blowing air into the baby's mouth. A short puff of breath about every 5 seconds is enough. As soon as the baby starts to breathe or cry, mouth-to-mouth breathing should be stopped.

Cutting the Cord

There should be no hurry to cut the cord. Take as much time as necessary to prepare the ties and sharp instruments.

You will need two pieces of sterile white cotton tape or two pieces of 1-inch wide sterile gauze bandage about 9 inches long to use to tie the cord. (If you do not have sterile material for tying the cord but do have facilities for boiling water, strips of sheeting—boiled for 15 to 20 minutes to make them sterile—can be used.) Tie the umbilical cord with the sterile tape in two places, one about 4 inches from the baby and the other 2 inches farther along the cord toward the mother, making two or more simple knots at each place. Cut the cord between

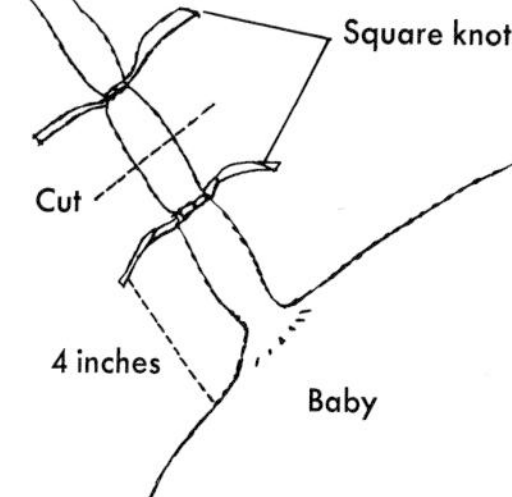

Cut between the square knots. Tie a square knot by bringing left tape over right tape for first loop and right tape over left for second loop. Tighten each loop firmly as tied. Use scissors or razor blade to cut cord.

these two ties with a clean sharp instrument such as a knife, razor blade, or scissors.

A sterile dressing about 4 inches square should be placed over the cut end of the cord at the baby's navel and should be held in place by wrapping a "belly band" or folded diaper around the baby. If a sterile dressing is not available, no dressing or belly band should be used. Regardless of whether a dressing is applied or not, no powder, solution, or disinfectant of any kind should be put on the cord or navel.

If the afterbirth has not yet been expelled, cover the end of the umbilical cord attached to it (and now protruding from the vagina) with a sterile dressing and tie it in place.

Third Stage of Labor

Usually a few minutes after the baby is born (although sometimes an hour or more will elapse) the mother will feel a brief return of the labor pains which had ceased with the birth. These are due to contractions of the uterus as it seeks to expel the afterbirth. *Do not pull on the cord to hurry this process.*

Some bleeding is to be expected at this stage. If there is a lot of bleeding before the afterbirth is expelled, the attendant should gently massage the mother's abdomen, just above the navel. This will help the uterus to tighten, help the afterbirth come out, and reduce bleeding.

It may be desirable to put the baby almost immediately to the mother's breast for a minute or two on each side even though the mother will have no milk as yet. This helps the uterus contract and reduce the bleeding.

Someone should stand by the mother and occasionally massage her abdomen gently for about an hour after the afterbirth is expelled. After that, the mother should feel the rounded surface of the uterus through the abdomen and squeeze firmly but gently with her fingers.

The bedding should be changed and the mother sponged. Washing and wiping of the vaginal area should always be done from the front to the back in order to avoid contamination. A sanitary napkin should be applied.

Keep the mother warm with blankets. She may have a slight chill. Giver her a warm (not hot) drink of sweetened tea, milk, or bouillon. Wipe her hands and face with a damp towel. She may drop off to sleep.

The mother's diet after delivery may include any available foods she wishes. She may eat or drink as soon as she wants to, and she should be encouraged to drink plenty of fluids, especially milk. Canned milk can be used and made more palatable by diluting with equal parts of water and adding sugar, eggs, chocolate, or other flavoring.

For the first 24 or 48 hours after delivery, the mother will continue to have some cramping pain in the lower abdomen which may cause a great deal of discomfort. Aspirin may help reduce these afterpains. She should empty her bladder every few hours for 2 days following the birth. If her bowels do not move within 3 days after delivery, she should be given an enema.

Miscarriage

If a pregnant woman shows evidence of bleeding, she should restrict her activities and rest in bed in an effort to prevent possible loss of the baby. If a miscarriage does occur, keep the patient flat with the foot of the bed elevated from 12 to 18 inches to retard vaginal bleeding. Keep her warm and quiet, and give her fluids.

Appendix B
Nutritive Values of the Edible Part of Foods

The following Table[1] is an alphabetic arrangement of items listed in the publication of the Consumer and Food Economics Research Division in 1970 *Nutritive Value of Foods.* A few additional items from Agriculture Handbook 8 *Composition of Foods—Raw, Processed, Prepared* are also included. The explanation provided in the bulletin for this table is reproduced here in part:[2]

Weight in grams—rounded to the nearest whole gram—is shown for an approximate measure of each food as it is described; if inedible parts are included in the description, both measure and weight include these parts.

The approximate measure shown for each food is in cups, ounces, pounds, some other well-known unit, or a piece of certain size. Usually, the measure shown can be calculated to larger or smaller amounts by multiplying or dividing. Because the measures are approximate (some are rounded for convenient use), calculated nutritive values for larger quantities of some food items may be less representative than those calculated for smaller quantities.

The cup measure refers to the standard measuring cup of 8 fluid ounces or ½ liquid pint. The ounce refers to $\frac{1}{16}$ of a pound avoirdupois, unless fluid ounce is indicated. The weight of a fluid ounce varies according to the food measured. . . .

The values for food energy (calories) and nutrients shown in the Table are the amounts present in the edible part of the item, that is, in only that portion of the weight of the item customarily eaten—corn without cob, meat without bone, potatoes without skin, European-type grapes without seeds. If additional parts are eaten—the skin of the potato, for example—amounts of some nutrients obtained will be somewhat greater than those shown.

For many of the prepared items, values have been calculated from the ingredients in typical recipes. Examples of such items are biscuits, corn muffins, oyster stew, macaroni and cheese, custard, and a number of other dessert-type items.

For toast and for vegetables, values are without fat added, either during preparation or at the table. Values for the thiamine content of toast are about 20 per cent lower than for fresh bread; it was impossible to show this loss adequately because of the small amount of thiamine present in a slice of bread. Some destruction of vitamins in vegetables, especially of ascorbic acid, may occur when foods are cut or shredded. Such losses are variable, and no deduction for these losses has been made.

For meat, values are for meat as cooked, drained, and without drippings. For many cuts, two sets of values are shown: Meat including the fat, and meat from which the fat has been trimmed off in the kitchen or on the plate.

A variety of manufactured items, such as some of the milk products, ready-to-eat breakfast cereals, imitation cream products, fruit drinks, and various mixes are included in the Table. Frequently these foods are fortified with one or more nutrients. If nutrients are added, this information is on the label. Values shown in this bulletin for these foods are usually based on products from several manufacturers and may differ somewhat from the values provided by any one source.

[1] Reprinted from Corinne H. Robinson, *Normal and Therapeutic Nutrition* (New York: Macmillan Publishing Co., Inc, 1972).

[2] Consumer and Food Economics Research Division, Agricultural Research Service: *Nutritive Value of Foods.* Home and Garden Bull. 72, U.S. Department of Agriculture, Washington, D.C., 1970.

Table A–1. Nutritive Values of the Edible Part of Foods*

[Dashes in the columns for nutrients show that no suitable value could be found although there is reason to believe that a measurable amount of the nutrient may be present]

	Food, Approximate Measure, and Weight (in grams)		gm	Water per cent	Food Energy calories	Protein gm	Fat gm	Fatty Acids: Saturated (total) gm	Fatty Acids: Unsaturated: Oleic gm	Fatty Acids: Unsaturated: Linoleic gm	Carbohydrate gm	Calcium mg	Iron mg	Vitamin A Value I.U.	Thiamine mg	Riboflavin mg	Niacin mg	Ascorbic Acid mg
	Milk, Cheese, Cream, Imitation Cream; Related Products																	
	Milk:																	
	Fluid:																	
1	Whole, 3.5% fat	1 cup	244	87	160	9	9	5	3	Trace	12	288	0.1	350	0.07	0.41	0.2	2
2	Nonfat (skim)	1 cup	245	90	90	9	Trace	—	—	—	12	296	0.1	10	0.09	0.44	0.2	2
3	Partly skimmed, 2% nonfat milk solids added	1 cup	246	87	145	10	5	3	2	Trace	15	352	0.1	200	0.10	0.52	0.2	2
	Canned, concentrated, undiluted:																	
4	Evaporated, unsweetened	1 cup	252	74	345	18	20	11	7	1	24	635	0.3	810	0.10	0.86	0.5	3
5	Condensed, sweetened	1 cup	306	27	980	25	27	15	9	1	166	802	0.3	1,100	0.24	1.16	0.6	3
	Dry, nonfat instant:																	
6	Low-density (1 1/3 cups needed for reconstitution to 1 qt)	1 cup	68	4	245	24	Trace	—	—	—	35	879	0.4	[1]20	0.24	1.21	0.6	5
7	High-density (7/8 cup needed for reconstitution to 1 qt)	1 cup	104	4	375	37	1	—	—	—	54	1,345	0.6	[1]30	0.36	1.85	0.9	7
	Buttermilk:																	
8	Fluid, cultured, made from skim milk	1 cup	245	90	90	9	Trace	—	—	—	12	296	0.1	10	0.10	0.44	0.2	2
9	Dried, packaged	1 cup	120	3	465	41	6	3	2	Trace	60	1,498	0.7	260	0.31	2.06	1.1	—
	Cheese:																	
	Natural:																	
	Blue or Roquefort type:																	
10	Ounce	1 oz.	28	40	105	6	9	5	3	Trace	1	89	0.1	350	0.01	0.17	0.3	0
11	Cubic inch	1 cu. in.	17	40	65	4	5	3	2	Trace	Trace	54	0.1	210	0.01	0.11	0.2	0
12	Camembert, packaged in 4-oz pkg. with 3 wedges per pkg.	1 wedge	38	52	115	7	9	5	3	Trace	1	40	0.2	380	0.02	0.29	0.3	0
	Cheddar:																	
13	Ounce	1 oz	28	37	115	7	9	5	3	Trace	1	213	0.3	370	0.01	0.13	Trace	0
14	Cubic inch	1 cu in	17	37	70	4	6	3	2	Trace	Trace	129	0.2	230	0.01	0.08	Trace	0
	Cottage, large or small curd:																	
	Creamed:																	
15	Package of 12 oz, net wt.	1 pkg	340	78	360	46	14	8	5	Trace	10	320	1.0	580	0.10	0.85	0.3	0
16	Cup, curd pressed down	1 cup	245	78	260	33	10	6	3	Trace	7	230	0.7	420	0.07	0.61	0.2	0
	Uncreamed:																	
17	Package of 12 oz net wt.	1 pkg	340	79	290	58	1	1	Trace	Trace	9	306	1.4	30	0.10	0.95	0.3	0
18	Cup, curd pressed down	1 cup	200	79	170	34	1	Trace	Trace	Trace	5	180	0.8	20	0.06	0.56	0.2	0
	Cream:																	
19	Package of 8 oz, net wt.	1 pkg	227	51	850	18	86	48	28	3	5	141	0.5	3,500	0.05	0.54	0.2	0
20	Package of 3 oz, net wt.	1 pkg	85	51	320	7	32	18	11	1	2	53	0.2	1,310	0.02	0.20	0.1	0
21	Cubic inch	1 cu in	16	51	60	1	6	3	2	Trace	Trace	10	Trace	250	Trace	0.04	Trace	0
	Parmesan, grated:																	
22	Cup, pressed down	1 cup	140	17	655	60	43	24	14	1	5	1,893	0.7	1,760	0.03	1.22	0.3	0
23	Tablespoon	1 tbsp	5	17	25	2	2	1	Trace	Trace	Trace	68	Trace	60	Trace	0.04	Trace	0
24	Ounce	1 oz	28	17	130	12	9	5	3	Trace	1	383	0.1	360	0.01	0.25	0.1	0
	Swiss:																	
25	Ounce	1 oz	28	39	105	8	8	4	3	Trace	1	262	0.3	320	Trace	0.11	Trace	0
26	Cubic inch	1 cu in	15	39	55	4	4	2	1	Trace	Trace	139	0.1	170	Trace	0.06	Trace	0

	Pasteurized processed cheese:																		
	American:																		
27	Ounce	1 oz	28	40	105	7	9	5	3	Trace	1	198	0.3	350	0.01	0.12	Trace	0
28	Cubic inch	1 cu in	18	40	65	4	5	3	2	Trace	Trace	122	0.2	210	Trace	0.07	Trace	0
	Swiss:																		
29	Ounce	1 oz	28	40	100	8	8	4	3	Trace	1	251	0.3	310	Trace	0.11	Trace	0
30	Cubic inch	1 cu in	18	40	65	5	5	3	2	Trace	Trace	159	0.2	200	Trace	0.07	Trace	0
	Pasteurized process cheese food, American:																		
31	Tablespoon	1 tbsp	14	43	45	3	3	2	1	Trace	1	80	0.1	140	Trace	0.08	Trace	0
32	Cubic inch	1 cu in	18	43	60	4	4	2	1	Trace	1	100	0.1	170	Trace	0.10	Trace	0
33	Pasteurized process cheese spread, American	1 oz	28	49	80	5	6	3	2	Trace	2	160	0.2	250	Trace	0.15	Trace	0
	Cream:																		
34	Half-and-half (cream and milk)	1 cup	242	80	325	8	28	15	9	1	11	261	0.1	1,160	0.07	0.39	0.1	2
35		1 tbsp	15	80	20	1	2	1	1	Trace	1	16	Trace	70	Trace	0.02	Trace	Trace
36	Light, coffee or table	1 cup	240	72	505	7	49	27	16	1	10	245	0.1	2,020	0.07	0.36	0.1	2
		1 tbsp	15	72	30	1	3	2	1	Trace	1	15	Trace	130	Trace	0.02	Trace	Trace
38	Sour	1 cup	230	72	485	7	47	26	16	1	10	235	0.1	1,930	0.07	0.35	0.1	2
		1 tbsp	12	72	25	Trace	2	1	1	Trace	1	12	Trace	100	Trace	0.02	Trace	Trace
40	Whipped topping (pressurized)	1 cup	60	62	155	2	14	8	5	Trace	6	67	—	570	—	0.04	—	—
		1 tbsp	3	62	10	Trace	1	Trace	Trace	Trace	Trace	3	—	30	—	Trace	—	—
	Whipping, unwhipped (volume about double when whipped):																		
42	Light	1 cup	239	62	715	6	75	41	25	2	9	203	0.1	3,060	0.05	0.29	0.1	2
43		1 tbsp	15	62	45	Trace	5	3	2	Trace	1	13	Trace	190	Trace	0.02	Trace	Trace
44	Heavy	1 cup	238	57	840	5	90	50	30	3	7	179	0.1	3,670	0.05	0.26	0.1	2
45		1 tbsp	15	57	55	Trace	6	3	2	Trace	1	11	Trace	230	Trace	0.02	Trace	Trace
	Imitation cream products (made with vegetable fat):																		
	Creamers:																		
46	Powdered	1 cup	94	2	505	4	33	31	1	0	52	21	0.6	[2]200	—	—	Trace	—
47		1 tsp	2	2	10	Trace	1	Trace	Trace	0	1	1	Trace	[2]Trace	—	—	—	—
48	Liquid (frozen)	1 cup	245	77	345	3	27	25	1	0	25	29	—	[2]100	0	0	—	—
49		1 tbsp	15	77	20	Trace	2	1	Trace	0	2	2	—	[2]10	0	0	—	—
50	Sour dressing (imitation sour cream) made with nonfat dry milk	1 cup	235	72	440	9	38	35	1	Trace	17	277	0.1	10	0.07	0.38	0.2	1
51		1 tbsp	12	72	20	Trace	2	2	Trace	Trace	1	14	Trace	Trace	Trace	Trace	Trace	Trace
	Whipped topping:																		
52	Pressurized	1 cup	70	61	190	1	17	15	1	0	9	5	—	[2]340	—	0	—	—
53		1 tbsp	4	61	10	Trace	1	1	Trace	0	Trace	Trace	—	[2]20	—	0	—	—
54	Frozen	1 cup	75	52	230	1	20	18	Trace	0	15	5	—	[2]560	—	0	—	—
55		1 tbsp	4	52	10	Trace	1	1	Trace	0	1	Trace	—	[2]30	—	0	—	—
56	Powdered, made with whole milk	1 cup	75	58	175	3	12	10	1	Trace	15	62	Trace	[2]330	0.02	0.08	0.1	Trace
57		1 tbsp	4	58	10	Trace	1	1	Trace	Trace	1	3	Trace	[2]20	Trace	Trace	Trace	Trace
	Milk beverages:																		
58	Cocoa, homemade	1 cup	250	79	245	10	12	7	4	Trace	27	295	1.0	400	0.10	0.45	0.5	3
59	Chocolate-flavored drink made with skim milk and 2% added butterfat	1 cup	250	83	190	8	6	3	2	Trace	27	270	0.5	210	0.10	0.40	0.3	3
	Malted milk:																		
60	Dry powder, approx. 3 heaping teaspoons per ounce	1 oz	28	3	115	4	2	—	—	—	20	82	0.6	290	0.09	0.15	0.1	0
61	Beverage	1 cup	235	78	245	11	10	—	—	—	28	317	0.7	590	0.14	0.49	0.2	2
	Milk desserts:																		
62	Custard	1 cup	265	77	305	14	15	7	5	1	29	297	1.1	930	0.11	0.50	0.3	1
	Ice cream:																		
63	Regular (approx. 10% fat)	1/2 gal	1,064	63	2,055	48	113	62	37	3	221	1,553	0.5	4,680	0.43	2.23	1.1	11
64		1 cup	133	63	255	6	14	8	5	Trace	28	194	0.1	590	0.05	0.28	0.1	1
65		3-fl-oz cup	50	63	95	2	5	3	2	Trace	10	73	Trace	220	0.02	0.11	0.1	1

**Nutritive Value of Foods*, Home and Garden Bulletin No. 72. U.S. Department of Agriculture, Washington, D.C., 1970.

[1]Value applies to unfortified product; value for fortified low-density product would be 1500 I.U. and the fortified high-density product would be 2290 I.U.

[2]Contributed largely from beta-carotene used for coloring.

Table A–1. (Cont.)

	Food, Approximate Measure, and Weight (in grams)		gm	Water per cent	Food Energy calories	Protein gm	Fat gm	Fatty Acids: Saturated (total) gm	Fatty Acids: Unsaturated: Oleic gm	Fatty Acids: Unsaturated: Linoleic gm	Carbohydrate gm	Calcium mg	Iron mg	Vitamin A Value I.U.	Thiamine mg	Riboflavin mg	Niacin mg	Ascorbic Acid mg
	Ice Cream (cont.)																	
66	Rich (approx. 16% fat)	1/2 gal	1,188	63	2,635	31	191	105	63	6	214	927	0.2	7,840	0.24	1.31	1.2	12
67		1 cup	148	63	330	4	24	13	8	1	27	115	Trace	980	0.03	0.16	0.1	1
	Ice milk:																	
68	Hardened	1/2 gal	1,048	67	1,595	50	53	29	17	2	235	1,635	1.0	2,200	0.52	2.31	1.0	10
69		1 cup	131	67	200	6	7	4	2	Trace	29	204	0.1	280	0.07	0.29	0.1	1
70	Soft-serve	1 cup	175	67	265	8	9	5	3	Trace	39	273	0.2	370	0.09	0.39	0.2	2
	Yoghurt:																	
71	Made from partially skimmed milk	1 cup	245	89	125	8	4	2	1	Trace	13	294	0.1	170	0.10	0.44	0.2	2
72	Made from whole milk	1 cup	245	88	150	7	8	5	3	Trace	12	272	0.1	340	0.07	0.39	0.2	2
	Eggs																	
	Eggs, large, 24 ounces per dozen:																	
	Raw or cooked in shell or with nothing added:																	
73	Whole, without shell	1 egg	50	74	80	6	6	2	3	Trace	Trace	27	1.1	590	0.05	0.15	Trace	0
74	White of egg	1 white	33	88	15	4	Trace	—	—	—	Trace	3	Trace	0	Trace	0.09	Trace	0
75	Yolk of egg	1 yolk	17	51	60	3	5	2	2	Trace	Trace	24	0.9	580	0.04	0.07	Trace	0
76	Scrambled with milk and fat	1 egg	64	72	110	7	8	3	3	Trace	1	51	1.1	690	0.05	0.18	Trace	0
	Meat, Poultry, Fish, Shellfish; Related Products																	
77	Bacon (20 slices per lb raw), broiled or fried crisp	2 slices	15	8	90	5	8	3	4	1	1	2	0.5	0	0.08	0.05	0.8	—
	Beef,[3] cooked:																	
	Cuts braised, simmered, or pot-roasted:																	
78	Lean and fat	3 ounces	85	53	245	23	16	8	7	Trace	0	10	2.9	30	0.04	0.18	3.5	—
79	Lean only	2.5 ounces	72	62	140	22	5	2	2	Trace	0	10	2.7	10	0.04	0.16	3.3	—
	Hamburger (ground beef), broiled:																	
80	Lean	3 ounces	85	60	185	23	10	5	4	Trace	0	10	3.0	20	0.08	0.20	5.1	—
81	Regular	3 ounces	85	54	245	21	17	8	8	Trace	0	9	2.7	30	0.07	0.18	4.6	—
	Roast, oven-cooked, no liquid added:																	
	Relatively fat, such as rib:																	
82	Lean and fat	3 ounces	85	40	375	17	34	16	15	1	0	8	2.2	70	0.05	0.13	3.1	—
83	Lean only	1.8 ounces	51	57	125	14	7	3	3	Trace	0	6	1.8	10	0.04	0.11	2.6	—
	Relatively lean, such as heel of round:																	
84	Lean and fat	3 ounces	85	62	165	25	7	3	3	Trace	0	11	3.2	10	0.06	0.19	4.5	—
85	Lean only	2.7 ounces	78	65	125	24	3	1	1	Trace	0	10	3.0	Trace	0.06	0.18	4.3	—
	Steak, broiled:																	
	Relatively, fat, such as sirloin:																	
86	Lean and fat	3 ounces	85	44	330	20	27	13	12	1	0	9	2.5	50	0.05	0.16	4.0	—
87	Lean only	2.0 ounces	56	59	115	18	4	2	2	Trace	0	7	2.2	10	0.05	0.14	3.6	—
	Relatively, lean, such as round:																	
88	Lean and fat	3 ounces	85	55	220	24	13	6	6	Trace	0	10	3.0	20	0.07	0.19	4.8	—
89	Lean only	2.4 ounces	68	61	130	21	4	2	2	Trace	0	9	2.5	10	0.06	0.16	4.1	—
	Beef, canned:																	
90	Corned beef	3 ounces	85	59	185	22	10	5	4	Trace	0	17	3.7	20	0.01	0.20	2.9	—
91	Corned beef hash	3 ounces	85	67	155	7	10	5	4	Trace	9	11	1.7	—	0.01	0.08	1.8	—
92	Beef, dried or chipped	2 ounces	57	48	115	19	4	2	2	Trace	0	11	2.9	—	0.04	0.18	2.2	—
93	Beef and vegetable stew	1 cup	235	82	210	15	10	5	4	Trace	15	28	2.8	2,310	0.13	0.17	4.4	15
94	Beef potpie, baked, 4 1/4-inch diam., weight before baking about 8 ounces	1 pie	227	55	560	23	33	9	20	2	43	32	4.1	1,860	0.25	0.27	4.5	7
	Chicken, cooked:																	
95	Flesh only, broiled	3 ounces	85	71	115	20	3	1	1	1	0	8	1.4	80	0.05	0.16	7.4	—
	Breast, fried, 1/2 breast:																	
96	With bone	3.3 ounces	94	58	155	25	5	1	2	1	1	9	1.3	70	0.04	0.17	11.2	—
97	Flesh and skin only	2.7 ounces	76	58	155	25	5	1	2	1	1	9	1.3	70	0.04	0.17	11.2	—

	Drumstick, fried:																	
98	With bone	2.1 ounces	59	55	90	12	4	1	2	1	Trace	6	0.9	50	0.03	0.15	2.7	—
99	Flesh and skin only	1.3 ounces	38	55	90	12	4	1	2	1	Trace	6	0.9	50	0.03	0.15	2.7	—
100	Chicken, canned, boneless	3 ounces	85	65	170	18	10	3	4	2	0	18	1.3	200	0.03	0.11	3.7	3
101	Chicken potpie, baked 4 1/4-inch diam., weight before baking about 8 ounces	1 pie	227	57	535	23	31	10	15	3	42	68	3.0	3,020	0.25	0.26	4.1	5
	Chili con carne, canned:																	
102	With beans	1 cup	250	72	335	19	15	7	7	Trace	30	80	4.2	150	0.08	0.18	3.2	—
103	Without beans	1 cup	255	67	510	26	38	18	17	1	15	97	3.6	380	0.05	0.31	5.6	—
104	Heart, beef, lean, braised	3 ounces	85	61	160	27	5	—	—	—	1	5	5.0	20	0.21	1.04	6.5	1
	Lamb,[3] cooked:																	
105	Chop, thick, with bone, broiled	1 chop 4.8 ounces	137	47	400	25	33	18	12	1	0	10	1.5	—	0.14	0.25	5.6	—
106	Lean and fat	4.0 ounces	112	47	400	25	33	18	12	1	0	10	1.5	—	0.14	0.25	5.6	—
107	Lean only	2.6 ounces	74	62	140	21	6	3	2	Trace	0	9	1.5	—	0.11	0.20	4.5	—
	Leg, roasted:																	
108	Lean and fat	3 ounces	85	54	235	22	16	9	6	Trace	0	9	1.4	—	0.13	0.23	4.7	—
109	Lean only	2.5 ounces	71	62	130	20	5	3	2	Trace	0	9	1.4	—	0.12	0.21	4.4	—
	Shoulder, roasted:																	
110	Lean and fat	3 ounces	85	50	285	18	23	13	8	1	0	9	1.0	—	0.11	0.20	4.0	—
111	Lean only	2.3 ounces	64	61	130	17	6	3	2	Trace	0	8	1.0	—	0.10	0.18	3.7	—
112	Liver, beef, fried	2 ounces	57	57	130	15	6	—	—	—	3	6	5.0	30,280	0.15	2.37	9.4	15
	Pork, cured, cooked:																	
113	Ham, light cure, lean and fat, roasted	3 ounces	85	54	245	18	19	7	8	2	0	8	2.2	0	0.40	0.16	3.1	—
	Luncheon meat:																	
114	Boiled ham, sliced	2 ounces	57	59	135	11	10	4	4	1	0	6	1.6	0	0.25	0.09	1.5	—
115	Canned, spiced or unspiced	2 ounces	57	55	165	8	14	5	6	1	1	5	1.2	0	0.18	0.12	1.6	—
	Pork, fresh,[3] cooked:																	
116	Chop, thick, with bone	1 chop, 3.5 ounces	98	42	260	16	21	8	9	2	0	8	2.2	0	0.63	0.18	3.8	—
117	Lean and fat	2.3 ounces	66	42	260	16	21	8	9	2	0	8	2.2	0	0.63	0.18	3.8	—
118	Lean only	1.7 ounces	48	53	130	15	7	2	3	1	0	7	1.9	0	0.54	0.16	3.3	—
	Roast, oven-cooked, no liquid added:																	
119	Lean and fat	3 ounces	85	46	310	21	24	9	10	2	0	9	2.7	0	0.78	0.22	4.7	—
120	Lean only	2.4 ounces	68	55	175	20	10	3	4	1	0	9	2.6	0	0.73	0.21	4.4	—
	Cuts, simmered:																	
121	Lean and fat	3 ounces	85	46	320	20	26	9	11	2	0	8	2.5	0	0.46	0.21	4.1	—
122	Lean only	2.2 ounces	63	60	135	18	6	2	3	1	0	8	2.3	0	0.42	0.19	3.7	—
	Sausage:																	
123	Bologna, slice, 3-in diam. by 1/8 inch	2 slices	26	56	80	3	7	—	—	—	Trace	2	0.5	—	0.04	0.06	0.7	—
124	Braunschweiger, slice 2-in diam. by 1/4 inch	2 slices	20	53	65	3	5	—	—	—	Trace	2	1.2	1,310	0.03	0.29	1.6	—
125	Deviled ham, canned	1 tbsp	13	51	45	2	4	2	2	Trace	0	1	0.3	—	0.02	0.01	0.2	—
126	Frankfurter, heated (8 per lb purchased pkg)	1 frank	56	57	170	7	15	—	—	—	1	3	0.8	—	0.08	0.11	1.4	—
127	Pork links, cooked (16 links per lb raw)	2 links	26	35	125	5	11	4	5	1	Trace	2	0.6	0	0.21	0.09	1.0	—
128	Salami, dry type	1 oz	28	30	130	7	11	—	—	—	Trace	4	1.0	—	0.10	0.07	1.5	—
129	Salami, cooked	1 oz	28	51	90	5	7	—	—	—	Trace	3	0.7	—	0.07	0.07	1.2	—
130	Vienna, canned (7 sausages per 5-oz can)	1 sausage	16	63	40	2	3	—	—	—	Trace	1	0.3	—	0.01	0.02	0.4	—
	Veal, medium fat, cooked, bone removed:																	
131	Cutlet	3 oz	85	60	185	23	9	5	4	Trace	—	9	2.7	—	0.06	0.21	4.6	—
132	Roast	3 oz	85	55	230	23	14	7	6	Trace	0	10	2.9	—	0.11	0.26	6.6	—
	Fish and shellfish:																	
133	Bluefish, baked with table fat	3 oz	85	68	135	22	4	—	—	—	0	25	0.6	40	0.09	0.08	1.6	—
	Clams:																	
134	Raw, meat only	3 oz	85	82	65	11	1	—	—	—	2	59	5.2	90	0.08	0.15	1.1	8
135	Canned, solids and liquid	3 oz	85	86	45	7	1	—	—	—	2	47	3.5	—	0.01	0.09	0.9	—
136	Crabmeat, canned	3 oz	85	77	85	15	2	—	—	—	1	38	0.7	—	0.07	0.07	1.6	—

[3]Outer layer of fat on the cut was removed to within approximately 1/2-inch of the lean. Deposits of fat within the cut were not removed.

Table A–1. (Cont.)

No.	Food, Approximate Measure, and Weight (in grams)		gm	Water per cent	Food Energy calories	Protein gm	Fat gm	Fatty Acids: Saturated (total) gm	Fatty Acids: Unsaturated: Oleic gm	Fatty Acids: Unsaturated: Linoleic gm	Carbohydrate gm	Calcium mg	Iron mg	Vitamin A Value I.U.	Thiamine mg	Riboflavin mg	Niacin mg	Ascorbic Acid mg
137	Fish sticks, breaded, cooked, frozen; stick 3 3/4 by 1 by 1/2 inch	10 sticks or 8 oz pkg.	227	66	400	38	20	5	4	10	15	25	0.9	—	0.09	0.16	3.6	—
138	Haddock, breaded, fried	3 oz	85	66	140	17	5	1	3	Trace	5	34	1.0	—	0.03	0.06	2.7	2
139	Ocean perch, breaded, fried	3 oz	85	59	195	16	11	—	—	—	6	28	1.1	—	0.08	0.09	1.5	—
140	Oysters, raw, meat only (13–19 med. selects)	1 cup	240	85	160	20	4	—	—	—	8	226	13.2	740	0.33	0.43	6.0	—
141	Salmon, pink, canned	3 oz	85	71	120	17	5	1	1	Trace	0	[4]167	0.7	60	0.03	0.16	6.8	—
142	Sardines, Atlantic, canned in oil, drained solids	3 oz	85	62	175	20	9	—	—	—	0	372	2.5	190	0.02	0.17	4.6	—
143	Shad, baked with table fat and bacon	3 oz	85	64	170	20	10	—	—	—	0	20	0.5	20	0.11	0.22	7.3	—
144	Shrimp, canned, meat	3 oz	85	70	100	21	1	—	—	—	1	98	2.6	50	0.01	0.03	1.5	—
145	Swordfish, broiled with butter or margarine	3 oz	85	65	150	24	5	—	—	—	0	23	1.1	1,750	0.03	0.04	9.3	—
146	Tuna, canned in oil, drained solids	3 oz	85	61	170	24	7	2	1	1	0	7	1.6	70	0.04	0.10	10.1	—
	Mature Dry Beans and Peas, Nuts, Peanuts; Related Products																	
147	Almonds, shelled, whole kernels	1 cup	142	5	850	26	77	6	52	15	28	332	6.7	0	0.34	1.31	5.0	Trace
	Beans, dry:																	
	Common varieties as Great Northern, navy and others:																	
	Cooked, drained:																	
148	Great Northern	1 cup	180	69	210	14	1	—	—	—	38	90	4.9	0	0.25	0.13	1.3	0
149	Navy (pea)	1 cup	190	69	225	15	1	—	—	—	40	95	5.1	0	0.27	0.13	1.3	0
	Canned, solids and liquid:																	
	White with—																	
150	Frankfurters (sliced)	1 cup	255	71	365	19	18	—	—	—	32	94	4.8	330	0.18	0.15	3.3	Trace
151	Pork and tomato sauce	1 cup	255	71	310	16	7	2	3	1	49	138	4.6	330	0.20	0.08	1.5	5
152	Pork and sweet sauce	1 cup	255	66	385	16	12	4	5	1	54	161	5.9	—	0.15	0.10	1.3	—
153	Red kidney	1 cup	255	76	230	15	1	—	—	—	42	74	4.6	10	0.13	0.10	1.5	—
154	Lima, cooked, drained	1 cup	190	64	260	16	1	—	—	—	49	55	5.9	—	0.25	0.11	1.3	—
155	Cashew nuts, roasted	1 cup	140	5	785	24	64	11	45	4	41	53	5.3	140	0.60	0.35	2.5	—
	Coconut, fresh, meat only:																	
156	Pieces, approx. 2 by 2 by 1/2 inch	1 piece	45	51	155	2	16	14	1	Trace	4	6	0.8	0	0.02	0.01	0.2	1
157	Shredded or grated, firmly packed	1 cup	130	51	450	5	46	39	3	Trace	12	17	2.2	0	0.07	0.03	0.7	4
158	Cowpeas or blackeye peas, dry, cooked	1 cup	248	80	190	13	1	—	—	—	34	42	3.2	20	0.41	0.11	1.1	Trace
159	Peanuts, roasted, salted, halves	1 cup	144	2	840	37	72	16	31	21	27	107	3.0	—	0.46	0.19	24.7	0
160	Peanut butter	1 tbsp	16	2	95	4	8	2	4	2	3	9	0.3	—	0.02	0.02	2.4	0
161	Peas, split, dry, cooked	1 cup	250	70	290	20	1	—	—	—	52	28	4.2	100	0.37	0.22	2.2	—
162	Pecans, halves	1 cup	108	3	740	10	77	5	48	15	16	79	2.6	140	0.93	0.14	1.0	2
163	Walnuts, black or native, chopped	1 cup	126	3	790	26	75	4	26	36	19	Trace	7.6	380	0.28	0.14	0.9	—
	Vegetables and Vegetable Products																	
	Asparagus, green:																	
	Cooked, drained:																	
164	Spears, 1/2-in. diam. at base	4 spears	60	94	10	1	Trace	—	—	—	2	13	0.4	540	0.10	0.11	0.8	16
165	Pieces, 1 1/2 to 2-in. lengths	1 cup	145	94	30	3	Trace	—	—	—	5	30	0.9	1,310	0.23	0.26	2.0	38
166	Canned, solids and liquid	1 cup	244	94	45	5	1	—	—	—	7	44	4.1	1,240	0.15	0.22	2.0	37

	Beans:																	
167	Lima, immature seeds, cooked, drained	1 cup	170	71	190	13	1	—	—	—	34	80	4.3	480	0.31	0.17	2.2	29
	Snap:																	
	Green:																	
168	Cooked, drained	1 cup	125	92	30	2	Trace	—	—	—	7	63	0.8	680	0.09	0.11	0.6	15
169	Canned, solids and liquid	1 cup	239	94	45	2	Trace	—	—	—	10	81	2.9	690	0.07	0.10	0.7	10
	Yellow or wax:																	
170	Cooked, drained	1 cup	125	93	30	2	Trace	—	—	—	6	63	0.8	290	0.09	0.11	0.6	16
171	Canned, solids and liquid	1 cup	239	94	45	2	1	—	—	—	10	81	2.9	140	0.07	0.10	0.7	12
172	Sprouted mung beans, cooked, drained	1 cup	125	91	35	4	Trace	—	—	—	7	21	1.1	30	0.11	0.13	0.9	8
	Beets:																	
	Cooked, drained, peeled:																	
173	Whole beets, 2-in. diam.	2 beets	100	91	30	1	Trace	—	—	—	7	14	0.5	20	0.03	0.04	0.3	6
174	Diced or sliced	1 cup	170	91	55	2	Trace	—	—	—	12	24	0.9	30	0.05	0.07	0.5	10
175	Canned, solids and liquid	1 cup	246	90	85	2	Trace	—	—	—	19	34	1.5	20	0.02	0.05	0.2	7
176	Beet greens, leaves and stems, cooked, drained	1 cup	145	94	25	3	Trace	—	—	—	5	144	2.8	7,400	0.10	0.22	0.4	22
	Blackeye peas. See Cowpeas																	
	Broccoli, cooked, drained:																	
177	Whole stalks, medium size	1 stalk	180	91	45	6	1	—	—	—	8	158	1.4	4,500	0.16	0.36	1.4	162
178	Stalks cut into 1/2-in pieces	1 cup	155	91	40	5	1	—	—	—	7	136	1.2	3,880	0.14	0.31	1.2	140
179	Chopped, yield from 10-oz frozen pkg	1 3/8 cups	250	92	65	7	1	—	—	—	12	135	1.8	6,500	0.15	0.30	1.3	143
180	Brussels sprouts, 7–8 sprouts (1 1/4 to 1 1/2 in diam.) per cup, cooked	1 cup	155	88	55	7	1	—	—	—	10	50	1.7	810	0.12	0.22	1.2	135
	Cabbage:																	
	Common varieties:																	
	Raw:																	
181	Coarsely shredded or sliced	1 cup	70	92	15	1	Trace	—	—	—	4	34	0.3	90	0.04	0.04	0.2	33
182	Finely shredded or chopped	1 cup	90	92	20	1	Trace	—	—	—	5	44	0.4	120	0.05	0.05	0.3	42
183	Cooked	1 cup	145	94	30	2	Trace	—	—	—	6	64	0.4	190	0.06	0.06	0.4	48
184	Red, raw, coarsely shredded	1 cup	70	90	20	1	Trace	—	—	—	5	29	0.6	30	0.06	0.04	0.3	43
185	Savoy, raw, coarsely shredded	1 cup	70	92	15	2	Trace	—	—	—	3	47	0.6	140	0.04	0.06	0.2	39
186	Cabbage, celery or Chinese raw, cut in 1-in pieces	1 cup	75	95	10	1	Trace	—	—	—	2	32	0.5	110	0.04	0.03	0.5	19
187	Cabbage, spoon (or pakchoy), cooked	1 cup	170	95	25	2	Trace	—	—	—	4	252	1.0	5,270	0.07	0.14	1.2	26
	Carrots:																	
	Raw:																	
188	Whole, 5 1/2 by 1 inch, (25 thin strips)	1 carrot	50	88	20	1	Trace	—	—	—	5	18	0.4	5,500	0.03	0.03	0.3	4
189	Grated	1 cup	110	88	45	1	Trace	—	—	—	11	41	0.8	12,100	0.06	0.06	0.7	9
190	Cooked, diced	1 cup	145	91	45	1	Trace	—	—	—	10	48	0.9	15,220	0.08	0.07	0.7	9
191	Canned, strained or chopped (baby food)	1 ounce	28	92	10	Trace	Trace	—	—	—	2	7	0.1	3,690	0.01	0.01	0.1	1
192	Cauliflower, cooked, flower-buds	1 cup	120	93	25	3	Trace	—	—	—	5	25	0.8	70	0.11	0.10	0.7	66
	Celery, raw:																	
193	Stalk, large outer, 8 by about 1 1/2 inches, at root end	1 stalk	40	94	5	Trace	Trace	—	—	—	2	16	0.1	100	0.01	0.01	0.1	4
194	Pieces, diced	1 cup	100	94	15	1	Trace	—	—	—	4	39	0.3	240	0.03	0.03	0.3	9
195	Collards, cooked	1 cup	190	91	55	5	1	—	—	—	9	289	1.1	10,260	0.27	0.37	2.4	87
	Corn sweet:																	
196	Cooked, ear 5 by 1 3/4 inches[5]	1 ear	140	74	70	3	1	—	—	—	16	2	0.5	[6]310	0.09	0.08	1.0	7
197	Canned, solids and liquid	1 cup	256	81	170	5	2	—	—	—	40	10	1.0	[6]690	0.07	0.12	2.3	13

[4]If bones are discarded, value will be greatly reduced.

[5]Measure and weight apply to entire vegetable or fruit including parts not usually eaten.

[6]Based on yellow varieties; white varieties contain only a trace of cryptoxanthin and carotenes, the pigments in corn that have biologic activity.

Table A–1. (Cont.)

	Food, Approximate Measure, and Weight (in grams)		gm	Water per cent	Food Energy calories	Protein gm	Fat gm	Fatty Acids: Saturated (total) gm	Fatty Acids: Unsaturated: Oleic gm	Fatty Acids: Unsaturated: Linoleic gm	Carbohydrate gm	Calcium mg	Iron mg	Vitamin A Value I.U.	Thiamine mg	Riboflavin mg	Niacin mg	Ascorbic Acid mg
198	Cowpeas, cooked immature seeds	1 cup	160	72	175	13	1	—	—	—	29	38	3.4	560	0.49	0.18	2.3	28
	Cucumbers, 10-ounce; 7 1/2 by about 2 inches:																	
199	Raw, pared	1 cucumber	207	96	30	1	Trace	—	—	—	7	35	0.6	Trace	0.07	0.09	0.4	23
200	Raw, pared, center slice 1/8-inch thick	6 slices	50	96	5	Trace	Trace	—	—	—	2	8	0.2	Trace	0.02	0.02	0.1	6
201	Dandelion greens, cooked	1 cup	180	90	60	4	1	—	—	—	12	252	3.2	21,060	0.24	0.29	—	32
202	Endive, curly (including escarole)	2 ounces	57	93	10	1	Trace	—	—	—	2	46	1.0	1,870	0.04	0.08	0.3	6
203	Kale, leaves including stems, cooked	1 cup	110	91	30	4	1	—	—	—	4	147	1.3	8,140	—	—	—	68
	Lettuce, raw:																	
204	Butterhead, as Boston types; head, 4-inch diameter	1 head	220	95	30	3	Trace	—	—	—	6	77	4.4	2,130	0.14	0.13	0.6	18
205	Crisphead, as Iceberg; head, 4 3/4 inch diameter	1 head	454	96	60	4	Trace	—	—	—	13	91	2.3	1,500	0.29	0.27	1.3	29
206	Looseleaf, or bunching varieties, leaves	2 large	50	94	10	1	Trace	—	—	—	2	34	0.7	950	0.03	0.04	0.2	9
207	Mushrooms, canned, solids and liquid	1 cup	244	93	40	5	Trace	—	—	—	6	15	1.2	Trace	0.04	0.60	4.8	4
208	Mustard greens, cooked	1 cup	140	93	35	3	1	—	—	—	6	193	2.5	8,120	0.11	0.19	0.9	68
209	Okra, cooked, pod 3 by 5/8 inch	8 pods	85	91	25	2	Trace	—	—	—	5	78	0.4	420	0.11	0.15	0.8	17
	Onions:																	
	Mature:																	
210	Raw, onion 2 1/2-inch diameter	1 onion	110	89	40	2	Trace	—	—	—	10	30	0.6	40	0.04	0.04	0.2	11
211	Cooked	1 cup	210	92	60	3	Trace	—	—	—	14	50	0.8	80	0.06	0.06	0.4	14
212	Young green, small, without tops	6 onions	50	88	20	1	Trace	—	—	—	5	20	0.3	Trace	0.02	0.02	0.2	12
213	Parsley, raw, chopped	1 tablespoon	4	85	Trace	Trace	Trace	—	—	—	Trace	8	0.2	340	Trace	0.01	Trace	7
214	Parsnips, cooked	1 cup	155	82	100	2	1	—	—	—	23	70	0.9	50	0.11	0.12	0.2	16
	Peas, green:																	
215	Cooked	1 cup	160	82	115	9	1	—	—	—	19	37	2.9	860	0.44	0.17	3.7	33
216	Canned, solids and liquid	1 cup	249	83	165	9	1	—	—	—	31	50	4.2	1,120	0.23	0.13	2.2	22
217	Canned, strained (baby food)	1 ounce	28	86	15	1	Trace	—	—	—	3	3	0.4	140	0.02	0.02	0.4	3
218	Peppers, hot, red, without seeds, dried (ground chili powder, added seasonings)	1 tablespoon	15	8	50	2	2	—	—	—	8	40	2.3	9,750	0.03	0.17	1.3	2
	Peppers, sweet:																	
	Raw, about 5 per pound:																	
219	Green pod without stem and seeds	1 pod	74	93	15	1	Trace	—	—	—	4	7	0.5	310	0.06	0.06	0.4	94
220	Cooked, boiled, drained	1 pod	73	95	15	1	Trace	—	—	—	3	7	0.4	310	0.05	0.05	0.4	70
	Potatoes, medium (about 3 per pound raw):																	
221	Baked, peeled after baking	1 potato	99	75	90	3	Trace	—	—	—	21	9	0.7	Trace	0.10	0.04	1.7	20
	Boiled:																	
222	Peeled after boiling	1 potato	136	80	105	3	Trace	—	—	—	23	10	0.8	Trace	0.13	0.05	2.0	22
223	Peeled before boiling	1 potato	122	83	80	2	Trace	—	—	—	18	7	0.6	Trace	0.11	0.04	1.4	20
	French-fried, piece 2 by 1/2 by 1/2 inch:																	
224	Cooked in deep fat	10 pieces	57	45	155	2	7	2	2	4	20	9	0.7	Trace	0.07	0.04	1.8	12
225	Frozen, heated	10 pieces	57	53	125	2	5	1	1	2	19	5	1.0	Trace	0.08	0.01	1.5	12
	Mashed:																	
226	Milk added	1 cup	195	83	125	4	1	—	—	—	25	47	0.8	50	0.16	0.10	2.0	19
227	Milk and butter added	1 cup	195	80	185	4	8	4	3	Trace	24	47	0.8	330	0.16	0.10	1.9	18
228	Potato chips, medium, 2-inch diameter	10 chips	20	2	115	1	8	2	2	4	10	8	0.4	Trace	0.04	0.01	1.0	3

229	Pumpkin, canned	1 cup	228	90	75	2	1	—	—	—	18	57	0.9	14,590	0.07	0.12	1.3	12
230	Radishes, raw, small, without tops	4 radishes	40	94	5	Trace	Trace	—	—	—	1	12	0.4	Trace	0.01	0.01	0.1	10
231	Sauerkraut, canned, solids and liquid	1 cup	235	93	45	2	Trace	—	—	—	9	85	1.2	120	0.07	0.09	0.4	33
	Spinach:																	
232	Cooked	1 cup	180	92	40	5	1	—	—	—	6	167	4.0	14,580	0.13	0.25	1.0	50
233	Canned, drained solids	1 cup	180	91	45	5	1	—	—	—	6	212	4.7	14,400	0.03	0.21	0.6	24
	Squash:																	
	Cooked:																	
234	Summer, diced	1 cup	210	96	30	2	Trace	—	—	—	7	52	0.8	820	0.10	0.16	1.6	21
235	Winter, baked, mashed	1 cup	205	81	130	4	1	—	—	—	32	57	1.6	8,610	0.10	0.27	1.4	27
	Sweetpotatoes:																	
	Cooked, medium, 5 by 2 inches, weight raw about 6 ounces:																	
236	Baked, peeled after baking	1 sweet-potato	110	64	155	2	1	—	—	—	36	44	1.0	8,910	0.10	0.07	0.7	24
237	Boiled, peeled after boiling	1 sweet-potato	147	71	170	2	1	—	—	—	39	47	1.0	11,610	0.13	0.09	0.9	25
238	Candied, 3 1/2 by 2 1/4 inches	1 sweet-potato	175	60	295	2	6	2	3	1	60	65	1.6	11,030	0.10	0.08	0.8	17
239	Canned, vacuum or solid pack	1 cup	218	72	235	4	Trace	—	—	—	54	54	1.7	17,000	0.10	0.10	1.4	30
	Tomatoes:																	
240	Raw, approx. 3-in diam. 2 1/8 in high; wt., 7 oz	1 tomato	200	94	40	2	Trace	—	—	—	9	24	0.9	1,640	0.11	0.07	1.3	[7]42
241	Canned, solids and liquid	1 cup	241	94	50	2	1	—	—	—	10	14	1.2	2,170	0.12	0.07	1.7	41
	Tomato catsup:																	
242	Cup	1 cup	273	69	290	6	1	—	—	—	69	60	2.2	3,820	0.25	0.19	4.4	41
243	Tablespoon	1 tbsp.	15	69	15	Trace	Trace	—	—	—	4	3	0.1	210	0.01	0.01	0.2	2
	Tomato juice, canned:																	
244	Cup	1 cup	243	94	45	2	Trace	—	—	—	10	17	2.2	1,940	0.12	0.07	1.9	39
245	Glass (6 fl oz)	1 glass	182	94	35	2	Trace	—	—	—	8	13	1.6	1,460	0.09	0.05	1.5	29
246	Turnips, cooked, diced	1 cup	155	94	35	1	Trace	—	—	—	8	54	0.6	Trace	0.06	0.08	0.5	34
247	Turnips greens, cooked	1 cup	145	94	30	3	Trace	—	—	—	5	252	1.5	8,270	0.15	0.33	0.7	68
	Fruits and Fruit Products																	
248	Apples, raw (about 3 per lb)[5]	1 apple	150	85	70	Trace	Trace	—	—	—	18	8	0.4	50	0.04	0.02	0.1	3
249	Apple juice, bottled or canned	1 cup	248	88	120	Trace	Trace	—	—	—	30	15	1.5	—	0.02	0.05	0.2	2
	Applesauce, canned:																	
250	Sweetened	1 cup	255	76	230	1	Trace	—	—	—	61	10	1.3	100	0.05	0.03	0.1	[8]3
251	Unsweetened or artificially sweetened	1 cup	244	88	100	1	Trace	—	—	—	26	10	1.2	100	0.05	0.02	0.1	[8]2
	Apricots:																	
252	Raw (about 12 per lb)[5]	3 apricots	114	85	55	1	Trace	—	—	—	14	18	0.5	2,890	0.03	0.04	0.7	10
253	Canned in heavy syrup	1 cup	259	77	220	2	Trace	—	—	—	57	28	0.8	4,510	0.05	0.06	0.9	10
254	Dried, uncooked (40 halves per cup)	1 cup	150	25	390	8	1	—	—	—	100	100	8.2	16,350	0.02	0.23	4.9	19
255	Cooked, unsweetened, fruit and liquid	1 cup	285	76	240	5	1	—	—	—	62	63	5.1	8,550	0.01	0.13	2.8	8
256	Apricot nectar, canned	1 cup	251	85	140	1	Trace	—	—	—	37	23	0.5	2,380	0.03	0.03	0.5	[8]8
	Avocados, whole fruit, raw:[5]																	
257	California (mid- and late-winter; diam. 3 1/8 in)	1 avocado	284	74	370	5	37	7	17	5	13	22	1.3	630	0.24	0.43	3.5	30
258	Florida (late summer, fall; diam. 3 5/8 in)	1 avocado	454	78	390	4	33	7	15	4	27	30	1.8	880	0.33	0.61	4.9	43
259	Bananas, raw, medium size[5]	1 banana	175	76	100	1	Trace	—	—	—	26	10	0.8	230	0.06	0.07	0.8	12
260	Banana flakes	1 cup	100	3	340	4	1	—	—	—	89	32	2.8	760	0.18	0.24	2.8	7
261	Blackberries, raw	1 cup	144	84	85	2	1	—	—	—	19	46	1.3	290	0.05	0.06	0.5	30
262	Blueberries, raw	1 cup	140	83	85	1	1	—	—	—	21	21	1.4	140	0.04	0.08	0.6	20
263	Cantaloups, raw; medium, 5-inch diameter about 1 2/3 pounds[5]	1/2 melon	385	91	60	1	Trace	—	—	—	14	27	0.8	[9]6,540	0.08	0.06	1.2	63

[5]Measure and weight apply to entire vegetable or fruit including parts not usually eaten.

[7]Year-round average. Samples marketed from November through May, average 20 milligrams per 200-gram tomato; from June through October, around 52 milligrams.

[8]This is the amount from the fruit. Additional ascorbic acid may be added by the manufacturer. Refer to the label for this information.

[9]Value for varieties with orange-colored flesh; value for varieties with green flesh would be about 540 I.U.

Table A–1. (Cont.)

No.	Food, Approximate Measure, and Weight (in grams)		gm	Water per cent	Food Energy calories	Protein gm	Fat gm	Fatty Acids: Saturated (total) gm	Fatty Acids: Unsaturated: Oleic gm	Fatty Acids: Unsaturated: Linoleic gm	Carbohydrate gm	Calcium mg	Iron mg	Vitamin A Value I.U.	Thiamine mg	Riboflavin mg	Niacin mg	Ascorbic Acid mg
264	Cherries, canned, red, sour, pitted, water pack	1 cup	244	88	105	2	Trace	—	—	—	26	37	0.7	1,660	0.07	0.05	0.5	12
265	Cranberry juice cocktail, canned	1 cup	250	83	165	Trace	Trace	—	—	—	42	13	0.8	Trace	0.03	0.03	0.1	[10]40
266	Cranberry sauce, sweetened, canned, strained	1 cup	277	62	405	Trace	1	—	—	—	104	17	0.6	60	0.03	0.03	0.1	6
267	Dates, pitted, cut	1 cup	178	22	490	4	1	—	—	—	130	105	5.3	90	0.16	0.17	3.9	0
268	Figs, dried, large, 2 by 1 in	1 fig	21	23	60	1	Trace	—	—	—	15	26	0.6	20	0.02	0.02	0.1	0
269	Fruit cocktail, canned, in heavy syrup	1 cup	256	80	195	1	Trace	—	—	—	50	23	1.0	360	0.05	0.03	1.3	5
	Grapefruit:																	
	Raw, medium, 3 3/4-in diam.[5]																	
270	White	1/2 grapefruit	241	89	45	1	Trace	—	—	—	12	19	0.5	10	0.05	0.02	0.2	44
271	Pink or red	1/2 grapefruit	241	89	50	1	Trace	—	—	—	13	20	0.5	540	0.05	0.02	0.2	44
272	Canned, syrup pack	1 cup	254	81	180	2	Trace	—	—	—	45	33	0.8	30	0.08	0.05	0.5	76
	Grapefruit juice:																	
273	Fresh	1 cup	246	90	95	1	Trace	—	—	—	23	22	0.5	(11)	0.09	0.04	0.4	92
	Canned, white:																	
274	Unsweetened	1 cup	247	89	100	1	Trace	—	—	—	24	20	1.0	20	0.07	0.04	0.4	84
275	Sweetened	1 cup	250	86	130	1	Trace	—	—	—	32	20	1.0	20	0.07	0.04	0.4	78
	Frozen, concentrate, unsweetened:																	
276	Undiluted, can, 6 fluid ounces	1 can	207	62	300	4	1	—	—	—	72	70	0.8	60	0.29	0.12	1.4	286
277	Diluted with 3 parts water, by volume	1 cup	247	89	100	1	Trace	—	—	—	24	25	0.2	20	0.10	0.04	0.5	96
278	Dehydrated crystals	4 oz	113	1	410	6	1	—	—	—	102	100	1.2	80	0.40	0.20	2.0	396
279	Prepared with water (1 pound yields about 1 gallon)	1 cup	247	90	100	1	Trace	—	—	—	24	22	0.2	20	0.10	0.05	0.5	91
	Grapes, raw:[5]																	
280	American type (slip skin)	1 cup	153	82	65	1	1	—	—	—	15	15	0.4	100	0.05	0.03	0.2	3
281	European type (adherent skin)	1 cup	160	81	95	1	Trace	—	—	—	25	17	0.6	140	0.07	0.04	0.4	6
	Grapejuice:																	
282	Canned or bottled	1 cup	253	83	165	1	Trace	—	—	—	42	28	0.8	—	0.10	0.05	0.5	Trace
	Frozen concentrate, sweetened:																	
283	Undiluted, can, 6 fluid ounces	1 can	216	53	395	1	Trace	—	—	—	100	22	0.9	40	0.13	0.22	1.5	(12)
284	Diluted with 3 parts water, by volume	1 cup	250	86	135	1	Trace	—	—	—	33	8	0.3	10	0.05	0.08	0.5	(12)
285	Grapejuice drink, canned	1 cup	250	86	135	Trace	Trace	—	—	—	35	8	0.3	—	0.03	0.03	0.3	(12)
286	Lemons, raw, 2 1/8-in diam., size 165.[5] Used for juice	1 lemon	110	90	20	1	Trace	—	—	—	6	19	0.4	10	0.03	0.01	0.1	39
287	Lemon juice, raw	1 cup	244	91	60	1	Trace	—	—	—	20	17	0.5	50	0.07	0.02	0.2	112
	Lemonade concentrate:																	
288	Frozen, 6 fl oz per can	1 can	219	48	430	Trace	Trace	—	—	—	112	9	0.4	40	0.04	0.07	0.7	66
289	Diluted with 4 1/3 parts water, by volume	1 cup	248	88	110	Trace	Trace	—	—	—	28	2	Trace	Trace	Trace	0.02	0.2	17
	Lime juice:																	
290	Fresh	1 cup	246	90	65	1	Trace	—	—	—	22	22	0.5	20	0.05	0.02	0.2	79
291	Canned, unsweetened	1 cup	246	90	65	1	Trace	—	—	—	22	22	0.5	20	0.05	0.02	0.2	52
	Limeade concentrate, frozen:																	
292	Undiluted, can, 6 fluid ounces	1 can	218	50	410	Trace	Trace	—	—	—	108	11	0.2	Trace	0.02	0.02	0.2	26
293	Diluted with 4 1/3 parts water, by volume	1 cup	247	90	100	Trace	Trace	—	—	—	27	2	Trace	Trace	Trace	Trace	Trace	5
294	Oranges, raw, 2 5/8-in diam., all commercial varieties[5]	1 orange	180	86	65	1	Trace	—	—	—	16	54	0.5	260	0.13	0.05	0.5	66
295	Orange juice, fresh, all varieties	1 cup	248	88	110	2	1	—	—	—	26	27	0.5	500	0.22	0.07	1.0	124

No.	Food	Measure																
296	Canned, unsweetened	1 cup	249	87	120	2	Trace	—	—	—	28	25	1.0	500	0.17	0.05	0.7	100
	Frozen concentrate:																	
297	Undiluted, can, 6 fluid ounces	1 can	213	55	360	5	Trace	—	—	—	87	75	0.9	1,620	0.68	0.11	2.8	360
298	Diluted with 3 parts water, by volume	1 cup	249	87	120	2	Trace	—	—	—	29	25	0.2	550	0.22	0.02	1.0	120
299	Dehydrated crystals	4 oz	113	1	430	6	2	—	—	—	100	95	1.9	1,900	0.76	0.24	3.3	408
300	Prepared with water (1 pound yields about 1 gallon)	1 cup	248	88	115	2	1	—	—	—	27	25	0.5	500	0.20	0.07	1.0	109
301	Orange-apricot juice drink	1 cup	249	87	125	1	Trace	—	—	—	32	12	0.2	1,440	0.05	0.02	0.5	[10]40
	Orange and grapefruit juice:																	
	Frozen concentrate:																	
302	Undiluted, can, 6 fluid ounces	1 can	210	59	330	4	1	—	—	—	78	61	0.8	800	0.48	0.06	2.3	302
303	Diluted with 3 parts water, by volume	1 cup	248	88	110	1	Trace	—	—	—	26	20	0.2	270	0.16	0.02	0.8	102
304	Papayas, raw, 1/2-inch cubes	1 cup	182	89	70	1	Trace	—	—	—	18	36	0.5	3,190	0.07	0.08	0.5	102
	Peaches:																	
	Raw:																	
305	Whole, medium, 2-inch diameter, about 4 per pound[5]	1 peach	114	89	35	1	Trace	—	—	—	10	9	0.5	[13]1,320	0.02	0.05	1.0	7
306	Sliced	1 cup	168	89	65	1	Trace	—	—	—	16	15	0.8	[13]2,230	0.03	0.08	1.6	12
	Canned, yellow-fleshed, solids and liquid:																	
	Syrup pack, heavy:																	
307	Halves or slices	1 cup	257	79	200	1	Trace	—	—	—	52	10	0.8	1,100	0.02	0.06	1.4	7
308	Water pack	1 cup	245	91	75	1	Trace	—	—	—	20	10	0.7	1,100	0.02	0.06	1.4	7
309	Dried, uncooked	1 cup	160	25	420	5	1	—	—	—	109	77	9.6	6,240	0.02	0.31	8.5	28
310	Cooked, unsweetened, 10–12 halves and juice	1 cup	270	77	220	3	1	—	—	—	58	41	5.1	3,290	0.01	0.15	4.2	6
	Frozen:																	
311	Carton, 12 ounces, not thawed	1 carton	340	76	300	1	Trace	—	—	—	77	14	1.7	2,210	0.03	0.14	2.4	[14]135
	Pears:																	
312	Raw, 3 by 2 1/2-inch diameter[5]	1 pear	182	83	100	1	1	—	—	—	25	13	0.5	30	0.04	0.07	0.2	7
	Canned, solids, and liquid:																	
	Syrup pack, heavy:																	
313	Halves or slices	1 cup	255	80	195	1	1	—	—	—	50	13	0.5	Trace	0.03	0.05	0.3	4
	Pineapple:																	
314	Raw, diced	1 cup	140	85	75	1	Trace	—	—	—	19	24	0.7	100	0.12	0.04	0.3	24
	Canned, heavy syrup pack, solids and liquids:																	
315	Crushed	1 cup	260	80	195	1	Trace	—	—	—	50	29	0.8	120	0.20	0.06	0.5	17
316	Sliced, slices and juice	2 small or 1 large	122	80	90	Trace	Trace	—	—	—	24	13	0.4	50	0.09	0.03	0.2	8
317	Pineapple juice, canned	1 cup	249	86	135	1	Trace	—	—	—	34	37	0.7	120	0.12	0.04	0.5	[8]22
	Plums, all except prunes:																	
318	Raw, 2-inch diameter, about 2 ounces[5]	1 plum	60	87	25	Trace	Trace	—	—	—	7	7	0.3	140	0.02	0.02	0.3	3
	Canned, syrup pack (Italian prunes):																	
319	Plums (with pits) and juice[5]	1 cup	256	77	205	1	Trace	—	—	—	53	22	2.2	2,970	0.05	0.05	0.9	4
	Prunes, dried, "softenized," medium:																	
320	Uncooked[5]	4 prunes	32	28	70	1	Trace	—	—	—	18	14	1.1	440	0.02	0.04	0.4	1
321	Cooked, unsweetened, 17–18 prunes and 1/3 cup liquid[5]	1 cup	270	66	295	2	1	—	—	—	78	60	4.5	1,860	0.08	0.18	1.7	2
322	Prune juice, canned or bottled	1 cup	256	80	200	1	Trace	—	—	—	49	36	10.5	—	0.03	0.03	1.0	[8]5

[5]Measure and weight apply to entire vegetable or fruit inc uding parts not usually eaten.

[8]This is the amount from the fruit. Additional ascorbic acid may be added by the manufacturer. Refer to the label for this information.

[10]Value listed is based on product with label stating 30 milligrams per 6-fl-oz serving.

[11]For white-fleshed varieties value is about 20 I.U. per cup; for red-fleshed varieties, 1,080 I.U. per cup.

[12]Present only if added by the manufacturer. Refer to the label for this information.

[13]Based on yellow-fleshed varieties; for white-fleshed varieties value is about 50 I.U. per 114-gm peach and 80 I.U. per cup of sliced peaches.

[14]This value includes ascorbic acid added by manufacturer.

Table A–1. (Cont.)

No.	Food, Approximate Measure, and Weight (in grams)		gm	Water per cent	Food Energy calories	Protein gm	Fat gm	Fatty Acids: Saturated (total) gm	Fatty Acids: Unsaturated: Oleic gm	Fatty Acids: Unsaturated: Linoleic gm	Carbohydrate gm	Calcium mg	Iron mg	Vitamin A Value I.U.	Thiamine mg	Riboflavin mg	Niacin mg	Ascorbic Acid mg
	Raisins, seedless:																	
323	Packaged, 1/2 oz or 1 1/2 tbsp per pkg.	1 pkg	14	18	40	Trace	Trace	—	—	—	11	9	0.5	Trace	0.02	0.01	0.1	Trace
324	Cup, pressed down	1 cup	165	18	480	4	Trace	—	—	—	128	102	5.8	30	0.18	0.13	0.8	2
	Raspberries, red:																	
325	Raw	1 cup	123	84	70	1	1	—	—	—	17	27	1.1	160	0.04	0.11	1.1	31
326	Frozen, 10-ounce carton, not thawed	1 carton	284	74	275	2	1	—	—	—	70	37	1.7	200	0.06	0.17	1.7	59
327	Rhubarb, cooked, sugar added	1 cup	272	63	385	1	Trace	—	—	—	98	212	1.6	220	0.06	0.15	0.7	17
	Strawberries:																	
328	Raw, capped	1 cup	149	90	55	1	1	—	—	—	13	31	1.5	90	0.04	0.10	1.0	88
329	Frozen, 10-ounce carton, not thawed	1 carton	284	71	310	1	1	—	—	—	79	40	2.0	90	0.06	0.17	1.5	150
330	Tangerines, raw, medium, 2 3/8-in diam., size 176[5]	1 tangerine	116	87	40	1	Trace	—	—	—	10	34	0.3	360	0.05	0.02	0.1	27
331	Tangerine juice, canned, sweetened	1 cup	249	87	125	1	1	—	—	—	30	45	0.5	1,050	0.15	0.05	0.2	55
332	Watermelon, raw, wedge, 4 by 8 inches (1/16 of 10 by 16-inch melon, about 2 pounds with rind)[5]	1 wedge	925	93	115	2	1	—	—	—	27	30	2.1	2,510	0.13	0.13	0.7	30
	Grain Products																	
	Bagel, 3-in diam.:																	
333	Egg	1 bagel	55	32	165	6	2	—	—	—	28	9	1.2	30	0.14	0.10	1.2	0
334	Water	1 bagel	55	29	165	6	2	—	—	—	30	8	1.2	0	0.15	0.11	1.4	0
335	Barley, pearled, light, uncooked	1 cup	200	11	700	16	2	Trace	1	1	158	32	4.0	0	0.24	0.10	6.2	0
336	Biscuits, baking powder from home recipe with enriched flour, 2-in diam.	1 biscuit	28	27	105	2	5	1	2	1	13	34	0.4	Trace	0.06	0.06	0.1	Trace
337	Biscuits, baking powder from mix, 2-in diam.	1 biscuit	28	28	90	2	3	1	1	1	15	19	0.6	Trace	0.08	0.07	0.6	Trace
338	Bran flakes (40% bran), added thiamine and iron	1 cup	35	3	105	4	1	—	—	—	28	25	12.3	0	0.14	0.06	2.2	0
339	Bran flakes with raisins, added thiamine and iron	1 cup	50	7	145	4	1	—	—	—	40	28	13.5	Trace	0.16	0.07	2.7	0
	Breads:																	
340	Boston brown bread, slice 3 by 3/4 in	1 slice	48	45	100	3	1	—	—	—	22	43	0.9	0	0.05	0.03	0.6	0
	Cracked-wheat bread:																	
341	Loaf, 1 lb	1 loaf	454	35	1,190	40	10	2	5	2	236	399	5.0	Trace	0.53	0.41	5.9	Trace
342	Slice, 18 slices per loaf	1 slice	25	35	65	2	1	—	—	—	13	22	0.3	Trace	0.03	0.02	0.3	Trace
	French or Vienna bread:																	
343	Enriched, 1-lb loaf	1 loaf	454	31	1,315	41	14	3	8	2	251	195	10.0	Trace	1.27	1.00	11.3	Trace
344	Unenriched, 1-lb loaf	1 loaf	454	31	1,315	41	14	3	8	2	251	195	3.2	Trace	0.36	0.36	3.6	Trace
	Italian bread:																	
345	Enriched, 1-lb loaf	1 loaf	454	32	1,250	41	4	Trace	1	2	256	77	10.0	0	1.32	0.91	11.8	0
346	Unenriched, 1-lb loaf	1 loaf	454	32	1,250	41	4	Trace	1	2	256	77	3.2	0	0.41	0.27	3.6	0
	Raisin bread:																	
347	Loaf, 1 lb	1 loaf	454	35	1,190	30	13	3	8	2	243	322	5.9	Trace	0.23	0.41	3.2	Trace
348	Slice, 18 slices per loaf	1 slice	25	35	65	2	1	—	—	—	13	18	0.3	Trace	0.01	0.02	0.2	Trace
	Rye bread:																	
	American, light (1/3 rye, 2/3 wheat):																	
349	Loaf, 1 lb	1 loaf	454	36	1,100	41	5	—	—	—	236	340	7.3	0	0.82	0.32	6.4	0
350	Slice, 18 slices per loaf	1 slice	25	36	60	2	Trace	—	—	—	13	19	0.4	0	0.05	0.02	0.4	0
351	Pumpernickel, loaf, 1 lb	1 loaf	454	34	1,115	41	5	—	—	—	241	381	10.9	0	1.04	0.64	5.4	0
	White bread, enriched:[15]																	
	Soft-crumb type																	
352	Loaf, 1 lb	1 loaf	454	36	1,225	39	15	3	8	2	229	381	11.3	Trace	1.13	0.95	10.9	Trace

353	Slice, 18 slices per loaf	1 slice	25	36	70	2	1	—	—	—	13	21	0.6	Trace	0.06	0.05	0.6	Trace
354	Slice, toasted	1 slice	22	25	70	2	1	—	—	—	13	21	0.6	Trace	0.06	0.05	0.6	Trace
355	Slice, 22 slices per loaf	1 slice	20	36	55	2	1	—	—	—	10	17	0.5	Trace	0.05	0.04	0.5	Trace
356	Slice, toasted	1 slice	17	25	55	2	1	—	—	—	10	17	0.5	Trace	0.05	0.04	0.5	Trace
357	Loaf, 1 1/2 lb	1 loaf	680	36	1,835	59	22	5	12	3	343	571	17.0	Trace	1.70	1.43	16.3	Trace
358	Slice, 24 slices per loaf	1 slice	28	36	75	2	1	—	—	—	14	24	0.7	Trace	0.07	0.06	0.7	Trace
359	Slice, toasted	1 slice	24	25	75	2	1	—	—	—	14	24	0.7	Trace	0.07	0.06	0.7	Trace
360	Slice, 28 slices per loaf	1 slice	24	36	65	2	1	—	—	—	12	20	0.6	Trace	0.06	0.05	0.6	Trace
361	Slice, toasted	1 slice	21	25	65	2	1	—	—	—	12	20	0.6	Trace	0.06	0.05	0.6	Trace
	Firm-crumb type:																	
362	Loaf, 1 lb	1 loaf	454	35	1,245	41	17	4	10	2	228	435	11.3	Trace	1.22	0.91	10.9	Trace
363	Slice, 20 slices per loaf	1 slice	23	35	65	2	1	—	—	—	12	22	0.6	Trace	0.06	0.05	0.6	Trace
364	Slice, toasted	1 slice	20	24	65	2	1	—	—	—	12	22	0.6	Trace	0.06	0.05	0.6	Trace
365	Loaf, 2 lb	1 loaf	907	35	2,495	82	34	8	20	4	455	871	22.7	Trace	2.45	1.81	21.8	Trace
366	Slice, 34 slices per loaf	1 slice	27	35	75	2	1	—	—	—	14	26	0.7	Trace	0.07	0.05	0.6	Trace
367	Slice, toasted	1 slice	23	35	75	2	1	—	—	—	14	26	0.7	Trace	0.07	0.05	0.6	Trace
	Whole-wheat bread, soft-crumb type:																	
368	Loaf, 1 lb	1 loaf	454	36	1,095	41	12	2	6	2	224	381	13.6	Trace	1.36	0.45	12.7	Trace
369	Slice, 16 slices per loaf	1 slice	28	36	65	3	1	—	—	—	14	24	0.8	Trace	0.09	0.03	0.8	Trace
370	Slice, toasted	1 slice	24	24	65	3	1	—	—	—	14	24	0.8	Trace	0.09	0.03	0.8	Trace
	Whole-wheat bread, firm-crumb type:																	
371	Loaf, 1 lb	1 loaf	454	36	1,100	48	14	3	6	3	216	449	13.6	Trace	1.18	0.54	12.7	Trace
372	Slice, 18 slices per loaf	1 slice	25	36	60	3	1	—	—	—	12	25	0.8	Trace	0.06	0.03	0.7	Trace
373	Slice, toasted	1 slice	21	24	60	3	1	—	—	—	12	25	0.8	Trace	0.06	0.03	0.7	Trace
374	Breadcrumbs, dry, grated	1 cup	100	6	390	13	5	1	2	1	73	122	3.6	Trace	0.22	0.30	3.5	Trace
375	Buckwheat flour, light, sifted	1 cup	98	12	340	6	1	—	—	—	78	11	1.0	0	0.08	0.04	0.4	0
376	Bulgur, canned, seasoned	1 cup	135	56	245	8	4	—	—	—	44	27	1.9	0	0.08	0.05	4.1	0
	Cakes made from cake mixes:																	
	Angel food:																	
377	Whole cake	1 cake	635	34	1,645	36	1	—	—	—	377	603	1.9	0	0.03	0.70	0.6	0
378	Piece, 1/12 of 10-in diam. cake	1 piece	53	34	135	3	Trace	—	—	—	32	50	0.2	0	Trace	0.06	0.1	0
	Cakes made from cake mixes (cont.)																	
	Cupcakes, small, 2 1/2 in diam.:																	
379	Without icing	1 cupcake	25	26	90	1	3	1	1	1	14	40	0.1	40	0.01	0.03	0.1	Trace
380	With chocolate icing	1 cupcake	36	22	130	2	5	2	2	1	21	47	0.3	60	0.01	0.04	0.1	Trace
	Devil's food, 2-layer, with chocolate icing:																	
381	Whole cake	1 cake	1,107	24	3,755	49	136	54	58	16	645	653	8.9	1,660	0.33	0.89	3.3	1
382	Piece, 1/16 of 9-in diam. cake	1 piece	69	24	235	3	9	3	4	1	40	41	0.6	100	0.02	0.06	0.2	Trace
383	Cupcake, small, 2 1/2-in diam	1 cupcake	35	24	120	2	4	1	2	Trace	20	21	0.3	50	0.01	0.03	0.1	Trace
	Gingerbread:																	
384	Whole cake	1 cake	570	37	1,575	18	39	10	19	9	291	513	9.1	Trace	0.17	0.51	4.6	2
385	Piece, 1/9 of 8-in square cake	1 piece	63	37	175	2	4	1	2	1	32	57	1.0	Trace	0.02	0.06	0.5	Trace
	White, 2-layer, with chocolate icing:																	
386	Whole cake	1 cake	1,140	21	4,000	45	122	45	54	17	716	1,129	5.7	680	0.23	0.91	2.3	2
387	Piece, 1/16 of 9-in diam. cake	1 piece	71	21	250	3	8	3	3	1	45	70	0.4	40	0.01	0.06	0.1	Trace
	Cakes made from home recipes:[16]																	
388	Boston cream pie; piece 1/12 of 8-in diam.	1 piece	69	35	210	4	6	2	3	1	34	46	0.3	140	0.02	0.08	0.1	Trace
	Fruitcake, dark, made with enriched flour:																	
389	Loaf, 1 lb	1 loaf	454	18	1,720	22	69	15	37	13	271	327	11.8	540	0.59	0.64	3.6	2
390	Slice, 1/30 of 8-in loaf	1 slice	15	18	55	1	2	Trace	1	Trace	9	11	0.4	20	0.02	0.02	0.1	Trace
	Plain sheet cake:																	
	Without icing:																	
391	Whole cake	1 cake	777	25	2,830	35	108	30	52	21	434	497	3.1	1,320	0.16	0.70	1.6	2
392	Piece, 1/9 of 9-in square cake	1 piece	86	25	315	4	12	3	6	2	48	55	0.3	150	0.02	0.08	0.2	Trace

[5]Measure and weight apply to entire vegetable or fruit including parts not usually eaten.

[15]Values for iron, thiamine, riboflavin, and niacin per pound of unenriched white bread would be as follows:

	Iron *mg*	Thiamine *mg*	Riboflavin *mg*	Niacin *mg*
Soft crumb	3.2	.31	.39	5.0
Firm crumb	3.2	.32	.59	4.1

[16]Unenriched cake flour used unless otherwise specified.

Table A–1. (Cont.)

No.	Food, Approximate Measure, and Weight (in grams)		gm	Water per cent	Food Energy calories	Protein gm	Fat gm	Fatty Acids: Saturated (total) gm	Fatty Acids: Unsaturated: Oleic gm	Fatty Acids: Unsaturated: Linoleic gm	Carbohydrate gm	Calcium mg	Iron mg	Vitamin A Value I.U.	Thiamine mg	Riboflavin mg	Niacin mg	Ascorbic Acid mg
393	With boiled white icing, piece, 1/9 of 9-in square cake	1 piece	114	23	400	4	12	3	6	2	71	56	0.3	150	0.02	0.08	0.2	Trace
	Pound:																	
394	Loaf, 8 1/2 by 3 1/2 by 3 in	1 loaf	514	17	2,430	29	152	34	68	17	242	108	4.1	1,440	0.15	0.46	1.0	0
395	Slice, 1/2-in thick	1 slice	30	17	140	2	9	2	4	1	14	6	0.2	80	0.01	0.03	0.1	0
	Sponge:																	
396	Whole cake	1 cake	790	32	2,345	60	45	14	20	4	427	237	9.5	3,560	0.40	1.11	1.6	Trace
397	Piece, 1/12 of 10-in diam. cake	1 piece	66	32	195	5	4	1	2	Trace	36	20	0.8	300	0.03	0.09	0.1	Trace
	Yellow, 2 layer, without icing:																	
398	Whole cake	1 cake	870	24	3,160	39	111	31	53	22	506	618	3.5	1,310	0.17	0.70	1.7	2
399	Piece, 1/16 of 9-in diam. cake	1 piece	54	24	200	2	7	2	3	1	32	39	0.2	80	0.01	0.04	0.1	Trace
	Yellow, 2-layer, with chocolate icing:																	
400	Whole cake	1 cake	1,203	21	4,390	51	156	55	69	23	727	818	7.2	1,920	0.24	0.96	2.4	Trace
401	Piece, 1/16 of 9-in diam. cake	1 piece	75	21	275	3	10	3	4	1	45	51	0.5	120	0.02	0.06	0.2	Trace
	Cake icings. See Sugars, Sweets																	
	Cookies:																	
	Brownies with nuts:																	
402	Made from home recipe with enriched flour	1 brownie	20	10	95	1	6	1	3	1	10	8	0.4	40	0.04	0.02	0.1	Trace
403	Made from mix	1 brownie	20	11	85	1	4	1	2	1	13	9	0.4	20	0.03	0.02	0.1	Trace
	Chocolate chip:																	
404	Made from home recipe with enriched flour	1 cookie	10	3	50	1	3	1	1	1	6	4	0.2	10	0.01	0.01	0.1	Trace
405	Commercial	1 cookie	10	3	50	1	2	1	1	Trace	7	4	0.2	10	Trace	Trace	Trace	Trace
406	Fig bars, commercial	1 cookie	14	14	50	1	1	—	—	—	11	11	0.2	20	Trace	0.01	0.1	Trace
407	Sandwich, chocolate or vanilla, commercial	1 cookie	10	2	50	1	2	1	1	Trace	7	2	0.1	0	Trace	Trace	0.1	0
	Corn flakes, added nutrients:																	
408	Plain	1 cup	25	4	100	2	Trace	—	—	—	21	4	0.4	0	0.11	0.02	0.5	0
409	Sugar-covered	1 cup	40	2	155	2	Trace	—	—	—	36	5	0.4	0	0.16	0.02	0.8	0
	Corn (hominy) grits, degermed, cooked:																	
410	Enriched	1 cup	245	87	125	3	Trace	—	—	—	27	2	0.7	[17]150	0.10	0.07	1.0	0
411	Unenriched	1 cup	245	87	125	3	Trace	—	—	—	27	2	0.2	[17]150	0.05	0.02	0.5	0
	Cornmeal:																	
412	Whole-ground, unbolted, dry	1 cup	122	12	435	11	5	1	2	2	90	24	2.9	[17]620	0.46	0.13	2.4	0
413	Bolted (nearly whole-grain) dry	1 cup	122	12	440	11	4	Trace	1	2	91	21	2.2	[17]590	0.37	0.10	2.3	0
	Degermed, enriched:																	
414	Dry form	1 cup	138	12	500	11	2	—	—	—	108	8	4.0	[17]610	0.61	0.36	4.8	0
415	Cooked	1 cup	240	88	120	3	1	—	—	—	26	2	1.0	[17]140	0.14	0.10	1.2	0
	Degermed, unenriched:																	
416	Dry form	1 cup	138	12	500	11	2	—	—	—	108	8	1.5	[17]610	0.19	0.07	1.4	0
417	Cooked	1 cup	240	88	120	3	1	—	—	—	26	2	0.5	[17]140	0.05	0.02	0.2	0
418	Corn muffins, made with enriched degermed cornmeal and enriched flour; muffin 2 3/8-in diam.	1 muffin	40	33	125	3	4	2	2	Trace	19	42	0.7	[17]120	0.08	0.09	0.6	Trace
419	Corn muffins, made with mix, egg, and milk; muffin 2 3/8-in diam.	1 muffin	40	30	130	3	4	1	2	1	20	96	0.6	100	0.07	0.08	0.6	Trace
420	Corn, puffed, presweetened, added nutrients	1 cup	30	2	115	1	Trace	—	—	—	27	3	0.5	0	0.13	0.05	0.6	0
421	Corn, shredded, added nutrients	1 cup	25	3	100	2	Trace	—	—	—	22	1	0.6	0	0.11	0.05	0.5	0

	Crackers:																	
422	Graham, 2 1/2-in square	4 crackers	28	6	110	2	3	—	—	—	21	11	0.4	0	0.01	0.06	0.4	0
423	Saltines	4 crackers	11	4	50	1	1	—	1	—	8	2	0.1	0	Trace	Trace	0.1	0
	Danish pastry, plain (without fruit or nuts):																	
424	Packaged ring, 12 ounces	1 ring	340	22	1,435	25	80	24	37	15	155	170	3.1	1,050	0.24	0.51	2.7	Trace
425	Round piece, approx. 4 1/4-in diam. by 1 in	1 pastry	65	22	275	5	15	5	7	3	30	33	0.6	200	0.05	0.10	0.5	Trace
426	Ounce	1 oz	28	22	120	2	7	2	3	1	13	14	0.3	90	0.02	0.04	0.2	Trace
427	Doughnuts, cake type	1 doughnut	32	24	125	1	6	1	4	Trace	16	13	[18]0.4	30	[18]0.05	[18]0.05	[18]0.4	Trace
428	Farina, quick-cooking, enriched, cooked	1 cup	245	89	105	3	Trace	—	—	—	22	147	[19]0.7	0	[19]0.12	[19]0.07	[19]1.0	0
	Macaroni, cooked:																	
	Enriched:																	
429	Cooked, firm stage (undergoes additional cooking in a food mixture)	1 cup	130	64	190	6	1	—	—	—	39	14	[19]1.4	0	[19]0.23	[19]0.14	[19]1.8	0
430	Cooked until tender	1 cup	140	72	155	5	1	—	—	—	32	8	[19]1.3	0	[19]0.20	[19]0.11	[19]1.5	0
	Unenriched:																	
431	Cooked, firm stage (undergoes additional cooking in a food mixture)	1 cup	130	64	190	6	1	—	—	—	39	14	0.7	0	0.03	0.03	0.5	0
432	Cooked until tender	1 cup	140	72	155	5	1	—	—	—	32	11	0.6	0	0.01	0.01	0.4	0
433	Macaroni (enriched) and cheese, baked	1 cup	200	58	430	17	22	10	9	2	40	362	1.8	860	0.20	0.40	1.8	Trace
434	Canned	1 cup	240	80	230	9	10	4	3	1	26	199	1.0	260	0.12	0.24	1.0	Trace
435	Muffins, with enriched white flour; muffin, 3-inch diam.	1 muffin	40	38	120	3	4	1	2	1	17	42	0.6	40	0.07	0.09	0.6	Trace
	Noodles (egg noodles), cooked:																	
436	Enriched	1 cup	160	70	200	7	2	1	1	Trace	37	16	[19]1.4	110	[19]0.22	[19]0.13	[19]1.9	0
437	Unenriched	1 cup	160	70	200	7	2	1	1	Trace	37	16	1.0	110	0.05	0.03	0.6	0
438	Oats (with or without corn) puffed, added nutrients	1 cup	25	3	100	3	1	—	—	—	19	44	1.2	0	0.24	0.04	0.5	0
439	Oatmeal or rolled oats, cooked	1 cup	240	87	130	5	2	—	—	1	23	22	1.4	0	0.19	0.05	0.2	0
	Pancakes, 4-inch diam.:																	
440	Wheat, enriched flour (home recipe)	1 cake	27	50	60	2	2	Trace	1	Trace	9	27	0.4	30	0.05	0.06	0.4	Trace
441	Buckwheat (made from mix with egg and milk)	1 cake	27	58	55	2	2	1	1	Trace	6	59	0.4	60	0.03	0.04	0.2	Trace
442	Plain or buttermilk (made from mix with egg and milk)	1 cake	27	51	60	2	2	1	1	Trace	9	58	0.3	70	0.04	0.06	0.2	Trace
	Pie (piecrust made with unenriched flour):																	
	Sector, 4-in, 1/7 of 9-in-diam. pie:																	
443	Apple (2-crust)	1 sector	135	48	350	3	15	4	7	3	51	11	0.4	40	0.03	0.03	0.5	1
444	Butterscotch (1-crust)	1 sector	130	45	350	6	14	5	6	2	50	98	1.2	340	0.04	0.13	0.3	Trace
445	Cherry (2-crust)	1 sector	135	47	350	4	15	4	7	3	52	19	0.4	590	0.03	0.03	0.7	Trace
446	Custard (1-crust)	1 sector	130	58	285	8	14	5	6	2	30	125	0.8	300	0.07	0.21	0.4	0
447	Lemon meringue (1-crust)	1 sector	120	47	305	4	12	4	6	2	45	17	0.6	200	0.04	0.10	0.2	4
448	Mince (2-crust)	1 sector	135	43	365	3	16	4	8	3	56	38	1.4	Trace	0.09	0.05	0.5	1
449	Pecan (1-crust)	1 sector	118	20	490	6	27	4	16	5	60	55	3.3	190	0.19	0.08	0.4	Trace
450	Pineapple chiffon (1-crust)	1 sector	93	41	265	6	11	3	5	2	36	22	0.8	320	0.04	0.08	0.4	1
451	Pumpkin (1-crust)	1 sector	130	59	275	5	15	5	6	2	32	66	0.7	3,210	0.04	0.13	0.7	Trace
	Piecrust, baked shell for pie made with:																	
452	Enriched flour	1 shell	180	15	900	11	60	16	28	12	79	25	3.1	0	0.36	0.25	3.2	0
453	Unenriched flour	1 shell	180	15	900	11	60	16	28	12	79	25	0.9	0	0.05	0.05	0.9	0
	Piecrust mix including stick form:																	
454	Package, 10 oz, for double crust	1 pkg.	284	9	1,480	20	93	23	46	21	141	131	1.4	0	0.11	0.11	2.0	0
455	Pizza (cheese) 5 1/2-in sector; 1/8 of 14-in diam. pie	1 sector	75	45	185	7	6	2	3	Trace	27	107	0.7	290	0.04	0.12	0.7	4

[17]This value is based on product made from yellow varieties of corn; white varieties contain only a trace.

[18]Based on product made with enriched flour. With unenriched flour, approximate values per doughnut are: iron, 0.2 mg; thiamine, 0.01 mg; riboflavin, 0.03 mg; niacin, 0.2 mg.

[19]Iron, thiamine, riboflavin, and niacin are based on the minimum levels of enrichment specified in standards of identity promulgated under the Federal Food, Drug, and Cosmetic Act.

Table A–1. (Cont.)

No.	Food, Approximate Measure, and Weight (in grams)		gm	Water per cent	Food Energy calories	Protein gm	Fat gm	Fatty Acids: Saturated (total) gm	Fatty Acids: Unsaturated: Oleic gm	Fatty Acids: Unsaturated: Linoleic gm	Carbohydrate gm	Calcium mg	Iron mg	Vitamin A Value I.U.	Thiamine mg	Riboflavin mg	Niacin mg	Ascorbic Acid mg
	Popcorn, popped:																	
456	Plain, large kernel	1 cup	6	4	25	1	Trace	—	—	—	5	1	0.2	—	—	0.01	0.1	0
457	With oil and salt	1 cup	9	3	40	1	2	1	Trace	Trace	5	1	0.2	—	—	0.01	0.2	0
458	Sugar coated	1 cup	35	4	135	2	1	—	—	—	30	2	0.5	—	—	0.02	0.4	0
	Pretzels:																	
459	Dutch, twisted	1 pretzel	16	5	60	2	1	—	—	—	12	4	0.2	0	Trace	Trace	0.1	0
460	Thin, twisted	1 pretzel	6	5	25	1	Trace	—	—	—	5	1	0.1	0	Trace	Trace	Trace	0
461	Sticks, small 2 1/4 inches	10 sticks	3	5	10	Trace	Trace	—	—	—	2	1	Trace	0	Trace	Trace	Trace	0
462	Stick, regular, 3 1/8 inches	5 sticks	3	5	10	Trace	Trace	—	—	—	2	1	Trace	0	Trace	Trace	Trace	0
	Rice, white:																	
	Enriched:																	
463	Raw	1 cup	185	12	670	12	1	—	—	—	149	44	[20]5.4	0	[20]0.81	[20]0.06	[20]6.5	0
464	Cooked	1 cup	205	73	225	4	Trace	—	—	—	50	21	[20]1.8	0	[20]0.23	[20]0.02	[20]2.1	0
465	Instant, ready to serve	1 cup	165	73	180	4	Trace	—	—	—	40	5	[20]1.3	0	[20]0.21	[20]—	[20]1.7	0
466	Unenriched, cooked	1 cup	205	73	225	4	Trace	—	—	—	50	21	0.4	0	0.04	0.02	0.8	0
467	Parboiled, cooked	1 cup	175	73	185	4	Trace	—	—	—	41	33	[20]1.4	0	[20]0.19	[20]—	[20]2.1	0
468	Rice, puffed, added nutrients	1 cup	15	4	60	1	Trace	—	—	—	13	3	0.3	0	0.07	0.01	0.7	0
	Rolls, enriched:																	
	Cloverleaf or pan:																	
469	Home recipe	1 roll	35	26	120	3	3	1	1	1	20	16	0.7	30	0.09	0.09	0.8	Trace
470	Commercial	1 roll	28	31	85	2	2	Trace	1	Trace	15	21	0.5	Trace	0.08	0.05	0.6	Trace
471	Frankfurter or hamburger	1 roll	40	31	120	3	2	1	1	1	21	30	0.8	Trace	0.11	0.07	0.9	Trace
472	Hard, round or rectangular	1 roll	50	25	155	5	2	Trace	1	Trace	30	24	1.2	Trace	0.13	0.12	1.4	Trace
473	Rye wafers, whole-grain, 1 7/8 by 3 1/2 inches	2 wafers	13	6	45	2	Trace	—	—	—	10	7	0.5	0	0.04	0.03	0.2	0
474	Spaghetti, cooked, tender stage, enriched	1 cup	140	72	155	5	1	—	—	—	32	11	[19]1.3	0	[19]0.20	[19]0.11	[19]1.5	0
	Spaghetti with meat balls, and tomato sauce:																	
475	Home recipe	1 cup	248	70	330	19	12	4	6	1	39	124	3.7	1,590	0.25	0.30	4.0	22
476	Canned	1 cup	250	78	260	12	10	2	3	4	28	53	3.3	1,000	0.15	0.18	2.3	5
	Spaghetti in tomato sauce with cheese:																	
477	Home recipe	1 cup	250	77	260	9	9	2	5	1	37	80	2.3	1,080	0.25	0.18	2.3	13
478	Canned	1 cup	250	80	190	6	2	1	1	1	38	40	2.8	930	0.35	0.28	4.5	10
479	Waffles, with enriched flour, 7-in diam.	1 waffle	75	41	210	7	7	2	4	1	28	85	1.3	250	0.13	0.19	1.0	Trace
480	Waffles, made from mix, enriched, egg and milk added, 7-in diam.	1 waffle	75	42	205	7	8	3	3	1	27	179	1.0	170	0.11	0.17	0.7	Trace
481	Wheat, puffed, added nutrients	1 cup	15	3	55	2	Trace	—	—	—	12	4	0.6	0	0.08	0.03	1.2	0
482	Wheat, shredded, plain	1 biscuit	25	7	90	2	1	—	—	—	20	11	0.9	0	0.06	0.03	1.1	0
483	Wheat flakes, added nutrients	1 cup	30	4	105	3	Trace	—	—	—	24	12	1.3	0	0.19	0.04	1.5	0
	Wheat flours:																	
484	Whole wheat, from hard wheats, stirred	1 cup	120	12	400	16	2	Trace	1	1	85	49	4.0	0	0.66	0.14	5.2	0
	Wheat flours (cont.)																	
	All-purpose or family flour, enriched:																	
485	Sifted	1 cup	115	12	420	12	1	—	—	—	88	18	[19]3.3	0	[19]0.51	[19]0.30	[19]4.0	0
486	Unsifted	1 cup	125	12	455	13	1	—	—	—	95	20	[19]3.6	0	[19]0.55	[19]0.33	[19]4.4	0
487	Self-rising, enriched	1 cup	125	12	440	12	1	—	—	—	93	331	[19]3.6	0	[19]0.55	[19]0.33	[19]4.4	0
488	Cake or pastry flour, sifted	1 cup	96	12	350	7	1	—	—	—	76	16	0.5	0	0.03	0.03	0.7	0
	Fats, Oils																	
	Butter:																	
	Regular, 4 sticks per pound:																	
489	Stick	1/2 cup	113	16	810	1	92	51	30	3	1	23	0	[21]3,750	—	—	—	0
490	Tablespoon (approx. 1/8 stick)	1 tbsp.	14	16	100	Trace	12	6	4	Trace	Trace	3	0	[21]470	—	—	—	0
491	Pat (1-in sq. 1/3-in high; 90 per lb)	1 pat	5	16	35	Trace	4	2	1	Trace	Trace	1	0	[21]170	—	—	—	0

	Whipped, 6 sticks or 2, 8-oz containers per pound:																	
492	Stick	1/2 cup	76	16	540	1	61	34	20	2	Trace	15	0	[21]2,500	—	—	—	0
493	Tablespoon (approx. 1/8 stick)	1 tbsp.	9	16	65	Trace	8	4	3	Trace	Trace	2	0	[21]310	—	—	—	0
494	Pat (1 1/4-in sq 1/3-in high; 120 per lb)	1 pat	4	16	25	Trace	3	2	1	Trace	Trace	1	0	[21]130	—	—	—	0
	Fats, cooking:																	
495	Lard	1 cup	205	0	1,850	0	205	78	94	20	0	0	0	0	0	0	0	0
496		1 tbsp.	13	0	115	0	13	5	6	1	0	0	0	0	0	0	0	0
497	Vegetable fats	1 cup	200	0	1,770	0	200	50	100	44	0	0	0	—	0	0	0	0
498		1 tbsp	13	0	110	0	13	3	6	3	0	0	0	—	0	0	0	0
	Margarine:																	
	Regular, 4 sticks per pound:																	
499	Stick	1/2 cup	113	16	815	1	92	17	46	25	1	23	0	[22]3,750	—	—	—	0
500	Tablespoon (approx. 1/8 stick)	1 tbsp	14	16	100	Trace	12	2	6	3	Trace	3	0	[22]470	—	—	—	0
501	Pat (1-in sq 1/3-in high; 90 per lb)	1 pat	5	16	35	Trace	4	1	2	1	Trace	1	0	[22]170	—	—	—	0
	Whipped, 6 sticks per pound:																	
502	Stick	1/2 cup	76	16	545	1	61	11	31	17	Trace	15	0	[22]2,500	—	—	—	0
	Soft, 2 8-oz tubs per pound:																	
503	Tub	1 tub	227	16	1,635	1	184	34	68	68	1	45	0	[22]7,500	—	—	—	0
504	Tablespoon	1 tbsp	14	16	100	Trace	11	2	4	4	Trace	3	0	[22]470	—	—	—	0
	Oils, salad or cooking:																	
505	Corn	1 cup	220	0	1,945	0	220	22	62	117	0	0	0	—	0	0	0	0
506		1 tbsp	14	0	125	0	14	1	4	7	0	0	0	—	0	0	0	0
507	Cottonseed	1 cup	220	0	1,945	0	220	55	46	110	0	0	0	—	0	0	0	0
508		1 tbsp	14	0	125	0	14	4	3	7	0	0	0	—	0	0	0	0
509	Olive	1 cup	220	0	1,945	0	220	24	167	15	0	0	0	—	0	0	0	0
510		1 tbsp	14	0	125	0	14	2	11	1	0	0	0	—	0	0	0	0
511	Peanut	1 cup	220	0	1,945	0	220	40	103	64	0	0	0	—	0	0	0	0
512		1 tbsp	14	0	125	0	14	3	7	4	0	0	0	—	0	0	0	0
513	Safflower	1 cup	220	0	1,945	0	220	18	37	165	0	0	0	—	0	0	0	0
514		1 tbsp	14	0	125	0	14	1	2	10	0	0	0	—	0	0	0	0
515	Soybean	1 cup	220	0	1,945	0	220	33	44	114	0	0	0	—	0	0	0	0
516		1 tbsp	14	0	125	0	14	2	3	7	0	0	0	—	0	0	0	0
	Salad dressing:																	
517	Blue cheese	1 tbsp	15	32	75	1	8	2	2	4	1	12	Trace	30	Trace	0.02	Trace	Trace
	Commercial, mayonnaise type:																	
518	Regular	1 tbsp	15	41	65	Trace	6	1	1	3	2	2	Trace	30	Trace	Trace	Trace	—
519	Special dietary, low calorie	1 tbsp	16	81	20	Trace	2	Trace	Trace	1	1	3	Trace	40	Trace	Trace	Trace	—
	French:																	
520	Regular	1 tbsp	16	39	65	Trace	6	1	1	3	3	2	0.1	—	—	—	—	—
521	Special dietary, low fat with artificial sweeteners	1 tbsp	15	95	Trace	Trace	Trace	—	—	—	Trace	2	0.1	—	—	—	—	—
522	Home cooked, boiled	1 tbsp	16	68	25	1	2	1	1	Trace	2	14	0.1	80	0.01	0.03	Trace	Trace
523	Mayonnaise	1 tbsp	14	15	100	Trace	11	2	2	6	Trace	3	0.1	40	Trace	0.01	Trace	—
524	Thousand island	1 tbsp	16	32	80	Trace	8	1	2	4	3	2	0.1	50	Trace	Trace	Trace	Trace

Sugars, Sweets

	Cake icings:																	
525	Chocolate made with milk and table fat	1 cup	275	14	1,035	9	38	21	14	1	185	165	3.3	580	0.06	0.28	0.6	1
526	Coconut (with boiled icing)	1 cup	166	15	605	3	13	11	1	Trace	124	10	0.8	0	0.02	0.07	0.3	0
527	Creamy fudge from mix with water only	1 cup	245	15	830	7	16	5	8	3	183	96	2.7	Trace	0.05	0.20	0.7	Trace
528	White, boiled	1 cup	94	18	300	1	0	—	—	—	76	2	Trace	0	Trace	0.03	Trace	0

[19]Iron, thiamine, riboflavin, and niacin are based on the minimum levels of enrichment specified in standards of identity promulgated under the Federal Food, Drug, and Cosmetic Act.

[20]Iron, thiamine, and niacin are based on the minimum levels of enrichment specified in standards of identity promulgated under the Federal Food, Drug, and Cosmetic Act. Riboflavin is based on unenriched rice. When the minimum level of enrichment specified in the standards of identity becomes effective the value will be 0.12 mg per cup of parboiled rice and of white rice.

[21]Year-round average.

[22]Based on the average vitamin A content of fortified margarine. Federal specifications for fortified margarine require a minimum of 15,000 I.U. of vitamin A per pound.

Table A–1. (Cont.)

No.	Food, Approximate Measure, and Weight (in grams)		gm	Water per cent	Food Energy calories	Protein gm	Fat gm	Fatty Acids: Saturated (total) gm	Fatty Acids: Unsaturated: Oleic gm	Fatty Acids: Unsaturated: Linoleic gm	Carbohydrate gm	Calcium mg	Iron mg	Vitamin A Value I.U.	Thiamine mg	Riboflavin mg	Niacin mg	Ascorbic Acid mg
	Candy:																	
529	Carmels, plain or chocolate	1 oz	28	8	115	1	3	2	1	Trace	22	42	0.4	Trace	0.01	0.05	0.1	Trace
530	Chocolate, milk, plain	1 oz	28	1	145	2	9	5	3	Trace	16	65	0.3	80	0.02	0.10	0.1	Trace
531	Chocolate-coated peanuts	1 oz	28	1	160	5	12	3	6	2	11	33	0.4	Trace	0.10	0.05	2.1	Trace
532	Fondant; mints, uncoated; candy corn	1 oz	28	8	105	Trace	1	—	—	—	25	4	0.3	0	Trace	Trace	Trace	0
533	Fudge, plain	1 oz	28	8	115	1	4	2	1	Trace	21	22	0.3	Trace	0.01	0.03	0.1	Trace
534	Gum drops	1 oz	28	12	100	Trace	Trace	—	—	—	25	2	0.1	0	0	Trace	Trace	0
535	Hard	1 oz	28	1	110	0	Trace	—	—	—	28	6	0.5	0	0	0	0	0
536	Marshmallows	1 oz	28	17	90	1	Trace	—	—	—	23	5	0.5	0	0	Trace	Trace	0
	Chocolate-flavored syrup or topping:																	
537	Thin type	1 fl oz	38	32	90	1	1	Trace	Trace	Trace	24	6	0.6	Trace	0.01	0.03	0.2	0
538	Fudge type	1 fl oz	38	25	125	2	5	3	2	Trace	20	48	0.5	60	0.02	0.08	0.2	Trace
	Chocolate-flavored beverage powder (approx. 4 heaping teaspoons per oz):																	
539	With nonfat dry milk	1 oz	28	2	100	5	1	Trace	Trace	Trace	20	167	0.5	10	0.04	0.21	0.2	1
540	Without nonfat dry milk	1 oz	28	1	100	1	1	Trace	Trace	Trace	25	9	0.6	—	0.01	0.03	0.1	0
541	Honey, strained or extracted	1 tbsp	21	17	65	Trace	0	—	—	—	17	1	0.1	0	Trace	0.01	0.1	Trace
542	Jams and preserves	1 tbsp	20	29	55	Trace	Trace	—	—	—	14	4	0.2	Trace	Trace	0.01	Trace	Trace
543	Jellies	1 tbsp	18	29	50	Trace	Trace	—	—	—	13	4	0.3	Trace	Trace	0.01	Trace	1
	Molasses, cane:																	
544	Light (first extraction)	1 tbsp	20	24	50	—	—	—	—	—	13	33	0.9	—	0.01	0.01	Trace	—
545	Blackstrap (third extraction)	1 tbsp	20	24	45	—	—	—	—	—	11	137	3.2	—	0.02	0.04	0.4	—
	Syrups:																	
546	Sorghum	1 tbsp	21	23	55	—	—	—	—	—	14	35	2.6	—	—	0.02	Trace	—
	Syrups (cont.)																	
547	Table blends, chiefly corn, light and dark	1 tbsp	21	24	60	0	0	—	—	—	15	9	0.8	0	0	0	0	0
	Sugars:																	
548	Brown, firm packed	1 cup	220	2	820	0	0	—	—	—	212	187	7.5	0	0.02	0.07	0.4	0
	White:																	
549	Granulated	1 cup	200	Trace	770	0	0	—	—	—	199	0	0.2	0	0	0	0	0
550		1 tbsp	11	Trace	40	0	0	—	—	—	11	0	Trace	0	0	0	0	0
551	Powdered, stirred before measuring	1 cup	120	Trace	460	0	0	—	—	—	119	0	0.1	0	0	0	0	0
	Miscellaneous Items																	
552	Barbecue sauce	1 cup	250	81	230	4	17	2	5	9	20	53	2.0	900	0.03	0.03	0.8	13
	Beverages, alcoholic:																	
553	Beer	12 fl oz	360	92	150	1	0	—	—	—	14	18	Trace	—	0.01	0.11	2.2	—
	Gin, rum, vodka, whiskey:																	
554	80 proof	1 1/2 fl oz jigger	42	67	100	—	—	—	—	—	Trace	—	—	—	—	—	—	—
555	86 proof	1 1/2 fl oz jigger	42	64	105	—	—	—	—	—	Trace	—	—	—	—	—	—	—
556	90 proof	1 1/2 fl oz jigger	42	62	110	—	—	—	—	—	Trace	—	—	—	—	—	—	—
557	94 proof	1 1/2 fl oz jigger	42	60	115	—	—	—	—	—	Trace	—	—	—	—	—	—	—
558	100 proof	1 1/2 fl oz jigger	42	58	125	—	—	—	—	—	Trace	—	—	—	—	—	—	—
	Wines:																	
559	Dessert	3 1/2 fl oz glass	103	77	140	Trace	0	—	—	—	8	8	—	—	0.01	0.02	0.2	—
560	Table	3 1/2 fl oz glass	102	86	85	Trace	0	—	—	—	4	9	0.4	—	Trace	0.01	0.1	—
	Beverages, carbonated, sweetened, nonalcoholic:																	
561	Carbonated water	12 fl oz	366	92	115	0	0	—	—	—	29	—	—	0	0	0	0	0
562	Cola type	12 fl oz	369	90	145	0	0	—	—	—	37	—	—	0	0	0	0	0
563	Fruit-flavored sodas and Tom Collins mixes	12 fl oz	372	88	170	0	0	—	—	—	45	—	—	0	0	0	0	0

564	Ginger ale	12 fl oz	366	92	115	0	0	—	—	—	29	—	—	0	0	0	0	0
565	Root beer	12 fl oz	370	90	150	0	0	—	—	—	39	—	—	0	0	0	0	0
566	Bouillon cubes, approx. 1/2 in	1 cube	4	4	5	1	Trace	—	—	—	Trace	—	—	—	—	—	—	—
	Chocolate:																	
567	Bitter or baking	1 oz	28	2	145	3	15	8	6	Trace	8	22	1.9	20	0.01	0.07	0.4	0
568	Semisweet, small pieces	1 cup	170	1	860	7	61	34	22	1	97	51	4.4	30	0.02	0.14	0.9	0
	Gelatin:																	
569	Plain, dry powder in envelope	1 envelope	7	13	25	6	Trace	—	—	—	0	—	—	—	—	—	—	—
570	Dessert powder, 3-oz package	1 pkg	85	2	315	8	0	—	—	—	75	—	—	—	—	—	—	—
571	Gelatin dessert, prepared with water	1 cup	240	84	140	4	0	—	—	—	34	—	—	—	—	—	—	—
	Olives, pickled:																	
572	Green	4 medium or 3 extra large or 2 giant	16	78	15	Trace	2	Trace	2	Trace	Trace	8	0.2	40	—	—	—	—
573	Ripe: Mission	3 small or 2 large	10	73	15	Trace	2	Trace	2	Trace	Trace	9	0.1	10	Trace	Trace	—	—
	Pickles, cucumber:																	
574	Dill, medium, whole, 3 3/4 in long, 1 1/4 in diam.	1 pickle	65	93	10	1	Trace	—	—	—	1	17	0.7	70	Trace	0.01	Trace	4
575	Fresh, sliced, 1 1/2 in diam., 1/4 in thick	2 slices	15	79	10	Trace	Trace	—	—	—	3	5	0.3	20	Trace	Trace	Trace	1
576	Sweet, gherkin, small, whole, approx. 2 1/2 in long, 3/4 in diam.	1 pickle	15	61	20	Trace	Trace	—	—	—	6	2	0.2	10	Trace	Trace	Trace	1
577	Relish, finely chopped, sweet	1 tbsp	15	63	20	Trace	Trace	—	—	—	5	3	0.1	—	—	—	—	—
	Popcorn. See Grain Products																	
578	Popsicle, 3-fl oz size	1 popsicle	95	80	70	0	0	0	0	0	18	0	Trace	0	0	0	0	0
	Pudding, home recipe with starch base:																	
579	Chocolate	1 cup	260	66	385	8	12	7	4	Trace	67	250	1.3	390	0.05	0.36	0.3	1
580	Vanilla (blanc mange)	1 cup	255	76	285	9	10	5	3	Trace	41	298	Trace	410	0.08	0.41	0.3	2
581	Pudding mix, dry form, 4-oz package	1 pkg	113	2	410	3	2	1	1	Trace	103	23	1.8	Trace	0.02	0.08	0.5	0
582	Sherbet	1 cup	193	67	260	2	2	—	—	—	59	31	Trace	120	0.02	0.06	Trace	4
	Soups:																	
	Canned, condensed, ready-to-serve:																	
	Prepared with an equal volume of milk:																	
583	Cream of chicken	1 cup	245	85	180	7	10	3	3	3	15	172	0.5	610	0.05	0.27	0.7	2
584	Cream of mushroom	1 cup	245	83	215	7	14	4	4	5	16	191	0.5	250	0.05	0.34	0.7	1
585	Tomato	1 cup	250	84	175	7	7	3	2	1	23	168	0.8	1,200	0.10	0.25	1.3	15
	Prepared with an equal volume of water:																	
586	Bean with pork	1 cup	250	84	170	8	6	1	2	2	22	63	2.3	650	0.13	0.08	1.0	3
587	Beef broth, bouillon consommé	1 cup	240	96	30	5	0	—	—	—	3	Trace	0.5	Trace	Trace	0.02	1.2	—
588	Beef noodle	1 cup	240	93	70	4	3	1	1	1	7	7	1.0	50	0.05	0.07	1.0	Trace
589	Clam chowder, Manhattan type (with tomatoes, without milk)	1 cup	245	92	80	2	3	—	—	—	12	34	1.0	880	0.02	0.02	1.0	—
590	Cream of chicken	1 cup	240	92	95	3	6	1	2	3	8	24	0.5	410	0.02	0.05	0.5	Trace
591	Cream of mushroom	1 cup	240	90	135	2	10	1	3	5	10	41	0.5	70	0.02	0.12	0.7	Trace
592	Minestrone	1 cup	245	90	105	5	3	—	—	—	14	37	1.0	2,350	0.07	0.05	1.0	—
593	Split pea	1 cup	245	85	145	9	3	1	2	Trace	21	29	1.5	440	0.25	0.15	1.5	1
594	Tomato	1 cup	245	90	90	2	3	Trace	1	1	16	15	0.7	1,000	0.05	0.05	1.2	12
595	Vegetable beef	1 cup	245	92	80	5	2	—	—	—	10	12	0.7	2,700	0.05	0.05	1.0	—
596	Vegetarian	1 cup	245	92	80	2	2	—	—	—	13	20	1.0	2,940	0.05	0.05	1.0	—
	Dehydrated, dry form:																	
597	Chicken noodle (2-oz package)	1 pkg	57	6	220	8	6	2	3	1	33	34	1.4	190	0.30	0.15	2.4	3
598	Onion mix (1 1/2-oz package)	1 pkg	43	3	150	6	5	1	2	1	23	42	0.6	30	0.05	0.03	0.3	6
599	Tomato vegetable with noodles (2 1/2-oz pkg)	1 pkg	71	4	245	6	6	2	3	1	45	33	1.4	1,700	0.21	0.13	1.8	18
	Frozen, condensed:																	
	Clam chowder, New England type (with milk, without tomatoes):																	
600	Prepared with equal volume of milk	1 cup	245	83	210	9	12	—	—	—	16	240	1.0	250	0.07	0.29	0.5	Trace

Table A–1. (Cont.)

No.	Food, Approximate Measure, and Weight (in grams)	Measure	gm	Water per cent	Food Energy calories	Protein gm	Fat gm	Fatty Acids: Saturated (total) gm	Unsaturated: Oleic gm	Unsaturated: Linoleic gm	Carbohydrate gm	Calcium mg	Iron mg	Vitamin A Value I.U.	Thiamine mg	Riboflavin mg	Niacin mg	Ascorbic Acid mg
	Soups, frozen (cont.)																	
	Clam chowder, New England type																	
601	Prepared with equal volume of water	1 cup	240	89	130	4	8	—	—	—	11	91	1.0	50	0.05	0.10	0.5	—
	Cream of potato:																	
602	Prepared with equal volume of milk	1 cup	245	83	185	8	10	5	3	Trace	18	208	1.0	590	0.10	0.27	0.5	Trace
603	Prepared with equal volume of water	1 cup	240	90	105	3	5	3	2	Trace	12	58	1.0	410	0.05	0.05	0.5	—
	Cream of shrimp:																	
604	Prepared with equal volume of milk	1 cup	245	82	245	9	16	—	—	—	15	189	0.5	290	0.07	0.27	0.5	Trace
605	Prepared with equal volume of water	1 cup	240	88	160	5	12	—	—	—	8	38	0.5	120	0.05	0.05	0.5	—
	Oyster stew:																	
606	Prepared with equal volume of milk	1 cup	240	83	200	10	12	—	—	—	14	305	1.4	410	0.12	0.41	0.5	Trace
607	Prepared with equal volume of water	1 cup	240	90	120	6	8	—	—	—	8	158	1.4	240	0.07	0.19	0.5	—
608	Tapioca, dry, quick cooking	1 cup	152	13	535	1	Trace	—	—	—	131	15	0.6	0	0	0	0	0
	Tapioca desserts:																	
609	Apple	1 cup	250	70	295	1	Trace	—	—	—	74	8	0.5	30	Trace	Trace	Trace	Trace
610	Cream pudding	1 cup	165	72	220	8	8	4	3	Trace	28	173	0.7	480	0.07	0.30	0.2	2
611	Tartar sauce	1 tbsp	14	34	75	Trace	8	1	1	4	1	3	0.1	30	Trace	Trace	Trace	Trace
612	Vinegar	1 tbsp	15	94	Trace	Trace	0	—	—	—	1	1	0.1	—	—	—	—	—
613	White sauce, medium	1 cup	250	73	405	10	31	10	10	1	22	288	0.5	1,150	0.10	0.43	0.5	2
	Yeast:																	
614	Bakers', dry, active	1 pkg	7	5	20	3	Trace	—	—	—	3	3	1.1	Trace	0.16	0.38	2.6	Trace
615	Brewers', dry	1 tbsp	8	5	25	3	Trace	—	—	—	3	17	1.4	Trace	1.25	0.34	3.0	Trace
	Yogurt. See Milk, Cheese, Cream, Imitation Cream																	

Index

Abelev, G., 229
Abortion, 107–111
  legality of, 109–110
  morality of, 110–111
  spontaneous, 100, 108
  therapeutic, 108–109, 116
Accidents, 380–401, 422
  automobile, 383–88
  children under five, 391–95
  deaths due to, 380
  electrical, 397–99
  epidemiological study of, 381–82
  in the home, 391–400
  old age and, 395–96
  spray can disposal, 400
Acidosis, 246
Acromegaly, 24
ACTH, 228, 248
Activity, physical, 123–24
Acupuncture, 422
Addicting drugs, 311–13, 315. *See also* Barbiturates; Methaqualone; Opiates; Tranquilizers
Adler, Alfred, 22
Adrenal glands, 25
Advertising
  Better Business Bureau's role in, 275–76
  cigarette, 275, 338–41
  countercommercials by consumer groups and health organizations, 275, 339, 340
  by drug industry, 263
  FCC controls of television advertising, 274–75
  food faddism, 162
  FTC controls of, 273–74
  health quackery, 261–62
Aerosols, in air pollution, 348–49
Afterbirth. *See* Placenta
Aged. *See* Old age
Agglutinins, 189
Aggressive behavior, 33, 44
Air pollution, 347–57
  control of, 352–57
  effects of, 250–51
  emphysema and, 350
  industry and, 351–52
  the pollutants, 348–49
  weather and, 349–50
Alcohol, 303, 305, 319–20
  abstinence, 322, 323
  and automobile accidents, 388
  as a drug, 323
  effects of, on the body, 324–27
  hangover "cures," 327, 328
  patterns of alcohol use, 321–23
Alcoholic beverages: basic types of, 323–24
Alcoholics, 320–23
  treatment of, 330–31
Alcoholics Anonymous, 330–31
Alcoholism, 10, 320
  causes of, 329
  Korsakoff's psychosis caused by, 46
  problem of, 327, 329–30
Allergies, 247–49
Amenorrhea, 93
American Academy of Pediatrics, 184, 193–94
American Cancer Society, 226
American College of Physicians, 280
American College of Surgeons, 280
American Dental Association, 276
American Heart Association, 215
American Medical Association (AMA), 276
  Committee on Alcoholism and Addiction, 316
  Directory of, 280
  on Dr. Atkins' diet, 160–61
American Osteopathic Association, 282

American Pharmaceutical Association, 265
American Public Health Association, 170–71, 284, 285
Amnesia, 38
Amniocentesis, 117–18, 237, 238, 239, 242, 243, 245
Amniotic sac, 95, 96, 102
Amphetamines, 303, 306–307, 314 *t.*, 316
Anger, 29, 36
Angina pectoris, 214–15
Animal bites, 469–70
Antibiotics: international standardization of, 434
Antibodies, 188, 189
  Rh factor and development of, 100–101
Antidepressants, 51
Antigen-antibody reaction, 188–89
Antigens, 188, 189
Anxiety, 28, 36, 37, 41
  mental mechanisms to cope with, 30–34
  neurotic, 38
Arbous, A. G., 380
Arteries: synthetic tubing for replacement of, 451
Arteriosclerosis, 45, 211, 212, 217, 245, 322
Arthritis, 156, 250–53
  osteoarthritis, 250–51
  quackery, 257–58
  rheumatoid, 250
Artificial heart, 447, 448
Artificial insemination, 116–17
Artificial respiration, 455–58, 459
Aspirin, 262, 272, 274, 303, 305
Asthma, 37, 247, 248, 335
Astronauts: heart muscles of, 125
Atheromas, 211, 212–13, 217
Artherosclerosis, 156, 211, 212
Athlete's foot, 187
Atkins, Robert C., 158, 160–61
Atomic Energy Commission, 378
Auditory nerve, 141
Automobiles. *See also* Motorbikes; Snowmobiles
  as accident factor, 383–87
  air bags in, 387
  air pollution and, 352, 354
  Ralph Nader, on unsafe construction of, 383, 385
  recalling of, 386
  safety belts in, 386–87

Babies
  blue babies, 220
  gonorrhea and blindness in, 207
  methadone-addicted, 318
  premature, 106–107, 108
  prenatal care, 96–100
  thalidomide, 264
Bacilli, 186
Bacteria, 186
Bacteriolysins, 189
Bandaging, 458, 460–61
Barbiturates, 307, 311–12, 314 *t.*, 316
Barnard, Christian, 448
Bartholin's glands, 92
Basic needs 18–22
BCG vaccine, 229, 430, 436
Beers, Clifford, 55
Behavior control, 444–46
Better Business Bureaus, 275–76
Beuren, Aloss J., 220
Bile, 172
Bilharziasis, 425–28, 435
Birth. *See* Childbirth
Birth control. *See* Contraception
Birth control clinics, 407
Birth defects, 85

Bites, 247, 469–70, 476–77
Blatz, William, 22
Bleeding: first aid for, 458, 460–61, 477
Blind spot of eye, 126–27, 133
Blindness, 137, 452
  corneal transplant for, 137, 450
  glaucoma and, 135
  gonorrhea and, in infants 204, 207
  legal, 137
  onchocerciasis and, 431
  in Tay-Sachs disease, 242
  trachoma and, 432
Blisters, 470–71
Blood
  leukemia, 221, 222, 226, 227, 243, 374, 376
  Rh factor in, 100–102
Blood clot, 113, 211, 212, 213, 215, 231, 334
Blood pressure, high, 216–17
Blue baby, 220
Bones: fractures of, 462–64
Botulism, 171
Brain, the, 23, 126, 141
  and cerebral palsy, 232
  and epilepsy, 231–32
  and mental retardation, 235
  and stroke, 215, 216
Brain death, 448 *n.*, 450
Bread, in balanced diet, 175, 178
Breast cancer, 222, 224–25, 229
Breast feeding, 100
Bronchitis, 335, 342, 350
Bronfenbrenner, Urie, 80
Buerger's disease, 334
Burkitt's lymphoma, 222
Burns, 392, 396
  first-aid for, 467–68
Caesarean section, 104, 247
Calderone, Mary S., 59
Cancer, 211, 221–31, 341, 422
  of the blood. *See* Leukemia
  of the breast, 222, 224–25, 229
  cervical, 86, 225
  choriocarcinoma, 228
  of the colon and rectum, 223–24
  danger signals for, 226
  factors contributing to, 221–23
  krebiozen case, 258
  of the lung, 4, 10, 222, 223, 308, 335–38, 341, 342, 351, 377, 453
  of the lymph glands, 222, 226
  of the prostate, 222, 225
  quackery, 258
  relationship of radiation exposure to, 221, 227, 377
  research, 228–30
  sites of, 223–26
  of the skin, 222, 223, 229
  of the stomach, 223, 229
  retinoblastoma, 222
  treatment for, 226–28
    chemotherapy, 227–28
    radiation, 227, 376
    surgery, 226–27
  of the uterus, 222, 225
  vaginal, 108, 222
Carbon monoxide, in air pollution, 348, 351
Cardiovascular disease, 211–15, 216
  angina pectoris, 214–15
  arteriosclerosis, 45, 211, 212, 217
  atherosclerosis, 156, 211, 212
  cholesterol and, 212
  coronary thrombosis, 212–15
  diet and, 156, 212

Cardiovascular disease (*Cont.*)
effect of smoking on, 212, 215
obesity and, 156
Russian research, 424
CARE/MEDICO, 439
Caries, dental, 145
Carroll, Herbert, 22–23
Carson, Rachel, 365, 368
Cataracts, 132, 135
Cereal, in balanced diet, 175, 178
Cerebellum, 23
Cerebral arteriosclerosis, 45
Cerebral palsy, 232–33, 234
Rh factor and, 100, 232
Cerebrovascular disease (stroke), 211, 215–16, 217, 231
Cerebrum, 23
Cervical cancer, 86, 225
Cervix, 92, 102, 103, 114
Cesium 137, 375
Chancre, 201
Cheese, 178
Chemotherapy, for treatment of cancer, 227–28
Chest: "sucking wounds" in, 462
Childbirth, 102–107
breech birth, 104
Caesarean section, 104
emergency, 480–84
multiple births, 105–106, 116
natural, 104–105
premature child, 106–107
stages of, 102–103
Children. *See also* Babies
accidents, 391–95
fluoridation of drinking water, 145–46
home pool drownings, 394–95
married couple's attitude toward having children, 86–87
Children (*Cont.*)
poisoning, 9, 391, 394, 395
premature, 106–107, 108
public health programs for, 406–407
recommended dietary allowances for, 176–77 *t.*
role of family in rearing of, 79–80
Chinese health care system, 422, 423–24
Chiropractic, 283–87
Choking: first aid for, 471
Cholera, 184, 430–31, 435
Cholesterol, 212
Choriocarcinoma, 228
Chronic disease control, 408
Cigarettes. *See also* Smoking
advertising, 275, 338–41
possible corrective measures in manufacture of, 343
Circumcision, 91
Cirrhosis of the liver, 325
Citizen's Board of Inquiry, 152, 153
Claustrophobia, 41, 42
Cleft palate, 147
Clemente, John A., 107
Clinics, free, 417–18
Clitoris, 92
Cloning, genetic, 442–44
Clubfoot, 149
Cocaine, 314 *t.*, 318
Cocci, 186
Codeine, 314 *t.*
Colds, 186
Colitis, 36–37
Colon: cancer of, 223–24
Color blindness, 135–36, 245
Communicable diseases, 183–209. *See also* specific diseases
defined, 184–85
disease-producing organisms, 186–87

Communicable diseases (*Cont.*)
transmission of, 187–88
health department, in control of, 406
immunity to, 188–94. *See also* Immunity
mortality rates, 183
terminology of, 184, 186
Community
health care centers for minority groups, 416–18
hospitals, 294, 413
interest and action of, for water conservation, 362–63
public health organization, 405–20
voluntary health agencies, 411–13
Community Mental Health Centers, 52–54
Compensation, as defense mechanism, 31
Condom, 114
Congenital diseases. *See also* Genetic diseases
cleft palate, 147
cystic fibrosis, 85, 237, 239
Down's syndrome (mongolism), 118, 222, 234, 243
foot problems, 148, 149
heart defects, 219–20. *See also* Hypervitaminosis
phenylketonuria (PKU), 235, 237, 240–42
sickle-cell anemia, 85, 237–39, 417
some forms of mental retardation, 235
syphilis, 204
Tay-Sachs disease, 85, 242–43
Constipation, 173
Constitutional diseases, 211–53. *See also* Disease: constitutional
Consumer protection, 269–76
Consumer quackery, 257–62
Consumer Reports, 278–79, 370
Contact lenses, 130–33
soft lenses, 132–33
Contagious diseases. *See* Communicable diseases
Contraception, 85, 111–16, 407
methods of, 111–16
Conversion reaction (or conversion hysteria), 40
Convulsions: first aid for, 471
Convulsive disorders, 231–32
COPD (chronic obstructive bronchopulmonary disease), 335, 342
Cornea, 126, 127, 128, 132, 137
Corneal transplant, 137, 450
Coronary risk profile, 217, 219. *See also* Heart disease
Coronary thrombosis, 212–15
Corpus luteum, 93
Cortisone, 219, 228, 248
Cretinism, 24
Crossed eye (strabismus), 8, 129, 133–34
Cystic fibrosis, 85, 237, 239

Darvon, 272
Daydreaming, 31
DDT, 369, 428–29, 432
Deafness. *See* Hearing loss
Death, 34–35
defined, 448 *n.*, 450
DeBakey, Michael, 448
Deficiency diseases
goiter, 25, 165
kwashiorkor, 424–25
night blindness, 136
Degenerative diseases, 211–53. *See also* Disease: constitutional and degenerative
Delirium tremens, 330
Demerol, 314 *t.*
Dental health, 145–47. *See also* Teeth
specialists, 282
utilization of X rays, 376
Depression, manic, 44–45

Depression, neurotic, 42
Diabetes, 9, 135, 156, 216, 245–47
  control of, 246–47
  diabetes insipidus, 245
  diabetes mellitus, 245
  emergency first aid, 471–72
Diarrhea, 435, 436
Diet(s), 156–57. *See also* Nutrition
  AMA criticism of Dr. Atkins' diet, 160–61
  balanced, 174, 178–79
  in cardiovascular disease, 156, 212
  in diabetes, 246
  during pregnancy, 97
  faddist, 158–59, 164
  in hypertension, 217
  in management of phenylketonuria, 240, 242
  for ulcers and gall bladder disease, 172
  for weight control, 156–57
Digestion: problems related to food and, 170–73
Diphtheria, 185, 192, 424
Disease(s). *See also* specific diseases
  communicable, 183–209. *See also* Communicable diseases
  constitutional and degenerative, 211–53. *See also* Allergies; Cancer; Cardiovascular disease; Cerebrovascular disease; Diabetes; Emphysema; Genetic diseases; Hypertension; Mental retardation; Neurological disorders; Rheumatic diseases; rheumatic fever
  of deficiency. See Deficiency diseases
  immunity, 188–94
  infectious, 186
  in underdeveloped countries, 424–32
Disease-producing organisms, 186–87
  transmission of, 187–88
DNA (deoxyribonucleic acid), 223, 237
Doctor. *See* Medical profession
Dohner, Alton, 303
Dooley, Tom, 439
Down's syndrome (mongolism), 118, 222, 234, 243
Drowning, 394–95
Drug addiction, 10, 301–302, 311–13, 315, 317, 423–24
  approaches to problem of, 317–19
  and drug abusers, 303–306
  signs and ssymtpoms of, 314 *t.*
  as social-health problem, 318–19
Drug habituation, 302
Drug industry, 262–69, 316
Drug therapy, for mental and emotional problems, 51
Drug traffic, 315–17
Drugs, 299–319. *See also* Cigarettes; Smoking
  addicting, 311–13, 315, 317
  alcohol as a drug, 323. *See also* Alcohol
  amphetamines, 303, 306–307, 316
  anticonvulsant, 232
  antituberculosis, 430
  in cancer treatment, 227–28
  in childbirth, 105
  contributions of, 299–300
  and driving, 388
  ethical (prescription), 262–65, 300
  FDA functions regarding, 271
  federal legislation, 270–75
  fertility drugs, 116
  generic *vs.* brand name, 262–63
  hallucinogenic, 43, 307–11
  health quackery, 258, 260
  high price of, 263, 265–66
  misleading advertising, 261–62
  Omnibus Drug Bill, 268–69
  proprietary, 301
  stimulants, 51
  therapy, 317
  tranquilizers, 51

Drugs (*Cont.*)
use of, during pregnancy, 98
use and abuse of, 314 *t.*
WHO control of, 434
Dubos, René, 7
Durkheim, Emil, 46
Dwarfism, 24
Dysentery, amebic, 187
Dysmenorrhea, 93, 113

Ear. *See also* Hearing
infections, 139–40
inner ear, 141
middle ear, 139–41
otosclerosis and its treatment, 140
outer ear, 138–39
tympanic membrane (eardrum), 139, 140
Egg cell (ovum), 91, 94, 112, 116
Ego: Freud on, 26–27
Ejaculation, 70, 90
Electrical safety, 397–99
ground-fault interrupter, 399
Ellis, Albert, 65
Embolism, 215
Emergency first aid, 455–84
Emotional problems, 86
and accident causation, 388–89
first aid in case of, 472–73
hearing loss and, 143
obesity, dieting and, 155–56, 157
treatment of, 49–51
Emotions, 29–30, 36–37, 40, 444
Emphysema, 10, 249–50, 308, 334, 341, 350, 453
air pollution and, 350
cigarette smoking and, 249–50, 334, 350–51
Endocrine system, 24–25
Endometrium, 93
Environment, 5–7, 347–78
and accidents, 382–83
factors of, responsible for cancer, 229
foot problems arising from, 149–50
and mental health, 18–22
and physical and emotional development, 443–44
provided by marriage, 74–75
Epidemiology
in cancer research, 229
in heart disease research, 217, 219
in safety research, 381–83
Epilepsy, 231–32
first aid for, 471
Episiotomy, 103
Estrogen, 92, 93, 94, 212, 225, 228
synthetic, 108
Eustachian tube, 139
Exercise, 123–26
weight control and, 154, 155
Eye. *See* also Vision
accommodation of, 127
artificial, research on, 452
blind spot, 126–27, 133
cataracts, 132, 135
devices responding to eyeball movement, 446–47
diseases of, 134–35
plastic or glass, 138
refractive errors of, 127–28, 130
structure of, 126–27
Eye banks, 137
Eyeglasses, 128, 130. *See also* Contact lenses
after surgical removal of the lens, 135
safety requirements for, 130
for strabismus, 133
sunglasses, 136

Fallopian tubes, 91, 95, 112, 116, 206
Fallout. *See* Radioactive fallout
Falls, among the aging, 395–96
False labor, 102
Family planning. *See* Contraception
FAO (Food and Agriculture Organization), 437–39
FDA. *See* Food and Drug Administration
Fear, 29, 30, 37
  phobic, 41–42
Federal Bureau of Narcotics, 316
Federal Communications Commission (FCC), 274–75
Federal Food, Drug, and Cosmetic Acts, 167–68, 269, 270, 300
Federal Trade Commission (FTC)
  consumer protection by, 273–74, 339
  criticized by Ralph Nader, 273–74
Federal Water Pollution Control Act, 360–61
Female reproductive system, 91–93
Femininity, 59, 60
Fenestration operation, 140–41
Fertility drugs, 116
Fetus, 96, 98, 100–101, 106, 108, 110, 117–18
Fires, 392, 396
First aid, 455–84
Fish, in balanced diet, 178
Fixation, as defense mechanism, 33
Flat feet, 150
Fluoridation of drinking water, 145–46
Food
  additives, 165–67
  FDA functions regarding, 270
  federal legislation concerning, 167–68
  health food-organic food movement, 163–65, 260
  nutritional misinformation about, 158–63
  nutritive values of edible part of, 485, 486–504 *t.*
  problems related to digestion and, 170–73
  processed, 162, 164
  supplements, 162–63, 260
Food and Agriculture Organization, 437–39
Food and Drug Administration, 167, 257, 258
  consumer protection by, 270–73
  criticized by Ralph Nader, 267
  role in combating food faddism, 168–69
Food and Nutrition Education Program, 169
Food poisoning, 163, 170–71
Food Stamp Program, 153–54
Foot problems, 147–50
Foreskin, 91
Fractures, 462–64
Framingham Study, The, 217
Free clinics, 417–18
Freud, Sigmund, 26–27
Frostbite, 473–75
Fruits, in balanced diet, 175, 178
Fungi, 187

Galactosemia, 243
Gall bladder disease, 172
Gamma globulin, 98, 189
Gamma rays, 373
Gay Liberation movement, 72–73
Genetic cloning, 442–44
Genetic counseling, 85, 117–18
Genetic diseases, 117–18, 237–45. *See also* Congenital diseases
  sex-linked, 243–45
Geritol, 274
German measles (Rubella), 189, 192–93
  during pregnancy, 98, 110, 135, 193, 220, 232, 235
Glands, endocrine, 24–25
Glaucoma, 8, 132, 135
Glucose tolerance tests, 246
Goddard, James, 5, 266, 269
Goiter, 25, 165
Gonads, the, 25

Gonorrhea, 198, 199, 205–207
Gout, 251
Group practice in medical profession, 288–89, 294
Group therapy, 50
Gurdon, John, 442
Guthrie blood test, 240
Guyon, René, 65

Hallucinogenic drugs, 43, 307–11. *See also* LSD; Marihuana; Mescaline; Psilocybin
  schizophrenia and, 43
Handicapped persons, 407
  foot care and rehabilitation of, 150
  visually handicapped, 137
Hand prints
  Down's syndrome, 243
  leukemia, 243
Hansen's Disease, 432
Hardening of the arteries. *See* Arteriosclerosis
Harris-Dodd Act, 307
Health agency, official, 405
Health care
  changing nature of, 287–89
  emergency first aid, 455–84
  financing cost of, 289–91
  future of, 294–97
  humanization of, 416–18
  inequities in, 291–93
Health careers, 418–20
Health centers, community, 416–18
Health departments
  at federal level, 409–11
  at local level, 406–408
  at state level, 408–409
Health food movement, 163–65, 260
Health insurance, 289–91, 293
  group practice and, 288–89
  Medicare, 290–91
  voluntary, 289–90
Health Maintenance Organizations, 297
Hearing, 138–45. *See also* Ear
  specialists, 143
Hearing aids, 143–44
Hearing loss, 8, 193
  diseases causing, 141
  due to inner ear malfunction, 141
  middle ear infection as cause of, 139–40
  noise and, 141–42
  otosclerosis, 140–41
  psychological aspects of, 144–45
  types of, 142–43
Heart
  artificial, 447, 448
  boosters, 448
  development of mechanism to aid heart muscles of astronauts, 125
  pacemakers, 451–52
  transplants, 448–50
Heart disease, 10, 94, 211, 217, 422. *See also* Cardiovascular disease
  angina pectoris, 214–15
  congenital defects, 219–20
  coronary thrombosis, 212–15
  damage in rheumatic heart disease, 219
  identification of high risk coronary person, 217, 219
  obesity and, 156
  open heart surgery, 294, 447–52
  relationship between hypertension and, 217
  Russian research, 424
  smoking and, 334, 342
Heart-lung machine, 219
Heat exhaustion and heat stroke, 475–76

Hemophilia, 243, 245
Hepatitis, 184, 186, 197–98
  infectious, 197–98, 435
  serum hepatitis, 186, 198
Heredity
  and atherosclerosis, 212
  and cancer, 222
  and color blindness, 135
  and cystic fibrosis, 239
  and diabetes, 246
  and galactosemia, 243
  as health factor, 11–12
  and hypertension, 216–17
  and malocclusion, 147
  and multiple births, 106
  and muscular dystrophy, 233
  and myopia, 127
  and obesity, 155
  and phenylketonuria, 240
  and sickle-cell anemia, 237, 238
  and strabismus, 133
  and Tay-Sachs disease, 242–43
Heroin, 303, 314 *t.*, 315–16, 317
Hettlinger, Richard F., 70–71
HEW (Department of Health, Education and Welfare), 409–10
High blood pressure, 216–17
HIP (New York City Health Insurance Plan), 289
Histamine, 247
Hives, 247
Hodgkin's disease, 226, 228
Hofmann, Albert, 310
Home accidents, 391–400
Homosexuality, 72–73
Hormones, 24–25
  cancer and, 222, 225, 228
  estrogen, 92, 93, 94
Hormones (*Cont.*)
  FSH and LH, 92–93
  progesterone, 92, 93
  testosterone, 90
Hospitals, 294, 413
  increased cost of care in, 293
  Medicare and, 290–91
  mental hospitals, 51–54
  of Veteran's Administration, 410
Hunger, 152–54, 437
Hyaline membrane disease (HMD), 106–107
  treatment and detection of, 106–107
Hydrocephalus, 235
Hymen, 60, 85, 92
Hypertension, 216–17
Hypervitaminosis, 152
Hypoglycemia, 246
Hysteria, conversion, 40

Id, the: Freud on, 26
Identification, as mental mechanism, 33
Immunity, 188–94. *See also* Vaccines
  to allergens, 248
  cancer research on, 229
  "herd immunity" approach, 193
  recommended schedule for immunization, 194 *t.*
  tuberculosis, 229, 430
  types of, 189
Immunotherapy, 229
Incidence of disease, defined, 186
Income and health, 5–6
Industrial safety, 400–401
Infant mortality, 86
Infectious disease, defined, 186
Infectious hepatitis, 197–98, 435

Infectious mononucleosis, 196–97
Infertility: aspects of, 116–17
Influenza, 184, 193, 194–96, 434
Ingraham, Hollis, S., 261
Injured persons: transportation of, 465–66
Insanity, 43
Insect bites, 247, 476–77
Insulin, 245, 246, 247, 472
Insurance. *See* Health insurance
Interferon, 209
International Boundary and Water Commission, 361
International Sanitary Regulations, 434
Interstate Commerce Commission, 388
Interstate highway system, 387–88
Intoxication. *See* Alcoholism
Intrauterine devices (IUD's), 113–14
Iodine, 165, 260
Ivy, Andrew, 258

Jaundice, 197
Jourard, Sidney, 22

Kantrowitz, Adrian, 448
Kaplan, Louis, 28, 37
Kefauver, Estes: investigation of drug industry by, 262, 263, 264–65
Kefauver-Harris Drug Amendments Act of 1962, 262, 269, 300
Keller, Mark, 327
Kelsey, Frances, 264
Kerr-Mills Medical Assistance program, 290–91, 415
Kidney transplants, 449, 450
Kirkendall, Lester, 64
Kleptomania, 41
Korsakoff's psychosis, 46
Krebiozen case, 258
Kwashiorkor, 424–25

Labor, in childbirth, 102, 481–82
Lahey Clinic (Boston), 288
Land pollution, 363–65
  solution for problems of, 364–65
Laparoscopy, 112
Lapp, Ralph E., 375
Laryngectomee, 457
  first aid for, 458
Laxatives, 173
Lens of the eye, 126, 127, 128, 135
Leprosy, 432, 435, 436
Leukemia, 221, 222, 226, 227, 243, 374, 376
Lightning accidents, 397
Linder, Forrest E., 3
Lindesmith, Dr., 302
Liver, 222, 229
  cirrhosis of, 325
Louria, Donald B., 306
Love, 18, 19, 29
  and marriage, 75, 76–77
  and sex, 67–69
LSD, 43, 303, 305, 306, 309–11, 314 *t.*
Luminal, 311
Lung diseases
  cancer, 4, 10, 222, 223, 308, 335–38, 341, 342, 351, 377, 453
  chronic obstructive bronchopulmonary disease (COPD), 335, 342
  as complication of cystic fibrosis, 239
  emphysema, 249–50, 308, 334, 341, 350, 453
  hyaline membrane disease, 106–107
  tuberculosis. *See* Tuberculosis
Lymph glands: cancer of, 222, 226

Mace, David, 64
Macrobiotic diet, 164
Malaria, 187, 428–29, 435, 436
  and sickle-cell anemia, 238
Male reproductive system, 89–91
Malnutrition, 152–54, 436
Malocclusion, 147, 148
Manic depressive psychosis, 44–45
Marihuana, 303, 305, 306, 307–309, 314 *t.*
Marriage. *See also* Reproduction; Sexuality
  engagement period prior to, 83–84
  motivations for, 74–76
  Nena and George O'Neill, on open marriage, 83
  premarital intercourse and, 71
  premarital physical examination, 85–86
  preparation for, 74–87
  question of having children, 86–87
  religion and, 80–81, 87
  role of economics in, 78–80
  role expectations in, 81–83
  sexual relationship in, 67, 80
Masculinity, 59–60, 82
Maslow, Abraham, 21
Masturbation, 68, 69–70, 90
Maternal health programs, 406–407
Maturity, defined, 74
Mayo Clinic (Rochester, Minn.), 288
Measles, 141, 186, 235, 424
  vaccine, 192, 194 *t.*, 237
Meat, in balanced diet, 175, 178
Medicaid, 290–91
Medical care. *See* Health care
Medical insurance. *See* Health insurance
Medical profession, 280–82
  education and training of physicians, 280
  group practice, 288–89, 294
  increasing specialization, 288, 294
  selection and evaluation of physician, 280
  types of specialists, 280–82
  utilization of X rays, 376
Medicare, 290–91
Medicine Show, The, 279
Memory, 23, 25–26, 38, 215
Meningitis, 235
Menninger, Karl, 17–18, 36, 55
Menopause, 93–94, 212
Menstruation, 92–93, 113, 114
  pregnancy and, 95
Mental health, 17–56
  bases of, 17–35
  changing attitudes toward, 55–56
  conscious and unconscious mind, 25–27
  defined, 22–23
  erosion of, 36–56
  methods of treating problems of, 49–51
  neuroses, 37–42. *See also* Neuroses
  psychoses, 42–46. *See also* Psychoses
  psychosomatic disorders, 36–37
  relationship of body systems to, 23–25
  specialists in, 49
  suicide, 46–49
  treatment facilities, 51–54
Mental hospitals, 51–54
Mental Hygiene Movement, 55
Mental mechanisms to cope with anxiety, 30–34
Mental retardation, 234–37, 240, 242
  attitudes toward the retarded, 235–36
  hypervitaminosis, vitamin D, 235
  programs for the retarded, 236
  Rh factor and, 100, 235
Mescaline, 309

Metabolism
  and obesity, 155
  thyroid gland and, 24
Metastasis, 221
Methadone, 314 *t.*
  maintenance programs, 317–18
Methaqualone, 312
Milk
  in balanced diet, 174, 175, 178
  fortified, 165–66
Minority groups: health care centers for, 416–18
Miscarriage, 108, 484
Modell, Walter, 267
Mongolism. *See* Down's syndrome
Mononucleosis, 196–97
Morbidity, defined, 186
Morehouse, Laurence E., 123
Morphine, 313, 314 *t.*
Mortality rates, 186
  accidents, 380, 389, 391
  cancer, 223, 224, 225
  communicable diseases, 183
  COPD, 335
  diabetes, 245
  emphysema, 249
  infant, 86
  overweight and, 156
  poliomyelitis, 183
Mosquitoes, as carriers of disease, 188, 428, 435
Motion sickness, 141
Motor vehicles. *See* Automobiles; Motorbikes; Snowmobiles
Motorbike accidents, 389
Multiple births, 105–106, 116
Multiple sclerosis, 233
Mumps, 98, 186
Muscular coordination, 23
Muscular dystrophy, 233–34
Myocardial infarction, 212–15
Myxedema, 24

Nader, Ralph, 267, 273–74, 383, 385
National Advisory Cancer Council, 223
National Cancer Institute, The, 228
National Center for Toxilogical Research, 271
National Commission on Marihuana and Drug Abuse, 309
National Health Survey, 5
National Highway Traffic Safety Administration, 386
National Institutes of Health, 410
National Safety Council, 396, 400
National School Lunch Act, 154
National Traffic and Motor Vehicle Safety Act, 385–86
Natural childbirth, 104–105
Naturopathy, 284–85
Needs, basic, 18–22
Nelson, Gaylord, 268
Nembutal, 311
Nephritis, 156
Nervous system, 23–24
  autonomic, 29, 30
  convulsive disorders, 231–32
  multiple sclerosis, 233
Neurological disorders, 231–34. *See also* Cerebral palsy; Epilepsy; Multiple sclerosis; Muscular dystrophy; Parkinson's disease
Neuroses, 37–42
  anxiety reaction, 38
  conversion reactions, 40
  depressive reactions, 42
  dissociative reaction, 38
  obsessive compulsive reaction, 40–41
  phobic reaction, 41–42
  vs. psychoses, 37

New York City Health Insurance Plan, 289
New York State: Chromosome Registry, 245
Night blindness, 136
Nocturnal emissions, 68, 70, 90
Noise: and hearing loss, 141–42
Nonmedical specialists, 283
Nosebleed, 477
Nuclear-powered plants
  and radiation, 377–78
  and water pollution, 359
Nursing homes, 415–16
Nutrition, 152–79. *See also* Diet; Food
  alcoholism and, 330
  balanced diet, 174, 178–79
  books on, 277–79
  during pregnancy, 97, 235, 237
  FAO and, 437
  Kwashiorkor, 424–25
  misinformation on, 158–63
  need for education in, 169–70
  nutritive values of edible part of foods, 485, 486–504 *t.*
  poverty, hunger, and malnutrition, 152–54
  quackery in, 157, 158, 260
  recommended daily dietary allowances, 176–77 *t.*

Obesity, 154–55
  and diabetes, 245, 246
  diseases and, 156
  heredity and, 155
  thyroid gland and, 24
Obsessive compulsive reactions, 40–41
Oculist, 127, 128, 130, 131, 281
Official health agency, 405
Old age
  eye disease, 135
  falling accidents, 395–96

Old age (*Cont.*)
  foot problems, 150
  medicinal use of alcohol, 322
Omnibus Drug Bill, 268–69
Onchocerciasis, 431–32
O'Neill, Nena and George, 83
Open heart surgery, 294, 447–52
Ophthalmologist, 127, 128, 130, 131, 281
Opiates, 313, 315
Opsonins, 189
Optic nerve, 126
Optician, 130, 283
Optometrist, 127, 128, 131, 283
Oral health, 145–47. *See also* Dental health; Teeth
Organic food movement, 163–65
Orgasm, 70, 90, 92
Osteoarthritis, 250–51
Osteopathy, 282–83
Otitis media (middle ear infection), 139–40
Otosclerosis, 140–41
Ovaries, 25, 91, 94
  transplant of, 452
Over-the-counter (OTC) drugs, 271–72
Overpopulation, 86
Overweight. *See* Obesity
Ovulation, 91, 92, 93, 95, 112, 114
Ovum. *See* Egg cell
Ozone, in air pollution, 348–49

Pacatal, 264
Pacemaker, heart, 451–52
Pan-American Health Organization, 435
Pandemic, 431
Papanicolaou (Pap) test, 86, 225
Paranoic schizophrenia, 44

Parasitic worms, 187
Parathyroid glands, 25
Paresis, 45–46
Parkinson's disease, 234
Pathogenic organisms, 186–87
Penicillin, 46, 198, 204, 207, 219, 247, 299, 300
Penis, 89, 90–91, 206
"Pep" pills. *See* Amphetamines
Peptic ulcers, 36, 171–72, 327
Periodontal diseases, 146–47
Personality, 18–21, 24, 25
  adjustment to marriage, 77–78
  disintegrated, 42
  dissociative reaction and, 38
  fixation of, 33
  hearing loss and, 144–45
  LSD effects and, 310
  psychological stress and, 27
Pertussis (whooping cough), 185, 186, 192, 193, 235
Pesticides, 163, 365, 368–73
  benefits of, 371–72
  effects on wildlife, 369
  federal control in use of, 370–71
  poisoning, 368–69
  proper personal use of, 372–73
  research, 371
  toxicity of, 369–70
Petting, 70–71
Phenobarbital, 311
Phenylalanine, 240, 242
Phenylketonuria (PKU), 235, 237, 240–42
Phobias, 41–42
Physical education needs, 125–26
Physical fitness, 123–25
Physician. *See* Medical profession
"Pill, the," 111, 112–13, 208
"Pink-eye," 134
  marihuana and, 308
Pituitary gland, 24
Placenta, 95, 98, 100, 102, 103, 107, 484
Pneumonia, 184, 194–96, 211, 239, 327
Podiatry, 150, 283
Poisoning, 399–400
  of children, 9, 391, 394, 395
  first aid for, 478–79
  food poisoning, 163, 170–71
  pesticide poisoning, 368–69
Poliomyelitis, 183–84, 185, 186, 192, 424
Pollution, 422. *See also* Air pollution; Land pollution; Water pollution
Polonium, 338
Popenoe, Paul, 68
Post Office Department, 275
Poverty, hunger, and malnutrition, 152–54
Pregnancy, 95–100. *See also* Abortion
  of diabetic woman, 247
  German measles during, 98, 110, 135, 193, 220, 232, 235
  gonorrhea during, 207
  and hearing loss, 140
  maternal health programs, 406–407
  prenatal care, 96–100, 237
  prenatal development, 96
  Rh factor, 100–102
  signs of, 95–96
  syphilis during, 204
Premarital sex, 68, 71
Premature child, 106–107, 108
  hyaline membrane disease, 106–107
Prenatal care, 96–100
Prescription drugs, 262–65, 300
Preservatives, 165, 166
Preventive medicine, 294–95, 417, 422, 424

Progesterone, 92, 93
Projection, as defense mechanism, 33–34
Proprietary drugs, 301
Prostaglandins, 108
  possible use of, in birth control, 116
Prostate gland, 89, 90
  cancer of, 222, 225
Protein, 164
  Kwashiorkor caused by deficiency of, 424–25
Protozoa, 187
Psilocybin, 309, 314 *t.*
Psychiatric social worker, 49
Psychiatrist, 49, 281
Psychoanalyst, 49
Psychogenic disorder, 40
Psychological factors
  hearing loss and, 144–45
  in mental health, 18, 21, 27–29, 49–50
  weight control and, 155–56
Psychologist, 49
Psychoses, 42–46
  as LSD effect, 310
  manic depressive, 44–45
  organic, 45–46
  schizophrenia. *See* Schizophrenia
  vs. neuroses, 37
Psychosomatic disorders, 36–37
Psychotherapy, 49–50
Puberty, 24, 90
Public health. *See also* Health departments
  community action and, 405–20
  environmental problems, 347–78
  nutrition education, 169–70
  venereal disease control, 208–209
Public Health Service, 5, 153, 183, 409, 418

Quackery, 8, 157–58, 257–62

Radiation, 373–78. *See also* X rays
  cancer, and overexposure to, 221, 227
  cosmic radiation, 373
  FDA functions regarding, 271
  Hiroshima–Nagasaki bombing studies, 374
  man-made, sources of, 375–78
  medical and dental, 376
  nature and effects of, 373–75
  as treatment for cancer, 227
Radioactive fallout, 375
Radioactive materials, 373, 376–77
  industrial accidents involving, 376
  waste disposal of, 377
Rank, Otto, 22
Rationalization, as defense mechanism, 33
Reaction-formation, as defense mechanism, 33
Rectum: cancer of, 223–24
Regression, as defense mechanism, 31
Religion, 80–81, 86–87
Repression, 32
Reproduction, 89–119. *See also* Abortion; Birth control; Childbirth; Pregnancy
  artificial insemination, 116–17
  female reproductive system, 91–93
  fertilization, 94–95
  genetic counseling, 85, 117–18
  infertility, 116–17
  male reproductive system, 89–91
  sex determination of children, 94–95
  social implication, 17
Reserpine, 51, 264, 299, 300
Respiration, artificial, 455–58, 459
Respiratory disease. *See* Bronchitis; Emphysema; Influenza; Lung disease; Pneumonia
Retardation. See Mental retardation
Retina, 126, 128, 135
  detached, 128, 134

Retinoblastoma, 222
Rh factor, 100–102, 107, 232, 233, 235, 237
anti-Rh immune globulin, 101
Rheumatic diseases, 250–53. *See also* Gout; Osteoarthritis; Rheumatoid arthritis
Rheumatic fever, 219
Rheumatic heart disease, 219
Rheumatoid arthritis, 250
Richmond, Julius B., 11
Rickets, 165
Rickettsia, 187, 188
Ringworm, 187
River blindness, 431–32
RNA (ribonucleic acid), 223
Rockey Mountain Spotted Fever, 187, 188
Roentgens, 373–74
Rubella. *See* German measles
Russia, 424

Sabin, Albert B., 183
Safety, 380–401. *See also* Accidents
electrical, 397–99
in the home, 391–400
industrial, 400–401
interstate highway system, 387–88
traffic safety, 383. *See also* Automobiles
Safety belts, automobile, 386–87
Salk, Jonas, 183
Salmonella contamination, 163, 170–71
Sanitation, 406
Scarlet fever, 141, 235
Schistosomiasis, 187, 425–28
Schizophrenia, 42–44
catatonic type, 44
hebephrenic type, 43
paranoid type, 44
simple type, 43
Schools: health and, 407, 413–15
Schubert, Jack, 375
Self-concept, 21–22
Semen, 90, 94, 115, 116
Sensitivity training, 50–51
Serum hepatitis, 186, 198
Sewage disposal and water pollution, 359–60, 361–62
Sex drive, 67, 68
Sex-linked genetic diseases, 243–45
Sexual intercourse, 71, 85, 94–95
Sexuality, 59–73. *See also* Marriage; Reproduction
changes in values concerning, 64–65, 71
homosexuality, 72–73
and love, 67–69
and marriage, 67, 80
masculinity and femininity, 59–61
menstruation and, 93
negative bases of sexual involvement, 66–67
Playboy philosophy, 65
premarital sexual outlets, 69–71
women's liberation movement, 61–64
Shettles, Landrum, 90, 94–95
Shock, from injury, 468–69
Shock therapy, 51, 445–46
Sickle-cell anemia, 85, 237–39, 417
Silent Spring (Rachel Carson), 365, 368
Silver nitrate, 207
Skin cancer, 222, 223, 229
Sleeping sickness, 187, 431
Smallpox, 435, 436
control of, 183, 184, 192
recent epidemics of, 183, 421
routine vaccinations discontinued in the United States, 183
steps in preparation of vaccine, 190–91
Smog, 350
Smoking, 10. *See also* Cigarettes
and cardiovascular disease, 212, 213, 215, 334, 342

Smoking (*Cont.*)
and COPD, 335, 342
educational programs, 343–44
and emphysema, 249, 250, 334–35, 350–51
growing militancy of nonsmokers, 344–45
and lung cancer, 4, 222
marihuana, 308–309
physiological effects of, 333–38
reasons for, 332–33
and strokes, 215–16
Surgeon General's report on, 335, 341
decade since, 341–42
Snail fever, 425–28
Snellen Visual Acuity Test, 128–30
Snowmobiles, 389
Solid Waste Disposal Act, 364
Space medicine, 125, 446–47
Sperm cells, 89, 90, 94, 112, 115
Spinal cord, 23–24
Spirochetes, 186, 200
Splinting, 462–64
Split personality, 42
Sprains, 465
Spray cans: danger from, 400
SS *Hope* (ship), 439–41
Stapes mobilization operation, 140, 141
Staphylococcal contamination, 170
State health departments, 408–409
Status needs, 20
Sterilization, for birth control, 111, 112
Stimulant drugs, 51. *See also* Amphetamines
Stokes, Walter, 64–65
Stomach
cancer of, 223, 229
gastric ulcers, 171–72
Strabismus, 8, 129, 133–34
Strang Cancer Clinic, 230
"Strep" throat, 186
Streptococcal infection, 219
Streptomycin, 141
Stress, psychological, 27–28
Stroke, 211, 215–16, 217, 231
Strontium 90, 373, 375
Styes, 134–35
Sublimation, as defense mechanism, 32
Substitution, as defense mechanism, 31–32
Sucking wounds, 462
Suffocation, 393–94
Suicide, 46–49
basic types of, 46–47
misconceptions about, 47–48
youthful, 47
Sulfanilamide drugs, 269
Sulfur dioxide, in air pollution, 352
Superego: Freud on, 26
Supression, as defense mechanism, 32
Surgeon General, 409
report on smoking, 335, 341
Syphilis, 45–46, 141, 198, 199–205

Taller, Herman, 158
Tay-Sachs disease, 85, 242–43
Teeth. *See also* Dental health
decay of, 98
factors in, 145
fluorides and, 145–46
pregnancy and, 98
malocclusion, 147, 148
and periodontal diseases, 146–47
Television
cigarette advertising on, 275, 339
health quackery on, 262
radiation from sets, 375
Temperature inversion and air pollution, 349–50

Testes, 25, 89–90, 225
Testosterone, 90
Tetanus, 193
Thalidomide, 98, 264, 269
Thanatology, 34
Thomas John L., 59
Thyroid gland, 24–25
Thyroxin, 24
Tobacco. *See* Cigarettes; Smoking
Today's Health, 280
Tourniquet application, 460–61
Toxemia, 107
Toxoids, 192
  diphtheria, 192, 194 *t.*
  tetanus, 192, 194 *t.*
Trachoma, 134, 432, 436
Traffic safety, 383
Tranquilizers, 51, 313, 314 *t.*
  in treatment of alcoholism, 330
Transmission of infectious organisms, 187–88
Transplanting organs, 448–51
Transportation of injured persons, 465–66
Travel safety. *See also* Automobiles
  interstate highway system, 387–88
Treponema pallida, 200
Trypanosomiasis, 431
Tsetse fly, 431
Tubal ligation, 112, 113
Tuberculin test, 194 *t.*, 221, 429, 430
Tuberculosis, 186, 193, 211, 229, 429–30, 435, 436
Twins, 105–106
Tympanic membrane (eardrum), 139, 140
Typhoid fever, 164, 186, 193, 435
Typhus, 187

Ulcers, 36, 171–72, 327
Umbilical cord, 95, 103, 483
Unconsciousness, 479–80
UNICEF (United Nations Children Fund), 436–37
United Nations. *See also* FAO; UNICEF; World Health Organization
  and narcotics trade, 316
United States, agreement on health cooperation, 424
United States Public Health Service, 5, 153, 183, 409, 418
Upper respiratory infection, 194–96
Urethra, 90, 206
Uric acid, 251
Uterus, 91, 92, 93, 95, 102, 103, 484 cancer of, 222, 225

Vaccines, 186, 192–94
  influenza, 195–96
  international standardization of, 434
  measles, 192, 194 *t.*, 237
  poliomyelitis, 183, 184, 192, 194 *t.*
  rubella (German measles), 193, 194 *t.*
  smallpox, 183, 190–91, 192
  tuberculosis, 430
  whooping cough, 192
Vagina, 91–92, 103, 206
Vaginal cancer, 108, 222
Vaginal douche, 115
Vaginitis, 115, 206
Varicose veins, 220–21
Vas deferens, 89, 90, 112
Vasectomy, 112
Vectors, 188
Vegetables, in balanced diet, 175, 178
Vegetarian diets, 164
Venereal disease, 11, 184, 198–209, 422, 423. *See also* Gonorrhea; Syphilis
  development in control of, 208–209
  "the pill" and, 113, 208
Veteran's Administration hospitals, 410

Veterinary medicine, 271
Vincent, Ronald G., 10
Virginity, 60, 70
Viruses, 186
  and cancer, 221–22
Vision, 126–38. *See also* Eye; Blindness
  astigmatism, 128, 130, 131, 132
  color blindness, 135–36, 245
  hyperopia (farsightedness), 128, 129
  myopia (nearsightedness), 127–28, 129, 131, 132
  night vision, 136
  presbyopia, 128
  proper lighting, 136–37
  strabismus, 8, 129, 133–34
  testing, 128–30
  tunnel vision, 137
  use of sunglasses, 136
Visually handicapped persons, 137
Vital statistics, 406
Vitamin(s)
  A, 136, 166, 178
  B vitamins, 166, 172, 178, 222
  C, 146, 166, 172, 178
  claims regarding, 162
  D, 165–66, 220, 235
  E, 233
Voluntary health organizations, 411–13

Walsh, William B., 439
Water pollution, 357–63
  control of, 359–60
  federal legislation, 360–61
  need for community interest and action, 362–63
  nuclear plants and, 359
Water pollution (*Cont.*)
  research, 361–62
  sewage disposal and, 359–60, 361–62
Water supply
  fluoridation of drinking water, 145–46
  industrial uses of water, 357, 360
  pollution of, 357
Weather, and air pollution, 349–50
Weight control, 154–58. *See also* Diet
  desirable weights of persons, 160 *t*.
  during pregnancy, 97
  physical fitness and, 123
  quackery in, 157–58
Wheeler-Lea Amendment of 1938, 273
White House Conference on Food, Nutrition, and Health, 169
WHO. *See* World Health Organization
Whooping cough (pertussis), 185, 186, 192, 193, 235
Withdrawal illness
  addicting drugs, 312, 313, 315
  alcoholism, 330
Women's liberation movement, 61–64
World Food Program, 438
World health, 421–41
  diseases found in underdeveloped countries, 424–32
  problems, 422–24
World Health Organization (WHO), 196, 301, 424, 428, 429, 432–36
  activities, 434–36
Wounds, 461–62
Wynder, Ernest L., 4

X rays, 98, 221, 373, 375, 376. *See also* Radiation

Yaws, 435, 436